Current Cancer Research

Series Editor
Wafik El-Deiry

More information about this series at http://www.springer.com/series/7892

Joseph R. Testa

Editor

Asbestos and Mesothelioma

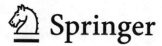 Springer

Editor
Joseph R. Testa
Cancer Biology Program
Fox Chase Cancer Center
Philadelphia, PA, USA

ISSN 2199-2584   ISSN 2199-2592   (electronic)
Current Cancer Research
ISBN 978-3-319-85183-9   ISBN 978-3-319-53560-9   (eBook)
DOI 10.1007/978-3-319-53560-9

Printed on acid-free paper

This Springer imprint is published by Springer Nature
The registered company is Springer International Publishing AG
The registered company address is: Gewerbestrasse 11, 6330 Cham, Switzerland

This monograph is inspired by and dedicated to patients afflicted with asbestos-related diseases, their families, medical caregivers, patient advocates, and researchers worldwide who are committed to advancing the understanding of the biological underpinnings of mesothelioma and its prevention, as well as the development of more effective therapies.
This volume is also dedicated to my wife, Priscilla, *for her unwavering support and my daughter,* Courtney, *for her indefatigable spirit and optimism about the future.*

Contents

Chapter 1
Malignant Mesothelioma: An Asbestos Legacy

Joseph R. Testa

Abstract With the advent of the industrial age, asbestos' unique properties, including its resistance to fire, tensile strength, softness and flexibility, resulted in its widespread commercial use. Decades later, its usage was shown to have tragic medical consequences, as these fibrous minerals became causally linked to malignant mesothelioma and other debilitating diseases. Malignant mesotheliomas are aggressive tumors that arise from serous membranes, such as the pleura and the peritoneum. Mesothelioma has a dismal prognosis due to its inherent chemo- and radio-resistance as well as to the general ineffectiveness of surgical intervention. Mesotheliomas account for approximately 3200 deaths per year in the USA, with more than 450,000 deaths predicted over the next 40 years in the USA, Europe, Australia, and Japan. Legal compensation alone is projected to amount to hundreds of billions of dollars worldwide over this time span, and this already enormous figure does not include health care costs. Currently, about 125 million people worldwide are exposed to asbestos in the workplace. Given such continued exposure to asbestos fibers, there is thus great public, medical, and legal interest in this malignancy. This introduction provides a general overview of the mesothelioma burden and a brief outline about the contents of this monograph, which includes a multidisciplinary assessment of the characteristics of asbestos along with the epidemiology, cell biology, pathology, and treatment of mesothelioma. Psychological aspects and legal challenges facing mesothelioma patients and their families are also presented.

Keywords History of asbestos usage • Health effects of asbestos • Malignant mesothelioma • Mesothelioma epidemiology • Pathology and treatment • Mesothelioma cell biology and genetics • Germline and somatic mutations • Rodent models of mesothelioma • Psychological and legal issues

J.R. Testa (✉)
Cancer Biology Program, Fox Chase Cancer Center,
Philadelphia, PA 19111, USA
e-mail: joseph.testa@fccc.edu

© Springer International Publishing AG 2017
J.R. Testa (ed.), *Asbestos and Mesothelioma*, Current Cancer Research,
DOI 10.1007/978-3-319-53560-9_1

1.1 Asbestos Usage Over the Years

Asbestos refers to a family of six silicate minerals that contain silicon and oxygen embodied as fibrous aggregates of long, thin crystals that can readily separate. Among its remarkably useful attributes are its resistance to fire, tensile strength, flexibility, softness, and affordability, with early usage of asbestos dating back at least two millennia. In their fascinating historical account of the ups-and-downs of asbestos' past, Alleman and Mossman alluded to the irony of the asbestos tragedy, i.e., that the medical catastrophe would never have become so severe had the industrial world not previously found the substance to be so valuable commercially (Alleman and Mossman 1997).

Over the years, asbestos has been used to weave cloaks, tablecloths, theater curtains, and flameproof suits for shielding against fires. Other everyday uses have included automobile brake shoes, air filters for military gas masks, hospital ventilators, and even cigarette filters. Mixed with rubber, asbestos permitted the development of durable steam engine components, such as steam gaskets. When melded into tar, burlap, and paper, asbestos fibers provided fire-resistant roofing material, thereby opening up a vast industry of asbestos-based construction products. Mixtures of asbestos and cement were heavily used for paneling in buildings and ships, as well as for pipes and synthetic slate roof shingles. When mixed with plastic, asbestos was used in everything from electrical boards to telephones, and vinyl-asbestos tiles became paramount in the flooring industry, including in schools. In skyscrapers, spray-on asbestos coating was used to protect steel structures against fire-induced buckling (Alleman and Mossman 1997).

1.2 Malignant Mesothelioma and Other Health Effects of Asbestos

In a seminal report published in 1960, Wagner and colleagues provided conclusive epidemiological evidence linking asbestos to malignant mesothelioma in individuals living and/or working in a crocidolite asbestos mining area of South Africa (Wagner et al. 1960). Malignant mesotheliomas are tumors derived from mesothelial cells that form the serosal membranes lining the chest and abdomen. Most mesotheliomas are highly aggressive neoplasms that have a median survival of about 9 months from the time of diagnosis. The incidence of malignant mesothelioma is several-fold higher in men than in women and is often diagnosed during the seventh and eighth decades of life, typically 20–50 years after initial exposure to asbestos. Mesothelioma currently accounts for 3200 deaths per year in the USA and about 5000 deaths in Western Europe (Henley et al. 2013; Ismail-khan et al. 2006).

In the late 1990s, it was estimated that 20% of homes and commercial buildings in the USA still contained products, e.g., shingles, cement pipes, and insulation, made from chrysotile asbestos (Alleman and Mossman 1997). Deaths due to mesothelioma are expected to increase by 5–10% per year in most industrialized countries until about 2020, and asbestos has also been shown to cause asbestosis, pleural fibrosis/ plaques, as well as lung and laryngeal cancer (Carbone et al. 2012). Notably, the incidence of mesothelioma has continued to increase despite various measures implemented in the 1970s and 1980s to reduce (U.S.) or eliminate (countries of the European Union) the use of products containing asbestos.

Both epidemiological studies and experimental work performed in vitro and in rodents have shown a strong link between mesothelioma and exposure to crocidolite asbestos, a needlelike (amphibole) form of asbestos, and erionite, a needlelike type of zeolite. Other forms of amphibole asbestos, such as tremolite, have also been associated with the development of mesothelioma, although the risk appears to be lower than for crocidolite fibers. Whether other amphibole types or the serpentine (snakelike) asbestos fiber, chrysotile, causes mesothelioma is still debated; however, the World Health Organization's International Agency for Research on Cancer (IARC) has concluded that all forms of asbestos can cause mesothelioma (IARC 2009; http://monographs.iarc.fr/ENG/Monographs/vol100C/mono100C-11.pdf).

Given that asbestos is virtually an inescapable carcinogen in industrialized societies, almost everyone may have some level of exposure. Although it has been hypothesized that there is a threshold level of exposure above which risk of developing mesothelioma increases significantly, the threshold is unknown, and individual genetic susceptibility likely influences this threshold (Testa and Carbone 2016). There does not appear to be a linear dose-response relationship between asbestos exposure and development of mesothelioma, and in addition to genetic differences, tumor risk may depend on the type of mineral fiber inhaled and exposure to certain cofactors.

Interestingly, while billions of dollars per year are spent on asbestos-related litigation and asbestos abatement, progress in understanding mesothelioma pathogenesis has been hampered by limited research funding—due in part to its lower incidence than other types of cancer, such as lung and breast carcinomas, but also because of the mistaken belief by some that the disease is disappearing. In fact, the incidence of mesothelioma in the USA has remained constant since the mid-1990s. Alarmingly, in countries that produce and/or are expanding their use of asbestos, including India, China, Russia, Zambia, Colombia, and Kazakhstan, a surge in disease incidence is expected to occur in these countries (see Chap. 4 by Røe and Stella in this volume), particularly in countries such as India, where little or no precautions are being taken to prevent exposure of workers (Burki 2010). In Western countries, exposure to high levels of asbestos in the workplace has been largely abolished, but the number of workers exposed to low, but above-background, levels of asbestos has increased; furthermore, use of asbestos in some products continues in the USA (Carbone et al. 2012).

In addition to mesothelioma, asbestos was shown to act as a carcinogen in lung carcinoma, and the combination of cigarette smoking and asbestos greatly increased the risk of lung cancer (Barrett et al. 1989). Moreover, inhalation of asbestos fibers was also found to induce other occupational lung diseases, including benign pleural plaques as well as two potentially deadly diseases: asbestosis, marked by chronic inflammation and scarring of the lungs, and a form of pneumoconiosis, a respiratory disease that restricts lung expansion. More recently, a comprehensive review by the IARC determined that there is *sufficient evidence* for the carcinogenicity of all forms of asbestos (chrysotile, crocidolite, amosite, tremolite, actinolite, and antho-phyllite) and that exposure to asbestos can cause not only mesothelioma and lung cancer, but also cancer of the larynx (IARC 2009; http://monographs.iarc.fr/ENG/Monographs/vol100C/mono100C-11.pdf). Additionally, IARC noted that positive associations have been observed between exposure to asbestos and cancers of the ovary and stomach.

Since asbestos has been shown to be the major cause of mesothelioma, with a history of asbestos exposure being documented in about 80% of individuals diagnosed with the pleural form of the tumor (Robinson and Lake 2005), and since no safe lower threshold of exposure has been identified, asbestos products have been banned in all the countries of the European Union, beginning January 1, 2005 (http://monographs.iarc.fr/ENG/Monographs/vol100C/mono100C-11.pdf;   EU 1999). Moreover, in addition to those exposed occupationally, family members can be at risk, e.g., as a result of washing contaminated work clothes, or simply by living in proximity to mining or asbestos cement processing factories (Magnani et al. 2001; Musti et al. 2009).

Patients with peritoneal mesothelioma, which comprise approximately 20% of all cases, tend to be younger than patients with pleural mesothelioma; moreover, a higher proportion of peritoneal mesothelioma cases, mostly women, are long-term survivors (Kindler 2013). Among patients eligible for surgery, a locoregional approach consisting of cytoreductive surgery and perioperative intraperitoneal chemotherapy—introduced over the last decade—achieved an overall 5-year survival rate of 30–60% (Mirarabshahii et al. 2012). Malignant pleural mesothelioma, on the other hand, is almost uniformly resistant to treatment. Cancer-directed surgery for malignant pleural mesothelioma is associated with a 5-year survival rate of only 15% (Wolf and Flores 2016), and chemotherapy-naive patients who were not eligible for curative surgery had a median survival of only about 12 months when treated with pemetrexed plus cisplatin, the current standard chemotherapeutic regimen (Vogelzang et al. 2003).

1.3   Outline of Monograph Contents

To understand how clinical outcomes may be improved in the future, it is necessary to better comprehend the biology of the disease. In recognition of the continuing global use of asbestos and its deadly legacy, this volume includes reviews on the various forms of asbestos and their relative carcinogenic potential, the epidemiology and biology of mesothelioma, and the current therapeutic options for this aggressive, therapy-resistant malignancy. In Chap. 2, Wylie describes the physical and chemical attributes of a group of very narrow fibrils that form bundles of parallel fibers characteristic of the "asbestiform habit." Included in this chapter are numerous photographs of the various types of asbestiform amphiboles, such as cro-cidolite, as well as the serpentine group of minerals that include chrysotile, the most widely used type of asbestos. Erionite, a fibrous zeolite, is also discussed.

Chapters 3, 4, and 5 discuss various aspects of the epidemiology of malignant mesothelioma, particularly in connection with exposure to asbestos or erionite. In addition to asbestos and other carcinogenic mineral fibers, Moolgavkar and cowork-ers point out that there is evidence for idiopathic mesotheliomas, i.e., those that arise spontaneously or from an obscure or unknown cause, as well as for other con-tributing factors, including germline and acquired, age-related gene mutations. Other risk factors, such as ionizing radiation, and the impact of non-occupational low levels of fiber exposure are also reviewed. Røe and Stella review the history of asbestos usage and its connection with mesothelioma causation as well as current unresolved questions and controversies regarding the epidemiology and biology of this dreaded disease. Additionally, these authors review recent studies indicating that man-made carbon nanofibers could pose dangers similar to those of asbestos in the coming years, and thus they urge regulatory bodies to be proactive in ensuring thorough evaluation of novel substances before commercial use. Emmett and Cakouros describe a diverse group of communities that have a high incidence of malignant mesothelioma and other asbestos-related diseases. They highlight lessons from communities where there is an elevated risk of mesothelioma due to asbestos mining, processing, and manufacturing as well as regions such as Cappadocia, Turkey, where asbestiform erionite occurs naturally in the local environment. They also describe a wide assortment of issues, including shortcomings in the regulatory definition of asbestos, diffuse administrative responsibilities, diverse community attitudes about disease risk and prevention, as well as difficulties in quantifying exposures and justifying remediation actions.

In Chap. 6, Pavlisko et al. describe in detail the gross pathology of mesothelioma arising from pleura, peritoneum, pericardium, and the tunica vaginalis. The authors provide an overview of the histomorphologic growth patterns, ranging from epithe-lioid to sarcomatoid, and discuss the importance of immunohistochemical stains in helping to assure the diagnosis of malignant mesothelioma. They also review the value of BAP1 immunohistochemistry together with fluorescence in situ hybridiza-tion for detection of homozygous loss of the gene encoding p16INK4A in distin-guishing benign/reactive from malignant mesothelial proliferations.

Chapters 7, 8, 9, 10, and 11 present overviews of various biological processes important in the development and progression of malignant mesothelioma. Thompson and Shukla review the role of asbestos-induced inflammation in meso-thelioma, fibrosis, and other lung diseases. They discuss the possibility that early inflammatory gene "signatures" might be exploited as novel predictive biomarkers and therapeutic targets to aid in early diagnosis and treatment of mesothelioma, respectively. Cheung and colleagues highlight our current understanding of the role of both germline and acquired (somatic) mutations in human malignant mesotheli-oma, as well as lessons learned from experimental studies of asbestos-exposed rodent models of mesothelioma. The authors review the body of literature about relevant genes, particularly the tumor suppressor genes *BAP1*, *CDKN2A* and *NF2*, which are frequently mutated somatically in human mesotheliomas and may serve as "drivers" of this lethal disease. They also explore recent research about familial risk of mesothelioma due to germline mutation of *BAP1* and potentially other genetic factors that may play a role in tumor predisposition (Testa et al. 2011). Evidence for gene–environment interaction, i.e., the convergence of germline *BAP1* mutation and exposure to asbestos fibers in the same individual, is also highlighted. De Rienzo et al. discuss recent efforts to discover gene signatures that might hold promise for personalized therapeutic decisions, with the goal of improving clinical outcome in patients with mesothelioma. They summarize findings using several different technologies such as sequencing, expression, and methylation arrays, and they discuss current challenges, including the need for large-scale validation before gene signatures can be implemented into the clinic. Mossman provides an overview of cell signaling and epigenetic mechanisms critically involved in the transformation of a mesothelial cell into a malignant mesothelioma. She reviews integrated genomic and proteomic analyses of mesothelioma, which have uncovered recurrent activation of multiple cell signaling cascades and transcription factors, as well as epigenetic mechanisms, with an emphasis on research that links such changes to key cell survival and proliferative pathways in tumor formation. Broaddus and coworkers discuss the value of three-dimensional, multicellular spheroid models for investigating mechanisms of cell survival in mesothelioma. They highlight areas in which in vitro multicellular spheroids and ex vivo tumor fragment spheroids have advanced the understanding of mesothelioma cell survival and other processes. As compared to conventional two-dimensional (monolayer) cultures, their findings with spheroid models appear to more closely mimic the therapeutic response in the actual tumor and could offer novel insights that can be subsequently tested in the clinic.

The review by Mesaros et al. (Chap. 12) focuses on recent advances in the identification of biomarkers of response to asbestos exposure, with the ultimate goal being to promote early diagnosis and timely clinical intervention. They evaluate various potential biomarkers of response to asbestos exposure, including the High Mobility Group Box 1 (HMGB1) protein, which has a regulatory role in inflammatory immune responses. Preliminary work has revealed that increased nonacetylated HMGB1 in serum may serve as a biomarker of asbestos exposure, whereas acetylated serum HMBG1 was associated with progression to mesothelioma. The potential merit of combined use of a multiplexed serum lipid biomarker panel with serum protein biomarkers is also discussed.

Chapters 13, 14, 15, and 16 contain comprehensive overviews of state-of-the-art therapies for mesothelioma. Wolf and Flores describe current surgical approaches for mesothelioma. They point out that although the role of surgical resection in malignant pleural mesothelioma is controversial, surgery has yielded long-term survivors, with a 15% 5-year survival in eligible patients. The authors summarize preoperative, perioperative, and postoperative management of mesothelioma patients as well as results of studies evaluating the two operations developed for surgical resection, extrapleural pneumonectomy and radical or extended pleurectomy/decortication (P/D), with the authors advocating the better tolerated P/D procedure for most pleural mesothelioma patients. Simone et al. discuss the role of both technologically sophisticated ionizing radiotherapy and non-ionizing radiotherapy (photodynamic therapy—a procedure that combines a photosensitizer, light, and oxygen) in both the palliative and definitive treatment of pleural mesothelioma, particularly in providing durable local control. The authors outline the mechanistic and logistical basics of radio- and photodynamic therapies and their use in the multidisciplinary care of mesothelioma patients. They also discuss the potential for future improvements in the use of these therapies. Zauderer summarizes standard chemotherapeutic approaches as well as clinical trials of novel molecularly targeted agents for malignant mesothelioma. She reviews challenges in conducting large randomized clinical trials in mesothelioma, including the scarcity and geographic distribution of patients, the intrinsic chemoresistance of the malignancy, as well as the limited interest and modest financial support from pharmaceutical companies and various funding agencies. Despite these drawbacks, standard cytotoxic chemotherapeutic regimens have been established, and clinical trials with multiple novel agents are ongoing. Thomas et al. review immunotherapeutic strategies to inhibit immune checkpoints and their ligands in mesothelioma. Furthest along currently are clinical investigations of the tumor differentiation antigen mesothelin, with immunotherapies developed that include immunotoxin, tumor vaccine, chimeric antigen receptor T cell, and antibody-based approaches. The authors also describe current work aimed at understanding the antitumor responses to immune-based approaches and ways to identify prospectively those patients most likely to respond to immunotherapy.

In addition to understanding the etiology, biology, and treatment of mesothelioma from a scientific and medical perspective, understanding the disease from the vantage point of the patient is critical. Thus, the final section of this volume focuses on the patient experience. Mesothelioma patients face enormous medical, stress-related, and financial challenges as emphasized in Chaps. 17 and 18. Hartley and Hesdorffer present an overview of medical and legal aspects of the disease, in particular lawsuits intended to seek compensation for patients who develop a mesothelioma potentially caused by exposure to asbestos fibers. Factors to consider when seeking legal advice—and the qualifications of prospective law firms—are presented. Pretrial discovery processes are discussed in detail, including possible requests for genetic testing to determine if an underlying heritable factor may have contributed to development of the disease. The authors also summarize new developments at the intersections between medicine and law, i.e., the possible use of molecular biomarkers, as well as genetic and epigenetic signatures, as potential indicators of asbestos exposure. Buchholz provides a compassionate overview of the complex experience of the mesothelioma patient. He delves into the psychological, sociological, and communicative elements of the individual patient's experience, with the aim being to help medical caregivers comprehend and better respond to that experience. Through interesting case studies, the author illustrates that mesothelioma patients are under great stress that is often unrecognized, but which may be alleviated, at least in part, when the nature of suffering is identified and integrated into a comprehensive treatment strategy.

Finally, the Editor thanks all of the chapter authors for their invaluable contributions to this volume on asbestos and mesothelioma. In the interest of transparency, the publisher has requested that all authors include a brief conflict of interest statement, because a diagnosis of mesothelioma often results in litigation, and many investigators are consulted about matters concerning disease causation—often with very different perspectives on such issues. In any case, the views and opinions expressed by authors of individual chapters do not necessarily reflect those of the Editor.

Acknowledgements The Editor is grateful to the many talented laboratory colleagues and collaborators he has been privileged to work with over the years in a collective effort to unravel the pathogenesis of mesothelioma. He gives special thanks to Fox Chase Cancer Center, NIH, and the Local #14 of the International Association of Heat and Frost Insulators and Allied Workers for their sustained financial support over the last three decades.

References

Alleman JE, Mossman BT (1997) Asbestos revisited. Sci Am 277:70–75

Barrett JC, Lamb PW, Wiseman RW (1989) Multiple mechanisms for the carcinogenic effects of asbestos and other mineral fibers. Environ Health Perspect 81:81–89.

Burki T (2010) Health experts concerned over India's asbestos industry. Lancet 375:626–627

Carbone C, Ly BH, Dodson RF et al (2012) Malignant mesothelioma: facts, myths and hypotheses. J Cell Physiol 227:44–58

Henley SJ, Larson TC, Wu M et al (2013) Mesothelioma incidence in 50 states and the district of Columbia, U.S., 2003–2008. Int J Occup Environ Health 19:1–10

International Agency for Research on Cancer (2009) Chrysolite, amosite, crocidolite, tremolite, actinolite, and anthophyllite. In: IARC monographs. arsenic, metals, fibres and dusts. International Agency for Research on Cancer, Lyon, pp 147–167

Ismail-Khan R, Robinson LA, Williams CC Jr et al (2006) Malignant pleural mesothelioma: a comprehensive review. Cancer Control 13:255–263

Kindler HL (2013) Peritoneal mesothelioma: the site of origin matters. Am Soc Clin Oncol Educ Book 33:182–188

Magnani C, Dalmasso P, Biggeri A et al (2001) Increased risk of malignant mesothelioma of the pleura after residential or domestic exposure to asbestos: a case-control study in Casale Monferrato, Italy. Environ Health Perspect 109:915–919

Mirarabshahii P, Pillai K, Chua TC et al (2012) Diffuse malignant peritoneal mesothelioma—an update on treatment. Cancer Treat Rev 38:605–612

Musti M, Pollice A, Cavone D et al (2009) The relationship between malignant mesothelioma and an asbestos cement plant environmental risk: a spatial case-control study in the city of Bari (Italy). Int Arch Occup Environ Health 82:489–497

Robinson BW, Lake RA (2005) Advances in malignant mesothelioma. N Engl J Med 353:1591–1603

Testa JR, Cheung M, Pei J et al (2011) Germline BAP1 mutations predispose to malignant mesothelioma. Nat Genet 43:1022–1025

Testa JR, Carbone M (2016) Mesothelioma. In: Schwab M (ed) Encyclopedia of cancer, 3rd edn. Springer, Heidelberg

Vogelzang N, Rusthoven JJ, Symanowski J et al (2003) Phase III study of pemetrexed in combination with cisplatin versus cisplatin alone in patients with malignant pleural mesothelioma. J Clin Oncol 21:2636–2644

Wagner JC, Sleggs CA, Marchand P (1960) Diffuse pleural mesothelioma and asbestos exposure in the North Western Cape province. Br J Ind Med 17:260–271

Wolf AS, Flores RM (2016) Current treatment of mesothelioma: extrapleural pneumonectomy versus pleurectomy/decortication. Thorac Surg Clin 26:359–375

Chapter 2
Asbestos and Fibrous Erionite

Ann G. Wylie

Abstract Very narrow fibrils forming bundles of parallel fibers characterize the asbestiform habit. The width of fibrils varies among asbestos types and among occurrences of the same type. The known asbestiform amphiboles have the composition of anthophyllite, tremolite-actinolite-ferroactinolite (prieskaite), cummingtonite-grunerite (amosite and montasite), magnesioarfvedsonite-arfedsonite, magnesioriebeckite-riebeckite (crocidolite), winchite (Libby amphibole), richterite, and fluoro-edenite-edenite. Amphiboles are common rock-forming minerals that normally occur in a prismatic or massive habit and are not asbestos. The most widely exploited type of asbestos is chrysotile, a member of the serpentine group of minerals. Erionite is a fibrous zeolite; when asbestiform, it is called woolly erionite. This chapter describes the characteristics of these minerals as they occur in an asbestiform habit.

Keywords Asbestos • Tremolite-asbestos • Actinolite-asbestos • Ferroactinolite-asbestos • Anthophyllite-asbestos • Amosite • Crocidolite • Edenite-asbestos • Winchite-asbestos • Richterite-asbestos • Chrysotile-asbestos • Woolly erionite

2.1 Introduction

Asbestos is a naturally occurring, heat-resistant, and chemically inert silicate material that can be readily separated into long, thin, strong fibers with sufficient flexibility to be woven. It may be formed from a number of different minerals that belong to the amphibole or serpentine mineral groups. For thousands of years, the unique properties of asbestos have made it a valuable commodity that has found applications in ceramics, whitewash, paint, fireproof fabrics, reinforced cement, insulation, brake pads, filters, and roofing tiles.

The author has served as a consultant on mineral occurrence, identification, and characterization.

A.G. Wylie (✉)
Laboratory for Mineral Deposits Research, Department of Geology, University of Maryland, College Park, MD 20742, USA
e-mail: awylie@umd.edu

© Springer International Publishing AG 2017
J.R. Testa (ed.), *Asbestos and Mesothelioma*, Current Cancer Research,
DOI 10.1007/978-3-319-53560-9_2

In the mid-twentieth century, it became clear that the inhalation of asbestos and asbestiform erionite could induce mesothelioma, stimulating extensive research into their physical and chemical characteristics and occurrences in nature. The research focused on relationships between the association of elevated levels of mesothelioma and (1) the size of fibers in the dust cloud, (2) mineral make-up of the fibers, including mineral alterations, intergrowths, and impurities, (3) the biodurability of the various fibers, (4) surface chemistry, particularly iron content, (5) surface area, and (6) reactivity in vivo. The research has demonstrated that all these characteristics can affect mesotheliomagenicity and that there is considerable variation in carcinogenic potential among asbestiform minerals.

While asbestos and erionite with asbestos-like dimensions are relatively rare, the minerals that form them exist most commonly in a form that is not asbestos. They are common rock-forming minerals and may also be found in soils. Amphiboles and serpentine are found in 6–10% of the land area of the USA and are probably similarly common elsewhere in the world (Wylie and Candela 2015). Erionite is found in geological environments that are common in the western USA and elsewhere; it is only rarely asbestiform (Van Gosen et al. 2013). When disturbed by recreational activities, mining, and excavation for road and building construction, both fragments and fibers of these minerals may become airborne. This chapter will describe the mineralogical characteristics thought to have relevance to biological activity of the major occurrences of commercially exploited amphibole- and serpentine-asbestos, of asbestiform erionite, and of unexploited naturally occurring asbestos and erionite.

2.2 Discussion of Terminology

In modern usage, *asbestos* is applied to a set of minerals from the amphibole and serpentine silicate mineral groups that were mined during the twentieth century and sold as asbestos. The term is also used for asbestiform amphibole that has not been exploited commercially, but is identified as asbestos because of its similarity in habit to commercially exploited asbestos. This would include, for example, the Na-Ca amphiboles that make up the asbestos gangue in the vermiculite deposit at Libby, Montana, some standard reference samples of asbestos, and many museum samples.

The formation of friable mineral fiber is restricted to particular physical and chemical conditions that are limited in their geographical extent. A discussion of geologic occurrences of asbestos in the USA has been provided by Van Gosen (2007). Rock must have been of the appropriate composition and subsequently altered by hot water-rich fluids, dissolving the mineral components until changing conditions resulted in crystallization of secondary minerals in a fibrous form. The *asbestiform habit* describes flexible mineral fibers, formed from parallel or nearly parallel bundles of very thin single crystals, called *fibrils* that are not otherwise regularly aligned. In asbestos, fibrils range in width from about 0.01 to about 0.5 μm. These very small fibrils give a silky luster to asbestos. Fibrils combine to

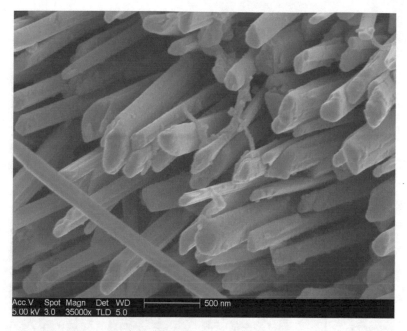

Fig. 2.1 Field emission scanning electron microscopy (FESEM) micrograph of fibril bundle of tremolite-asbestos from North Carolina. Note typical irregularity of the cross section. Photo courtesy R.J. Lee Group

form *fibers* (Fig. 2.1). Asbestos and asbestiform erionite fibers are easily separable with hand pressure, but the ease of *disaggregation* or *separation* into individual fibrils varies among occurrences (Fig. 2.1).

Glassy, brittle fibrils, with width of about 0.5–10 μm or more may accompany asbestos and asbestiform-erionite, or may occur separately. Such glassy brittle fibers of amphibole are referred to as *byssolite* and brittle fibers of serpentine are sometimes referred to as *picrolite* (Fig. 2.2).

In the USA, *regulatory criteria* for counting airborne particles as "fibers" during exposure monitoring are: (1) longer than 5 μm, (2) an aspect ratio of at least 3:1, and (3) visible by optical microscopy. Some portion of a population of airborne asbestos fibers will meet these criteria, but a large portion is below the resolution of the light microscopy (≈0.25 μm) or is ≤5 μm in length. A portion of airborne fragmented amphibole, erionite and serpentine particles will also meet these criteria. The National Institute of Occupational Safety and Health has recently clarified that what is being measured are optically visible *Elongated Mineral Particles* (EMP), which are not necessarily fibers in the mineralogical sense (NIOSH 2011). An *EMP* is, therefore, any particle with a length to width ratio of at least 3:1 whether it is a fiber or fragment; for purposes of occupational exposure monitoring, EMPs must be >5 μm.

In this chapter, the term "*fiber*" means an EMP that is a single or twinned crystal bounded by growth surfaces or *crystal faces* (a fibril) or a bundle of such crystals (*fiber bundle*). The term "*fragment*" applies to a particle that is bounded by broken

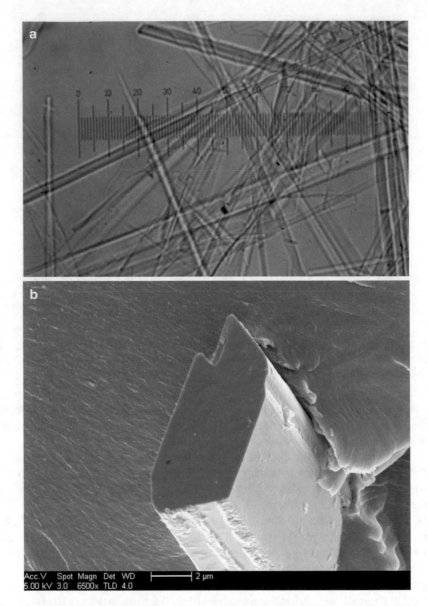

Fig. 2.2 Micrographs of actinolitic byssolite fibers from Austria. (**a**) Photograph of fiber sizes (smallest scale division = 2 μm). (**b**) FESEM micrograph of single fiber (Courtesy R.J. Lee Group). The largest prismatic surfaces that flatten the fiber are {100}

surfaces, originating when rock or brittle fiber is crushed. Fragments may be shaped by geometrically related planes if they possess *cleavage*, defined as the regular way a mineral breaks. Cleavage planes are planes of weakness within the ordered atomic structure of a mineral. In amphiboles, perfect *cleavage* in two directions forms prismatic EMPs, called *cleavage fragments*. Because cleavage arises from weak structural bonds, the potential for cleavage is the same in every sample of a given mineral. *Parting* resembles cleavage, but the planes of weakness arise from structural defects or inclusions, which are not necessarily present in every sample.

2.3 Amphiboles

There are many *amphibole* minerals, but all are built on double chains of Si_4O_{11} groups linked to each other by a variety of cations. Amphiboles occur in one of two crystal systems: monoclinic and orthorhombic. For both, modern nomenclature is based on the atomic proportions of the major elements assigned to the A, B, C, and T structural sites, following the rules of Leake et al. (1997, 2004) and Hawthorne et al. (2012). The general formula for amphibole is: $AB_2C_5T_8O_{22}(OH)_2$ where $A = \square$,[1] Na, K; B = Na, Ca, Mg, Fe2+, Mn2+ Li and rarer ions of similar size; $C = Mg$, $Fe^{2+,}$ Mn^{2+}, Li, Fe^{3+}, Al, Mn^{3+} Cr^{3+}, Zr^{4+}, Ti^{4+}; T = Si, Al, Ti^{4+}; and (OH) may be replaced by F, Cl, and O. The A-site is in 10–12-fold coordination, the B- and C-sites are octahedrally coordinated, and the T-site is tetrahedrally coordinated. The structure of amphibole suggests that the A-, B-, and T-sites come in contact with bodily fluids, which would have only limited access to C cations. For this reason, the amphibole formulae in this chapter are written to make the distinctions between A, B, C, and T.

Other systems of nomenclature have been used in the past. The earliest relied primarily on optical properties. Despite changes, there is general agreement among all nomenclature systems used for the last 50 years, although there are notable exceptions, such as the nomenclature of Na-Ca amphiboles, the chemical boundary between tremolite and actinolite, and the nomenclature within the large group of amphiboles generally known as hornblende. Because nomenclature is now strictly tied to crystal system and chemical composition, it may be useful to refer to amphibole-asbestos within solid solutions as, for example, tremolitic-asbestos instead of tremolite-asbestos or actinolitic-asbestos instead of actinolite-asbestos when the exact composition is inferred from qualitative or semi-quantitative chemical analyses or optical properties.

Amphibole minerals and mineral solid solutions known to have formed asbestos are: magnesioriebeckite-riebeckite (crocidolite), cummingtonite-grunerite (amosite and montasite), magnesioarfvedsonite, tremolite-actinolite-ferroactinolite, winchite, richterite, fluoro-edenite-edenite, and anthophyllite. Sometimes, dynamic physical and chemical conditions result in the formation of fibers with several amphibole compositions from the same location. For example, at Libby, MT, and Biancaville, Italy, winchite-asbestos, richterite-asbestos, tremolite-asbestos and edenite-asbestos have been reported (Meeker et al. 2003; Gianfagna et al. 2007). Actinolite-asbestos and crocidolite occur together in South Africa.

Not all amphibole compositions can form asbestos. In particular, Al substitution for Si in the T-site >0.5 atoms per formula unit (apfu) appears to limit the development

---

[1] $A_\square$ means the structural site A is empty.

of the asbestiform habit. The highest ^{T}Al is found in the fluoroedenite-asbestos fibers from Sicily, a region of active volcanism and high heat flow. The generally low ^{T}Al in asbestos is likely due to the requirement of a temperature for its incorporation into the structure higher than is common in most environments where asbestos forms (Dorling and Zussman 1987).

Amphiboles are well studied, and much is known about their occurrences and the natural variability they show in chemical composition and atomic structure. The optical properties of the common amphiboles are also well known. The reader is referred to major reference works for detailed discussions. These include Hawthorne et al. (2007), Guthrie and Mossman (1993), and Deer et al. (1997).

2.4 Amphibole Fibers and Fragments

Fibers form in open, often fluid-filled spaces or from hydrothermal alteration of pre-existing material in low-pressure environments. Fiber surfaces are often striated from vicinal faces associated with the rapid growth and metastability that arise from rapid precipitation from supersaturated hot water-rich fluids. Prolonged favorable conditions during growth or slow nucleation and crystal growth may result in larger fibril widths. Most fibrils of high quality amphibole asbestos range from 0.03 to <0.5 μm in width. In some asbestos occurrences, there are several generations of fibril growth, some of which are byssolite fibers of several micrometers in width. Some occurrences of asbestos may be referred to as *mountain leather* or *mountain cork*, when they have been subject to weathering on the earth's surface for long periods of time.

Fibrils are irregular in cross section, only occasionally displaying the expected crystal faces, {110}, {100} and {010},[2] as is evident in Fig. 2.1. However, many analysts report that amphibole fibers encountered in transmission electron microscopy (TEM) and optical studies are frequently flattened near {100}. A general relationship between width and thickness of fibers of crocidolite and amosite was established by Wylie et al. (1982) from TEM and scanning electron microscopy (SEM) measurements of fibers. It predicts that a fiber 0.1 μm in width would have a thickness of about 0.06 μm, while one that is 0.5 μm in width would have a thickness of about 0.2 μm.

Amphibole fragments are generally smooth as they are bounded by perfect {110} cleavage. They may also be bounded by {010} and/or {100} parting planes; offsets of faces parallel to cleavage are common (Fig. 2.3).

Structural studies of amphibole asbestos have shown that chain width defects parallel to {010} (e.g., a triple chain instead of the double chain characteristic of amphibole), known as Wadsley defects, and twinning or stacking faults parallel to {100} are both common. These are particularly well developed in anthophyllite-asbestos but have been reported in all amphibole asbestos and in many samples of common amphibole. Defects may explain the development of large {100} surfaces

---

[2] Miller Indices, e.g., {110}, are used to designate the orientation of planes within a crystal structure. A detailed discussion can be found in Bloss (1971) or other mineralogy textbooks.

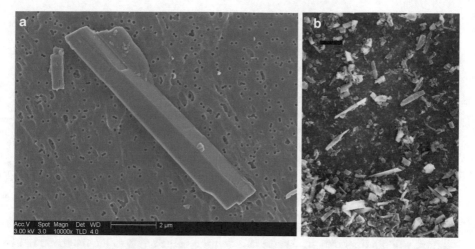

Fig. 2.3 (**a**) FESEM micrograph of a cleavage fragment of tremolite from Shininess, Scotland (Courtesy R.J. Lee Group). The EMP is formed by perfect {110} cleavage. Note offsets on prism surfaces and notched terminus. (**b**) SEM micrograph of cleavage fragments of grunerite from Homestake Mine, South Dakota (scale bar = 10 μm)

on fibrils. When defects are abundant, parting on {100} and {010} develops, enhancing the elongation (aspect ratio) of cleavage fragments.

Amphibole surfaces react to some extent with lung fluids, providing varying amounts of Ca, Na, Mg, K, Fe, and Si to the fluid. Some small chemical alterations have been observed on fibers retained in the human lung and there is some evidence for preferential dissolution on {100}. However, dissolution rates are very slow and fibers persist in the lung many years after exposure. In general, iron and aluminum reduce amphibole solubility in neutral to acidic solutions. Armoring by other minerals, such as talc, might also reduce solubility. In contrast, chrysotile is very soluble in lung fluid (Hume and Rimstidt 1992).

All amphiboles and serpentine would be expected to have tensile strength enhanced by the stable silicon-oxygen chains or sheets that characterize them. However, tensile strength has been shown to increase as the diameter of a fiber decreases (O'Hanley 1986); thus, given its extremely small fibril widths, it is not surprising that the tensile strength of crocidolite from Cape Asbestos Belt in South Africa and from the Hamersley Range in Western Australia has been measured at about 25–48,000 kg/cm^2 (Hodgson 1979) at room temperature; Hodgson (1979) reports tensile strength for amosite as 20–25,000 kg/cm^2. These compare to the tensile strength of steel piano wire, which is usually given as 25,000 kg/cm^2. The measured tensile strength of other amphibole-asbestos varies widely, and measurements of tremolitic, actinolitic, and anthophyllite-asbestos, which characteristically have fibrils wider than crocidolite, are usually much lower than that of crocidolite, amosite, and chrysotile. In addition to fibril size, a high frequency of planar defects may also result in an increase in tensile strength.

Surface area of amphibole-asbestos used in manufacturing is quite high, approaching 90,000 cm^2/g as measured by nitrogen absorption, while unprocessed ore may have a surface area an order of magnitude smaller. After ore is mined, it is normally "fiberized" in the mill to differing degrees, depending on its intended use. Fiberization liberates fibrils, affects fiber size, and increases surface area. In comparing lung fibrosis after exposure to Cape crocidolite, Hamersley crocidolite, amosite, and Paakkila anthophyllite-asbestos, Lippmann and Timbrell (1990) have concluded that it is the surface area of inhaled fibers that controls the degree of lung fibrosis, not mineral type per se, so surface area is an important variable in characterizing asbestos.

The magnetic properties of asbestos have been studied by Timbrell (1975). Amphiboles are paramagnetic and will align in a magnetic field if suspended in air or a liquid. The higher the iron content, in general the lower the field strength required for alignment. Crocidolite, chrysotile, and other fibers generally align with fiber axis parallel to the field. These are referred to as P-fibers. Amosite fibers may be P fibers, but some may align perpendicular to the magnetic field, referred to as N-fibers. Magnetite does not account for the alignment in amphiboles, although it does for some chrysotile. Timbrell reported that a synthetic fluoro-amphibole aligned with its fiber axis transverse at a definite acute angle to the magnetic field (T-fibers), but the relevance to natural mineral fiber is unknown. Variations from P-type fibers might be explained by structural defects such as twinning or by intergrowth of a second mineral phase.

Amphibole fibers and fragments carry a negative charge on their surfaces and a positive charge at their ends. Repulsive forces between fibers, however, are small and settled fibers form an open latticework with many voids. Because surface charge has been shown to be a function of aspect ratio, long narrow fibers will carry a higher charge than shorter or wider ones.

The optical properties of minerals occurring in an asbestiform habit are normally anomalous. Fibrils smaller than about 0.25 µm are not individually resolvable by polarized light microscopy, so it is the properties of a bundle that are observed. In their common form, amphiboles, serpentine, and erionite are birefringent with three principal indices of refraction: *gamma*, *alpha*, and *beta*. Because of the fibrillar habit of asbestos, however, only two indices of refraction can be measured, one parallel and one perpendicular to the fiber axis. Because of this, asbestos is characterized by *parallel extinction* or near parallel extinction. In monoclinic nonasbestiform amphiboles, the vibration directions make an angle with the axis of elongation; they are said to have *oblique extinction*. The anomalous optical properties are described in more detail by Wylie (1979) and by Verkouteren and Wylie (2002).

Generally speaking, each occurrence of amphibole has a distinct chemical composition and has experienced a distinctive geologic history, which determined its habit and the particle sizes it forms when disaggregated (asbestiform habit) and/or fragmented (common mineral forms). Habit and composition of the same mineral can be similar across locations, e.g., crocidolite from Western Australia and the Cape Asbestos Belt of South Africa, but they are more commonly quite different, e.g., crocidolite from other locations differ in both composition and size of fibrils. For occurrences of asbestos of tremolite-actinolite-ferroactinolite composition, the range in properties is quite large. In summary, with few exceptions, generalizations about the nature of asbestos across occurrences and among types without specifying the source location should be made with great care.

2.5 Amphibole-Asbestos

2.5.1 Sodic Amphibole Group

Riebeckite-magnesioriebeckite is a solid solution in the sodic group of amphiboles represented by the end member formula $^A\square^B Na_2\ ^C(Mg, Fe^{2+})_3\ ^C Fe^{3+}_2\ ^T Si_8O_{22}(OH)_2$, where the following apfu restrictions apply to substitutions: $^T Al < Fe^{3+}$, $^B Na > 1.5$, $^A(Na + K) < 0.50$, $Si > 7.5$, $Al < 0.5$, and $(Mn^{2+} + Mn^{3+}) < {}^C(Al + Fe^{3+} + Fe^{2+} + Mg)$, $Li < 0.5$. If $^A(Na + K) > 0.50$, the amphiboles are called *magnesioarfvedsonite-arfvedsonite*. $Mg/(Mg + Fe^{2+}) = 0.5$ separates magnesioriebeckite from riebeckite and magnesioarfvedsonite from arfvedsonite. Magnesioriebeckite-riebeckite and magnesioarfvedsonite-arfvedsonite are normally blue in color.

The asbestiform variety of magnesioriebeckite-riebeckite is known as crocidolite, or blue asbestos. Cross fiber veins have been mined in the Hamersley Range, Western Australia, and in the Cape Asbestos Belt, north central South Africa. Cross fiber crocidolite has also been mined from the Transvaal Asbestos Belt, northeast South Africa, and from Cochabamba, Bolivia (Redwood, 1993). Crocidolite from any locality may be expected to be accompanied by small amounts of magnetite, iron-rich biotite, carbonate, and quartz. In the mines in the Transvaal, kerogen has been reported.

Crocidolite mines in Hamersley Range and Cape Asbestos Belt have provided most of the world's crocidolite; in both places, its composition is riebeckite. Fibril widths <0.1 μm are characteristic as illustrated by Fig. 2.4a and by the frequency distribution of width from the mining and milling aerosol in Fig. 2.4b. The smallest fibrils are on the order of 0.02 μm in width, but rarely 0.5 μm single fibrils occur. The high frequency of airborne fibers of all lengths with widths <0.1 μm is unique among the varieties of commercially important amphibole-asbestos (Table 2.1). Cape and Hammersley crocidolite disaggregates into component fibrils readily, as reflected by the insensitivity of modal width to length (Table 2.1; Shedd 1985). Frequency distributions derived from bulk samples of long fiber products may be quite different from that of aerosols, reflecting either sampling protocols, removal of the finest fibrils during air processing, or sample preparation protocols, as illustrated in Fig. 2.4c.

Transvaal crocidolite fibers are coarser and harsher than Cape fiber. Compositionally, they are riebeckite but in some ore, grunerite (amosite) asbestos fiber may be intergrown. Cochabamba crocidolite fibers are typically light blue, long, and silky. Compositionally, they are magnesioriebeckite, but small amounts of another amphibole may be found intergrown. Frequency distributions of the width of crocidolite fibers from the Transvaal or from Cochabamba are more likely to resemble those of amosite (Fig. 2.5) than the crocidolite depicted in Fig. 2.4. They contain a smaller proportion of fibers less than 0.25 μm and widths extend over a wider range. Modal fiber widths are approximately 0.5 μm and 0.3 μm for Cochabamba, and Transvaal crocidolite, respectively (Shedd 1985).

Massive, nonfibrous, common riebeckite is found in the rock that encloses crocidolite veins in the asbestos mining regions of South Africa, the Hammersley

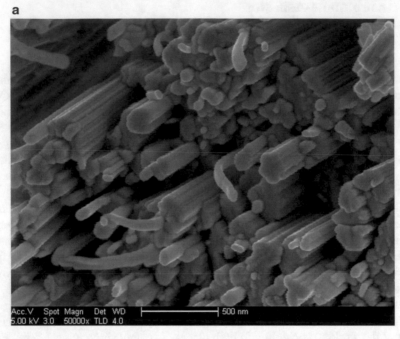

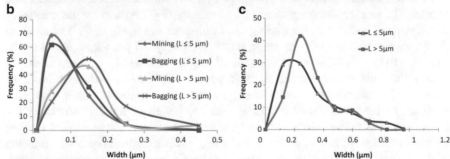

Fig. 2.4 Crocidolite characteristics. (**a**) FESEM micrograph showing fibrillar structure of crocidolite from the Cape asbestos province, South Africa (Courtesy R.J. Lee Group). (**b**) Frequency of width of airborne crocidolite EMPs from the mining and milling environments. Data are taken from Gibbs and Hwang (1980). Magnitude of the largest category of width (w >0.3 μm) is plotted at 0.45 μm. Lengths range from ≤2.5 to 10 μm: 96% of the fibers from mining and 93% of the fibers from bagging are less than 5 μm in length; the modal length for both mining and bagging is ≤ 2.5 μm. (**c**) Frequency of width of EMPs from bulk crocidolite used as a Standard Reference Material (SRM) by the National Institute of Standards and Technology (NIST). Data are from TEM measurements by Beard et al. (2007); sampling protocol is described by Harper et al. (2008). 23% of fibers measured are ≤5 μm. The range is 2 – 28 μm, and the modal length is 9.5 ± 2 μm. Note that the fibers measured in the bulk material are slightly wider and much longer than those found in the mining and milling aerosol

Range of Australia, and Cochabamba, Bolivia. It is also associated with certain igneous rocks in the western USA and elsewhere. Dimensional characterizations of common riebeckite can be found in Wylie (in press).

Table 2.1 Selected length and width measurements of amphibole-asbestos and amphibole cleavage fragments

	(a) Amosite and crocidolite				(b) Tremolite-ferroactinolite asbestos				Construction[a]
	Airborne amosite[b]		Airborne crocidolite[c]		Asbestos mine[d]	Asbestos mine[b]	raw-NIST SRM	Asbestos mine[a] / Asbestos mine[b]	raw-NIST SRM
	Electrical Co.	Shipyard	Mine	Eagging	Tremolite	Tremolite	Tremolite	Prieskaite	Actinolite
					Korea	India	CA	South Africa	VA
$L \leq 5\ \mu m > =1$									
Number measured	90	406			788	125	129	371	91
Width mode (μm)	0.20 ± 0.05	0.20 ± 0.05	<0.06	0.15 ± 0.05	0.07 ± 0.02	0.22 ± 0.06	0.48 ± 0.06	0.22 ± 0.06	0.72 ± 0.06
Mean width ± SD (μm)	0.31 ± 0.22	0.31 ± 0.22			0.20 ± 0.19	0.36 ± 0.21	0.68 ± 0.28	0.30 ± 0.15	0.71 ± 0.25
$5 < L \leq 10\ \mu m$									
Number	121	265			396	30	77	34	32
Width mode (μm)	0.30 ± 0.05	0.35 ± 0.10	0.15 ± 0.05	0.15 ± 0.05	0.07 ± 0.02	0.33 ± 0.06	1.50 ± 0.24	0.22 ± 0.06	0.66 ± 0.12
Mean width ± SD (μm)	0.40 ± 0.23	0.41 ± 0.24			0.26 ± 0.33	0.71 ± 0.44	1.48 ± 0.57	0.45 ± 0.20	1.06 ± 0.48
$10 < L \leq 15\ \mu m$									
Number measured	55	70			136	3	19	9	9
Width mode (μm)	0.30 ± 0.05	0.20 ± 0.05	0.15 ± 0.05[e]	0.15 ± 0.05[e]	0.14 ± 0.05	Undefined	Undefined	Undefined	1.14 ± 0.06
Mean width ± SD (μm)	0.42 ± 0.29	0.47 ± 0.35			0.39 ± 0.42	1.12 ± 0.64	2.55 ± 0.64	0.45 ± 0.18	1.28 ± 0.52

	(c) Amphibole-asbestos from Libby Montana			(d) Airborne fragments of common amphibole			
	Airborne	Extracted	Extracted	Stone quarry	Taconite mine	Gold mine	El Dorado Co.
	town[f]	Mine products[g]	Exfoliation products[g]	VA[b]	Mn[b]	SD[b]	CA[h]
$L \leq 5\ \mu m > =1$							
Number measured	1448	245	311	236	58	202	1545
Width mode (μm)	0.25 ± 0.05	0.16 ± 0.06	0.16 ± 0.06	0.55 ± 0.06	0.55 ± 0.06	0.55 ± 0.06	0.3 ± 0.1

(continued)

Table 2.1 (continued)

	(a) Amosite and crocidolite				(b) Tremolite-ferroactinolite asbestos				
	Airborne amosite[b]		Airborne crocidolite[c]		Asbestos mine[d]	Asbestos mine[b]	Asbestos mine[a]		Construction[a]
							raw-NIST SRM	Asbestos mine[b]	raw-NIST SRM
	Electrical Co.	Shipyard	Mine	Bagging	Tremolite	Tremolite	Tremolite	Prieskaite	Actinolite
					Korea	India	CA	South Africa	VA
Mean width ± SD (µm)	0.35 ± 0.20	0.28 ± 0.23		0.27 ± 0.19	0.71 ± 0.32	0.70 ± 0.29	0.77 ± 0.29	0.59 ± 0.31	
5 < L ≤ 10 µm									
Number measured	1044	83		151	128	23	126	1080	
Width mode (µm)	0.25 ± 0.05	0.28 ± 0.06		0.28 ± 0.06	1.16 ± 0.06	Undefined	1.10 ± 0.06	0.7 ± 0.1	
Mean width ± SD (µm)	0.59 ± 0.40	0.51 ± 0.33		0.47 ± 0.28	1.48 ± 0.80	1.59 ± 0.44	1.28 ± 0.54	1.29 ± 0.67	
10 < L ≤ 15 µm									
Number measured	429	34		49	40	2	27	367	
Width mode	0.25 ± 0.05	0.27 ± 0.06		0.27 ± 0.06	Undefined	Undefined	Undefined	2.5 ± 0.1	
Mean width ± SD (µm)	0.73 ± 0.56	0.49 ± 0.22		0.54 ± 0.30	2.32 ± 0.93	2.05 ± 1.34	1.91 ± 0.76	2.17 ± 1.14	

[a]Beard et al. (2007)
[b]Wylie et al. (2015)
[c]Gibb and Hwang (1980)
[d]Jenny Verkouteren (personal communication)
[e]The mode is for fibers between 10 and 20 µm in length
[f]EPA (2006)
[g]Atkinson et al. (1981)
[h]Ecology and the Environment (2005)

2.5.2   *Magnesium-Iron-Manganese-Lithium Amphibole Group*

2.5.2.1   Cummingtonite-Grunerite

Cummingtonite-grunerite is a solid solution in the magnesium-iron-manganese-lithium group of monoclinic amphiboles represented by the end member formula $^A\square^B(Mg, Fe^{2+})_2 \, ^C(Mg, Fe^{2+})_5 \, ^T(Si)_8O_{22}(OH)_2$; the following restrictions to substitutions apply: $^B(Ca + Na) < 1.0$, $^B(Mg, Fe, Mn, Li) \geq 1.0$, $^BLi < 1.00$, $Si > 7.0$. Mg/$(Mg + Fe^{2+}) = 0.5$ divides cummingtonite from grunerite. Cummingtonite-grunerite is light to dark brown in color.

The asbestiform variety of cummingtonite-grunerite is known as *amosite* or *brown asbestos*. The silky variety is sometimes called *montasite*. The name amosite

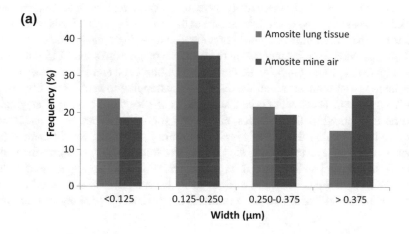

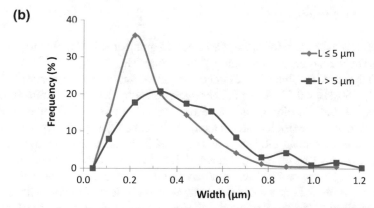

Fig. 2.5 Characteristics of amosite. (**a**) Frequency of width of amosite EMPS from lungs of miners and the mine aerosol, Transvaal, South Africa. Data for fibers of all lengths are taken from TEM measurements of Pooley and Clark (1980). Fibers ranged from <1 to >10 μm in length. Modal length is 2-3 μm, with 8-9% >10 μm and with 32% of airborne and 40% of lung burden fibers longer than 4 μm. (**b**) Frequency of width of amosite EMPS from shipyard aerosol. Fibers range from about 1.5 to >100 μm. Modal length is 2.5 ± 1 μm and about 23% are longer than 5 μm. Particle measurements can be found in Wylie et al. (2015). Many more long fiber bundles are found in the aerosol surrounding the construction of ships than in the mine

is not a proper mineral name; it was derived from the Asbestos Mines of South Africa located in the Transvaal Asbestos Belt. These mines have been the only important source of amosite worldwide.

Small amounts of ferroactinolite-asbestos, sometimes referred to as prieskaite, occur in association with amosite in the Transvaal. Magnetite and quartz are common accessory minerals, and minor biotite, pyrite, carbonate, stilpnomelane, kerogen, graphite, and magnesite have been reported in raw asbestos.

Amosite is sometimes described as "harsh." When the Bureau of Mines was trying to reduce the size of amosite in an air jet mill, the amosite blew a hole through hard-surfaced stainless steel (Campbell et al. 1980). Harshness results when fibrils resist disaggregation, forming larger fibers with less flexibility. Some level of coherence or semi-coherence in the amphibole structure across fibril boundaries has been observed in amosite, and sheet silicates, such as iron-rich talc, serpentine, and chlorite, are normally intergrown with the fibrils; these likely increase amosite's resistance to disaggregation.

Like crocidolite, frequency distributions of the width of amosite fibrils found in lung tissue and the air of mines and mills normally display a single modal value, as depicted in Fig. 2.5a. Modal widths reported in the literature range from about 0.15 μm for short fibers up to 0.5 μm for fibers longer than 5 μm. Unlike Cape and Hammersley crocidolite, there is a prominent tail on the distribution extending toward larger fiber widths. Such a tail is consistent with fibrils that adhere to one another, resisting disaggregation and resulting in wider fiber bundles, particularly for longer fibers. Of course, amosite may undergo varying degrees of fiberization during processing for different applications, which would be reflected in the size and structure of the tails; some distributions may be multimodal as illustrated in Fig. 2.5b, which shows the frequency of width of amosite fibers in the aerosol of a shipyard. The distribution displays the characteristic increase in the width of longer fibers formed from the bundles of many smaller fibrils.

2.5.2.2 Anthophyllite

Anthophyllite is a solid solution in the Mg-Fe-Mn-Li group of orthorhombic amphiboles represented by the endmember formula $^A\square^B$ $(Mg, Fe)_2$ $^C(Mg, Fe)_5Si_8O_{22}(OH)_2$. Iron-rich anthophyllite is rare. The following restrictions apply to atomic substitutions: $^B(Mg,Fe^{+2}, Mn^{+2}, Li) \geq 1.50$, $^BLi < 0.50$, $^TSi > 7.0$. The largest anthophyllite-asbestos mine is found at Paakkila, Finland. Smaller deposits have been mined in the USA, Sweden, Russia, India, and Pakistan. The risk for mesothelioma from anthophyllite-asbestosis generally is considered to be among the lowest among amphibole-asbestos exposures, and its mineralogical characteristics readily distinguish it from crocidolite and amosite.

Unlike amosite and crocidolite, anthophyllite-asbestos does not normally occur in cross-fiber veins. It is found in pods, masses, and clusters of fibers. Within clusters, parallel fibrils form bundles, but the clusters are not aligned. Its mode of formation results in a less homogeneous material than is characteristic of cross fiber veins.

Talc is always present with anthophyllite-asbestos. It is intergrown in such a way that its structural elements are parallel to those of anthophyllite (the growth is said to be *epitaxial*), and fibers composed only of the mineral talc are commonly associated with anthophyllite-asbestos. Talc is so pervasive that most fiber surfaces are covered

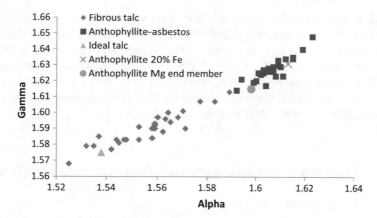

Fig. 2.6 Indices of refraction of fibrous talc, anthophyllite-asbestos, and intergrowths of talc and anthophyllite. Alpha is the smallest principal index of refraction, measured near perpendicular to elongation; gamma is the largest principal index of refraction measured near parallel to elongation. Data for fibrous talc are from Greenwood (1998). Data for anthophyllite-asbestos are from Watson (1999). Indices of refraction vary regularly with water content, $(Mg + Fe)/SiO2$ and Mg/Fe

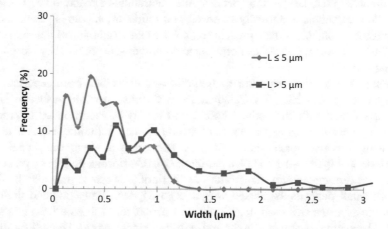

Fig. 2.7 Frequency of width of anthophyllite-asbestos EMPs from Udaipur, India. Data are from TEM measurements by Beard et al. (2007); sampling protocol is described by Harper et al. (2008). About 56% of the fibers measured are ≤5 μm in length. Lengths ranged from 1 to 40 μm, with a broad mode centered around 4 μm

by it. Some chemical compositions reported for anthophyllite with compositions of $Mg/(Mg + Fe)$ between 1.0 and 0.8 may be due primarily to intergrown talc (Watson 1999). Because of similarities in the atomic structure and the close association of these two minerals, a continuum in indices of refraction, birefringence, and chemical composition of fibers exists between end member fibrous talc and anthophyllite-asbestos (Fig. 2.6). Chlorite and serpentine in a variety of forms may also be associated with the anthophyllite-asbestos, and magnetite is a frequent accessory mineral.

A typical width distribution for anthophyllite-asbestos is shown in Fig. 2.7. The distribution shows the presence of very thin fibrils, both long and short, but fibers with wider widths are very common. Width distributions are frequently multimodal, a characteristic that arises from different generations of fiber growth, or the separation of discrete bundles of fibrils, and/or the incorporation of elongated particles formed by fragmentation. Timbrell et al. (1970) found a multimodal width distribution for anthophyllite-asbestos from Paakkila, Finland, as well. The frequency and size of modal widths will vary among anthophyllite-asbestos occurrences, sampling protocols, and degree of fiberization during processing (Fig. 2.7).

2.5.3 Magnesium-Iron-Manganese-Lithium Amphibole Group

2.5.3.1 Calcic Amphibole Group

Tremolite—Actinolite-Ferroactinolite is a solid solution in the calcic group of monoclinic amphibole represented by the endmember formula: $^A\square^B(Ca)_2$ $^C(Mg, Fe^{2+})_5$ $^TSi_8O_{22}(OH)_2$ with the following restrictions applied to substitutions: $^BCa \geq 1.50$, $^A(Na + K) < 0.50$, $^ACa < 0.50$, and $Si \geq 7.5$. $Mg/(Mg + Fe^{2+}) > 0.9$ defines the tremolite-actinolite boundary; <0.5 defines the actinolite-ferroactinolite boundary. Tremolitic amphibole is normally colorless, actinolitic amphibole is green, and ferroactinolitic amphibole is dark green in color. A general discussion of the characteristics of asbestiform and nonasbestiform calcic amphiboles is provided by Dorling and Zussman (1987).

Mesothelioma from exposure to tremolitic-asbestos has been reported from Turkey, Greece, Corsica, New Caledonia, and Cyprus. Tremolite-asbestos is also found associated with chrysotile-asbestos, and it may be incorporated in products containing chrysotile. Small deposits of tremolite- and actinolite-asbestos associated with iron and magnesium-rich rock were mined along the Appalachian Mountains and in the Western USA, particularly in California, during the nineteenth and early twentieth century. Tremolite- and actinolite-asbestos may also be found there in small deposits associated with altered Mg-rich limestone and dolomite. Actinolite-asbestos was used in antiquity in Europe, and asbestos from this series has also been mined in India, Russia, and elsewhere in the world. Tremolite-asbestos makes up a small proportion of the asbestiform amphibole in the vermiculite deposit in Libby, MT (discussed below). Consistent with older terminology, the amphibole-asbestos there was once referred to as tremolite or soda tremolite. Ferroactinolite-asbestos occurs in the Transvaal Asbestos Belt, where it is known as prieskaite.

Because members of this series are among the most common amphiboles, occurrences in the asbestiform habit are widespread although their exploitation as asbestos has been limited. Samples from many locations have been studied, and although asbestiform, they display a wide range in the size of the fibrils that make them up. Width and length data from five members of this series are provided in Table 2.1. Fibrils range from less than 0.1 to as much 0.66 μm. Only the asbestos from Korea has dimensions that are comparable to amosite and crocidolite. Mean widths for tremolite-asbestos that accompanies chrysotile-asbestos from Thetford, Quebec, have been reported from about 0.21–0.25 μm for fibers less than 5 μm and about 0.3–0.35 μm for longer fibers. This asbestos is likely more similar to Indian tremolite-asbestos in Table 2.1 than to Korean asbestos or the raw-NIST-SRM. The range in habits is also illustrated in Fig. 2.8, which depicts three tremolite-asbestos samples: Korea, the raw-NIST SRM from California, and the asbestos found in the Whitewash at Metsovo, Greece. The dimensions and the macroscopic appearance of the raw-NIST SRM are consistent with wide glassy fibers, so this asbestos appears to have characteristics that grade into byssolite.

Fluoro-edenite. Edenite-ferroedenite is a solid solution in the calcic group of monoclinic amphiboles represented by the end member formula $^A(Na,K)^B(Ca, Mg, Fe^{2+})_2 (Mg, Fe^{2+}, Mn, Li)_5 ^T(Si,Al)_8O_{22}(OH,F)_2$ with the following restrictions applied to substitutions: $^BCa \geq 1.50$, $^A(Na + K) \geq 0.50$, $6.5 < Si < 7.5$, and $Ti < 0.50$. The addition of the prefix fluoro- means that $F > 1.0$ in substitution for (OH). Mesothelioma from exposure to fluoro-edenite asbestos has been reported from Biancavilla, Sicily, Italy, where it is accompanied by small amounts of winchite-, richterite-, and tremolite-asbestos (Gianfagna et al. 2007). Minor feldspar, pyroxene, apatite, and magnetite are common. The widths of fibers with $L > 5$ μm from Biancavilla follow a frequency distribution similar to that of Indian tremolite-asbestos 2 shown in Fig. 2.8, with a modal width of 0.2–0.4 for fibers >5 μm (Paoletti and Bruni 2009).

2.5.3.2 Sodic-Calcic Amphibole Group

The *sodic-calcic amphibole* group contains several monoclinic amphiboles that are known to occur as asbestos including members of the solid solutions *richterite-ferrorichterite* represented by the endmember formula $^ANa ^B(CaNa)^C(Mg,Fe)_5^T Si_8O_{22}(OH)_2$ and *winchite-ferrowinchite*, represented by the end member formula $^A\square^B(CaNa)^C(Mg,Fe^{2+})_4^C(Al,Fe^{3+})^TSi_8O_{22}(OH)_2$. The following restrictions apply to substitutions for richterite-ferrorichterite: $^A(Na + K) \geq 0.50$, $^B (Ca + Na) \geq 1.00$, $0.50 < ^BNa < 1.50$ and $Si > 7.5$; for winchite-ferrowinchite: $^A(Na + K) < 0.50$, $^B (Ca + Na) \geq 1.00$, $0.50 < ^BNa < 1.50$ and $Si > 7.5$.

Amphibole-asbestos is abundant as gangue in the vermiculite ore mined at Libby, MT. Studies of its mineralogy have shown that winchite-asbestos is by far the most abundant, followed by richterite-asbestos and tremolite-asbestos; a small amount of edenite-asbestos may also be present (Meeker et al. 2003). The asbestos occurs in unaligned masses and clusters of parallel fibril bundles. The same amphibole-asbestos types are found at Biancavilla, Italy, although at that location edenite-asbestos is the most abundant.

Representative frequency distributions of the width of asbestos fibrils from Libby are shown in Fig. 2.9 and dimensional data are also provided in Table 2.1. Short fibers are dominated by particles that are 0.1–0.2 μm in width with very few wider particles. Long fibers are characterized by modal width of about 0.3 μm, with another distinctive mode at about 0.55 μm.

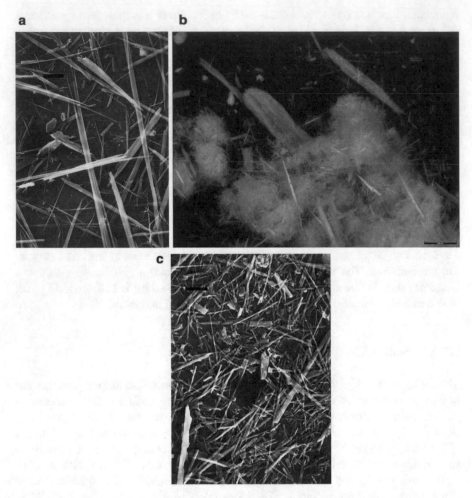

Fig. 2.8 Variability in the habits of asbestiform amphiboles are illustrated by three occurrences of tremoliteasbestos. (**a**) SEM micrograph of tremolite-asbestos from Korea (scale bar = 5 μm). (**b**) Macrophotograph of tremolite-asbestos from Condo Deposit, CA, NIST SRM 1867a (Courtesy R.J. Lee Group). This material contains many glassy fibers, more characteristic of byssolite than asbestos. (**c**) SEM micrograph of tremolite-asbestos from whitewash used in Metsovo, Greece, where exposure is associated with excess mesothelioma (scale bar = 5 μm)

2.5.4 Dimensional Characteristics of Common Amphibole

Many studies have examined common amphibole in mining aerosols. Others have looked at common amphibole dusts derived from comminution in the laboratory or directly measured in dusty environments. Populations of airborne and bulk cleavage fragments share dimensional characteristics, which are generalized in Fig. 2.10.

The frequencies of width for both long and short cleavage fragments of amphibole are multimodal. The smallest mode is normally <0.2 μm, but none of these

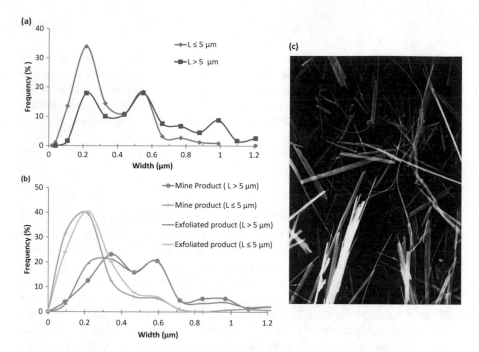

Fig. 2.9 Amphibole-asbestos from Libby, Montana. (**a**) Frequency of width of airborne amphi-bole asbestos EMPs collected from the town of Libby, MT. Data are from TEM measurements by the Environmental Protection Agency (Data courtesy R.J. Lee). Fibers range from about 1.5 to 95 μm in length, with modal lengths of 3.5 ± 1 μm and 9.5 ± 2 μm. (**b**) Frequency of width of amphi-bole-asbestos EMPs extracted from mined and exfoliated vermiculite, Grace Mine, Libby, MT. Data are from TEM measurements by Atkinson et al. (1981). Fibers ranged from 1 to 80 μm for mine products and <1 to >50 μm in exfoliated materials. Modal length for both populations was about 2.5 ± 1 μm. Approximately 64% of fibers from untreated vermiculite and 59% of the fibers extracted from the exfoliated vermiculite were ≤5 μm in length. (**c**) SEM micrograph of amphi-bole-asbestos from Libby (scale bar = 10 μm). The bimodal width and length distributions suggest several periods of fiber growth. This is reflected in the micrograph, which shows that wide fibers, narrow fibers and fiber bundles compose the material

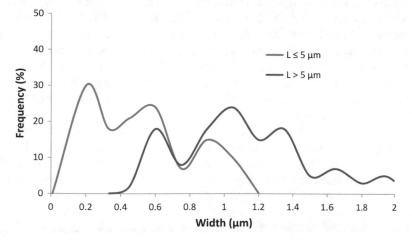

Fig. 2.10 Frequency of width typical of common amphibole cleavage fragment EMPs. Data can be found in Wylie et al. (2015). Between 20 and 50% of the EMPs in most populations are longer than 5 μm. Typical ranges of length are 1–50 μm

narrow particles are longer than 5 µm. Table 2.1 provides data on dimensions of airborne amphibole cleavage fragments. Amphibole particles that are longer than 5 µm are characteristically wider than 0.33 µm, and longer particles are characterized by even larger widths. For any length range, the variance in width can be quite large as indicated by the large standard deviations associate with mean width.

2.6 Serpentine

There are three types of structurally distinct *serpentine minerals: antigorite, lizardite, and chrysotile*. The structure of the serpentine minerals is based on a 1:1 layer motif, comprising tetrahedral $[Si_2O_5]$ and octahedral $[Mg_3O_2(OH)_4]$ sheets. Variation in stacking sequences of this composite layer results in multiple polytypes. There is a mismatch between the lateral dimensions of the silicate and hydroxide layers, which can be accommodated by curvature of the composite layer, with the octahedral layer on the outside. Two of the serpentine minerals involve curved layers. Antigorite possesses a modulated layered structure that alternates the sense of bending, producing a corrugated sheet. In chrysotile, the composite layers roll up into spiral or helical scrolls, resulting in tubular fibers. The lizardite structure can perhaps accommodate the structural misfit by a small crystallite size, slight curvature, chemical substitutions, and/or structural defects, but a full explanation is lacking. The three minerals have the same nominal, ideal chemical composition $Mg_3Si_2O_5(OH)_4$, although antigorite contains more Mg and hydroxyl and less Si than the ideal composition.

Serpentine minerals occur together. Chrysotile-asbestos is commonly found with lizardite, but all three polymorphs may occur together. In some cases, they are intergrown on the molecular scale. In others, one type dominates. Most serpentine-asbestos is chrysotile, although antigorite-asbestos has been reported from Australia (Keeling et al. 2008). A triple-chain mineral with a chemical composition similar to serpentine, $(Mg, Fe^{2+}, Fe^{3+}, Mn2^+)_{42}Si_{16}O_{54}(OH)_{40}$, and associated with massive serpentine and chrysotile-asbestos, has been mined as asbestos in Balangero, Italy, which gives the mineral its name, *balangeroite*. Serpentine also exists in splintery veins in a habit referred to as *picrolite*. Picrolite is composed of chrysotile and/or antigorite, but chrysotile fibrils are normally not liberated when the picrolite is fragmented. *Carlosturanite*, a double- and triple-chain silicate is found intergrown with antigorite and/or chrysotile in picrolite.

The most common chemical substitutions are Fe and Ni for Mg (*pecoraite* is the name used for the naturally occurring nickel analogue of chrysotile) and Al and Fe^{+3} for Si. Where found together in nature, the polymorphs may differ in their Al_2O_3 and FeO contents. While small amounts of Al and Fe^{+3} are common, iron-free occurrences of all three polymorphs are known. Chrysotile with FeO > 4 weight % has been reported. For a detailed discussion of the chemistry, structure and occurrences of serpentine, the reader is referred to Deer et al. (2009) and Guthrie and Mossman (1993).

2.6.1 Chrysotile-Asbestos

Chrysotile-asbestos occurs as veins or masses of parallel fibers in massive serpentine. An example is shown in Fig. 2.11a. In veins, chrysotile appears gold to light green, but when it is fiberized, it is almost colorless and may be referred to as *white asbestos*. Most chrysotile-asbestos comes from mines that exploit cross-fiber veins with magnetite, talc, chlorite, anthophyllite and tremolite-asbestos as accessory minerals. However, slip fiber veins have also been exploited such as in the Carey deposit in Quebec, Canada. The abundance of associated tremolite-asbestos varies significantly; Addison and Davies (1990) reported that the tremolite content (both fibers and fragments) of chrysotile-asbestos varies from undetected (<0.01%) to 0.6%. In Canada, it is a minor but ubiquitous component of the asbestos mined at Thetford Mines, but it is less common in the ore bodies at Asbestos, Quebec. Some attribute the higher rate of mesothelioma among miners and millers at Thetford to the tremolite-asbestos alone, and many have proposed that chrysotile-asbestos is not mesotheliomagenic. For a discussion of the health effects of chrysotile-asbestos, the reader is referred to Nolan et al. (2001).

The Coalinga asbestos deposit in California is a mass fiber deposit that did not produce a long fiber product, although fiber bundles as long as 30–40 μm occur. Small cross fiber veins were present but were inconsequential in ore tonnage (Mumpton and Thompson 1975.)

The structural scroll of chrysotile provides an interior tube that is normally hollow, but some fibrils have material filing their cores, which may account for observed variations in density and surface area measurements. These tubes are on the order of 70–80 Å in diameter; the diameter of a typical fibril is 220–270 Å but may range up to 650 Å. Fig. 2.11b shows the frequency distribution of width of a highly disaggregated chrysotile-asbestos from the Coalinga deposit. Fig. 2.11c depicts the frequency distribution of a bulk sample of an air-classified long fiber chrysotile-asbestos from Quebec (Fig. 2.11).

The very small diameter of chrysotile fibers promotes high tensile strength, which approaches that of crocidolite (Hodgson 1979). Like other high tensile strength asbestos, when ground in a mortar and pestle, fibers form matted aggregates and do not readily reduce to a powder.

Chrysotile contains a negligible amount of iron, yet its fibers normally align parallel to magnetic fields, indicating small magnetite particles among the fibers. If the material is well fiberized, it may be possible to use magnetic separation techniques to remove the associated magnetite.

A hexagonal array of hydroxyl groups of $Mg(OH)_2$ forms the surface of chrysotile. It will likely form at least transient hydrogen bonds to water, so chrysotile is hydrophilic. Lung fluid is normally undersaturated with respect to Mg and Si, and chrysotile will dissolve with time (Hume and Rimstidt 1992). Surface charge is strongly positive and settled dusts can form dense sediments.

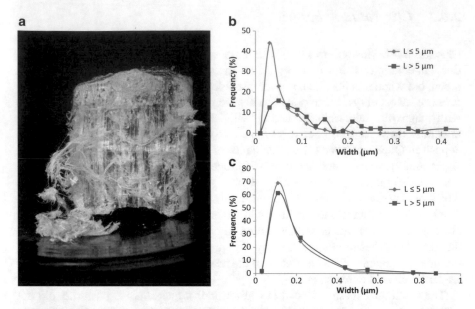

Fig. 2.11 (a) Chrysotile. Cross fiber vein, Quebec, Canada. Frequency distributions of width from two chrysotile populations are shown in (b) and (c). Samples prepared as reference materials for the National Institute of Environmental Health Sciences (NIEHS) (Campbell et al. 1980). Particle measurements can be found in Wylie and Virta (2016). (a) Frequency of width of chrysotile EMPs from Coalinga Deposit, CA, measured by TEM. The range of lengths measured is 0.1– 45 μm. The modal length is ≤1 μm, and 92% of the fibers have L ≤5 μm. (b) Frequency of width of a long fiber chrysotile EMPs from a mill product of the Jeffrey Mine, Quebec, Canada, measured by SEM. Lengths range from 0.4 to almost 1000 μm, with a broad mode at about 2 μm. 68% of fibers have L ≤5 μm

2.6.2   Other Serpentine EMPs

Keeling et al. (2008) report that about 18% of the antigorite-asbestos fibers from Australia that are longer than 5 μm are less than 0.25 μm in width, consistent with other forms of commercially available asbestos. Laths as wide as 4 μm are also present.

Picrolite is a splintery habit of serpentine. It occurs in veins and may have formed following thermal metamorphism of cross-fiber chrysotile veins. Under the optical microscopy, picrolite forms splinter lath-shaped EMPs but dimensional data on aerosol-sized particles are lacking.

2.7 The Zeolite Erionite

Erionite is one of a large group of silicate minerals called zeolites, microporous aluminosilicates, commonly found in altered volcanic tuffs, volcanic ash and muds derived from them. Zeolite-bearing volcanic tuff is widely used as a building stone. Many zeolites are used in water treatment, as a soil additive for horticulture and soil remediation, as a catalyst in hydrocarbon cracking, and in solar energy heating, cooling, and storage. For a detailed discussion of the mineralogy of the zeolites, the reader is referred to Deer et al. (2004) and Bish and Ming (2001).

Erionite belongs to a class of zeolites that is built on six-member rings of $[SiO_4]^{-4}$ tetrahedra in which Al substitutes for Si in a ratio of approximately 1:3. There are three species in the erionite series: erionite-Na, erionite-K, and erionite-Ca. The chemical composition of the series is represented by the formula $K_2(Na, K, Ca_{0.5})_7Al_9Si_{27}O_{72}\cdot30H_2O$. A compilation of the chemistry of many occurrences of the erionite series can be found in Dogan and Dogan (2008).

Zeolites are known for their ion exchange capacities, and complete replacement of Na by K, Rb, Cs, and Ca in erionite has been attained in the laboratory. Erionite is nominally iron free, but iron may be captured on its surface (Fe^{3+}) or by ion exchange (Fe^{2+}) in vivo (Eborn and Aust 1995). The density of erionite is low for silicate minerals, about 2 gm/cm^3, which can be attributed to a water content of almost 20 wt.% H_2O, rendering erionite unstable under an electron beam under normal operating conditions and making chemical analysis by EDS problematic.

Erionite frequently occurs with other zeolites, notably clinoptilolite, phillipsite, and chabazite, and may be epitaxially intergrown with the zeolite offretite or overgrown on the zeolite levyne. Iron oxides, iron hydroxides, and iron-rich clay (nontronite) have been reported as nanoparticles on fiber surfaces. Quartz, feldspar, and clay are commonly associated minerals. The detection limit for erionite in altered volcanic rocks by XRD is estimated to be 0.1–0.5% (Bish and Chipera 1991).

Most zeolites are not fibrous, although some form EMPs when crushed, but erionite is notable for a fibrous habit. The zeolite *mordenite* is also commonly fibrous, and ferrierite and phillipsite may sometimes occur as fibers, but none of these occurs in an asbestiform habit.

The type locality for erionite is Durkee Oregon, where it occurs in the asbestiform habit and is known as *woolly erionite* (Fig. 2.12). This material has been well characterized by Cametti et al. (2013). *Woolly erionite* has also been found in Lander County and Churchill County, Nevada (Gude and Sheppard 1981).

Woolly erionite has been shown to be a potent animal carcinogen, and exposure to fibrous erionite found in building stone and white wash in the Cappadocia region of Turkey is associated with a marked excess of mesothelioma. Similar occurrences and disease excess have recently been reported from Mexico and Nevada. Photographs, descriptions, and size and shape characterizations of erionite and other zeolites have been provided by Shedd et al. (1982). Van Gosen et al. (2013) have summarized erionite occurrences in the USA.

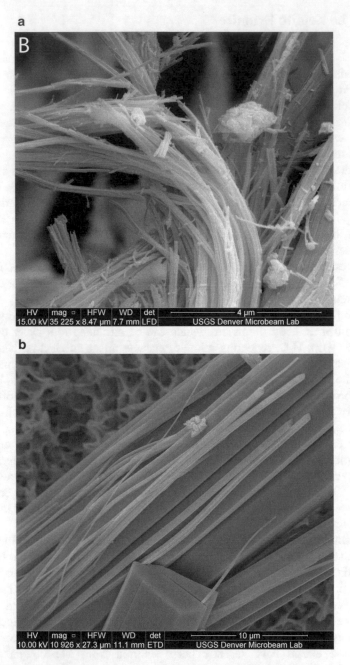

Fig. 2.12 Erionite. (**a**) Woolly erionite from Rome, Oregon, displaying an asbestiform habit. (**b**) Fibrous erionite from Pima County, Arizona. Most fibers are a few micrometers or more in width, although very fine, asbestiform fibers are also present. The two habits likely represent two periods of fiber formation. SEM micrographs courtesy of Van Gosen et al. (2013)

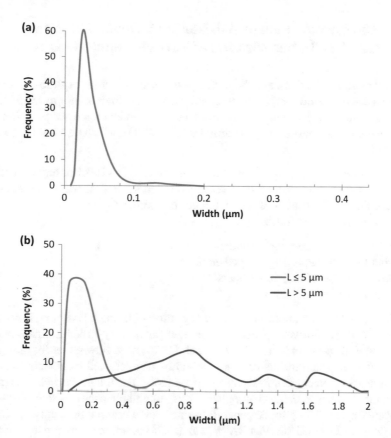

Fig. 2.13 Frequency of width of two erionite samples from Shedd et al. (1982). (**a**) Woolly erionite from Lander County, Nevada. The longest fiber included in the distribution in 9.7 μm and 6% are ≥ 5 μm in length. In this asbestiformerionite, width increases only slightly with length. (**b**) Fibrous, nonasbestiform erionite from Pershing County, Nevada. The longest common erionite particle measured is 20.6 μm; width increases systematically with length

Not all erionite is asbestiform. It may be found in prismatic or acicular particles and in more massive amygdaloidal form. Erionite in different habits may be found at the same location as shown in Fig. 2.12b. Elongated particles of nonasbestiform erionite may resemble those of common amphibole.

Figure 2.13a illustrates the frequency distribution of the width of woolly erionite fibers from Nevada (after Shedd et al. 1982). The variance in width is very small, with most fibers between 0.03 and 0.05 μm. The modal width of woolly erionite from Durkee, Oregon, is reported to be 0.016 μm (Matassa et al. 2015). The disaggregated fibrils from both locations are commonly less than 5 μm in length, although fibers and fiber bundles of 50 μm or more may occur. Gude and Sheppard (1981) reported fibers up to 10 mm in length. Other minerals intergrown with erionite fibers may inhibit disaggregation into the component fibrils. In Fig. 2.13b, the width frequency distribution typical of common erionite from Nevada is depicted. The modal width of short common erionite EMPS is 0.1–0.2 μm; longer particles have widths that range widely.

2.8 The Identification of Asbestos and Woolly Erionite, and the Characterization of Particle Populations

Mineral occurrences that have the potential to form long thin respirable fibers can be recognized in hand samples by their silky luster and their ability to readily separate into visible fibers by hand pressure. Under the optical microscope, asbestos is recognized by the following characteristics (EPA 1993), which also hold for woolly erionite:

1. Mean aspect ratios (length/width) ranging from 20:1 to 100:1 or higher for fibers longer than 5 μm (aspect ratio determined for individual fibers, not bundles)
2. Very thin fibrils, usually less than 0.5 μm in width, and
3. Two or more of the following:

a. Parallel fibers occurring in bundles
b. Fiber bundles displaying splayed ends
c. Matted masses of individual fibers
d. Fibers showing curvature

Under the electron microscope, the designation of a single EMP that is not composed of multiple fibrils as a fiber or a fragment can be very difficult. This is particularly true if the particle is short. Wylie et al. (1985) have shown that for amphibole EMPs of a few micrometers or less, the widths of fibers and fragments converge, and dimensions become unreliable discriminators. For longer particles, there are sufficient dimension data on populations of amphibole-asbestos and amphibole cleavage fragments to provide general discriminating criteria, but applying them to a single particle is difficult. Van Orden et al. (2008) describe characteristics of fibers and fragments that may be helpful for narrow EMPs (≈0.5 μm or less) that are not fiber bundles. A summary is provided in Table 2.2.

While it is accepted that dimensions of mineral particles are important factors in determining carcinogenicity, representation of those dimensions in ways that are meaningful for a quantitative assessment of risk is challenging. These challenges arise for many reasons, but important among them are: (1) the distributions of length and width are not normal, (2) short fibers are much more abundant than long fibers, but it is the long fibers that are of the most interest biologically, (3) fibers disaggregate into their component fibrils differently depending on their history and degree of manipulation, (4) the range of length may be several orders of magnitude greater than the range in width, and (5) with only a few exceptions, longer fibers contain a higher proportion of the mass of the population than shorter fibers. During preparation of bulk samples for characterization, grinding of the material has been used. For the higher tensile strength fibers, such as crocidolite, amosite, chrysotile and woolly erionite, hand grinding has limited impact on length distributions, but for the more brittle materials, fiber lengths can be significantly reduced by even a small amount of grinding. Grinding rarely breaks asbestos fibrils longitudinally, but may contribute to their disaggregation. The instrumentation used to characterize a mineral par-

Table 2.2 Representative magnitudes of the frequency of width of amphibole fibers and fragments with length >5 μm (Wylie 2016)

Mineral name and location	% ≤0.25 μm	% ≤0.33 μm	% ≤0.5 μm
1. Airborne and lung burden			
Crocidolite, cape asbestos province, South Africa	75	90	99
Amosite, Transvaal asbestos range, South Africa	20	45	70
Na-Ca amphibole-asbestos, Libby and Italy	20	45	70
Anthophyllite-asbestos, Finland	5	15	45
Brittle amphibole mining aerosol	Trace	2	7
2. Laboratory-prepared samples			
Tremolite-asbestos, Korea	50	70	80
Preskaite, Transvaal asbestos range, South Africa	20	45	70
Tremolite-asbestos, Udaipur, India	7	15	30
Brittle amphibole	Trace	2	6

ticle population is also an important factor. The very narrow width of asbestos and woolly erionite fibrils limits the use of optical microscopy. The full range of length may be impossible to characterize by TEM, while the smallest fibril widths may be difficult to measure by SEM. Ultrasound disaggregates fibers into their component fibrils, but the degree to which this happens varies among samples and with time of sonication. Sampling protocols may or may not designate a minimum aspect ratio or length. Accessory minerals, sometime fibrous, may or may not be included. Samples are sometimes dispersed in water and selectively sampled by settling times or column depth. In comparing population characterizations, it is important that protocols be considered.

Length distributions can be modeled by the relationship $\log N = -D \log L + C$, where N is the number of fibers with a length greater than L, C is a constant, and D is the fractal dimension (Wylie, 1993). Turcotte (1986) concluded that the fractal dimension is a measure of the resistance of the material to fragmentation. While this is true of fragmented material, in the case of high tensile strength asbestos fibrils that do not fragment, D reflects the ease of disaggregation into component fibrils over the range of length measured.

The relationship between log length and log width in particle populations can be expressed by the relationship: $\log width = F \log length + b$, where F is the fibrosity index (Siegrist and Wylie 1980). Small values of F are characteristic of greater fibrosity, as they are derived from populations in which the aspect ratios are high and widths are nearly constant; larger values of F imply more brittle behavior, with lower aspect ratios and variable widths that increase with length. For asbestos and woolly erionite, the fibrosity index is normally less than 0.2; for populations that contain both byssolite and asbestos, F as large as 3.4 has been reported.

The fibrosity indices characteristic of fragments of common amphibole and common erionite are greater than 0.7 (Siegrist and Wylie 1980, Shedd 1985).

The arithmetic means of width and length are not recommended as population parameters for describing asbestiform fiber. The geometric mean may be somewhat useful for width, but it has limitations for length, especially for characterization of bulk samples. Modal width for specific length segments may be the most useful descriptive statistic for comparing populations. This approach has been used in Table 2.2, which provides data on selective amphibole EMPs from a variety of sources.

2.9   Summary

Amphibole and erionite are biodurable. Their surface area (per unit weight) is largely controlled by width. Among asbestiform minerals, woolly erionite is composed of the narrowest fibrils, followed by commercially produced chrysotile, crocidolite, amosite and anthophyllite-asbestos, in that order. Asbestiform amphibole in the tremolite-actinolite-ferroactinolite, edenite, richterite, and winchite series occur with fibrils that range in size from crocidolite to anthophyllite-asbestos to byssolite; many occurrences are characterized inhomogeneous fibrils sizes.

Width frequency data from Wylie (in press) for EMPs >5 μm in length are summarized in Table 2.2. While widths for asbestos range widely, narrow widths are uncommon among cleavage fragment populations. Width ultimately controls the penetration of an EMP into the lung while length may be the major factor (other than biodurability) in controlling its residence time. Both dimensions are important in understanding mesotheliomagenicity of minerals.

References

Addison J, Davies LST (1990) Analysis of amphibole asbestos in chrysotile and other minerals. Ann Occup Hyg 34:159–175

Atkinson GR, Rose D, Thomas K, et al. (1981) Collection, analysis and characterization of vermiculite samples for fiber content and asbestos contamination. Midwest Research Institute report for the US Environmental Protection Agency Project 4901-A32 under EPA Contract 68-01-5915, Washington, DC

Beard ME, Ennis JT, Crankshaw OS, et al. (2007) Preparation of nonasbestiform amphibole minerals for method evaluation and Health Studies Summary Report and appendices. Prepared for Martin, Harper, NIOSH, Morgantown, WV by RTI International. (Hearl F, Personal communication, CDC/NIOSH/OD)

Bish DL, Chipera SJ (1991) Detection of trace amounts of erionite using X-ray powder diffraction: erionite in tuffs of Yucca Mountain, Nevada, and central Turkey. Clay Clay Miner 39:437–445

Bish DL, Ming DW (eds) (2001) Natural zeolites: occurrence, properties, applications, Reviews in mineralogy and geochemistry, vol 45. Mineralogical Society of America, Washington, DC

Bloss FD (1971) Crystallography and crystal chemistry: an introduction. Holt, Rinehart and Winston, New York, NY

Cametti G, Pacella A, Mura F et al (2013) New morphological chemical and structural data of woolly erionite-Na from Durkee, Oregon, USA. Am Mineral 98:2155–2163

Campbell WJ, Huggins CW, Wylie AG (1980) Chemical and physical characterization of amosite, chrysotile, crocidolite, and nonfibrous tremolite for oral ingestion studies by the National Institute of Environmental Health Sciences. US Bureau of Mines Report of Investigations 8452. United States Department of the Interior.

Deer WA, Howie RA, Zussman J (1997) Rock forming minerals. Volume 2B: double-chain silicates, 2nd edn. The Geological Society, London

Deer WA, Howie RA, Wise WS et al (2004) Rock forming minerals. Volume. 4B: framework silicates; silica minerals, feldspathoids and the Zeolites, 2nd edn. The Geological Society, London

Deer WA, Howie RA, Zussman J (2009) Rock forming minerals. Volume 3B: layered silicates; excluding micas and clay minerals. The Geological Society, London

Dogan AU, Dogan M (2008) Re-evaluation and reclassification of erionite. Environ Geochem Health 30:355–366

Dorling M, Zussman J (1987) Characteristics of asbestiform and nonasbestiform calcic amphiboles. Lithos 20:469–489

Eborn SK, Aust AE (1995) Effect of iron acquisition on induction of DNA single-strand breaks by erionite, a carcinogenic mineral fiber. Arch Biochem Biophys 316:507–154

Ecology and Environment, Inc (EEI) (2005) El Dorado Hills naturally occurring asbestos multimedia exposure assessment. El Dorado Hills, California Preliminary Assessment and Site Inspection Report Interim Final, LabCor Contract No. 68-W-01-012; TDD No.: 09-04-01-0011; Job No.: 001275.0440.01CP (Lee RJ, personal communication)

EPA (1993) Test Method: method for the determination of asbestos in bulk building materials. Perkins RL, Harvey BW. EPA/600/R-93/116

EPA US (2006) U.S. Environmental Protection Agency Produced Access Database, Libby Montana airborne particles; in the matter of United States of America vs. WR Grace, et al, CR-05-070 M-DWM (D. Montana), 2005–2006 (Lee RJ, personal communication)

Gianfagna A, Andreozzi B, Ballirano P et al (2007) Structural and chemical contrasts between prismatic and fibrous fluoro-edenite from Biancavilla, Sicily, Italy. Can Mineral 45:249–262

Gibb GW, Hwang CY (1980) Dimensions of airborne asbestos fibers. In: Wagner JC (ed) Biological effects of mineral fibers, vol 1. IARC Scientific Publication #30, Lyon, pp 69–77

Greenwood WS (1998) A mineralogical analysis of fibrous talc. Master of Science Thesis, Department of Geology, University of Maryland, College Park, MD

Gude AJ, Sheppard RA (1981) Woolly erionite from the Reese River zeolite deposit, Lander County Nevada and its relations to other erionites. Clay Clay Miner 29:378–384

Guthrie G, Mossman B (eds) (1993) Health effects of mineral dusts, Reviews in mineralogy, vol 28. Mineralogical Society of America, Washington

Harper M, Lee EG, Doorn SS et al (2008) Differentiating non-asbestiform amphibole and amphibole asbestos by size characteristics. J Occup Environ Hyg 5:761–770

Hawthorne FC, Oberti R, Ventura GD, Mottana A eds (2007) Amphiboles: Crystal Chemistry, Occurrence, and Health Issues. Reviews in Mineralogy. Vol. 67. Mineralogical Society of America, Washington DC

Hawthorne FC, Oberti R, Harlow GE, Maresch WV, Martin RF, Schumacher SC, Welch MD (2012) Nomenclature of the amphibole supergroup. Am Miner 97:2031–2048.

Hodgson AA (1979) Chemistry and physics of asbestos. In: Michaels L, Chissick SS (eds) Asbestos. Vol. 1. Applications and Hazards. Wiley, New York, pp 67–114

Hume LA, Rimstidt JD (1992) The biodurability of chrysotile asbestos. Am Mineral 77: 1125–1128

Keeling JL, Raven MD, Self PG, et al. (2008) Asbestiform antigorite occurrence in South Australia. Proc 9th Int Conf Applied Mineralogy, Brisbane, Australia, pp 329–336

Leake BE, Woolley AR, Arps CES et al (1997) Nomenclature of amphiboles: report of the Subcommittee on Amphiboles of the International Mineralogical Association, Commission on New Minerals and Mineral Names. Can Mineral 35:219–246

Leake BE, Woolley AR, Birch WD et al (2004) Nomenclature of amphiboles: additions and revisions to the International Mineralogical Association's amphibole nomenclature. Am Mineral 89:883–887

Lippmann M, Timbrell V (1990) Particle loading in the human lung: human experience and implications for exposure limits. J Aerosol Med 3:S155–S168

Matassa R, Familiari G, Relucenti M et al (2015) A deep look into erionite fibres: an electron microscopy investigation of their self-assembly. Sci Report 5:16757

Meeker GP, Bern AM, Brownfield IK et al (2003) The composition and morphology of amphiboles from the Rainy Creek Complex, near Libby Montana. Am Mineral 88:1955–1969

Mumpton FA, Thompson CS (1975) Mineralogy and origin of the Coalinga asbestos Deposit. Clay Clay Miner 23:131–143

NIOSH (2011) Asbestos fibers and other elongate mineral particles: state of the science and roadmap for research. Current Intelligence Bulletin 62. DHHS:CDC Pub. No. 2011–159

Nolan RP, Langer AM, Ross M et al (eds) (2001) Health effects of chrysotile asbestos: contribution of science to risk-management decisions. Mineralogical Society of Canada, Ontario. Special publication 5

O'Hanley DS (1986) The origin and mechanical properties of asbestos. Master of Science thesis, University of Minnesota, Twin Cities, MN

Paoletti L, Bruni BM (2009) Caratterizzazione dimensionale di fibre anfiboliche nel polmone e nella pleura di cassi di mesothelioma da esposizione ambientale. Med Lav 100:11–20

Pooley FD, Clark N (1980) A comparison of fibre dimensions in chrysotile, crocidolite and amosite particles from sampling of airborne dust and from post mortem lung tissue. IARC Sci Publ 30:79–86

Redwood SD (1993) Crocidolite and magnesite associated with lake superior-type banded iron formation in Chapare Group of eastern Andes, Bolivia. Institution of Mining and Metallurgy. Section B: Appl Earth Sci 102:114–122

Shedd KB (1985) Fiber dimensions of crocidolites from Western Australia, Bolivia, and the Cape and Transvaal Provinces of South Africa. US Bureau of Mines Report of Investigations 8998. US Department of the Interior

Shedd KB, Virta RL, Wylie AG (1982) Size and shape characterization of fibrous zeolites by electron microscopy. Bureau of Mines Report of Investigations 8674. US Department of the Interior

Siegrist HG, Wylie AG (1980) Characterizing and discriminating the shape of asbestos particles. Environ Res 23:348–361

Timbrell V (1975) Alignment of respirable asbestos fibres by magnetic fields. Ann Occup Hyg 18:299–311

Timbrell V, Pooley F, Wagner JC (1970) Characteristics of respirable asbestos fibers. Proc Int Conf Pneumoconiosis, Shapiro HA (ed), Oxford University Press, pp 120–125

Turcotte DL (1986) Fractals and Fragmentation. J Geophys Res 91:1921–1926

Van Gosen B (2007) The geology of asbestos in the United States and its practical applications. Environ Eng Geosci 13:55–68

Van Gosen BS, Blitz TA, Plumlee GS et al (2013) Geologic occurrences of erionite in the United States: an emerging national public health concern for respiratory disease. Environ Geochem Health 35:419–413

Van Orden DR, Allison KA, Lee RJ (2008) Differentiating amphibole asbestos from non-asbestos in a complex mineral environment. Indoor Built Environ 17:58–68

Verkouteren JR, Wylie AG (2002) Anomalous optical properties of fibrous tremolite, actinolite and ferro-actinolite. Am Mineral 87:1090–1095

Watson MB (1999) The effect of intergrowths on the properties of fibrous anthophyllite. Master of Science thesis, Department of Geology, University of Maryland, College Park, MD

Wylie AG (1979) Optical properties of the fibrous amphiboles. Ann N Y Acad Sci 330:600–605

Wylie AG (1993) Modeling asbestos populations: a fractal approach. Can Mineral 30:437–446

Wylie AG (2016). Amphibole dust: asbestos fibers, fragments, and mesothelioma. Canadian Mineral (in revision)

Wylie AG, Candela PA (2015) Methodologies for determining the sources, characteristics, distribution and abundance of asbestiform and nonasbestiform amphibole and serpentine in ambient air and water. J Toxicol Environ Health Part B: Crit Rev 18:1–42

Wylie, AG, Virta, RL (2016) Size distribution measurements of amosite, crocidolite, chrysotile, and nonfibrous tremolite: digital Repository at the University of Maryland, College Park, MD. http://dx.doi.org/10.13016/M2798Z

Wylie AG, Shedd KB, Taylor ME (1982) Measurement of the thickness of amphibole asbestos fibers with the scanning electron microscope and transmission electron microscope. In: Heinrich KFJ (ed) Microbeam Analysis. San Francisco Press, San Francisco, CA, pp 181–187

Wylie AG, Virta R, Russek E (1985) Characterizing and discriminating airborne amphibole cleavage fragments and amosite fibers: implications for the NIOSH Method. Am Ind Hyg Assoc J 46:197–201

Wylie AG, Virta RL, Shedd KB, et al. (2015) Size and shape characteristics of airborne amphibole asbestos and amphibole cleavage fragments. Digital Repository at the University of Maryland, http://dx.doi.org/10.13016/M2HP87

Chapter 3
Epidemiology of Mesothelioma

Suresh H. Moolgavkar, Ellen T. Chang, Gabor Mezei, and Fionna S. Mowat

Abstract While malignant mesothelioma has generally been associated with exposure to asbestos, several lines of evidence suggest strongly that, like all other cancers, it can and does occur spontaneously and that age is a strong risk factor for its development. This includes not only pleural mesothelioma, the most common site for this disease, but also extra-pleural sites (peritoneum, pericardium, tunica vaginalis testis). Recent epidemiologic studies show that ionizing radiation is another risk factor. The discovery of a germline mutation in the BRCA1 associated protein 1 (*BAP1*) gene, the inheritance of which increases greatly the risk of developing mesothelioma, may provide the first step in the understanding of the underlying genetic events in the pathogenesis of mesothelioma. Whether and how inheritance of this mutation interacts with other risk factors remains an open question. The diminution of the impact of asbestos on mesothelioma incidence in western countries due to its phase-out may enable the discovery of more modest risk factors. Exposure-response relationships are probably determined by the entire temporal history of exposure, not just the cumulative exposure to fibers. The concept of latency is more nuanced than appears at first sight.

Keywords Mesothelioma • Spontaneous tumors • Risk factors • Epidemiology • *BAP1* mutation • Age • Temporal trends • Asbestos • Carcinogenesis

S.H. Moolgavkar (✉)
Exponent, Inc., 15375 SE 30th Place, Suite 250, Bellevue, WA 98007, USA

Fred Hutchinson Cancer Research Center, Seattle, WA 98109, USA
e-mail: smoolgavkar@exponent.com

E.T. Chang
Exponent, Inc., 149 Commonwealth Drive, Menlo Park, CA 94025, USA

Department of Health Research and Policy (Epidemiology), Stanford University School of Medicine, Stanford, CA 94305, USA

G. Mezei • F.S. Mowat
Exponent, Inc., 149 Commonwealth Drive, Menlo Park, CA 94025, USA

© Springer International Publishing AG 2017
J.R. Testa (ed.), *Asbestos and Mesothelioma*, Current Cancer Research,
DOI 10.1007/978-3-319-53560-9_3

3.1   Introduction

Although malignant mesothelioma has generally been associated with exposure to asbestos and, rarely or in specific geographical regions, other fibers such as erionite/zeolites (e.g., Simonato et al. 1989; Baris and Grandjean 2006), ophiolites (e.g., Constantopoulos et al. 1985; Ross and Nolan 2003), and fluoro-edenite (e.g., Paoletti et al. 2000; Bruno et al. 2014), there is ample and growing evidence that, like all other cancers, it can occur spontaneously as a consequence of naturally occurring biological processes. As the use of asbestos declines, one should expect to see a larger fraction of spontaneously occurring cases among patients with mesothelioma. The pioneering investigations of Nordling (1953) and Armitage and Doll (1954) established that the age-specific incidence of human cancers is consistent with the sequential acquisition of mutations at critical gene loci in stem cells. While there is debate regarding the quantitative contribution of environmental risk factors to cancer in human populations (Tomasetti and Vogelstein 2015; Wu et al. 2016), there is general agreement that a substantial fraction of human cancers is attributable to the accumulation of random mutations in normally dividing stem cells without any contributing exposure by environmental agents.

While the specific gene loci involved in carcinogenesis are not known for most cancers, recent work in molecular genetics has shed some light on a tumor suppressor gene, BRCA1 associated protein 1 (*BAP1*), involved in some cases of mesothelioma (Testa et al. 2011). A germline mutation at this locus confers a high risk of developing mesothelioma, uveal melanoma, and possibly other tumors (Testa et al. 2011; Carbone et al. 2012) in individuals who inherit it. The dominant inheritance of this mutation explains the high incidence of mesothelioma in some families; however, germline mutation of *BAP1* appears to be rare in the general population (Rusch et al. 2015; Sneddon et al. 2015), suggesting that the population burden of mesothelioma imposed by the inheritance of this mutation is small. Nonetheless, the discovery of this susceptibility locus does suggest that a final common pathway for mesothelioma pathogenesis in both hereditary and sporadic (non-hereditary) cases involves either direct mutation at the locus or disruption of cellular signaling pathways involving the locus. Other genetic conditions, such as familial Mediterranean fever, and chromosomal abnormalities have also possibly been linked to mesothelioma, though studies are limited (e.g., Gentiloni et al. 1997; Musti et al. 2002; Hershcovici et al. 2006).

This chapter is not a comprehensive review of the epidemiology of asbestos and mesothelioma. Many such reviews have been published that describe asbestos-exposed worker cohorts (e.g., Nicholson 1986; Stayner et al. 1996; Hodgson and Darnton 2000; Berman and Crump 2008a, b; IARC 2012). Rather, this review focuses on not just asbestos and other fibers, but also other risk factors for the development of mesothelioma, such as age and ionizing radiation. With the continuing decline in the use of asbestos, these other risk factors will play an increasing role in the etiology of malignant mesothelioma. With respect to asbestos, we discuss mainly the literature appearing after the year 2000, with particular emphasis on the epidemiologic studies that have investigated the impact of low exposure levels, including take-home and environmental exposures, on the development of mesothelioma. We discuss also extra-pleural mesothelioma. As is well known, mesothelial tissue is present at four anatomical sites: pleura, peritoneum, pericardium, and tunica vaginalis testis (TVT). Malignant mesothelioma occurs at each of these sites, most commonly in the pleura, and only rarely in the pericardium and TVT.

3.2 Trends and the Impact of Age

Investigation of disease trends, particularly when a single environmental exposure is considered to be the dominant cause of the disease under investigation, can offer useful insights into etiology. Since asbestos is the single most prominent environmental exposure associated with mesothelioma, one would expect trends in the commercial use of asbestos to be reflected, with appropriate latency, in the trends in the incidence rates of malignant mesothelioma in the population. In the USA, trends in the commercial use of asbestos between the 1900s and the early 2000s are available from the United States Geological Survey (USGS); trends in mesothelioma incidence are available from the Surveillance, Epidemiology, and End Results (SEER) registries maintained by the National Cancer Institute (NCI). Of these registries, the longest series of data (1973–2013) are available from SEER 9 (i.e., the original nine SEER cancer registries) (SEER 2016). These data have been analyzed by us (Moolgavkar et al. 2009) and others (Price and Ware 2004, 2009; Teta et al. 2008; Henley et al. 2013).

We recently updated the trend analyses in Moolgavkar et al. (2009); the results are presented in Fig. 3.1. Trends in the incidence of pleural mesothelioma among men over the period 1973–2013 clearly reflect trends in the commercial use of asbestos in the USA with an approximately 30- to 40-year lag. By contrast, trends in incidence rates of pleural mesotheliomas among women and peritoneal mesotheliomas among both men and women show little or no association with commercial asbestos use trends in the USA, suggesting strongly that asbestos exposure plays a far smaller role in the etiology of these tumors than it does in the etiology of pleural mesothelioma among men in the USA. Using combined data from the National Program for Cancer Registries (NPCR) and SEER, Henley et al. (2013) confirmed that between 2003 and 2008, female pleural mesothelioma rates were flat, whereas male rates continued to decline. Trends in some European countries also indicate that a large fraction of peritoneal mesotheliomas is unrelated to asbestos exposure, with flat age-adjusted incidence rates in both men and women (e.g., Hemminki and Li 2003; Burdorf et al. 2007).

The small numbers of mesotheliomas of the pericardium and the TVT in SEER 9 preclude formal trend analyses. It is of interest to note, however, that the total numbers of pericardial mesotheliomas over the period 1973–2013 were similar in men and women. Since men are much more likely to have been exposed to asbestos

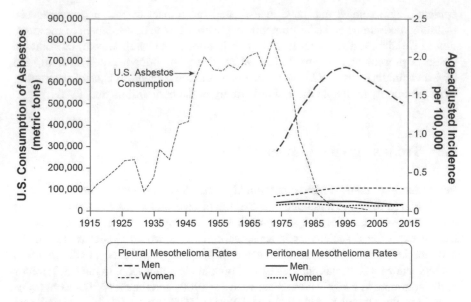

Fig. 3.1 Age-adjusted incidence rates of pleural and peritoneal mesothelioma among males and females in SEER 9 cancer registries (1973–2013). This figure extends the results reported in Moolgavkar et al. (2009) to include SEER data through 2013 (the most recent update). Note the strong increase in rates of pleural mesothelioma until the mid-1990s, with a subsequent decline, which mimics the trend in the use of commercial asbestos in the USA with a 30- to 40-year lag. Note also that the trend in pleural mesothelioma incidence rates among women and peritoneal mesothelioma incidence rates among women and men are flat, indicating that the commercial use of asbestos in the USA had little impact on these mesothelioma rates

occupationally, this observation suggests strongly that pericardial mesotheliomas are unrelated to asbestos exposure.

A more formal statistical analysis of time-series cancer registry data involves the use of age-period-cohort models (Holford 1983, 1991; Luebeck and Moolgavkar 2002; Meza et al. 2008a; Jeon et al. 2006; Rosenberg and Anderson 2011). These analyses allow the estimation of the age-specific incidence of the disease under study after adjustment for temporal trends. Moolgavkar et al. (2009) and others (La Vecchia et al. 2000; Cree et al. 2009; Schonfeld et al. 2014) have applied these methods to the analysis of mesothelioma incidence in cancer registries in the USA, Canada, and Europe. Results show that the age-specific incidence rates of both pleural and peritoneal mesothelioma increase continuously with age. Every doubling of age increases the risk of pleural mesothelioma approximately 30-fold and that of peritoneal mesothelioma approximately eightfold (Moolgavkar et al. 2009), as shown in Fig. 3.2.

Although similar age-period-cohort analyses cannot be performed for mesotheliomas of the pericardium and TVT because of the small number of cases of these diseases, examination of the data in SEER 9 indicates that the risk of mesothelioma at both sites increases with age.

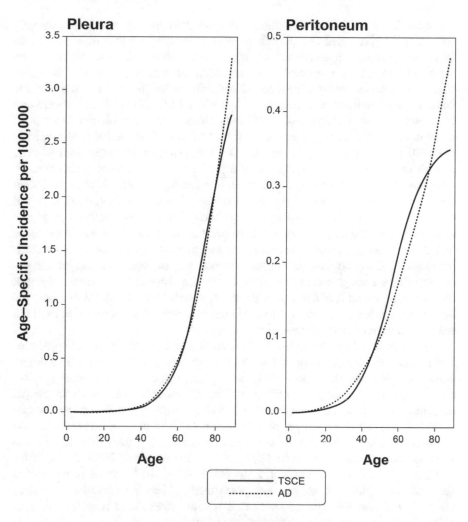

Fig. 3.2 Age-specific incidence curves generated by the Armitage-Doll (AD) and two-stage clonal expansion (TSCE) models. These curves represent the hazard functions (×100,000) estimated from age-period-cohort analyses with non-specific age effects replaced by the hazard functions of the AD and TSCE models for pleural mesothelioma (*left panel*) and peritoneal mesothelioma (*right panel*). Adapted from Moolgavkar et al. (2009)

3.3   Exposure-Response Analyses and Risks at Low Levels of Exposure to Asbestos

As in most epidemiologic studies of environmental risk factors, quantitative assessment of exposure to asbestos is difficult and imprecise. Most epidemiologic studies of asbestos-associated disease have relied on one of two measures of exposure to asbestos. Some occupational cohort studies have used direct measurements of concentration in various work locations. Many of these measurements are relatively crude and rely on converting particle or dust concentrations into fiber concentrations using simple conversion factors. Moreover, concentration measurements are often available only for selected years, and oftentimes pre- or post-date the exposures of the cohort being evaluated. This approach has formed the basis of the United States Environmental Protection Agency (USEPA)'s cancer risk assessment for mesothelioma (see Nicholson 1986) and of a recent site-specific risk assessment in the cohort of vermiculite workers at Libby, Montana (USEPA 2011; Moolgavkar et al. 2014). The occupational cohort studies with exposure estimates deemed to be reliable enough for exposure-response analyses have been thoroughly reviewed by Hodgson and Darnton (2000) and Berman and Crump (2008a, b). In some recent case-control studies, expert elicitation in conjunction with job-exposure matrices (JEM) has been used to estimate past exposures. While these methods may give more precise estimates of exposures for subjects in the study, there is little evidence that these measures are more accurate and less prone to error than other methods employed. The second common approach to assessing exposure is to use job categories or titles as surrogate measures of exposure. This approach has commonly been used in case-control studies of mesothelioma, which have confirmed that occupations with high levels of exposure to amphibole or mixed-fiber asbestos confer high risk for the development of mesothelioma.

Our focus here is on the review and discussion of exposure-response epidemiologic studies of mesothelioma at low levels of exposure to asbestos. There are no epidemiologic exposure-response studies of extra-pleural mesothelioma at low levels of exposure. Therefore, the discussion in this section applies only to pleural mesothelioma. For mixed-fiber exposures, studies conducted in Europe with exposures estimated either by using expert elicitation and JEM or by occupation are most informative. Most of these are case-control studies using data from the French mesothelioma registry (Iwatsubo et al. 1998; Rolland et al. 2005, 2006, 2010; Goldberg et al. 2006; Lacourt et al. 2010, 2012, 2013, 2014a, b); one case-control study of low exposure levels has been performed in Germany (Rödelsperger et al. 2001). In addition, there is one Dutch cohort study of exposure-response relationships at low exposure levels (Offermans et al. 2014).

The French case-control studies fall into two categories. In the first category are studies that investigated the risk of mesothelioma in occupations and industries (Rolland et al. 2005, 2010; Goldberg et al. 2006). These studies confirmed the increased risk of mesothelioma in occupations and industries such as shipbuilding, asbestos products manufacturing, and construction, long known to be associated with increased risk of mesothelioma. Notably, these studies did not report an increased risk of mesothelioma among vehicle mechanics, a well-studied occupation that was exposed to low levels of chrysotile asbestos as part of their work (e.g., Finley et al. 2007).

The second category of studies (Iwatsubo et al. 1998; Lacourt et al. 2010, 2012, 2014a, b) used the same or overlapping cases and controls as the studies in the first category, but instead of using occupation as a measure of exposure, relied on quantitative measures of exposure based on expert elicitation and JEM. The quantitative estimates of exposure-response relationships reported in these studies are not reliable, in our opinion, for the following reasons. First, the investigators had no direct information on actual exposure levels in the various jobs held by the subjects of the study. Second, quantitative measures of exposure were based in part on estimates of intensity of exposure in broad exposure ranges and on probability of exposure in a given job. Marchand et al. (2000) state, "As the cumulative levels were computed by weighting the exposure levels by the probabilities of exposure, they must not be interpreted as fibers/mL-year" (i.e., cumulative exposure). Iwatsubo et al. (1998) acknowledged the limitations inherent in their exposure estimates by calling them cumulative exposure indices and putting the estimates in quotes. The later French studies dispensed with the quotes and reported the estimates as f/mL-years. Rödelsperger et al. (2001) and Offermans et al. (2014) used a similar approach to quantifying exposures. As shown in a detailed simulation study by Burstyn et al. (2012), using the product of intensity and probability of exposure as a quantitative estimate of exposure results in aggregation of exposure across exposed and non-exposed individuals and can yield risk estimates that are seriously biased upwards.

Teschke (2016) has noted that occupation is an imprecise measure of exposure to asbestos or any other environmental agent; however, problems of exposure measurement error and exposure misclassification occur whether either occupation or expert elicitation with JEM is used as a surrogate measure of exposure. While occupation is probably a crude measure of exposure, it has the virtue of being easily remembered; this measure also allows for group-level of analyses of risk to be performed in the absence of refined exposure information (Garabrant et al. 2016a). Intuitively, individuals are less likely to forget specific occupations than the details of specific job locations, on which expert elicitations rely. Additionally, there is a widely held misperception that the estimate of risk is always lower than the true value in the presence of non-differential exposure measurement error. While this result is asymptotically true, in any given study, the estimated risk may be lower or higher than the true value (e.g., Jurek et al. 2005).

The European case-control studies of low exposure levels share some of the same limitations. Furthermore, the results are not consistent across studies. For example, the Rödelsperger study reports an odds ratio (OR) (a measure of relative risk) of 9.2 in the group exposed to less than 0.15 f/mL-years, whereas Iwatsubo et al. (1998) report an OR of 8.7 in the group exposed to more than 10 f/mL-years. In every exposure category, Rödelsperger et al. (2001) report risks that are far larger than those reported in Iwatsubo et al. (1998) or in Lacourt et al. (2010). Offermans et al. (2014), applying a JEM developed for Finnish workers to a Dutch population, also report a hazard ratio (another measure of relative risk) of 2.7 at a median exposure of 0.20 f/mL-years. The huge discrepancies in risk estimates among these studies cannot be attributed simply to chance. They suggest fundamental problems with the exposure estimates in the studies. Furthermore, the results of the French studies, although based on the same or overlapping data, are not consistent. Thus, for example, the results of the two case-control studies in Lacourt et al. (2010) are not consistent with each other. The risks associated with specific cumulative exposure are much larger in Lacourt et al. (2014a) than those reported in Iwatsubo et al. (1998).

Surprisingly, publications based on overlapping data, appearing in the same year and by the same group of investigators (Lacourt et al. 2014a, b), report highly discrepant risks, with the risks in Lacourt et al. (2014a) being substantially larger than those reported in Lacourt et al. (2014b). Finally, the results of the French studies in the first category, as defined above (i.e., Rolland et al. 2005, 2010; Goldberg et al. 2006), appear to be inconsistent with the results reported in the studies in the second category (Iwatsubo et al. 1998; Lacourt et al. 2010, 2012, 2013, 2014a, b). In view of these inconsistencies, interpretation of the results of this collection of studies is difficult at best.

Historically, vehicle mechanics were exposed to low levels of chrysotile asbestos as a consequence of their work with brakes, clutches, and gaskets. Therefore, for exposure to low levels of chrysotile asbestos, the epidemiologic studies of vehicle mechanics are informative. The most important of these studies are 13 case-control studies (McDonald and McDonald 1980; Teta et al. 1983; Spirtas et al. 1985, 1994; Woitowitz and Rödelsperger 1994; Teschke et al. 1997; Agudo et al. 2000; Hansen and Meersohn 2003; Hessel et al. 2004; Welch et al. 2005; Rolland et al. 2006, 2010; Rake et al. 2009; Aguilar-Madrid et al. 2010), all of which concluded that vehicle mechanics are not at increased risk of mesothelioma. In fact, the study by Teschke et al. (1997) concluded that vehicle mechanics are at no greater risk of mesothelioma than accountants and schoolteachers.

In addition to the 13 case-control studies cited above, five cohort studies of vehicle mechanics in Europe (Hansen 1989; Järvholm and Brisman 1988; Gustavsson et al. 1990; Merlo et al. 2010; Van den Borre and DeBoosere 2015) likewise provide no evidence of an association between work as a vehicle mechanic and mesothelioma. A recent review and quantitative meta-analysis (Garabrant et al. 2016a, b) also concluded that vehicle mechanics are not at increased risk of mesothelioma as a consequence of occupational exposure to chrysotile asbestos.

Most quantitative exposure-response analyses of asbestos exposure and mesothelioma have relied on cumulative exposure as the measure of interest. It is now becoming abundantly clear that temporal patterns of exposure, such as duration of exposure and time since cessation of exposure, are important in determining cancer risk and that the same cumulative exposure accrued in different ways may not impose the same risk (Hazelton et al. 2005; Meza et al. 2008b; Richardson 2009; Peto 2012; Thomas 2014). For mesothelioma specifically, the model first developed by Peto et al. (1982) and used by the USEPA for its risk assessment in 1986 (Nicholson 1986) and then in an extended form by Berman and Crump (2008a, b) explicitly addresses duration of exposure to asbestos and time since cessation in exposure-response analyses. We refer to this model as the Peto–Nicholson model. Recent articles note that early, high-intensity exposures may be most important when evaluating mesothelioma risk (e.g., Rake et al. 2009; La Vecchia and Boffetta 2012), while others note that the risk for pleural cancer plateaus when a sufficiently long time since first exposure (>40–50 years) has elapsed (Barone-Adesi et al. 2008). The importance of early exposure to asbestos is consistent with the predictions of the Peto–Nicholson model, but the plateauing of risk is not. The evidence on the role of early exposure is mixed, with some studies showing that it increases risk, as noted above; however, a study by Reid et al. (2007) suggests that individuals exposed early may be at lower risk of developing mesothelioma. In one of their analyses of the French case-control studies, Lacourt et al. (2012) showed that cumulative exposure is a poor predictor of risk and that patterns of exposure need to be considered–a finding that is in agreement with the Peto–Nicholson model.

3.4   Asbestos Fiber Type and Mesothelioma Risk

3.4.1   Pleural Mesothelioma

There continues to be debate in the literature on whether exposure to "pure" chrysotile, i.e., chrysotile uncontaminated with amphibole asbestos, can increase the risk of mesothelioma (e.g., Kanarek 2011; Yarborough 2006, 2007). In our view, this debate is largely irrelevant because chrysotile epidemiology is based on exposures to commercial chrysotile, which is generally contaminated with tremolite.

Whether or not "pure" chrysotile causes mesothelioma, there is little disagreement that even if it does, amphiboles are more potent as mesotheliogens. Various estimates of differential potency have been offered. Hughes and Weill (1986) suggested that it could be as low as five. The most complete reviews of the epidemiologic evidence have been undertaken by Hodgson and Darnton (2000) and Berman and Crump (2003, 2008a, b), which demonstrate that exposure to amphiboles is far more potent than exposure to chrysotile as a cause of mesothelioma. Hodgson and Darnton (2000) concluded that amosite is 100 times and crocidolite 500 times as potent as chrysotile in causing mesothelioma. Berman and Crump (2008b) considered various measures of exposure as they relate to the risk of mesothelioma in 11 cohorts occupationally exposed to asbestos, concluding that the hypothesis that chrysotile and amphibole asbestos are equally toxic was strongly rejected no matter which measure of exposure was used. The estimates of the potency of chrysotile relative to that of amphibole ranged from zero to about 0.005, depending on the measure of exposure used. Epidemiologic studies of vehicle mechanics exposed to low levels of commercial chrysotile asbestos have failed to reveal an increased risk of mesothelioma, as discussed above.

Given the problems of exposure assessment discussed above in the occupational cohort studies of asbestos and mesothelioma, the estimates of differential potency reported in Hodgson and Darnton (2000) and Berman and Crump (2008b) must be viewed as ball-park estimates. In fact, these authors readily acknowledge that there are problems with accurate assessment of exposure. While these two estimates of differential potency are based on overlapping datasets, they use quite different statistical approaches. Whereas Hodgson and Darnton (2000) draw their conclusions regarding relative potency on the fraction of mesothelioma deaths in an occupational cohort as a function of mean cumulative exposure in that cohort, followed by exposure-response analyses across cohorts, Berman and Crump (2008b) consider individual-level exposures for each member of a given cohort and model the risk of mesothelioma as a function of both intensity and duration of exposure within that cohort using an extended version of the Peto–Nicholson model. The fact that these two completely different methods of analyses yield broadly similar estimates of relative potency—i.e., showing that amphiboles are approximately two orders of magnitude more potent than chrysotile—suggests strongly that the potency estimates are at least broadly reliable.

Case-control studies involving direct lung fiber measurements among cases and controls lend strong support to the conclusion that mesothelioma is much more strongly associated with amphiboles than with chrysotile asbestos (e.g., McDonald et al. 2001a, b; Gilham et al. 2015). Toxicological evidence also supports the conclusion that chrysotile has much lower carcinogenic potency than amphiboles. Recent work (e.g., Bernstein et al. 2005, 2006, 2013, 2014, 2015) shows that chrysotile is more rapidly cleared from tissues than amphibole asbestos, suggesting that it can be more effectively dealt with by the defense mechanisms of the body and is less biopersistent. Analyses of toxicological data on fiber biopersistence have shown that biopersistence is strongly correlated with carcinogenicity (e.g., Moolgavkar et al. 2001). Other experimental work (e.g., Shukla et al. 2004, 2009; Barlow et al. 2013; Bernstein et al. 2013, 2015) shows that chrysotile is less potent than other types of asbestos in triggering critical biological events thought to be important in the carcinogenic process.

3.4.2   Extra-Pleural Mesothelioma

3.4.2.1   Peritoneal Mesothelioma

The investigation of trends in mesothelioma incidence *pari passu* with trends in the commercial use of asbestos in the USA suggests strongly that inhalation exposure to asbestos plays much less of a role in the development of peritoneal than pleural mesothelioma, a conclusion that is supported by trends analyses in Europe. The analyses in Hodgson and Darnton (2000) confirm that peritoneal mesothelioma is associated with heavier exposure to asbestos than pleural mesothelioma and that, furthermore, when peritoneal mesothelioma is associated with asbestos exposure, it is associated with heavy exposure to amphibole asbestos.

Marinaccio et al. (2010) examined the incidence of extra-pleural mesothelioma based on the Italian national mesothelioma register. They identified a total of 614 peritoneal cases between 1993 and 2004, representing 6.7% of all mesotheliomas. Of these, 59% were men and 41% women. Based on the authors' assessments, about 76% of male and 34% of female peritoneal mesothelioma cases were occupationally exposed to asbestos. The authors reported that they observed about twice as many peritoneal mesothelioma cases in the 25–44-year age group as expected, with correspondingly fewer cases aged ≥ 45 years, assuming no differences in the age distribution of mesotheliomas between pleural and extra-pleural sites. Thus, peritoneal mesothelioma incidence rates in this study did not increase as strongly with age as did pleural mesothelioma rates, an observation consistent with results reported in the USA (Moolgavkar et al. 2009).

In a review of the epidemiology of peritoneal mesothelioma, Boffetta (2007) identified 34 cohort studies that reported the occurrence of peritoneal mesothelioma among workers exposed to asbestos or among asbestosis patients. Boffetta (2007) reported a strong correlation between the percentage of peritoneal mesothelioma deaths and the percentage of pleural mesothelioma deaths in these studies. The author identified five occupational cohorts that were exposed to "pure" chrysotile. One of these studies, a Chinese cohort study (Yano et al. 2010), reported a single case of peritoneal mesothelioma, while the other four reported none. Later investigations, however, revealed that the Chinese chrysotile is contaminated with amphibole asbestos (Tossavainen et al. 2001; Courtice et al. 2016).

In their review and analyses of occupational cohorts exposed to asbestos, Hodgson and Darnton (2000) were unable to establish an exposure-response relationship between chrysotile and peritoneal mesothelioma because they found only a single case of peritoneal mesothelioma in what they called a pure chrysotile cohort (South Carolina Textile cohort). Hodgson and Darnton (2000) suggested that there could have been amphibole contamination in this cohort,[1] and, in fact, small quantities of crocidolite were used at this plant between the 1950s and 1975 (Yarborough 2006, 2007). Lung burden analyses (Green et al. 1997; Case et al. 2000) indicated also that this cohort was exposed to commercial amphiboles.

Several other studies offer evidence that even heavy exposure to commercial chrysotile asbestos is not associated with peritoneal mesothelioma. In a cohort of asbestos miners and millers in Quebec exposed to high levels of chrysotile asbestos contaminated with tremolite, with the average exposure level being 600 f/mL-year, there were 33 cases of pleural mesotheliomas, but not a single case of peritoneal mesothelioma (Hodgson and Darnton 2000). Similarly, in the Balangero cohort, Hodgson and Darnton (2000) reported two mesotheliomas, both of them pleural, with the average exposure in the cohort being 300 f/mL-year. In an update of the Balangero cohort, Pira et al. (2009) reported an increased risk of pleural cancer in the cohort, but not of peritoneal cancer.

In a cohort of French workers exposed to chrysotile alone and to mixed fibers, three cases of peritoneal mesothelioma occurred among men and five among women, all with more than 80 f/mL-year of exposure (Clin et al. 2009). The authors suggested that the higher risk among women was a consequence of the fact that more women (when compared to men) received mixed fiber exposure. Further support comes from a large case-control study of 657 peritoneal cancers, in which Cocco and Dosemeci (1999) reported no association between measures of asbestos exposure and peritoneal cancer among women, suggesting strongly that asbestos exposure was not involved in the etiology of these tumors. Among men, they showed

---

[1] The review by Boffetta (2007) considered this cohort, but reported no cases of peritoneal mesothelioma in the cohort.

an association only in the highest exposure group, which contained individuals in traditional high-risk asbestos occupations, suggesting that the peritoneal cancers occurring in men in exposure categories other than the highest were not attributable to asbestos exposure, and that risk was attributable to occupations with high levels of mixed fiber exposures.

3.4.2.2   Mesothelioma of the Pericardium and TVT

The pericardium and the TVT—thin, serous membranes that surround the heart and the testis, respectively—are uncommon sites of malignant mesothelioma. In Italy, malignant mesotheliomas of the pericardium and TVT each accounted for 0.3% of all malignant mesotheliomas diagnosed between 1993 and 2008 (Marinaccio et al. 2015). In the SEER 18 registries between 2000 and 2013, pericardial mesothelioma comprised 0.2% of all malignant mesotheliomas, while testicular mesothelioma comprised 0.6% (SEER 2016). Due to the rarity of these malignancies, they are generally described only sporadically in case reports and case series, rather than in epidemiologic studies, and little is known about their risk factors.

The descriptive epidemiology of malignant mesothelioma of the pericardium and TVT was examined in Italy between 1993 and 2004 by Marinaccio et al. (2015). Extra-pleural mesothelioma had a lower male:female ratio than pleural mesothelioma (1.57:1 for all extra-pleural cases, including peritoneal, vs. 2.75:1 for pleural cases), and extra-pleural cases tended to be diagnosed at a younger age, on average, than pleural cases (11.1% of pericardial cases and 3.2% of testicular cases <45 years vs. 1.9% of pleural cases). Based on direct or indirect interviews with 56% of cases, the authors determined that 11 (92%) of 12 male patients with pericardial mesothelioma had been occupationally exposed to asbestos and 1 (8%) had unknown or improbable exposure, whereas 1 (11%) of 9 female patients had occupational exposure, 2 (11%) had environmental exposure, and 7 (78%) had unknown or improbable exposure. Among the 65% of TVT mesothelioma cases interviewed, the authors classified 13 (65%) of 20 as having occupational exposure to asbestos, 1 (5%) as having leisure-related exposure, and 6 (30%) as having unknown or improbable exposure. These exposure distributions were not compared with those in a control population without malignant mesothelioma, so relative risks could not be estimated, nor is it possible to determine with certainty whether the mesotheliomas with asbestos exposure were associated with that exposure.

A comparable study has not been published in the USA, but based on SEER 18 cancer registry data between 2000 and 2013 in the USA, the incidence rate of pericardial mesothelioma did not differ significantly between males and females (rate ratio in males vs. females = 1.15, 95% confidence interval [CI] = 0.42–3.10) (SEER 2016). In both sexes combined, the nationally age-standardized incidence rate of pericardial mesothelioma increased with age, from 0.01 per million at <50 years to 0.03 per million at 50–59 and 60–69 years and 0.04 per million at ≥70 years. Likewise, the incidence rate of mesothelioma of the TVT in males rose from 0.04 per million at <50 years to 0.2 per million at 50–59 and 60–69 years and 0.9 per million at ≥70 years. Patients diagnosed under age 50 years represented 45% of pericardial cases and 22% of TVT cases, compared with 3.3% of pleural cases. In the SEER 9 registries between 1973 and 2013, the incidence rate of pericardial mesothelioma decreased by decade, from 0.08 per million in 1973–1979 to 0.05 per million in 1980–1989, 0.03 per million in 1990–1999, 0.01 per million in 2000–2009, and 0.03 per million in 2010–2013 (rate ratio for 2000–2009 vs. 1973–1979 = 0.19, 95% CI = 0.04–0.69; rate ratio for 2010–2013 vs. 1973–1979 = 0.44, 95% CI = 0.10, 1.64) (SEER 2016). The incidence rate of mesothelioma of the TVT among males exhibited no significant temporal trend (0.07, 0.11, 0.11, 0.15, and 0.13 per million, respectively; rate ratios for 2000–2009 and 2010–2013 vs. 1973–1979 = 2.28, 95% CI = 0.76–7.90 and 1.96, 95% CI = 0.50–7.86, respectively).

The declining or flat temporal trends for these extra-pleural mesotheliomas contrast with the striking increase in the incidence of pleural mesothelioma among US males from 1973 to the early 1990s (Moolgavkar et al. 2009). The latter trend is widely acknowledged to reflect temporal trends in asbestos use in the USA, with a lag of 20–40 years (Price and Ware 2004). Correspondingly, the lack of a comparable trend in the incidence of pericardial and TVT mesothelioma, as well as the relatively young average age at diagnosis and the lack of a male predominance of pericardial mesothelioma, suggests a minor etiologic role, if any, of asbestos exposure in these malignancies.

Mesothelioma of the pericardium or TVT also has not been observed to occur in the context of heavy asbestos exposure. In particular, Hodgson and Darnton (2000) identified 17 occupational cohort mortality studies as having quantified data on asbestos exposure as an average for the cohort or for individual subgroups. Yarborough (2006) identified 18 cohorts occupationally exposed to amphibole asbestos, 39 cohorts occupationally exposed to mixed asbestos fibers, and 14 cohorts occupationally exposed to non-amphibole asbestos only (with amphibole contamination possible in some cohorts). Berman and Crump (2008a, b) identified 20 cohort studies from 18 locations that enabled quantitative estimates of potency factors for lung cancer or malignant mesothelioma related to occupational asbestos exposure by fiber type. Among all of these cohorts (several of which overlapped among the three publications), none reported any cases of malignant mesothelioma of the pericardium or the TVT (n = 0, unknown, or not reported). Subsequently published cohort studies of asbestos workers also have not reported any cases of pericardial or testicular mesothelioma (Loomis et al. 2009; Pira et al. 2009). This evidence further reinforces the conclusion that these malignancies are not a common outcome of inhalation asbestos exposure, even at high cumulative levels.

In conclusion, epidemiologic studies show that there is a site-specific gradient in the mesothelioma risk associated with inhalation exposure to asbestos. Pleural mesothelioma is most strongly associated with asbestos exposure. Peritoneal mesothelioma is less strongly associated with asbestos exposure, and when it is, it is associated with high exposure to amphibole asbestos. There is no evidence that mesotheliomas of the pericardium and the TVT are associated with inhalation exposure to asbestos, a conclusion that is supported by a recent analysis of SEER data (Lowry and Weiss, 2016).

3.5   Ionizing Radiation and Mesothelioma Risk

Ionizing radiation is a multi-site carcinogen; therefore, it is not surprising that recent epidemiological literature has shown quite convincingly that exposure to ionizing radiation, particularly for the treatment of a first primary cancer, increases the risk of developing mesothelioma (Andersson et al. 1995; van Kaick et al. 1999; Travis et al. 2003, 2005; Tward et al. 2006; Teta et al. 2007; Deutsch et al. 2007; Hodgson et al. 2007; De Bruin et al. 2009; Goodman et al. 2009; Berrington de Gonzalez et al. 2010; Gibb et al. 2013; Farioli et al. 2013, 2016; Schubauer-Berigan et al. 2015). The risk of mesothelioma appears to be increased even if mesothelial tissue is not directly in the field of radiation (Farioli et al. 2013, 2016). This may be due to the unavoidable scatter (e.g., Diallo et al. 1996; Hall 2006; Purdy 2008; Taylor and Kron 2011; Farioli et al. 2013, 2016) of radiation outside the targeted area during radiation therapy. An intriguing possibility is that a part of the increased risk could be due to abscopal effects, i.e., radiation action at a distance, though data on such effects are sparse (UNSCEAR 2008).

3.6   Genetic Factors and Inter-Individual Variation in Susceptibility

Inter-individual variations in susceptibility to cancer in general and mesothelioma specifically may arise in three ways that are not mutually exclusive (Moolgavkar 2015). The highest risks for cancer are conferred by rare conditions involving the inheritance of "cancer genes." Quintessential examples of such conditions are familial retinoblastoma, in which inheritance of a mutated retinoblastoma gene (*RB1*) confers a greatly increased risk for the development of an otherwise rare childhood tumor of the eye; and familial adenomatous polyposis (FAP), in which inheritance of a mutated adenomatous polyposis coli gene (*APC*) confers an enormous risk of colon cancer. The susceptibility to retinoblastoma is inherited in a dominant fashion, and virtually every child born with this mutation develops the disease. Many children with the mutated *RB1* gene develop bilateral retinoblastoma. The elegant "two-hit" model proposed by Knudson (1975), which provided a unified biological explanation for both hereditary and sporadic cases of retinoblastoma (Knudson et al. 1975, 1976; Moolgavkar and Knudson 1981; Knudson 2001), led ultimately to the concept of the tumor suppressor gene. For colon cancer, FAP, a dominantly inherited condition involving mutation of one allele of the tumor suppressor gene *APC*, confers a greatly increased risk of colon cancer. Although there is no direct estimate of the relative risk associated with FAP, it can be surmised to be several thousand and is strongly age-dependent (Luebeck and Moolgavkar 2002). Inactivation of both alleles of a tumor suppressor gene, or equivalently abrogation of cellular signaling pathways controlled by its gene product, is thought to be an important obligatory step in carcinogenesis, although the tissue specificity of individual tumor-suppressor genes is not understood.

The discovery that germline mutation of the *BAP1* tumor suppressor gene confers a very high risk of mesothelioma, uveal melanoma, and a few other tumors (Testa et al. 2011; Carbone et al. 2012) could be the single most important development in understanding the sequence of steps involved in the pathogenesis of mesothelioma. Somatic inactivation of the *BAP1* locus has been reported in up to ~60% of cases of sporadic mesothelioma (e.g., Testa et al. 2011; Bott et al. 2011; Jean et al. 2012; Nasu et al. 2015; Yoshikawa et al. 2012). This observation suggests that the development of sporadic mesothelioma and mesothelioma in individuals with a germline *BAP1* mutation may follow similar pathways.

Whether and how asbestos exposure interacts with a germline *BAP1* mutation to modify the risk of mesothelioma is not known. Recent toxicological studies (Xu et al. 2014; Napolitano et al. 2015) indicate that mice that are heterozygous for a *Bap1* mutation are particularly sensitive to crocidolite injected directly into the peritoneal cavity, with the relative risk of peritoneal mesothelioma among heterozygous mice being approximately 3–5 when compared to wild-type mice. These studies did not yield any information on risks among *Bap1*-heterozygous or wild-type mice without crocidolite exposure, since none of the mice in these experimental groups developed any tumors. However, subsequent work by Testa and colleagues (Kadariya et al. 2016) assessed spontaneous tumor development in three mouse models with different germline heterozygous mutations in *Bap1*, including two models in which the knock-in mutations were identical to those reported in BAP1 cancer syndrome families. Notably, all three *Bap1*-mutant models showed a high incidence of neoplasms at various sites, including mesothelioma in 2 of 93 *Bap1*-mutant mice, but not in any wild-type animals. The relative risk of mesothelioma associated with *Bap1* heterozygosity among the crocidolite-exposed mice is rather modest compared to the relative risks associated with the *Rb* or *Apc* gene mutation. This study provides no support for the hypothesis (Carbone et al. 2013; Napolitano et al. 2015) that an environmental exposure, such as low-exposure chrysotile, not known to increase the risk of sporadic mesothelioma in human populations can increase the risk of mesothelioma among individuals carrying the *BAP1* mutation. We note also that route of exposure should be taken into account in the interpretation of the results of these studies. Many animal species are particularly sensitive to direct instillation of agents into the peritoneal cavity, an exposure route that is not relevant to human exposure.

While germline mutations of major cancer genes confer very high risks of cancer upon individuals who inherit them, such mutations are rare and account for only a small fraction of cancers in the population. Other factors contribute to heterogeneity in the susceptibility to cancer, including mesothelioma. Stochasticity is an underappreciated factor leading to heterogeneity. The concept of stochastic heterogeneity is best understood by means of an example. Toxicology experiments are often conducted on highly inbred strains of animals that presumably are genetically identical. Yet, when treated with an identical dose of a carcinogen, these animals exhibit considerable heterogeneity of response. Not all animals develop tumors, and those that do, develop tumors at different ages. Thus, even with identical "nature" and "nurture," the tumor response is heterogeneous. Heterogeneity appears to arise from purely stochastic sources. The third source of heterogeneity in cancer susceptibility, besides major germline mutations and stochasticity, arises from inter-individual variations in myriad biological factors, such as polymorphisms in metabolizing enzymes, efficiency of DNA repair, and rates of cell division, that are important in the carcinogenic process (Moolgavkar 2015).

3.7 Spontaneous Mesothelioma

Mesothelioma has often been called the sentinel tumor for asbestos exposure. This statement has often been misinterpreted to mean that asbestos exposure is the *sine qua non* for mesothelioma development. With the wide recognition of the hazards associated with asbestos exposure and the consequent substantial decline in its use, however, an increasing fraction of mesotheliomas is not attributable to asbestos exposure. A small fraction of the mesotheliomas not attributable to asbestos exposure are probably attributable to other external risk factors, such as ionizing radiation; however, the major fraction of mesotheliomas not attributable to asbestos exposure is spontaneous.

As we have noted above, the current paradigm for carcinogenesis is that it is a process of mutation accumulation with clonal expansion of partially altered cells on the pathway to malignancy. Since mutations can occur spontaneously during cell division, they accumulate with age, and therefore cancers can and do occur spontaneously. As a consequence, the risk of most cancers, including mesothelioma, increases with age. In addition to this general biological argument, several lines of evidence support the conclusion that mesothelioma can occur without asbestos exposure. Mesothelioma is known to occur in individuals with no history of exposure to asbestos. Epidemiologic studies (e.g., Pelnar 1988; Peterson et al. 1984; Spirtas et al. 1994; Agudo et al. 2000; Teschke et al. 1997; Rake et al. 2009) report that a significant fraction of mesothelioma cases has no history of exposure to asbestos, with a larger fraction of female cases reporting no exposure. Spirtas et al. (1994) reviewed the literature and reported that estimates of the fraction of mesothelioma cases exposed to asbestos in epidemiologic studies have varied from a low of 13% to a high of 100%.

Many epidemiological studies have estimated population-attributable fractions (PAFs) for asbestos and mesothelioma. The PAF is a measure of the fraction of disease in a population attributable to exposure to an environmental agent, and depends on the risk associated with the exposure and the fraction of the population exposed to the agent. The PAF in a population depends upon two factors: the risk associated with the exposure (which clearly depends upon the fiber type and the level of exposure) and the fraction of the population that is exposed. Since these factors vary from population to population, it is to be expected that the PAF would vary from population to population. Spirtas et al. (1994) undertook a formal analysis to estimate the fraction of mesothelioma cases that could be attributed to asbestos exposure. They concluded that in their study, 88% of pleural mesotheliomas and 58% of peritoneal mesotheliomas among men could be attributed to asbestos exposure. Among women, they could not estimate the PAF separately for pleural and peritoneal mesotheliomas, but they reported that only 23% of all mesotheliomas were attributable to asbestos exposure. This study provides strong evidence that both pleural and peritoneal mesothelioma can occur without asbestos exposure, and that the fraction of peritoneal mesothelioma occurring without asbestos exposure is larger than the fraction of pleural mesothelioma occurring without asbestos exposure. A recent large case-control study of mesothelioma in Great Britain (Rake et al. 2009) concluded that 86% of male and 38% of female cases were attributable to either occupational or domestic asbestos exposure. Price and Ware (2009) estimated that approximately 70–75% of mesotheliomas among males and only 3–10% of mesotheliomas among females in the USA in 2008 were attributable to asbestos exposure. Offermans et al. (2014) reported that only about 32% of pleural mesotheliomas occurring in the Netherlands were attributable to asbestos exposure. Other studies (Aguilar-Madrid et al. 2010; Lacourt et al. 2010) showed that a substantial fraction of mesotheliomas in Mexico and France, respectively, could not be attributed to asbestos exposure.

Mesothelioma, including peritoneal mesothelioma, has also been reported to occur in young children and even congenitally (e.g., WTO 2000; Huncharek 2002; Kobayashi et al. 2014; Taylor et al. 2015; Wolff-Bar et al. 2015). Such cases are manifestly not associated with asbestos exposure. Thus, mesothelioma can clearly occur spontaneously.

Finally, examination of time trends in mesothelioma incidence provides strong evidence that mesothelioma can and does occur in the absence of asbestos exposure, as we have discussed above.

3.8 Discussion

3.8.1 Time Trends and Projections

As discussed above, mesothelioma incidence rates in the USA and elsewhere are declining, reflecting the decreasing use of asbestos worldwide. In the USA, these trends are most clearly observed in the incidence rates of pleural mesothelioma among men. Formal age-period-cohort analyses (Moolgavkar et al. 2009) show that pleural mesothelioma incidence rates among men increased strongly in a cohort-wise fashion starting with the birth cohorts of the 1890s, as successive birth cohorts entered the work force. The risk reached a peak for men born in the late 1920s and early 1930s, and has been declining since. For men born in the mid-1960s, the risk of pleural mesothelioma is similar to that for men born in the 1890s. In the USA at least, the epidemic of asbestos-associated mesothelioma appears to be ending, and one should expect a convergence of male and female mesothelioma rates. Any projections of mesothelioma rates and numbers into the future must explicitly recognize that these will be soon dominated by mesotheliomas that are unrelated to asbestos exposure.

3.8.2   Exposure-Response Relationships and Thresholds

The most comprehensive analyses of exposure-response relationships of mesothelioma in cohorts occupationally exposed to asbestos have been undertaken by Hodgson and Darnton (2000) and Berman and Crump (2008a, b) using very different approaches. Hodgson and Darnton (2000) used average cumulative exposure as the measure of exposure in a cohort, and conducted non-linear regression analyses of the fraction of mesothelioma deaths across cohorts separately for pleural and peritoneal mesotheliomas. That is, their exposure-response analyses used the fraction of deaths due to mesothelioma in an entire cohort together with the average cumulative exposure in the cohort as a single unit of observation. They reported supra-linear exposure-response relationships between each of the three asbestos types (chrysotile, amosite, and crocidolite) and pleural mesothelioma, and a sublinear relationship between cumulative amphibole exposure and peritoneal mesothelioma. They were unable to estimate an exposure-response relationship between chrysotile and peritoneal mesothelioma, as only a single case was identified.

Berman and Crump (2008a, b) used exposure estimates for each member of a cohort and estimated hazard functions within single cohorts using the Peto–Nicholson model, which is loosely based on ideas of multistage carcinogenesis and which explicitly considers the individual roles of fiber concentration, duration of exposure, and time since exposure ceased in determining risk. Under the Peto–Nicholson model, cumulative exposure does not uniquely define risk. For example, the risk of mesothelioma associated with 10 f/mL-years will depend on the pattern of exposure: the risk associated with 2 f/mL sustained over 5 years will be quite different from the risk associated with 5 f/mL sustained over 2 years.

It is now becoming increasingly clear that the entire pattern of exposure to a carcinogen is important in determining risk (e.g., Hazelton et al. 2005; Meza et al. 2008b; Richardson 2009; Peto 2012; Thomas 2014); therefore, the Peto–Nicholson model is biologically the better approach to exposure-response analyses. Both the Hodgson–Darnton and the Peto–Nicholson models share a limitation in that they assume that mesothelioma can occur only as a consequence of asbestos exposure. This is not an unreasonable assumption for analyses of occupational cohorts exposed to substantial quantities of asbestos, because the vast majority of mesotheliomas in these cohorts are attributable to asbestos exposure.

Thresholds cannot be estimated from epidemiologic studies because identification of a threshold is inextricably linked with the power of a study. While a practical threshold can be based on epidemiologic principles, e.g., when multiple epidemiologic studies fail to show an increase in the risk of mesothelioma in certain occupations in which asbestos exposure occurs, the concept of an absolute threshold must be based on biological considerations.

3.8.3   The Concept of Latency

While the concept of latency period or latency has been defined in different, not necessarily mutually consistent, ways (e.g., Langholz et al. 1999; Richardson et al. 2011; Porta 2014), in this chapter we adopt the definition often used in cancer epidemiology, i.e., latency is the interval between the start of exposure to a causal agent and the appearance of clinical manifestations of the disease. The U.S. Centers for Disease Control and Prevention (CDC) adopts this definition for exposure to putative carcinogens, declaring that the latency period is "…the time between first exposure to a cancer-causing agent and clinical recognition of the disease", and opines, "…latency periods vary by cancer type, but usually are 15 to 20 years, or longer."

This seemingly simple definition of latency masks a number of complexities having to do with temporal factors in exposure and the temporal evolution of risk during and following exposure (e.g., Langholz et al. 1999; Richardson et al. 2011; Moolgavkar et al. 2015). For chronic diseases, such as cancer, additional complications are introduced by the fact the diseases have multifactorial etiologies and arise even in the absence of the putative exposure for which latency is being investigated. Thus, for example, lung cancer can occur in the absence of tobacco smoking, acute myeloid leukemia can occur without exposure to benzene, and mesothelioma can occur without exposure to asbestos. It is not possible to distinguish the cancer that occurred due to exposure from one that simply occurred following exposure. Therefore, for chronic diseases, latency as defined above cannot be interpreted to be the time between an exposure and disease *caused* by that exposure.

A rigorous approach to the analysis of latency is based on considerations of the hazard functions for various exposure scenarios and is outside the scope of this chapter. We are not aware that such an analysis has been undertaken for mesothelioma, although a beginning has been made (e.g., Frost 2013; Farioli et al. 2014). Practically, latency is often estimated by taking the mean (or the median) of the time between beginning of exposure to asbestos and the diagnosis of mesothelioma among those cohort members who actually develop mesothelioma. Clearly, this quantity will depend on a number of factors. First, it will depend upon how long the cohort is followed up. The longer the follow-up, the longer the estimated latency will be. The estimate of latency will depend also on competing causes of death because the distribution of times to the development of mesothelioma depends upon the changing composition of the cohort over time. Latency will depend also on age at start of exposure and, therefore, on the age distribution of the cohort members. If a cohort is exposed at age 20, members of the cohort have virtually an entire lifetime to develop mesothelioma and, therefore, the latency will be longer than if cohort members are exposed at age 70. In the latter case, the latency has to be less than 30 years because the cohort will have died out. One of the widespread misconceptions regarding latency is that it is shorter for higher exposures. This is by no means clear, not least because the definition of higher (or equal) exposure is ambiguous. The latency associated with exposure to 2 f/mL for 5 years will be different from the latency associated with 5 f/mL for 2 years, yet these patterns amount to "equal" cumulative exposure.

In summary, the concept of latency is much subtler than it appears to be on first sight.

3.8.4   The Role of Cigarette Smoking and Other Risk Factors

One consequence of the declining rates of asbestos-associated mesothelioma is that it may be easier to investigate other, more modest, potential risk factors for pleural mesothelioma, such as diet (Schiffman et al. 1988) and cigarette smoking. Cigarette smoking is a multi-site carcinogen, but there appears to be consensus that it is not associated with mesothelioma; however, a review of the epidemiological literature shows that this conclusion is based on evidence of questionable scientific reliability. Many of the case-control studies that have addressed this issue were conducted in the 1970s, when the principles for the proper conduct of case-control studies were not generally understood. For example, an early study by McEwen et al. (1971) used two sets of controls, one consisting of patients with cardiovascular disease, the other consisting of patients with either lung cancer or gastric cancer. Both sets of controls clearly included more smokers than would be expected in the source population, since both cardiovascular disease and lung cancer are known to be strongly associated with cigarette smoking. Therefore, it is not surprising that these authors reported no association between smoking and mesothelioma. Similarly, the case-control study by Zielhuis et al. (1975) also used controls with cardiovascular disease, and therefore could not be expected to find an association between smoking and mesothelioma. Other studies reported a positive association between heavy smoking and mesothelioma (Hain et al. 1974), an association among females but not males (McDonald and McDonald 1980), and no association (Muscat and Wynder 1991). Thus, the evidence on which the conclusion that there is no association between smoking and mesothelioma is based is mixed at best. If there is an increased risk of mesothelioma among smokers, it is likely to be modest, and therefore difficult to discern in the presence of asbestos exposure.

3.8.5   Non-Occupational Exposure to Asbestos

In addition to exposures experienced in the workplace, asbestos exposures can occur in non-occupational settings. These include (1) neighborhood exposures, which involve asbestos emissions from nearby point sources (e.g., manufacturing facilities or mines); (2) environmental exposures, which result from naturally occurring asbestos or asbestos-like minerals; (3) household exposures from use of asbestos-containing materials, such as tremolite-containing whitewash; and (4) domestic exposures as a result of asbestos fibers brought into the home on workers' clothing or body, and interaction with these workers and their personal belongings. Domestic exposures are discussed here. Inhalation of asbestos fibers within the home due to living with and/or handling clothing of workers directly exposed to asbestos has been established as a possible contributor to disease. To formally evaluate the relationship between disease and exposures in domestic contacts, in conjunction with the Workers' Family Protection Act of 1992, the National Institute of Occupational Safety and Health (NIOSH) in the USA produced the Report to Congress on workers' home contamination study conducted under the Workers' Family Protection Act (NIOSH 1995). At the time, this was the most comprehensive report regarding health effects associated with take-home exposure for many different substances, including asbestos. The report concluded that domestic asbestos exposures may pose an increased risk of disease, primarily among wives who laundered clothes and children who played with their father's shoes, but the report did not provide analyses regarding the type of asbestos exposure, level, frequency, or duration needed to produce specific asbestos-related diseases. As a follow-up to this report, NIOSH published a research agenda focused on protecting workers' families (NIOSH 2002); to date, NIOSH has not published any studies based on this agenda.

In 2000, Bourdès and colleagues published a meta-analysis of studies reporting on domestic exposure, reporting an approximately eightfold greater risk of developing pleural mesothelioma in spouses who experience take-home exposure to asbestos (Bourdès et al. 2000). The eight underlying studies were conducted in populations where the primary workers experienced high occupational exposures (e.g., miners, cement workers), and in all but one study, exposures included either predominant or concomitant amphibole exposure. More recently, Goswami et al. (2013) published a review and meta-analysis of the available exposure data and epidemiologic studies pertaining to take-home exposure. In this analysis, the summary relative risk estimate for mesothelioma among persons domestically exposed to asbestos was 5.02 (95% CI: 2.48–10.13) based on 10 case-control studies and two cohort studies published between 1960 and 2012. This estimate pertains to persons domestically exposed via workers involved in occupations with traditionally high risk of disease from exposure to asbestos, such as asbestos product manufacturers, insulators, shipyard workers, and asbestos miners. When reported, the domestically exposed individuals were nearly always exposed to amphibole asbestos (crocidolite, amosite, or tremolite) and the mesothelioma was primarily pleural. These findings are consistent with lung burden studies of domestic exposure, most of which reported that domestically exposed persons with mesothelioma were typically wives or daughters of insulators, boilermakers, or shipyard workers (Huncharek et al. 1989; Gibbs et al. 1990; Roggli and Longo 1991; Giarelli et al. 1992; Roggli 1992; Dodson et al. 2003). All six of these studies identified the fiber type detected in the lung tissue examined as amphibole asbestos, the fiber type often associated with these types of occupations.

3.9   Conclusions

The epidemic of asbestos-associated mesotheliomas in the USA, driven largely by pleural mesotheliomas among men, appears to have reached a peak in the mid-1990s. Mesothelioma rates have been declining since. Men born after the 1960s have not had the opportunity for substantial asbestos exposure, and the SEER data are consistent with the view that these men, who are now in their mid-fifties or younger, are at only minimal risk of developing asbestos-induced mesothelioma. The decreasing impact of asbestos on the risk of mesothelioma in the US population may lead to the discovery of other more modest risk factors for mesothelioma, the impacts of which have been masked by asbestos.

Conflict of Interest   SHM, ETC, GM, and FSM have been involved in asbestos litigation.

References

Agudo A, González CA, Bleda MJ et al (2000) Occupation and risk of malignant pleural mesothelioma: a case-control study in Spain. Am J Ind Med 37:159–168

Aguilar-Madrid G, Robles-Perez E, Juarez-Perez CA et al (2010) Case-control study of pleural mesothelioma in workers with social security in Mexico. Am J Ind Med 53:241–251

Andersson M, Wallin H, Jönsson M et al (1995) Lung carcinoma and malignant mesothelioma in patients exposed to Thoratrast: incidence, histology and p53 status. Int J Cancer 63:330–336

Armitage P, Doll R (1954) The age distribution of cancer and a multistage theory of carcinogenesis. Br J Cancer 8:1–12

Baris YI, Grandjean P (2006) Prospective study of mesothelioma mortality in Turkish villages with exposure to fibrous zeolite. J Natl Cancer Inst 98:414–417

Barlow CA, Lievense L, Gross S et al (2013) The role of genotoxicity in asbestos-induced mesothelioma: an explanation for the differences in carcinogenic potential among fiber types. Inhal Toxicol 25:553–567

Barone-Adesi F, Ferrante D, Bertolotti M et al (2008) Long-term mortality from pleural and peritoneal cancer after exposure to asbestos: possible role of asbestos clearance. Int J Cancer 123:912–916

Berman DW, Crump KS (2003) Environmental Protection Agency. Final draft: technical support document for a protocol to assess asbestos-related risk. EPA# 9345.4-06. U.S. Environmental Protection Agency (EPA), Office of Solid Waste and Emergency Response, Washington, DC

Berman DW, Crump KS (2008a) Update of potency factors for asbestos-related lung cancer and mesothelioma. Crit Rev Toxicol 38(S1):1–47

Berman DW, Crump KS (2008b) A meta-analysis of asbestos-related cancer risk that addresses fiber size and mineral type. Crit Rev Toxicol 38(S1):49–73

Bernstein DM, Rogers R, Smith P (2005) The biopersistence of Canadian chrysotile asbestos following inhalation: final results through one year after cessation of exposure. Inhal Toxicol 17:1–14

Bernstein DM, Rogers R, Smith P et al (2006) The toxicological response of Brazilian chrysotile asbestos: a multi-dose sub-chronic 90-day inhalation toxicology study with 92 day recovery to assess cellular and pathological response. Inhal Toxicol 18:313–332

Bernstein D, Dunnigan J, Hesterberg T et al (2013) Health risk of chrysotile revisited. Crit Rev Toxicol 43:154–183

Bernstein DM, Rogers R, Sepulveda R et al (2014) Evaluation of the deposition, translocation and pathological response of brake dust with and without added chrysotile in comparison to crocidolite asbestos following short-term inhalation: interim results. Toxicol Appl Pharmacol 276:28–46

Bernstein DM, Rogers R, Sepulveda R et al (2015) Evaluation of the fate and pathological response in the lung and pleura of brake dust alone and in combination with added chrysotile compared to crocidolite asbestos following short-term inhalation exposure. Toxicol Appl Pharmacol 283:20–34

Berrington de Gonzalez A, Curtis RE, Gilbert E et al (2010) Second solid cancers after radiotherapy for breast cancer in SEER cancer registries. Br J Cancer 102:220–226

Boffetta P (2007) Epidemiology of peritoneal mesothelioma: a review. Ann Oncol 18:985–990

Bott M, Brevet M, Taylor BS et al (2011) The nuclear deubiquitinase BAP1 is commonly inactivated by somatic mutations and 3p21.1 losses in malignant pleural mesothelioma. Nat Genet 43:668–672

Bourdès V, Boffetta P, Pisani P (2000) Environmental exposure to asbestos and risk of pleural mesothelioma: review and meta-analysis. Eur J Epidemiol 16:411–417

Bruno C, Tumino R, Fazzo L et al (2014) Incidence of pleural mesothelioma in a community exposed to fibres with fluoro-edenitic composition in Biancavilla (Sicily, Italy). Ann Ist Super Sanita 50:111–118

Burdorf A, Järvholm B, Siesling S (2007) Asbestos exposure and differences in occurrence of peritoneal mesothelioma between men and women across countries. Occup Environ Med 64:839–842

Burstyn I, Lavoué J, Van Tongeren M (2012) Aggregation of exposure level and probability into a single metric in job-exposure matrices creates bias. Ann Occup Hyg 56:1038–1050

Carbone M, Ferris LK, Baumann F et al (2012) BAP1 cancer syndrome: malignant mesothelioma, uveal and cutaneous melanoma, and MBAITs. J Transl Med 10:179

Carbone M, Yang H, Pass HI et al (2013) BAP1 and cancer. Nat Rev Cancer 13:153–159

Case BW, Dufresne A, McDonald AD et al (2000) Asbestos fiber type and length in lungs of chrysotile textile and production workers: fibers longer than 18 μm. Inhal Toxicol 12(Suppl 3):411–415

Clin B, Moralis F, Dubois B et al (2009) Occupational asbestos exposure and digestive cancers—a cohort study. Aliment Pharmacol Ther 30:364–374

Cocco P, Dosemeci M (1999) Peritoneal cancer and occupational exposure to asbestos: results from the application of a job-exposure matrix. Am J Ind Med 35:9–14

Constantopoulos SH, Goudevenos JA, Saratzis N et al (1985) Metsovo lung: pleural calcification and restrictive lung function in northwestern Greece. Environmental exposure to mineral fiber as etiology. Environ Res 38:319–331

Courtice MN, Berman WD, Yano E et al (2016) Size- and type-specific exposure assessment of an asbestos products factory in China. J Expo Sci Environ Epidemiol 26:63–69

Cree M, Lalji M, Jiang B et al (2009) Explaining Alberta's rising mesothelioma rates. Chronic Dis Can 29:144–152

De Bruin ML, Burgers JA, Baas P et al (2009) Malignant mesothelioma following radiation treatment for Hodgkin's lymphomas. Blood 113:3679–3681

Deutsch M, Land SR, Begovic M et al (2007) An association between postoperative radiotherapy for primary breast cancer in 11 National Surgical Adjuvant Breast and Bowel Project (NSABP) studies and the subsequent appearance of pleural mesothelioma. Am J Clin Oncol 30:294–296

Diallo I, Lamon A, Shamsaldin A et al (1996) Estimation of the radiation dose delivered to any point outside the target volume per patient treated with external beam radiotherapy. Radiother Oncol 38:269–271

Dodson RF, O'Sullivan M, Brooks DR et al (2003) Quantitative analysis of asbestos burden in women with mesothelioma. Am J Ind Med 43:188–195

Farioli A, Violante FS, Mattioli S et al (2013) Risk of mesothelioma following external beam radiotherapy for prostate cancer: a cohort analysis of SEER database. Cancer Causes Control 24:1535–1545

Farioli A, Mattioli S, Curti S et al (2014) Comment on "The latency period of mesothelioma among a cohort of British asbestos workers (1978–2005)": the effect of left censoring. Br J Cancer 111:2197–2198

Farioli A, Ottone M, Morganti AG et al (2016) Radiation-induced mesothelioma among long-term solid cancer survivors: a longitudinal analysis of SEER database. Cancer Med 5:950–959

Finley BL, Richter RO, Mowat FS et al (2007) Cumulative asbestos exposure for U.S. automobile mechanics involved in brake repair (circa 1950s–2000). J Exp Sci Environ Epidemiol 17:644–665

Frost G (2013) The latency period of mesothelioma among a cohort of British asbestos workers (1978–2005). Br J Cancer 109:1965–1973

Garabrant DH, Alexander DD, Miller PE et al (2016a) Mesothelioma among motor vehicle mechanics: an updated review and meta-analysis. Ann Occup Hyg 60:8–26

Garabrant DH, Alexander DD, Miller PE et al (2016b) Response to Kay Teschke re: mesothelioma among motor vehicle mechanics: an updated review and meta-analysis. Ann Occup Hyg 21(2016):1–2. [Epub ahead of print]. doi:10.1093/annhyg/mew038

Gentiloni N, Febbraro S, Barone C et al (1997) Peritoneal mesothelioma in recurrent familial peritonitis. J Clin Gastroenterol 24:276–279

Giarelli L, Bianchi C, Grandi G (1992) Malignant mesothelioma of the pleura in Trieste, Italy. Am J Ind Med 22:521–530

Gibb H, Fulcher K, Nagarajan S et al (2013) Analyses of radiation and mesothelioma in the US Transuranium and Uranium Registries. Am J Public Health 103:710–716. Response in Am J Public Health 104:e1–2

Gibbs AR, Griffiths DM, Pooley FD et al (1990) Comparison of fibre types and size distributions in lung tissues of paraoccupational and occupational cases of malignant mesothelioma. Br J Ind Med 47:621–626

Gilham C, Rake C, Burdett G et al (2015) Pleural mesothelioma and lung cancer risks in relation to occupational history and asbestos lung burden. Occup Environ Med 73:290–299

Goldberg M, Imbernon E, Rolland P et al (2006) The French national mesothelioma surveillance program. Occup Environ Med 63:390–395

Goodman JE, Nascarella MA, Valberg PA (2009) Ionizing radiation: a risk factor for mesothelioma. Cancer Causes Control 20:1237–1254

Goswami E, Craven V, Dahlstrom D et al (2013) Domestic asbestos exposure: a review of epidemiologic and exposure data. Int J Environ Res Public Health 10:5629–5670

Green FH, Harley R, Vallyathan V et al (1997) Exposure and mineralogical correlates of pulmonary fibrosis in chrysotile asbestos workers. Occup Environ Med 54:549–559

Gustavsson P, Plato N, Lidstrom EB et al (1990) Lung cancer and exposure to diesel exhaust among bus garage workers. Scand J Work Environ Health 16:348–354

Hain E, Dalquen P, Bohlig H et al (1974) Katamnestische Untersuchungen zur Genese des Mesothelioms: bericht uber 150 Falle aus dem Hamburger Raum [Retrospective study of 150 cases of mesothelioma in Hamburg area]. Int Arch Arbeitsmed 33:15–37

Hall EJ (2006) Intensity-modulated radiation therapy, protons, and the risk of second cancers. Int J Radiat Oncol Biol Phys 65:1–7

Hansen ES (1989) Mortality of auto mechanics: a ten-year follow-up. Scand J Work Environ Health 15:43–46

Hansen J, Meersohn A (2003) Kræftsygelighed blandt danske lønmodtagere (1970–1997) fordelt på Arbejdstilsynets 49 branchegrupper. Sections 4–4.2.2 [Materials and Methods]. Institut for Epidemiologisk Kræftforskning, Kræftens Bekæmpelse, København [Copenhagen]

Hazelton WD, Clements MS, Moolgavkar SH (2005) Multistage carcinogenesis and lung cancer mortality in three cohorts. Cancer Epidemiol Biomark Prev 14:1171–1181

Hemminki K, Li X (2003) Time trends and occupational risk factors for peritoneal mesothelioma in Sweden. J Occup Environ Med 45:451–455

Henley SJ, Larson T, Wu M et al (2013) Mesothelioma incidence in 50 states and the District of Columbia, United States, 2003–2008. Int J Occup Environ Health 19:1–10

Hershcovici T, Chajek-Shaul T, Hasin T et al (2006) Familial Mediterranean fever and peritoneal malignant mesothelioma: a possible association? Isr Med Assoc J 8:509–510

Hessel PA, Teta MJ, Lau E et al (2004) Mesothelioma among brake mechanics: an expanded analysis of a case-control study. Risk Anal 24:547–552

Hodgson JT, Darnton A (2000) The quantitative risks of mesothelioma and lung cancer in relation to asbestos exposure. Ann Occup Hyg 44:565–601

Hodgson DC, Gilbert ES, Dores GM et al (2007) Long-term solid cancer risk among 5-year survivors of Hodgkin's lymphoma. J Clin Oncol 25:1489–1497

Holford TR (1983) The estimation of age, period and cohort effects for vital rates. Biometrics 39:311–324

Holford TR (1991) Understanding the effects of age, period, and cohort on incidence and mortality rates. Annu Rev Public Health 12:425–457

Hughes JM, Weill H (1986) Asbestos exposure-quantitative assessment of risk. Am Rev Respir Dis 133:5–13

Huncharek M (2002) Non-asbestos related diffuse malignant mesothelioma. Tumori 88:1–9

Huncharek M, Capotorto JV, Muscat J (1989) Domestic asbestos exposure, lung fibre burden, and pleural mesothelioma in a housewife. Br J Ind Med 46:354–355

International Agency for Research on Cancer (IARC) (2012) IARC Monographs on the Evaluation of Carcinogenic Risks to Humans. Volume 100C: Arsenic, Metals, Fibres and Dusts. Lyon, France: IARC

Iwatsubo Y, Pairon JC, Boutin C et al (1998) Pleural mesothelioma: dose-response relation at low levels of asbestos exposure in a French population-based case-control study. Am J Epidemiol 148:133–142

Järvholm B, Brisman J (1988) Asbestos associated tumors in car mechanics. Br J Ind Med 45:645–646

Jean D, Daubriac J, Le Pimpec-Barthes F et al (2012) Molecular changes in mesothelioma with an impact on prognosis and treatment. Arch Pathol Lab Med 136:277–293

Jeon J, Luebeck EG, Moolgavkar SH (2006) Age effects and temporal trends in adenocarcinoma of the esophagus and gastric cardia (United States). Cancer Causes Control 17:971–981

Jurek AM, Greenland S, Maldonado G et al (2005) Proper interpretation of non-differential misclassification effects: expectations vs observations. Int J Epidemiol 34:680–687

Kadariya Y, Cheung M, Xu J et al (2016) Bap1 is a bona fide tumor suppressor: genetic evidence from mouse models carrying heterozygous germline Bap1 mutations. Cancer Res 76:2836–2844

Kanarek MS (2011) Mesothelioma from chrysotile asbestos: update. Ann Epidemiol 21:688–697

Knudson AG Jr (1975) The genetics of childhood cancer. Cancer 35(3 suppl):1022–1026

Knudson AG Jr (2001) Two genetic hits (more or less) to cancer. Nat Rev Cancer 1:157–162

Knudson AG Jr, Hethcote HW, Brown BW (1975) Mutation and childhood cancer: a probabilistic model for the incidence of retinoblastoma. Proc Natl Acad Sci U S A 72:5116–51120

Knudson AG Jr, Meadows AT, Nichols WW et al (1976) Chromosomal deletion and retinoblastoma. N Engl J Med 295:1120–1123

Kobayashi S, Waragai T, Sano H et al (2014) Malignant peritoneal mesothelioma in a child: chemotherapy with gemcitabine and platinum was effective for the disease unresponsive to other treatments. Anti-Cancer Drugs 25:1102–1105

La Vecchia C, Boffetta P (2012) Role of stopping exposure and recent exposure to asbestos in the risk of mesothelioma. Eur J Cancer Prev 21:227–230. Erratum in: Eur J Cancer Prev (2015); 24:68

La Vecchia C, Decarli A, Peto J et al (2000) An age, period and cohort analysis of pleural cancer mortality in Europe. Eur J Cancer Prev 9:179–184

Lacourt A, Rolland P, Gramond C et al (2010) Attributable risk in men in two French case-control studies on mesothelioma and asbestos. Eur J Epidemiol 25:799–806

Lacourt A, Leffondre K, Gramond C et al (2012) Temporal patterns of occupational asbestos exposure and risk of pleural mesothelioma. Eur Respir J 39:1304–1312

Lacourt A, Gramond C, Audignon S et al (2013) Pleural mesothelioma and occupational coexposure to asbestos, mineral wool, and silica. Am J Respir Crit Care Med 187:977–982

Lacourt A, Rinaldo M, Gramond C et al (2014a) Co-exposure to refractory ceramic fibres and asbestos and risk of pleural mesothelioma. Eur Respir J 44:725–733

Lacourt A, Gramond C, Rolland P et al (2014b) Occupational and non-occupational attributable risk of asbestos exposure for malignant pleural mesothelioma. Thorax 69:532–539

Langholz B, Thomas D, Xiang A et al (1999) Latency analysis in epidemiologic studies of occupational exposures: application to the Colorado Plateau uranium miners cohort. Am J Ind Med 35:246–256

Loomis D, Dement JM, Wolf SH et al (2009) Lung cancer mortality and fibre exposures among North Carolina asbestos textile workers. Occup Environ Med 66:535–542

Luebeck EG, Moolgavkar SH (2002) Multistage carcinogenesis and the incidence of colorectal cancer. Proc Natl Acad Sci U S A 99:15095–15100

Lowry SJ, Weiss NS (2016) Geographic distribution of incidence of pericardial and paratesticular mesotheliomas in the USA. Cancer Causes Control 27:1487–1489. doi 10.1007/s10552-016-0825-3.

Marchand JL, Luce D, Leclerc A et al (2000) Laryngeal and hypopharyngeal cancer and occupational exposure to asbestos and man-made vitreous fibers: results of a case-control study. Am J Ind Med 37:581–589

Marinaccio A, Binazzi A, Di Marzio D et al (2010) Incidence of extrapleural malignant mesothelioma and asbestos exposure, from the Italian national register. Occup Environ Med 67:760–765

Marinaccio A, Binazzi A, Bonafede M et al (2015) Malignant mesothelioma due to non-occupational asbestos exposure from the Italian national surveillance system (ReNaM): epidemiology and public health issues. Occup Environ Med 72:648–655

McDonald AD, McDonald JC (1980) Malignant mesothelioma in North America. Cancer 46:1650–1656

McDonald JC, Edwards CW, Gibbs AR et al (2001a) Case-referent survey of young adults with mesothelioma: I. Lung fibre analyses. Ann Occup Hyg 45:513–518

McDonald JC, Edwards CW, Gibbs AR et al (2001b) Case-referent survey of young adults with mesothelioma: II. Occupational analyses. Ann Occup Hyg 45:519–523

McEwen J, Finlayson A, Mair A et al (1971) Asbestos and mesothelioma in Scotland: an epidemiological study. Int Arch Arbeitsmed 28:301–311

Merlo DF, Stagi E, Fontana V et al (2010) A historical mortality study among bus drivers and bus maintenence workers exposed to urban air pollutants in the city of Genoa, Italy. Occup Environ Med 67:611–619

Meza R, Jeon J, Moolgavkar SH et al (2008a) Age-specific incidence of cancer: phases, transitions, and biological implications. Proc Natl Acad Sci U S A 105:16284–11629

Meza R, Hazelton WD, Colditz GA et al (2008b) Analysis of lung cancer incidence in the Nurses' Health and the Health Professionals' Follow-Up Studies using a multistage carcinogenesis model. Cancer Causes Control 19:317–328

Moolgavkar SH (2015) Commentary: multistage carcinogenesis and epidemiological studies of cancer. Int J Epidemiol 45:645–649. doi:10.1093/ije/dyv204

Moolgavkar SH, Knudson AG (1981) Mutation and cancer: a model for human carcinogenesis. J Natl Cancer Inst 66:1037–1052

Moolgavkar SH, Brown RC, Turim J (2001) Biopersistence, fiber length, and cancer risk assessment for inhaled fibers. Inhal Toxicol 13:755–772

Moolgavkar SH, Meza R, Turim J (2009) Pleural and peritoneal mesotheliomas in SEER: age effects and temporal trends, 1973–2005. Cancer Causes Control 20:935–944

Moolgavkar SH, Anderson EL, Chang ET et al (2014) A review and critique of U.S. EPA's risk assessments for asbestos. Crit Rev Toxicol 44:499–522

Moolgavkar SH, Chang ET, Luebeck G et al (2015) Diesel engine exhaust and lung cancer mortality: time-related factors in exposure and risk. Risk Anal 35:663–675

Muscat JE, Wynder EL (1991) Cigarette smoking, asbestos exposure, and malignant mesothelioma. Cancer Res 51:2263–2267

Musti M, Cavone D, Aalto Y et al (2002) A cluster of familial malignant mesothelioma with del(9p) as the sole chromosomal anomaly. Cancer Genet Cytogenet 138:73–76

Napolitano A, Pellegrini L, Dey A et al (2015) Minimal asbestos exposure in germline BAP1 heterozygous mice is associated with deregulated inflammatory response and increased risk of mesothelioma. Oncogene 35:1996–2002

Nasu M, Emi M, Pastorino S et al (2015) High incidence of somatic BAP1 alterations in sporadic malignant mesothelioma. J Thorac Oncol 10:565–576

National Institute for Occupational Safety and Health (NIOSH) (1995) Report to Congress on workers' home contamination study conducted under the Workers' Family Protection Act (29 USC 671a). DHHS (NIOSH) Pub. No. 95-123. US Department of Health and Human Services (HHS), Public Health Service, Centers for Disease Control and Prevention (CDC), NIOSH, Cincinnati, Ohio

National Institute for Occupational Safety and Health (NIOSH) (2002) Protecting workers' families: a research agenda. DHHS (NIOSH) Pub. No. 2002-113. Department of Health and Human Services, Centers for Disease Control and Prevention (CDC), National Institute for Occupational Safety and Health, Cincinnati, Ohio

Nicholson WJ (1986) Airborne asbestos health assessment update. EPA/600/8–84/003F. U.S. Environmental Protection Agency (EPA), Office of Health and Environmental Assessment

Nordling CO (1953) A new theory on cancer-inducing mechanism. Br J Cancer 7:68–72

Offermans NSM, Vermeulen R, Burdorf A et al (2014) Occupational asbestos exposure and risk of pleural mesothelioma, lung cancer, and laryngeal cancer in the prospective Netherlands Cohort Study. J Occup Environ Med 56:6–19

Paoletti L, Batisti D, Bruno C et al (2000) Unusually high incidence of malignant pleural mesothelioma in a town of eastern Sicily: an epidemiological and environmental study. Arch Environ Health 55:392–398

Pelnar PV (1988) Further evidence of nonasbestos-related mesothelioma: a review of the literature. Scand J Work Environ Health 14:141–144

Peterson JT, Greenberg SD, Buffler PA (1984) Non-asbestos-related malignant mesothelioma: a review. Cancer 54:951–960

Peto J (2012) That the effects of smoking should be measured in pack-years: misconceptions. Br J Cancer 107:406–407

Peto J, Seidman H, Selikoff IJ (1982) Mesothelioma mortality in asbestos workers: implications for models of carcinogenesis and risk assessment. Br J Cancer 45:124–135

Pira E, Pelucchi C, Piolatto PG et al (2009) Mortality from cancer and other causes in the Balangero cohort of chrysotile asbestos miners. Occup Environ Med 66:805–809

Porta M (2014) Latency period. In: A dictionary of epidemiology, 5th edn. Oxford University Press, New York, NY, pp 165–166

Price B, Ware A (2004) Mesothelioma trends in the United States: an update based on surveillance, epidemiology, and end results data for 1973 through 2003. Am J Epidemiol 159:107–112

Price B, Ware A (2009) Time trend of mesothelioma incidence in the United States and projection of future cases: an update based on SEER data for 1973 through 2005. Crit Rev Toxicol 39:576–588

Purdy JA (2008) Dose to normal tissues outside the radiation therapy patient's treated volume: a review of different radiation therapy techniques. Health Phys 95:666–676

Rake C, Gilham C, Hatch J et al (2009) Occupational, domestic and environmental mesothelioma risks in the British population: a case-control study. Br J Cancer 100:1175–1183

Reid A, Berry G, de Klerk N et al (2007) Age and sex differences in malignant mesothelioma after residential exposure to blue asbestos (crocidolite). Chest 131:376–382

Richardson DB (2009) Lung cancer in chrysotile asbestos workers: analyses based on the two-stage clonal expansion model. Cancer Causes Control 20:917–923

Richardson DB, MacLehose RF, Langholz B et al (2011) Hierarchical latency models for dose-time-response associations. Am J Epidemiol 173:695–702

Rödelsperger K, Jockel KH, Pohlabeln H et al (2001) Asbestos and man-made vitreous fibers as risk factors for diffuse malignant mesothelioma: results from a German hospital-based case-control study. Am J Ind Med 39:262–275

Roggli VL (1992) Quantitative and analytical studies in the diagnosis of mesothelioma. Semin Diagn Pathol 9:162–168

Roggli VL, Longo WE (1991) Mineral fiber content of lung tissue in patients with environmental exposures: household contacts vs. building occupants. Ann N Y Acad Sci 643:511–518

Rolland P, Gramond C, Berron H et al (2005) Pleural mesothelioma: professions and occupational areas at risk among humans. [Mesotheliome pleural: professions et secteurs d'activite a risque chez les hommes]. Institute de Veille Sanitaire, Departement Sante Travai, Saint-Maurice, France. October. Available at http://www.invs.sante.fr

Rolland P, Ducamp S, Gramond C et al (2006) Risk of pleural mesothelioma: a French population-based case-control study (1998–2002). Lung Cancer 54(Suppl 1):S9–S10. Abstracts of the 8th International Conference of the International Mesothelioma Interest Group, Chicago, IL

Rolland P, Gramond C, Lacourt A et al (2010) Occupations and industries in France at high risk for pleural mesothelioma: a population-based case-control study (1998–2002). Am J Ind Med 53:1207–1219

Rosenberg PS, Anderson WF (2011) Age-period-cohort models in cancer surveillance research: ready for prime time? Cancer Epidemiol Biomark Prev 20:1263–1268

Ross M, Nolan RP (2003) History of asbestos discovery and use and asbestos-related disease in context with the occurrence of asbestos within ophiolite complexes. In: Ophioloite concept and the evolution of geological thought, vol 373. Geological Society of America Special Papers, Boulder, CO, pp 447–470

Rusch A, Ziltener G, Nackaerts K et al (2015) Prevalence of BRCA-1 associated protein 1 germ-line mutation in sporadic malignant pleural mesothelioma cases. Lung Cancer 87:77–79

Schiffman MH, Pickle LW, Fontham E et al (1988) Case-control study of diet and mesothelioma in Louisiana. Cancer Res 48:2911–2915

Schonfeld SJ, McCormack V, Rutherford MJ et al (2014) Regional variations in German mesothelioma mortality rates: 2000–2010. Cancer Causes Control 25:615–624

Schubauer-Berigan MK, Daniels RD, Bertke SJ et al (2015) Cancer mortality through 2005 among a pooled cohort of U.S. nuclear workers exposed to external ionizing radiation. Radiat Res 183:620–631

Shukla A, Vacek P, Mossman BT (2004) Dose-response relationships in expression of biomarkers of cell proliferation in in vitro assays and inhalation experiments. Nonlin Biol Toxicol Med 2:117–128

Shukla A, MacPherson MB, Hillegass J et al (2009) Alterations in gene expression in human meso-thelial cells correlate with mineral pathogenicity. Am J Respir Cell Mol Biol 41:114–123

Simonato L, Baris R, Saracci R et al (1989) Relation of environmental exposure to erionite fibres to risk of respiratory cancer. IARC Sci Publ 90:398–405

Sneddon S, Leon JS, Dick IM et al (2015) Absence of germline mutations in BAP1 in sporadic cases of malignant mesothelioma. Gene 563:103–105

Spirtas R, Keehn R, Wright W et al (1985) Mesothelioma risk related to occupational or other asbestos exposure: preliminary results from a case-control study. Am J Epidemiol 122:518

Spirtas R, Heineman EF, Bernstein L et al (1994) Malignant mesothelioma: attributable risk of asbestos exposure. Occup Environ Med 51:804–811

Stayner LT, Dankovic DA, Lemen RA (1996) Occupational exposure to chrysotile asbestos and cancer risk: a review of the amphibole hypothesis. Am J Public Health 86:179–186

Surveillance, Epidemiology, and End Results (SEER) Program (2016) SEER*Stat Database: incidence—SEER 9/13/18 Reg. Research Data, Nov 2015 Sub (1973–2013, varying)<Katrina/Rita Population Adjustment>Linked To County Attributes Total U.S., 1969–2014 Counties, National Cancer Institute, DCCPS, Surveillance Research Program, Surveillance Systems Branch, released April 2016, based on the November 2015 submission

Taylor ML, Kron T (2011) Consideration of the radiation dose delivered away from the treatment field to patients in radiotherapy. J Med Phys 36:59–71

Taylor S, Carpentieri D, Williams J et al (2015) Malignant peritoneal mesothelioma in an adolescent male with BAP1 deletion. J Pediatr Hematol Oncol 37:e323–e327

Teschke K (2016) Thinking about occupation-response and exposure-response relationships: vehicle mechanics, chrysotile, and mesothelioma. Ann Occup Hyg 60:528–530

Teschke K, Morgan MS, Checkoway H et al (1997) Mesothelioma surveillance to locate sources of exposure to asbestos. Can J Public Health 88:163–168

Testa JR, Cheung M, Pei J et al (2011) Germline BAP1 mutations predispose to malignant mesothelioma. Nat Genet 43:1022–1025

Teta MJ, Lewinsohn HC, Meigs JW, Vidone RA, Mowad LZ, Flannery JT et al (1983) Mesothelioma in Connecticut, 1955–1977 Occupational and Geographic Associations. J Occup Med 25:749–756

Teta MJ, Lau E, Sceurman BK et al (2007) Therapeutic radiation for lymphoma: risk of malignant mesothelioma. Cancer 109:1432–1438

Teta MJ, Mink PJ, Lau E et al (2008) US mesothelioma patterns 1973–2002: indicators of change and insights into background rates. Eur J Cancer Prev 17:525–534

Thomas DC (2014) Invited Commentary: is it time to retire the "pack-years" variable? Maybe not! Am J Epidemiol 179:299–302

Tomasetti C, Vogelstein B (2015) Variation in cancer risk among tissues can be explained by the number of stem cell divisions. Science 347:78–81

Tossavainen A, Kotilainen M, Takahashi K et al (2001) Amphibole fibres in Chinese chrysotile asbestos. Ann Occup Hyg 45:145–152

Travis LB, Hauptmann M, Gaul LK et al (2003) Site-specific cancer incidence and mortality after cerebral angiography with radioactive Thorotrast. Radiat Res 160:691–706

Travis LB, Fossa SD, Schonfeld SJ et al (2005) Second cancers among 40,576 testicular cancer patients: focus on long-term survivors. J Natl Cancer Inst 97:1354–1365

Tward JD, Wendland MM, Shrieve DC et al (2006) The risk of secondary malignancies over 30 years after the treatment of non-Hodgkin lymphoma. Cancer 107:108–115

United Nations Scientific Committee on the Effects of Atomic Radiation (UNSCEAR) (2008) Effects of ionizing radiation. UNSCEAR 2006 Report. Volume I. Report to the General Assembly with Scientific Annexes A and B. New York: United Nations

United States Environmental Protection Agency (USEPA) (2011) Toxicological review of libby amphibole asbestos. In: Support of summary information on the integrated risk information system (IRIS). External Review Draft. EPA/635/R-11/002A. Washington, DC: USEPA

Van den Borre L, Deboosere P (2015) Enduring health effects of asbestos use in Belgian industries: a record-linked cohort study of cause-specific mortality (2001–2009). BMJ Open 5:e007384

Van Kaick G, Dalheimer A, Hornik S et al (1999) The German Thoratrast Study: recent results and assessment of risks. Radiat Res 152:S64–S71

Welch LS, Acherman YIZ, Haile E et al (2005) Asbestos and peritoneal mesothelioma among college-educated men. Int J Occup Environ Health 11:254–258

Woitowitz H-J, Rödelsperger K (1994) Mesothelioma among car mechanics? Ann Occup Hyg 38:635–638

Wolff-Bar M, Dujovny T, Vlodavsky E et al (2015) An 8-year-old child with malignant deciduoid mesothelioma of the abdomen: report of a case and review of the literature. Pediatr Dev Pathol 18:327–330

World Trade Organization (WTO) (2000) European communities–measures affecting asbestos and asbestos-containing products. Report of the panel WT/DS135/R. World Trade Organization (WTO)

Wu S, Powers S, Zhu W et al (2016) Substantial contribution of extrinsic risk factors to cancer development. Nature 529:43–47

Xu J, Kadariya Y, Cheung M et al (2014) Germline mutation of Bap1 accelerates development of asbestos-induced malignant mesothelioma. Cancer Res 74:4388–4397

Yano E, Wang X, Wang M et al (2010) Lung cancer mortality from exposure to chrysotile asbestos and smoking: a case-control study within a cohort in China. Occup Environ Med 67:867–871

Yarborough CM (2006) Chrysotile as a cause of mesothelioma: an assessment based on epidemiology. Crit Rev Toxicol 36:165–187

Yarborough CM (2007) The risk of mesothelioma from exposure to chrysotile asbestos. Curr Opin Pulm Med 13:3

Yoshikawa Y, Sato A, Tsujimura T et al (2012) Frequent inactivation of the BAP1 gene in epithelioid–type malignant mesothelioma. Cancer Sci 103:868–874

Zielhuis RL, Versteeg JPJ, Planteijdt HT (1975) Pleural mesothelioma and exposure to asbestos. Int Arch Occup Environ Health 36:1–18

Chapter 4
Malignant Pleural Mesothelioma: History, Controversy, and Future of a Man-Made Epidemic

Oluf Dimitri Røe and Giulia Maria Stella

Abstract Asbestos (Greek, *inextinguishable*) is the term of a family of naturally occurring minerals that have been used in small scale since ancient times. Industrialization demanded increased mining and refining in the twentieth century, and in 1960, Wagner, Sleggs, and Marchand from South Africa linked asbestos to mesothelioma, paving the way to the current knowledge about the epidemiology, etiology, and biology of malignant pleural mesothelioma. Pleural mesothelioma is one of the most lethal cancers with increasing incidence worldwide. This review provides some snapshots of the history of mesothelioma discovery and the body of epidemiological and biological research including some of the controversies and unresolved questions. Molecular high-throughput profiling is currently unravelling novel biomarkers for earlier diagnosis and novel treatment targets. Current break-through discoveries of clinically promising non-invasive biomarkers such as meso-thelin, the 13-protein signature in serum, fibulin-3, circulating microRNAs and the recently discovered BAP1 cancer syndrome are highlighted. The asbestos history is a lesson not be repeated, but here we also review recent in vivo and in vitro studies showing that man-made carbon nanofibers could pose a similar danger to human health. This should be taken seriously by regulatory bodies to ensure thorough testing of novel materials before release into society.

O.D. Røe (✉)
Department of Cancer Research and Molecular Medicine, Norwegian University of Science and Technology (NTNU), Erling Skjalgssons gt. 1, Trondheim 7491, Norway

Cancer Clinic, Levanger Hospital, Nord-Trøndelag Health Trust,
Kirkegata 2, Levanger 7600, Norway

Clinical Cancer Research Center, Department of Clinical Medicine,
Aalborg University Hospital, Hobrovej 18-22, Aalborg 9000, Denmark
e-mail: oluf.roe@ntnu.no

G.M. Stella
Laboratory of Biochemistry and Genetics Pneumology Unit,
Fondazione IRCCS Policlinico, San Matteo, Pavia 27100, Italy

© Springer International Publishing AG 2017
J.R. Testa (ed.), *Asbestos and Mesothelioma*, Current Cancer Research,
DOI 10.1007/978-3-319-53560-9_4

Keywords Malignant mesothelioma • Asbestos • Biopersistent fibers • Molecular oncology • Biomarkers • Molecular targets • Carbon nanotubes

Abbreviations

AGGF1	Angiogenic factor with G patch and FHA domains 1 gene
BAP1	Breast cancer associated protein 1
BKV	Human polyoma virus named by the first patient's initials
BMI	Body mass index
BRCA2	Breast cancer 2, early onset gene
CHEK1	Checkpoint kinase 1 gene
Circadian rhythm genes	Genes expressed in cycles of 24 hours
CNT	Carbon nano-tubes, man-made fibers
EGFR	Epidermal growth factor receptor
GO	Gene ontology, grouping of genes in functional entities
GSTM1	Glutathione S-transferase M1 gene
IARC	International Agency for Research on Cancer
JCV	Human polyoma virus named by the first patient's initials
KEGG PATHWAYS	Computerized system of identifying genes relation to signaling, metabolic and cancer pathways
KEGG	Kyoto Encyclopedia of Genes and Genomes, a large digital database
MWCNT	Multi-wall carbon nanotube
NQO1	NAD(P)H dehydrogenase, quinone 1, gene and protein
OR	Odds ratio (statistical term)
PCA	Principal Component Analysis (unsupervised statistical method)
PET-CT	Positron emission computed tomography
PLS	Partial Least Squares regression model (statistical method)
RAD21	RAD21 homolog (S.pombe), involved in double-strand break repair
SMRP	Soluble mesothelin-related protein
SV40	Simian (monkey) vacuolating virus 40
SWCNT	Single-wall carbon nanotube
TYMS	Thymidylate synthase gene
VP1	Viral capsid protein of polyoma virus
WHO	World Health Organization

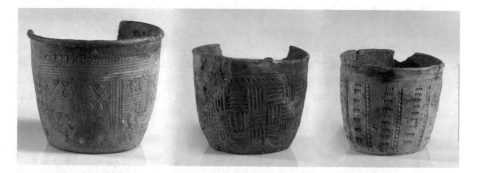

Fig. 4.1 Bucket-shaped pottery from Telemark, Norway and also found in several other areas in Norway, from the Bronze Age to the Roman Empire period (400–575 AD) (Dilek and Newcomb 2003). Such pottery was used for cooking and storage of food, with estimated asbestos content of 65–80%. (Photo with permission from Asbjørn Engevik, Bucket-shaped pots: style, chronology and regional diversity in Norway in the late Roman and migration periods, University of Bergen 2007)

4.1   Background

4.1.1   History of Asbestos Use and of Mesothelioma Discovery

Asbestos (Greek, *inextinguishable*) is the term used for a family of naturally occurring minerals that readily separate into thin fibers and are found in many parts of the world. The term *amiantus* (Greek, *untaintable*, currently used in modern Greek for asbestos) was used by Pliny the Elder (23–79 AD) who described that this material was mined in the mountains of Arcadia, could be spun and woven into material, and was resistant to fire (Dilek and Newcomb 2003). The Greek geographer Strabo (63/64 BC–ca. 24 AD) described similar use of the so-called Karystian stone from the ancient quarry in Evvia island of Greece, and Dioscorides (ca. 40–90 AD) described in his *Materia Medica* the use of this stone for weaving napkins that could be cleaned and whitened by fire (Dilek and Newcomb 2003). In Finland, asbestos was used in pottery 4500 years ago and in Norway, bucket-shaped pottery tempered with crushed asbestos was used for storing and making food in the Late Roman and Migration periods (ca. 350–475 AD) (Fig. 4.1). Marco Polo (1254–1324 AD) also described asbestos mining in China, so there is clear evidence for asbestos use among various cultures since ancient times (Rapp 2009). However, massive mining and use started in the twentieth century, due to asbestos' properties as insulation against heat, fire, corrosion and its tensile strength. Asbestos was widely used for insulation of water and combustion pipes, materials used for house construction and shipbuilding, car brakes and gaskets, as well as in toys, jewelry, and cigarette filters, and at its peak, 3000 products were registered (National Toxicology Program 2004).

The first report of a pleural tumor was in 1767 by Joseph Lieutand; however, mesothelioma was first characterized as an entity by Klemperer and Rabin in 1931

(Ribak et al. 2008). It took almost a further 30 years to become widely accepted as a separate cancer entity. The definite epidemiological study linking mesothelioma with asbestos came from South Africa, published in 1960 by J.C. Wagner, C.A. Sleggs, and P. Marchand, showing that mesothelioma was very prevalent in people, white or indigenous, living or working in a crocidolite asbestos mine area (Wagner et al. 1960). Later several studies from the USA, Europe, Australia, and Japan verified asbestos inhalation as an etiological cause of mesothelioma (Ribak et al. 2008; Armstrong et al. 1984; Gennaro et al. 1994; Musk and de Klerk 2004; http://monographs.iarc.fr/ENG/Monographs/vol100C/mono100C-11.pdf; Morinaga et al. 2001). The role of asbestos as a separate carcinogen in lung cancer was also described and even more dramatic, combining cigarette smoking with asbestos increased the risk of lung cancer from ten to almost 100-fold versus non-exposed (Barrett et al. 1989). Asbestos inhalation also induces pleural plaques, which are benign and not predictive of mesothelioma, asbestosis, a pneumoconiosis that may be fatal, and recently it was shown to increase the risk of cancer of the pharynx, stomach, colon and ovaries, as reviewed in the IARC 2012 monograph (http://monographs.iarc.fr/ENG/Monographs/vol100C/mono100C-11.pdf). Pleural mesothelioma is a relatively chemo- and radiation-resistant cancer that is usually diagnosed in a late stage and has a median survival of 12 months with current state-of-the-art treatment by pemetrexed and platinum.

4.1.2   Asbestos and Non-Asbestos Fiber Types, Exposure and Mesothelioma Epidemiology

Asbestos is classified into two main families, the serpentines and the amphiboles. The serpentines consist of one type, chrysotile, with characteristic short and curly fibers, also designated "white asbestos" due to its color, which accounts for 95% of asbestos in commercial use. The amphiboles, with straight and longer fibers, include crocidolite or "blue asbestos," amosite, tremolite, actinolite, and anthophyllite, and a thorough review of their physical and biological properties has recently been published and are also described in detail in Chap. 2 of this volume.

The risk of mesothelioma has previously been correlated to fiber type, where shorter fibers (chrysotile) were assumed to be less carcinogenic. This was mainly due to some research findings of high levels of long (amphibole) fibers in the lungs of the deceased patients and the animal experiments by Stanton leading to the "Stanton fiber hypothesis" (Stanton and Wrench 1972). Moreover, some researchers claimed that chrysotile could generate mesothelioma only if it was contaminated with an amphibole, the "tremolite contamination hypothesis" (Lippmann 1994). Nevertheless several animal models, including early work of Wagner from 1974 (Wagner et al. 1974), have pointed to the conclusion that chrysotile clearly is an important carcinogen and risk factor, not only for mesothelioma, but also for lung cancer and the current international perception according to the WHO and the IARC is that all types of asbestos are classified as class I carcinogens (IARC 2009) and that exposure to asbestos is the major cause of mesothelioma (Robinson et al. 2005). These findings resulted in banning of asbestos production and import in several European countries at various time points after 1970, and in all the EU as late as in 2005   (http://monographs.iarc.fr/ENG/Monographs/vol100C/mono100C-11.pdf; EU 1999).

There is a known dose-response pattern of asbestos exposure with mesothelioma as well as lung cancer, but as stated by the IARC and the WHO, no safe lower threshold has been identified. Moreover, it was discovered that not only people working with asbestos were at risk, but also their families due to cleaning of contaminated work clothes, and also people living close to places were asbestos was mined or processed (Ferrante et al. 2007; Langhoff et al. 2014). In Italy, in Casale Monferrato (Eternit factory) and Bari (Fibronit factory) an epidemic of mesothelioma was registered among inhabitants who never worked in the local asbestos factories where 25–33% of cases had only one risk factor: living to an asbestos cement factory. The calculated risk was very high (OR = 27.1 and OR = 5.29, respectively) for those living <500 m from the factory, and the fiber burden in the lungs of deceased cases was tenfold greater than in those from other areas (Magnani et al. 2001; Musti et al. 2009; Mirabelli et al. 2010).

In most epidemiological surveys, mesothelioma is more common in men, typically with a male to female ratio of 5:1, and some have inferred that susceptibility is correlated to gender. However, other studies showed this to be related to exposure and typically there is low asbestos exposure in women because the occupations that confer exposure traditionally are men's work. In occupations where women were most exposed, the majority of the victims were women (Wagner et al. 1974; Gao et al. 2015).

The extent of import and use of asbestos in a country is closely correlated with mesothelioma incidence. Norway, a small country but with solid cancer registry and asbestos statistics, exemplifies this point; in that country, the peak of asbestos import was 1970–1975 and the apparent mesothelioma peak is today, 40 years later (Fig. 4.2). International epidemiological surveys have estimated that the incidence peak in Europe will be reached around 2020 (Peto et al. 1999).

Asbestos may also cause lung cancer and up to 20,000 asbestos-related lung cancers and 10,000 mesotheliomas are estimated to occur annually across the population of Western Europe, Scandinavia, North America, Japan, and Australia (Tossavainen 2004), while registrations are not available in areas that still use asbestos, including Eastern Europe, South America, Africa and the rest of Asia, including China. The WHO reports that 125 million people encounter asbestos in the workplace. In 2004, asbestos-related lung cancer, mesothelioma, and asbestosis from occupational exposures resulted in 107,000 deaths and 1,523,000 Disability Adjusted Life Years (DALYs) and we know that those figures are increasing. In addition, several thousands of deaths can be attributed to other asbestos-related diseases, as well as to non-occupational exposures to asbestos (http://whqlibdoc.who.int/hq/2006/WHO_SDE_OEH_06.03_eng.pdf). Currently, the incidence of the disease is still increasing in most countries of the world, and only in countries in which

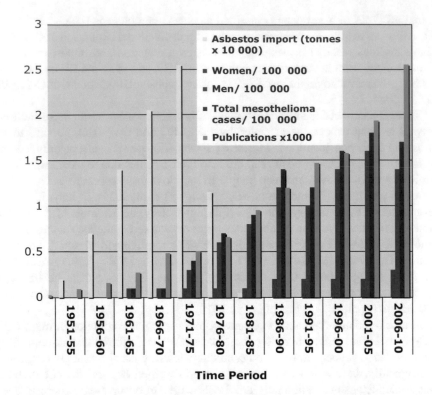

Fig. 4.2 Cumulative amounts of asbestos imports and incidence of mesothelioma in Norway over 5-year periods from 1946 to 2010. Histograph depicts import of raw asbestos to Norway in tons × 10,000 (*yellow bars*), based on Statistics Norway, 2002, incidence rates of mesothelioma per 100,000 (*dark red bars*) among Norwegian men (*blue*) and women (*light*) (Diagnosis Code C45 of the ICD10, based on data from the from Norwegian Cancer Registry, kreftregisteret.no), and cumulative number of publications in PubMed with the key word "mesothelioma" (×1000)

asbestos control measures were taken during the 1970s, such as Sweden and United Kingdom, has this increase leveled off (Bianchi and Bianchi 2007). Thus, the world-wide epidemic is in its beginning (Gaafar and Eldin 2005; Takahashi and Karjalainen 2003), and in countries that produce and/or use asbestos, including China, India, Russia, Zambia, Colombia, and Kazakhstan, a sharp rise in incidence could be expected (Luo et al. 2003; Joshi et al. 2006; Baris et al. 1978; http://minerals.usgs. gov/minerals/pubs/commodity/asbestos/mcs-2013-asbes.pdf).

Environmental exposure to carcinogenic fibers that exist on the earth surface is another, more uncontrollable risk factor. An old tradition of whitewashing houses with soft tremolite in the village of Metsovo, Greece was the reason for a cluster of mesotheliomas in young women, as women used to do this work (Sakellariou et al. 1996). Another important study by Luo et al. (Luo et al. 2003) documented that farmers exposed to crocidolite-containing soil in Da-Yao, a province in China, had a death rate of mesothelioma of 365/million, in contrast to e.g., Norway with 14 cases/million. Erionite, an asbestos-like mineral from the soil, was revealed as the main factor contributing to mesothelioma in young people in some villages in Cappadocia, Turkey, where more than 50% have died from mesothelioma (Roushdy-Hammady et al. 2001). The study of family trees in these villages showed a strong linkage to certain families, suggesting a genetic susceptibility for developing this disease, probably in an autosomal dominant way (Metintas et al. 2002). Recently, a breakthrough in the study of mesothelioma susceptibility showed that mutations in the gene *BAP1* is strongly associated with mesothelioma (Testa et al. 2011), which is discussed below.

4.1.3 Ionizing Radiation and Mesothelioma

Long-term effects of ionizing radiation have also been etiologically linked to meso-thelioma, even if it is a much smaller group of individuals than the asbestos exposed. The risk of developing mesothelioma is significantly higher in cases previously exposed to alpha particle-emitting agents, such as the radioactive contrast agent Thorotrast. It is also well documented that mesothelioma is over-represented in tes-ticular cancer and Hodgkin's lymphoma survivors who were treated with external radiotherapy (EU 1999; Travis et al. 2005; Goodman et al. 2009; Hodgson et al. 2007). However, today due to the knowledge of secondary cancer formation and improved alternatives for these cancers, these treatments are rarely used.

4.1.4 SV40 and Mesothelioma

There has been a controversy whether the simian virus SV40 could play a role in mesothelioma pathogenesis. The story is outlined in several papers, but currently the general belief is that it does not play an important role in human mesothelioma (Kjærheim et al. 2007; Røe and Stella 2015).

4.2 Pathophysiology

4.2.1 Normal Pleura Physiology and Fiber Clearance

The pleura is a thin, elastic membrane that covers the entire inner surface of the thoracic cavity. It is almost continuous, so it constitutes an expandable sac with a small amount of lubricating fluid for smooth movement of the thoracic cage, lungs, heart, and inner organs. The parietal pleura covers the thoracic wall, mediastinum, heart and diaphragm, and the visceral pleura covers the lungs (Fig. 4.3).

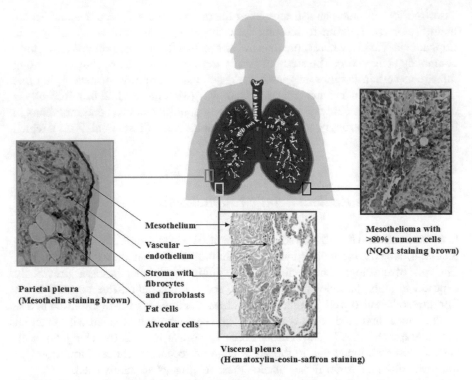

Fig. 4.3 Cartoon of normal parietal pleura, visceral pleura, and pleural mesothelioma. Most abundant cell types are shown (Courtesy of Oluf D. Røe)

Pleura is of mesodermal origin, is present at the 7th week of gestation, and comprises five layers: (1) a single layer of mesothelial cells; (2) a thin mesothelial connective tissue layer with a basal lamina; (3) a thin superficial elastic layer; (4) a loose connective tissue layer containing adipose tissue, fibrocytes, fibroblasts, mast cells, and other mononuclear cells including telocytes (Hinescu et al. 2011), blood vessels, nerves, and lymphatics; and (5) a deep fibroelastic layer that adheres tightly to the underlying structures (lung, thoracic muscle, etc.) (Light and Lee 2003). Studies of mesothelial cells have shown a variety of functions, among them inflammatory responses and phagocytosis of fibers (Mutsaers 2004).

Parietal and visceral pleura are similar, but they also have significant differences in structure and function (Table 4.1). Interestingly, genome-wide analysis of parietal versus visceral pleura from the same non-cancer patients reflected this as described previously in our study (Fig. 4.4; Røe et al. 2009).

Why is the pleura, and especially the parietal pleura, the target of asbestos disease? Inhaled fibers enter the visceral pleura and the pleural space to the parietal pleura through the alveolae, or retrograde through the lymphatics (Taskinen et al. 1973). This may be the reason why fibers of different sizes are more abundant in various segments, with the vast majority of chrysotile, the shorter asbestos fibers, being found in parietal pleura (Sebastien et al. 1980; Boulanger et al. 2014), while crocidolite and other amphibole fibers are mostly found in the lung parenchyma

Table 4.1 Structural and functional differences of the parietal and visceral pleura. Based on Light RW, Lee YCG, eds. Textbook of Pleural Diseases. 1st Edn. London, Arnold, 2003

Biological parameters	Parietal pleura	Visceral pleura
Mesothelial microvilli	Less (least on the costal surface)	More abundant
Mesothelial cell form	Flat	Cuboidal
Elasticity	Low	High
Permeability	High	Low
Tight junctions	Less	More
Intramembranous organization	Loose	Complex and tight
Innervation	Somatic, intercostals nerves	Vagus, sympathetic trunk
Pain receptors	Yes	No
Vascularization	Abundant	Poor
Drainage of pleural fluid and particles	Most	Little
Pleural fluid origin	Most	Little
Stomas	Yes, basal part	No
Lymphatic drainage	Abundant (mostly intercostals spaces)	Less, closer to alveolae than the mesothelium
Kampmeier's foci	Yes	No

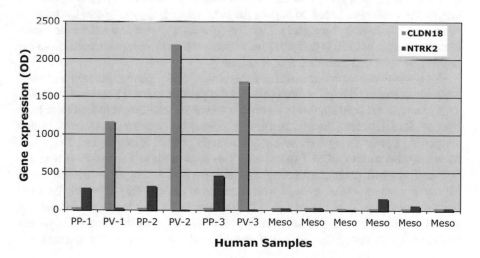

Fig. 4.4 Differential gene expression between parietal pleura (PP), visceral pleura (PV), and mesothelioma (Meso). Parietal and visceral pleura from the same non-cancer patients were analyzed with genome-wide mRNA array. Tight junctions are much more abundant in visceral pleura, and several claudins including the claudin 18 gene, *CLDN18*, was highly expressed in visceral pleura. The neurotrophic tyrosine kinase receptor, type 2 gene, *NTRK2*, which is abundant in nerve cells is also highly expressed in parietal pleura. Both genes were expressed at low levels in most of the mesotheliomas analyzed (Courtesy of Oluf D. Røe)

(McDonald et al. 2001). Moreover, the chronic inflammatory reaction believed to precede mesothelioma is mostly around the stomata and the lymphoid patches called Kampmeier's foci located in the basal part of the parietal pleura, which is the most common site of mesothelioma.

4.2.2   Origin and Site of the Mesothelioma Cell

Mesothelioma is derived from cells of the pleura, peritoneum, or tunica vaginalis, of which pleural location accounts for about 70% of cases (Bridda et al. 2007). Epithelial mesothelioma with its cuboidal cells is the most common subtype, while the sarcomatous type, with spindle-like cells, and the mixed subtype, are more rare.

Until recently it has been taken for granted that the mesothelial cell is the mesothelioma progenitor cell. However, when normal mesothelial cells are damaged, both regeneration from normal mesothelium and development from submesothelial multipotential stem cells are possible mechanisms of repair (Herrick and Mutsaers 2004; Bolen et al. 1986). Moreover, recent studies showed that adipocytes, circulating multipotent fibrocytes, and adult bone marrow-derived stem cells are able to transform to both epithelial and mesenchymal cells (Kettunen et al. 2001; Kim et al. 2004; Kothmaier et al. 2008). Interestingly, the mesothelial cell also has the ability to change its phenotype, to become smooth muscle cells and fibroblasts to internal organs and their vasculature, so normal mesothelial cells are multipotent, similar to stem cells (Rinkevich et al. 2012). Thus, the question arising is whether the mesothelioma progenitor cell is derived from a submesothelial multipotent cell, from the highly differentiated mesothelial cell, or both?

An obvious dilemma that remains unresolved is why pleural plaques and most probably mesothelioma primarily evolve in the parietal pleura (Boutin et al. 1998). This issue has not been studied in depth, but the above-mentioned factors have been hypothesized. However, there is not a general consensus on this point. Documentation supporting a parietal origin is that cases with only parietal affection, i.e., Stage T1a, have a median survival of 32.7 versus only 7 months in Stage T1b that involves parietal *and* visceral pleura, indicating that the parietal lesion is an earlier event. Moreover, to our knowledge, cases with affection of the visceral pleura only have not been reported. The current concept is that tumor grows in a loco-regional pattern, spreading from the parietal to the visceral pleura and invading the surrounding structures that induce the clinical picture of pleural fluid, thoracic pain, and dyspnea.

4.2.3   Mesothelioma Carcinogenesis and Molecular Profiling

Knowledge of the cytogenetic and molecular aspects of mesothelioma has progressed substantially in recent years and high-throughput analyses have revolutionized molecular characterization and our understanding of the underlying biological complexity. However, the carcinogenic mechanism of asbestos is not fully understood. Here a short overview is presented.

The currently accepted concept is that inhaled asbestos or other carcinogenic fibers end up in the pleura, inducing cytotoxicity, DNA damage, frustrated phagocytosis, and chronic inflammation (Jaurand and Fleury-Feith 2005; Jean et al. 2011). Through the latency period of 20–60 years, several key mechanisms affect the mesothelium such as chromosomal aberrations, epigenetic changes caused by promoter hypermethylation at tumor suppressor loci which result in functional disturbances measured by gene, microRNA, and protein expressions (Fennell 2011; Christensen et al. 2009; Røe et al. 2010; Gee et al. 2010; Hosako et al. 2012). Asbestos fibers are clastogenic and cytotoxic in vitro, induce abnormal segregation at mitosis, and their in vitro and in vivo transforming activity has been related to fiber dimensions, durability, and surface properties (reviewed in Barrett et al. 1989). Based on the epidemiological data, the long, thin amphiboles (crocidolite, amosite) have been regarded as the most carcinogenic, while the short and curly serpentines (chrysotile) are regarded as less dangerous, but undoubtedly carcinogenic, and as noted previously, more recent data point out that they probably should not be considered as less dangerous (Jaurand et al. 1986; Bignon and Jaurand 1983; Suzuki et al. 2005).

Cytogenetic studies have shown that mesotheliomas have highly complex and variable chromosomal aberrations (Murthy and Testa 1999; Ashburner et al. 2000), and only few features are shared between patients. Loss of heterozygosity (LOH) analyses have demonstrated frequent deletions of specific sites within chromosome arms 1p, 3p, 6q, 9p, 13q, 15q, and 22q. Two of these regions are most frequently altered, the tumor suppressors p16INK4A/p14ARF (encoded by the *CDKN2A* locus at chromosome band 9p21) and merlin, encoded by the *NF2* gene at 22q12. Homozygous deletion appears to be the major mechanism affecting *CDKN2A*, whereas inactivating mutations coupled with allelic loss occur at the *NF2* locus (Murthy and Testa 1999). Mesothelioma, as opposed to most other cancers, rarely has mutated p53, but loss of p14ARF indirectly inactivates p53 (Assoian and Yung 2008). Restoring p14ARF in a mouse model suppressed tumor growth significantly, showing the importance of this mechanism (Yang et al. 2000). Furthermore, pRb and p53 can be inactivated by the SV40 Large T-Antigen, which has been a suggested mechanism for mesothelioma progression (Giacinti and Giordano 2006). NF-κB (nuclear factor kappa-light-chain-enhancer of activated B cells) has been shown to be a survival factor in transformed human mesothelial cells and human mesothelioma cells. It acts as a survival factor in human mesothelial cells exposed to asbestos fibers (Yang et al. 2006). Proteasome genes are overexpressed in human mesothelioma, and proteasome inhibition was shown to suppress NF-κB activity in malignant mesothelioma cells and induce cell cycle blockade and apoptosis in vitro as well as tumor growth inhibition in vivo (Sartore-Bianchi et al. 2007). Recently, *Kras* and *Tp53* missense mutations were shown to induce not only lung carcinomas but also aggressive mesotheliomas in mice (Zeng et al. 2007), demonstrating that only two gene alterations can induce this tumor. Cell surface heparan sulfate proteoglycans, particularly syndecans, have recently been shown to be expressed in mesotheliomas, interact with growth factors and matrix components, and play a role in epithelial to mesenchymal transition of epithelial mesothelioma of the sarcomatous type (Dobra et al. 2003).

Extracellular signal-regulated kinases (ERK) are a family of molecules with distinct roles in cell injury, repair, differentiation, and carcinogenesis. In several cell line and animal studies, members of this family and especially ERK2 were critical to transformation and homeostasis of human malignant mesothelioma of the epithelial type (Shukla et al. 2011). The transcription factor, activator protein-1 (AP-1), a target of asbestos-induced signaling pathways, was also shown to be critical to the transformation of mesothelial cells through ERK-dependent Fra-1 elevation (Ramos-Nino et al. 2002). Hepatocyte growth factor/scatter factor (HGF) ligand and its receptor, the tyrosine kinase c-Met, are highly expressed in most human malignant mesotheliomas, and recently it was shown that HGF mediated cell proliferation of human mesothelioma cells through a PI3K/MEK5/Fra-1 pathway (Ramos-Nino et al. 2008). Moreover, c-Met was shown to be a relevant experimental treatment target as well as a negative prognostic factor (Jagadeeswaran et al. 2006; Levallet et al. 2012). Survival pathways such as the PI3K/Akt/mTOR are involved in cell growth and resistance to apoptosis and are often activated in mesothelioma. mTOR was shown to mediate survival signals in many mesothelioma tumors, and inhibition of mTOR was also proposed as a nontoxic adjunct to therapy directed against mesothelioma (Wilson et al. 2012). Inflammation has also been incriminated in mesothelioma tumorigenesis, and it was recently shown that inflammation precedes mesothelioma formation. Moreover, asbestos induced priming and activation of the NLRP3 inflammasome triggered an autocrine feedback loop modulated via the interleukin-1 receptor in mesothelial cells targeted in pleural infection, fibrosis, and carcinogenesis (Hillegass et al. 2013; Hillegass et al. 2010). A similar mechanism has been shown for carbon nanotubes (see Sect. 4.4).

High-throughput profiling of mRNA by various array platforms has indicated many interesting features of mesothelioma biology, but the results have not been concordant. This may be due to several factors including the use of different array platforms with various numbers of genes, and the fact that some researchers used cell lines, others correlated human tissue with cell lines, and others examined tumor tissue with parietal pleura from lung cancer patients or from non-cancer patients (Acevedo-Duncan et al. 2002; Hashimoto et al. 2004; Hassan and Ho 2008; Hoang et al. 2004; Jacquemont and Taniguchi 2007; Jackson 2003; Huang et al. 2005; Jung et al. 2007; Kanehisa et al. 2008). All these factors may have contributed separately and together to their largely incongruent results.

However, in our genome-wide analysis of six tumor and seven parietal pleura samples, we demonstrated dysregulation of several cellular systems, overexpression and down-regulation of genes reflecting several important biological functions among them, DNA replication and repair, as well as microtubule cytoskeleton organization and biogenesis (Røe et al. 2009; Røe et al. 2010). Of the DNA repair entity, genes related to double-strand break repair were over-represented. Several key genes encoding proteins known to be targets, but also to confer chemo-resistance (e.g., *NQO1*, *TOP2A*, *TYMS*, *BIRC5*/survivin, and proteasome) and radio-resistance by several DNA repair and damage checkpoint genes (e.g., *BRCA2*, *CHEK1*, *FANCA*,

FANCD2, *RAD21*, *RAD50*) were over-expressed in tumors (Kauffmann et al. 2008). A novel angiogenic gene *AGGF1* was also significantly overexpressed. Several genes encoding detoxifying enzymes, among them the multidrug resistance gene *ABCB1* (ATP-binding cassette sub-family B member 1), were down-regulated as were leukocyte transendothelial migration pathway and signal transduction genes.

Despite the low numbers of cases and controls, the differential gene expression detected was highly significant. Genes with previously known overexpression in mesothelioma were over-expressed here (e.g., genes for Ki67, syndecan 1, survivin and vitronectin). *FUT4* and *ST6GALNAC3*, genes coding for CD15 and sialyltransferase, respectively, and negative markers of mesothelioma were down-regulated. Unexpectedly, genes encoding calretinin, VEGFR, and mesothelin proteins, which are over-expressed in mesothelioma, were not differentially expressed in our study. However, recent studies showed that these are also expressed in normal mesothelial cells (Kettunen et al. 2005; Kennedy and D'Andrea 2006; Thickett et al. 1999)

mRNA profiling studies also resulted in the discovery of a novel biomarker, osteopontin (Pass et al. 2008), and the proteasome as a novel treatment target (Sun et al. 2006; Borczuk et al. 2007), as well as a gene signature for prognostication (Gordon et al. 2005), although the latter has not gained general acceptance yet (Lopez-Rios et al. 2006).

Recently, next-generation sequencing (NGS) of the whole genome uncovered massive genomic damage in mesothelioma versus normal tissue reflected in significant aneuploidy and novel, large-scale, inter- and intra-chromosomal deletions, inversions, and translocations. Nearly all candidate point mutations appeared to be previously unknown SNPs. One large deletion in *DPP10* resulted in altered transcription, and expression of *DPP10* transcripts correlated with survival in a set of 53 mesotheliomas. Three point mutations were observed in the coding regions of *NKX6-2*, which encodes a transcription regulator, and *NFRKB*, encoding a DNA-binding protein involved in modulating NFKB1, as well as amplification of genes such as *PCBD2* and *DHFR*, which are involved in growth factor signaling and nucleotide synthesis (Bueno et al. 2010). In a recent NGS study of 11 patients, the most common genes mutated were *BAP1* (36%), *CDKNA2A/B* (27%) and *NF2* (27%), but interestingly, in 27% no reportable genomic alterations were detected (Ugurluer et al. 2016). Exome sequencing of 21 tumor tissues of mesothelioma showed a similar pattern, but with additional discovery of novel mutations in BAP1, COPG1, INPP4A, MBD1, SDK1, SEMA5B, TTLL6, and XAB2 exclusively in asbestos-exposed patients (Mäki-Nevala et al. 2016). Further genomic profiling will increase the insight of the molecular basis and drivers of mesothelioma.

4.2.4 Mesothelioma Susceptibility and the BAP1 Cancer Syndrome

Mesothelioma develops in a minority of asbestos exposed individuals. This implies some kind of susceptibility to asbestos fiber carcinogenesis. Previous genome-wide association studies (GWAS) on polymorphisms failed to identify a single gene or even a signature of genes that were reproducible (reviewed in Neri et al. 2008). However, some gene polymorphisms showed increased risks of mesothelioma in a subset of studies, including cases not expressing the glutathione S-transferase M1 (*GSTM1*-null genotype), as well as two variant alleles of the DNA repair genes *XRCC1* and *XRCC3*. The GSTM1 protein is important for the detoxification of elec-trophilic compounds, including carcinogens, drugs, environmental toxins, and products of oxidative stress, and its down-regulation has been associated with several cancer forms. More recently, the largest GWAS to date on pleural mesothe-lioma did not reveal any significant new information other than indicating that genetic risk factors may play a role in the asbestos associated mesothelioma (Matullo et al. 2008).

Clustering of mesothelioma cases in some families has been observed by several researchers, and some have argued that this is not only due to shared asbestos expo-sure (Ugolini et al. 2013). A nuclear protein, BAP1 (BRCA1-Associated Protein 1), has several proposed functions, including transcriptional regulation, chromatin reg-ulation, and involvement in multi-protein complexes that regulate cellular differen-tiation, gluconeogenesis, cell cycle checkpoints, transcription, and apoptosis (Carbone et al. 2013). The *BAP1* gene is located on chromosome 3p21, a region that shows loss or deletion in numerous malignant tumors, including 30–60% of meso-theliomas. In the *BAP1* mutation families, there is a dramatically increased inci-dence of malignant tumors, often developed in an earlier age than observed in the general population. Currently, a BAP1 cancer syndrome has been proposed, includ-ing mesothelioma, uveal melanoma, cutaneous melanoma, and possibly other malignant tumors (Testa et al. 2011). Germline *BAP1* mutations are described in families with extraordinary high incidence of mesothelioma and in 25% of sporadic mesotheliomas (Testa et al. 2011), pointing to *BAP1* as the first gene reported to predispose for mesothelioma, but its role in mineral fiber carcinogenesis has not been established. Furthermore, subsequent reports indicate that about 60% of spo-radic mesotheliomas have alterations of the *BAP1* gene, when both deletions and sequence-level mutations are included (Yoshikawa et al. 2012) and that *BAP1* muta-tions are significantly more common in epithelial than sarcomatous and biphasic mesotheliomas (Bott et al. 2011; Yoshikawa et al. 2012). The discovery of a suscep-tibility gene will probably be of major importance for defining high-risk versus low risk groups when it comes to screening of asbestos exposed individuals with novel non-invasive biomarkers. A detailed summary of the role of *BAP1* in human and murine mesothelioma is presented in Chap. 8 of this volume.

4.3   Biomarkers

Diagnostic, prognostic, and predictive mesothelioma biomarkers is a rapidly evolv-ing field where several single molecules and signatures have been proposed (Panou et al. 2015). In this section we will focus not only on some of the most promising but also on some of the controversial novel biomarkers.

4.3.1 SMRP in Serum

Mesothelioma has a long latency period; 20–60 years may elapse between asbestos or other oncogenic exposure and the clinical presentation of disease, and the disease is usually diagnosed in a late stage. Non-invasive diagnostic biomarkers aiding early diagnosis and follow-up of patients have not been available.

The first potential mesothelioma tumor biomarker in serum was SMRP (Soluble Mesothelin-Related Protein), also called mesothelin (Beyer et al. 2007), which emerged as a marker for mesothelioma diagnosis (Robinson et al. 2003). Mesothelin is a family of proteins that are mainly membrane-bound, expressed in mesothelial cells, as well as various cancers such as pancreatic and ovarian cancer. The SMRP assay can detect three mesothelin variants, with Variant 1 being the predominant form in serum. SMRP is elevated in patients with epithelial mesothelioma, the most common subtype (Grigoriu et al. 2007). Robinson et al. (2003) also found SMRP elevated 1–5 years before clinical disease in some individuals exposed to asbestos, suggesting that SMRP could be used as a screening test. In addition, elevated SMRP level in serum was recently suggested as an independent negative prognostic factor of mesothelioma (Robinson et al. 2003). Pass et al. (2008) found a significant elevation in mesothelioma versus lung cancer, but also between Stage I and Stage II–IV mesothelioma, and importantly higher in Stage I than in non-cancer asbestos exposed individuals. The biological function of mesothelin is largely unknown and possibly plays a role in cell–cell adhesion. Interestingly it may also play a role in peritoneal metastasis of ovarian cancer, as CA125 expressed on ovarian cancer cell membranes adhere to mesothelin expressed on normal peritoneal cell membranes (Gubbels et al. 2006), facilitating local progression along the mesothelium. Mesothelioma cells also co-express CA125 (Rump et al. 2004), so the typical growth pattern with local progression and even tumor spread from the parietal to the visceral mesothelium could partly be explained by this mechanism.

The SMRP/mesothelin in serum is a non-invasive marker that can be helpful in making the diagnosis of mesothelioma, as the assay in the pivotal study had a sensitivity of 84% for mesothelioma, 100% specificity in differentiating mesothelioma from other pleural diseases, 95% against other lung cancers, and 100% against apparently healthy subjects (Robinson et al. 2005). However, in another study the best combination of sensitivity and specificity against controls was 66 and 70.9%, respectively (Azim et al. 2008). Moreover, as evaluation of response and recurrence by imaging techniques is difficult in mesothelioma, SMRP level is a sensitive measure of tumor burden as it is increased in more advanced disease. However, this assay failed as an early diagnostic biomarker, as we and others showed no significant difference in pre-clinical serum levels of cases and controls (Røe et al. 2008). Importantly, trials are ongoing with drugs targeting mesothelin in ovarian cancer, pancreatic cancer and mesothelioma, based on the quite unique expression of mesothelin in these tumors and non-expression in vital organs (Hassan and Ho 2008). Thus, mesothelin is currently an important molecule for follow-up of treatment and a putative treatment target for mesothelioma.

4.3.2   A 13-Protein Classifier in Serum

Proteomic technology has evolved rapidly, and a novel assay based on Slow Off-rate Modified Aptamers (SOMAmers) is used as capture reagents in order to achieve highly selective protein detection for biomarker identification (Kraemer et al. 2011). The SOMAmers are short, single stranded deoxynucleotides with an ability to bind discrete molecular targets. The use of SOMAmers as capture reagents carries many advantages over traditional antibody-based immunoassays, including high sensitivity and specificity, dynamic range, accurate quantification and reproducibility, and has the ability to measure thousands of human proteins in small volumes of biological samples with low limits of detection. Recently, a 13-protein signature was discovered in a cohort of 117 mesothelioma cases and 142 asbestos-exposed control individuals with a diagnostic area under the curve (AUC) of 0.99 in the training, 0.98 in the independent blinded verification, and 0.95 in the blinded validation studies. Sensitivity and specificity was 97%/92% in the training and 90%/95% in blinded verification studies, respectively. Sensitivity also correlated with pathologic stage: 77%/93%/96%/96% in Stages I–IV, respectively. An alternative decision threshold in the validation study yielding 98% specificity would still detect 60% of mesothelioma cases. When compared to mesothelin in a paired sample set, the 13-protein classifier AUC of 0.99 and 91%/94% sensitivity/specificity was superior to that of mesothelin with an AUC of 0.82 and a 66%/88% sensitivity/specificity. The candidate biomarker panel consisted of both inflammatory and proliferative proteins that could be associated with asbestos-induced malignancy (Ostroff et al. 2012). However, there have been no prospective studies on asbestos exposed cohorts to verify their value for early diagnosis and survival.

4.3.3   Fibulin-3 in Plasma

One recently published paper of very high interest in mesothelioma early diagnosis showed that the presence in plasma of a previously little studied protein, fibulin-3, could separate asbestos exposed mesothelioma individuals from those without mesothelioma with a sensitivity of 100% and specificity of 94.1%, and blinded validation study showed an AUC of 0.87 for plasma specimens from 96 asbestos-exposed persons as compared with 48 patients with mesothelioma. Moreover, fibulin-3 levels in plasma and pleural effusions were significantly different in patients with effusions from mesothelioma versus other malignant and benign effusions. Tumor tissue was examined for fibulin-3 by immunohistochemical analysis, and 26 of 26 cases was positive (Pass et al. 2012). However, in recent work by Creaney et al. (2014), these data could not be reproduced, and a comparative study found that SMRP was actually a more potent diagnostic serum marker than fibulin-3. In the same study, fibulin-3 in pleural effusion was proven a more potent prognostic marker than mesothelin, disconcordant with the previous study (Creaney et al. 2014). Thus, fibulin-3 is currently an unreliable marker as these studies did not point to the same direction.

4.3.4 Circulating MicroRNAs

MicroRNA is a novel class of non-coding RNA with several control functions and high stability in serum and plasma that was found to discriminate cases from controls in several cancer forms. Currently, there is evidence that increased circulating plasma miR-625-3p could serve as a potential diagnostic biomarker for patients with malignant pleural mesothelioma (Kirschner et al. 2012). A later study showed the promising prognostic value of a novel 6-microRNA signature (miR-Score) in operated pleural mesothelioma patients (miR-21-5p, -23a-3p, -30e-5p, -221-3p, -222-3p, and -31-5p) enabled prediction of long survival with an accuracy of 92.3% for EPP and 71.9% for palliative P/D. This may prove very valuable from the point of view that many patients are overtreated and may pay a high price to go through an extensive surgery with associated morbidity and mortality, when only a few can increase their survival (Kirschner et al. 2015). MicroRNAs not only can become the future biomarkers for mesothelioma but also promising treatment targets, reviewed (Reid 2015).

4.4 Man-Made Carbon Nanotubes

4.4.1 Man-Made Carbon Nanotubes and Disease; the Asbestos of the Future?

Among nanostructured materials, carbon nanotubes (CNT) are becoming the best known and studied due to their large-scale applications as structural materials in electronics, heating elements, batteries, production of stain resistant fabric, protection of aerospace materials against lighting strikes, water desalinization and purification, bone grafting, dental implants as well as targeted drug delivery and imaging diagnostics (Buzea et al. 2007; Lu et al. 2009; Prato et al. 2008). The interest in CNT is a direct consequence of the synthesis of buckminsterfullerene (C_{60}) and its derivatives in 1985. Fullerene is the third allotropic form of carbon (Krätschmer et al. 1990) after graphite and diamond. C_{60}, a 60-atom carbon molecule in the shape of a polyhedral cage made of 12 pentagons and 20 hexagons, can be considered the paradigm of a family of carbon nanostructures characterized by spherical or tubular shape. The diameter of a nanotube varies from few nanometers up to several micrometers. CNT are essentially of two types, namely, single-walled carbon nanotubes (SWCNT) and multi-walled nanotubes (MWCNT) (Iijima and Ichihashi 1993;

Kwon and Tomanek 1998). Although CNT are widely used in several applications, little is known about their potential toxicity in humans. The main exposure routes in occupational settings are known to be inhalation and dermal contact. Ingestion could also occur as a consequence of swallowing of the inhaled materials following mucociliary clearance or as a result of hand-to-mouth contact (Kwon and Tomanek 1998).

4.4.2 Current Evidence for CNT Carcinogenesis in the Lung and Pleura

Even if the literature on CNT health effects on development of mesothelioma is scarce, several lines of evidence indicate that CNT behave as biopersistent fibers in vivo and have a carcinogenic potential similar to that of asbestos (Fig. 4.5). By inhalation, a significant fraction of CNT can remain within the lungs for up to several months (Elgrabli et al. 2008), and in mice it was shown that the MWCNT migrate and reach the subpleural tissue after a single inhalation of CNT (Ryman-Rasmussen et al. 2009). In mice, Porter et al. showed that MWCNT of about 4 μm in length are able to reach the pleura and induce pleural inflammation 56 days after a single aspiration inducing an "asbestos-like pathogenicity" (Porter et al. 2010). In a very recent publication, rats inhaling sprayed MWCT weekly for 24 weeks were found to have CNT translocated into the pleural cavity, deposited in the parietal pleura and induced fibrosis and patchy parietal mesothelial proliferation lesions, very similar to the route and effects of inhaled asbestos (Xu et al. 2014). Intraperitoneal injection of MWCT in heterozygous $Tp53\pm$ mice that were followed for 1 year showed a dose-dependent development of mesothelioma, i.e., in 5/20, 17/20, and 19/20 mice by increasing the dose, a proof of principle that MWCT can produce mesothelioma and at a very high rate (Takagi et al. 2012). Moreover, chronic exposure to CNT showed invasive potential of human pleural mesothelial cells, through an increased expression of matrix metalloproteinase-2 (MMP-2) (Lohcharoenkal et al. 2013) and recently it was demonstrated that respiratory exposure to MWCNT in vivo and in vitro induced length-dependent pulmonary fibrosis and epithelial-derived fibroblasts via the TGF-β/Smad pathway (Chen et al. 2014). The CNT also could induce metastatic progression of lung carcinoma in mice, mediated by increased local and systemic accumulation of myeloid-derived suppressor cells, as their depletion abrogated pro-tumor activity in vivo (Shvedova et al. 2013). One of the theories on asbestos fiber toxicity and carcinogenicity is the "fiber paradigm" (Varga and Szendi 2010), where the geometry of fibers contributes their biopersistence (Donaldson et al. 2011). Similarly, it has been shown that CNT also have a length-dependent toxicity and carcinogenicity (Donaldson et al. 2011). Finally, changes of gene expression signature in mouse lungs following pharyngeal aspiration of MWCNT were associated with human lung cancer risk and progression signatures (Guo et al. 2012; Pacurari et al. 2011).

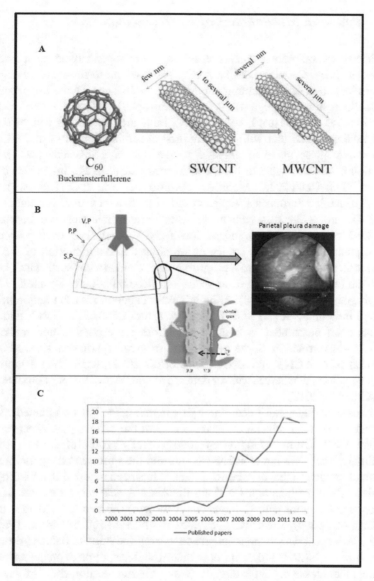

Fig. 4.5 Pleural hazard of exposure to CNT. (**a**) Structures of SWCNT and MWCNT derived from buckminsterfullerene (C_{60}). The structure of SWCNT (~0.4 nm in diameter) can be conceptualized by wrapping a 1-atom-thick layer of graphite (or graphene) into a seamless cylinder. MWCNT consists of multiple layers of graphite rolled upon themselves to form a tube shape with interlayer spacing of 3.4 Å, whereas their diameter ranges from 1 to 50 nm. (**b**) Schematic sequence of steps leading to pleural damage and/or malignant transformation due to exposure to biopersistent fibers. Long fibers and CNT are retained at stomatal openings and induce inflammatory oxidative stress response that leads to aberrant reactions at parietal pleura. Accordingly, the primary lesion caused by biopersistent fibers might form at the parietal pleural; this fact is reflected in MPM staging, where early mesothelioma is confined to parietal pleura, whereas more advanced MPM involves visceral layer. V.P, visceral pleura; P.P, parietal pleura; S.P, pleural space. (**c**) Increasing literature on lung and pleura toxicity induced by CNT (data from PubMed, by sorting CNT and pleural toxicity + CNT and mesothelioma) (Courtesy of Giulia Stella)

4.4.3   Potential Mechanisms of CNT Oncogenesis

As reviewed, several years of studies on asbestos carcinogenicity have not elucidated this process fully. Certainly, the knowledge is even more rudimentary regarding CNT, but induction of inflammation and gene toxicity seems to be important components. Interestingly, a significant acute neutrophilic influx into the lungs was demonstrated in animals just 1 day after CNT inhalation coexisting with histopathological findings consistent with bronchiolitis/alveolitis (Bonner et al. 2013). The epithelial damage seems to be mediated by reactive oxygen species (ROS), whose production has been related to the metallic contamination and impurities of CNT (Pacurari 2008; Stella 2011). Moreover, chronic exposure to CNT affects immune response, since it determines a sequestration of surfactant proteins A and D (SP-A and SP-D) and collectins, which, in turn, induce macrophages impairments (Salvador-Morales et al. 2007). Indeed, lowered SP-A and SP-D levels reduce resistance to some infections and induce an emphysema-like alteration of the lungs. Moreover these changes lead to a progressive accumulation of surfactant phospholipid in the lung tissue and alveolar space and accumulation of apoptotic alveolar macrophages (Botas et al. 1998). Although indirect genotoxic CNT action might be related to inflammation and ROS formation, direct CNT-related DNA damage of cells has been postulated as being responsible for epithelial and mesothelial malignant transformation. Some in vitro and in vivo experiments showed a direct interaction of MWCNT and DNA (Kato et al. 2013), suggesting a genotoxic/mutagenic potential, whereas weaker data are available on SWCNT (Lindberg et al. 2009; Kim et al. 2015).

Genotoxic damage can occur through direct interaction of retained asbestos fibers and mesothelial cells around the stomata of the parietal pleura as previously described. CNT feature a length-dependent toxicity profile of the mesothelium. Accordingly, long CNT could be retained around the stomata at the parietal pleura, in a similar fashion to that of asbestos fibers. It has been reported that macrophages recognize asbestos fibers and CNT via the class A scavenger receptor MARCO (Macrophage Receptor with Collagenous Structure) (Hirano et al. 2011), and that the uptake of both types of fibers activates the NLPR3 inflammasome (Palomaki et al. 2011). Recent data demonstrate that asbestos and erionite induce priming and activation of the NLRP3 inflammasome that modulates, through an autocrine feedback loop, the release of IL-1β, IL-6, IL-8, and Vascular Endothelial Growth Factor (VEGF). Production of such critical cytokines and growth factors probably is involved in the initiation of pleural injury and infection, pleural fibrosis, and mesothelioma (Hillegass et al. 2013). Moreover, when exposed to biopersistent fibers, mesothelial cells might avoid apoptosis when stimulated by TNFα secreted by the activated macrophages. This mechanism has been reported for asbestos and could theoretically be applicable to CNT (Bhattacharya et al. 2013).

4.4.4   Regulation of Health Hazards Posed by CNT and Future Aspects

During the past decade, CNT-related production capacity has increased at least tenfold and many companies are investing in diverse applications of CNT, from microelectronics and biotechnology to environment and energy storage (De Violder et al. 2013). Overall the production capacity for all CNT products is expected to exceed 12,300 tons in 2015, with the total production value expected to reach a value of $1.3 billion in 2015 (data from Innovative Research and Products (iRAP); website at www.innoresearch.net). With such a multitude of applications, a thorough understanding of associated toxicity is thus mandatory. The evaluation of CNT toxic profile might take in consideration exposure during manufacturing steps as well as their interaction with biological systems. Preliminary data have demonstrated that the main risk for humans is related to chronic occupational inhalation, mainly during those activities involving high CNT release and uncontrolled exposure. There is an urgent need to deeply test these materials and understanding their potential role in causing mesothelioma. In 2013, the National Institute for Occupational Safety and Health (NIOSH) carefully reviewed the animal and other toxicological data relevant to assessing the potential non-malignant adverse respiratory effects of CNT and proposed a recommended exposure limit (REL) of 1 $\mu g/m^3$ elemental carbon as a respirable mass 8-h time-weighted average (TWA) concentration (website at www.cdc.goc/NIOSH). The NIOSH REL is expected to reduce the risk for pulmonary inflammation and fibrosis. However, given the uncertainty about CNT-associated cancer risk, continued efforts should be made to reduce exposures as much as possible, and a number of strategies for controlling workplace exposures and implementing a medical surveillance program should be designed. Above all, CNT doses associated with genotoxicity should be determined by in vitro and in vivo studies. To avoid differences in inter-laboratory research protocols contributing to conflicting data in the literature, consortium research programs are emerging to reduce variability and validate findings (Xia et al. 2013). In parallel, a number of workplaces should be monitored: from research laboratories to CNT manufacturing, manipulating, and recycling plants. Surveillance programs should be extended worldwide, given that manufacturers in North America focused more on SWCNT, whereas Europe and Asia, with Japan on top and China second, are leading the production of MWCNT (Thiele and Das 2009). Exposure control challenges involved both the evaluation of exposure control techniques and the management of populations at risk through the identification of work practice recommendations and secondary prevention measures (Castranova et al. 2013; Shulte et al. 2012). Due to the probable latency, follow-up analysis should be performed on CNT-exposed people. It should be noted that preliminary reports suggest that functionalization allowing CNT solubilization and enhancing their biocompatibility by water-soluble nanoconjugates seems to emerge as a safe and effective procedure, with no cytotoxicity on macrophages and epithelial cells (Dvash et al. 2013; Mehara and Jain 2013). Therefore, the above observations allow relevant implications: (1) although promising in several fields, including pharmaceutics and biomedicine, CNT could exert a toxic and potentially tumorigenic effect; (2) based on a similar length-dependent pathogenicity, CNT may pose an asbestos-like mesothelioma hazard; and (3) nanotoxicology requires a multidisciplinary approach to these kinds of problems in order to achieve effective risk control.

4.5　Conclusions

Malignant pleural mesothelioma is a global, man-made cancer problem with increasing death tolls due to sustained mining and use of asbestos. Preventive measures including a global ban on asbestos should be mandatory. Awareness of the potential danger of new man-made fibers with similar carcinogenic properties, exemplified by CNT, should be high with thorough and relevant testing before further release into society. Novel diagnostic biomarkers are currently being tried for clinical use, but still we do not have markers for early diagnosis, prognosis or prediction of therapy. Molecular high-throughput profiling of tumor, blood and pleural fluids is currently unravelling novel biomarker candidates for earlier diagnosis and novel targets for improved treatment in the future.

Conflict of Interest　The authors have no conflicts of interest to disclose.

References

Armstrong BK, Musk AW, Baker JE et al (1984) Epidemiology of malignant mesothelioma in Western Australia. Med J Aust 141:86–88

Ashburner M, Ball CA, Blake JA et al (2000) Gene ontology: tool for the unification of biology. The Gene Ontology Consortium. Nat Genet 25:25–29

Assoian RK, Yung Y (2008) A reciprocal relationship between Rb and Skp2: implications for restriction point control, signal transduction to the cell cycle and cancer. Cell Cycle 7:24–27

Azim HA, Gaafar R, Abdel Salam I et al (2008) Soluble mesothelin-related protein in malignant pleural mesothelioma. J Egypt Natl Canc Inst 20:224–229

Baris YI, Sahin AA, Ozesmi M et al (1978) An outbreak of pleural mesothelioma and chronic fibrosing pleurisy in the village of Karain/Urgup in Anatolia. Thorax 33:181–192

Barrett JC, Lamb PW, Wiseman RW (1989) Multiple mechanisms for the carcinogenic effects of asbestos and other mineral fibers. Environ Health Perspect 81:81–89

Beyer HL, Geschwindt RD, Glover CL et al (2007) MESOMARK: a potential test for malignant pleural mesothelioma. Clin Chem 53:666–672

Bhattacharya K, Andón FT, El-Sayed R et al (2013) Mechanisms of carbon nanotube-induced toxicity: focus on pulmonary inflammation. Adv Drug Deliv Rev 65:2087–2097

Bianchi C, Bianchi T (2007) Malignant mesothelioma: global incidence and relationship with asbestos. Ind Health 45:379–387

Bignon J, Jaurand MC (1983) Biological in vitro and in vivo responses of chrysotile versus amphiboles. Environ Health Perspect 51:73–80

Bolen JW, Hammar SP, McNutt MA (1986) Reactive and neoplastic serosal tissue. A light-microscopic, ultrastructural, and immunocytochemical study. Am J Surg Pathol 10:34–47

Bonner JC, Silva RM, Taylor AJ et al (2013) Interlaboratory evaluation of rodent pulmonary responses to engineered nanomaterials: the NIEHS Nano GO Consortium. Environ Health Perspect 121:676–678

Borczuk AC, Cappellini GC, Kim HK et al (2007) Molecular profiling of malignant peritoneal mesothelioma identifies the ubiquitin-proteasome pathway as a therapeutic target in poor prognosis tumors. Oncogene 26:610–617

Botas C, Poulain F, Akiyama J et al (1998) Altered surfactant homeostasis and alveolar type II cell morphology in mice lacking Surfactant protein D. Proc Natl Acad Sci U S A 95:11869–11874

Bott M, Brevet M, Taylor BS et al (2011) The nuclear deubiquitinase BAP1 is commonly inactivated by somatic mutations and 3p21.1 losses in malignant pleural mesothelioma. Nat Genet 43:668–672

Boulanger G, Andujar P, Pairon JC et al (2014) Quantification of short and long asbestos fibers to assess asbestos exposure: a review of fiber size toxicity. Environ Health 13:59

Boutin C, Schlesser M, Frenay C et al (1998) Malignant pleural mesothelioma. Eur Respir J 12:972–981

Bridda A, Padoan I, Mencarelli R et al (2007) Peritoneal mesothelioma: a review. Med Gen Med 9:32

Bueno R, De Rienzo A, Dong L et al (2010) Second generation sequencing of the mesothelioma tumor genome. PLoS One 5:e10612

Buzea C, Pacheco II, Robbie K (2007) Nanomaterials and nanoparticles: sources and toxicity. Biointerphases 2:MR17–MR71

Carbone M, Yang H, Pass HI et al (2013) BAP1 and cancer. Nat Rev Cancer 13:153–159

Castranova V, Schulte PA, Zumwalde RD (2013) Occupational nanosafety considerations for carbon nanotubes and carbon nanofibers. Acc Chem Res 46:642–649

Chen T, Nie H, Gao X et al (2014) Epithelial-mesenchymal transition involved in pulmonary fibrosis induced by multi-walled carbon nanotubes via TGF-beta/Smad signaling pathway. Toxicol Lett 226:150–162

Christensen BC, Houseman EA, Godleski JJ et al (2009) Epigenetic profiles distinguish pleural mesothelioma from normal pleura and predict lung asbestos burden and clinical outcome. Cancer Res 69:227–234

Creaney J, Dick IM, Robinson BW et al (2014) Comparison of fibulin-3 and mesothelin as markers in malignant mesothelioma. Thorax 69:895–902

De Violder MF, Tawfick SH, Baughman RH et al (2013) Carbon nanotubes:present and future commercial applications. Science 339:535–539

Dilek Y, Newcomb S (2003) Geological Society of America Meeting. Ophiolite concept and the evolution of geological thought, vol XII. Geological Society of America, Boulder, CO, 504 pp

Dobra K, Nurminen M, Hjerpe A (2003) Growth factors regulate the expression profile of their syndecan co-receptors and the differentiation of mesothelioma cells. Anticancer Res 23:2435–2444

Donaldson K, Murphy F, Schinwald A et al (2011) Identifying the pulmonary hazard of high aspect ratio nanoparticles to enable their safety-by-design. Nanomedicine 6:143–156

Dvash R, Khatchatouriants A, Solmesky LJ et al (2013) Structural and biological performance of phospholipid-hyalutonan functionalized single-walled carbon nanotubes. J Control Dis 170:295–305

Elgrabli D, Floriani M, Abella-Gallart S et al (2008) Biodistribution and clearance of instilled carbon nanotubes in rat lung. Part Fibre Toxicol 5:20. Rapp GR (2009) Archaeomineralogy, vol. XV. Springer, Berlin/London, 348 pp

EU (1999) Commission Directive 1999/77/EC of 26 July 1999. Official Journal of the European Communities [L207/18L207/20]

Fennell DA (2011) Genetics and molecular biology of mesothelioma. Recent Results Cancer Res 189:149–167

Ferrante D, Bertolotti M, Todesco A et al (2007) Cancer mortality and incidence of mesothelioma in a cohort of wives of asbestos workers in Casale Monferrato, Italy. Environ Health Perspect 115:1401–1405

Gaafar RM, Eldin NH (2005) Epidemic of mesothelioma in Egypt. Lung Cancer 49(Suppl 1):S17–S20

Gao Z, Hiroshima K, Wu X et al (2015) Asbestos textile production linked to malignant peritoneal and pleural mesothelioma in women: analysis of 28 cases in Southeast China. Am J Ind Med 58:1040–1049

Gee GV, Koestler DC, Christensen BC et al (2010) Downregulated microRNAs in the differential diagnosis of malignant pleural mesothelioma. Int J Cancer 127:2859–2869

Gennaro V, Ceppi M, Boffetta P et al (1994) Pleural mesothelioma and asbestos exposure among Italian oil refinery workers. Scand J Work Environ Health 20:213–215

Giacinti C, Giordano A (2006) RB and cell cycle progression. Oncogene 25:5220–5227

Goodman JE, Nascarella MA, Valberg PA (2009) Ionizing radiation: a risk factor for mesothelioma. Cancer Causes Control 20:1237–1254

Gordon GJ, Rockwell GN, Godfrey PA et al (2005) Validation of genomics-based prognostic tests in malignant pleural mesothelioma. Clin Cancer Res 11:4406–4414

Grigoriu BD, Scherpereel A, Devos P et al (2007) Utility of osteopontin and serum mesothelin in malignant pleural mesothelioma diagnosis and prognosis assessment. Clin Cancer Res 13:2928–2935

Gubbels JA, Belisle J, Onda M et al (2006) Mesothelin-MUC16 binding is a high affinity, N-glycan dependent interaction that facilitates peritoneal metastasis of ovarian tumors. Mol Cancer 5:50

Guo NL, Murphy F, Schinwald A et al (2012) Multiwalled carbon nanotube-induced gene signatures in the mouse lung: potential predictive value for human lung cancer risk and prognosis. J Toxicol Environ Health A 75:1129–1153

Hashimoto K, Araki K, Osaki M et al (2004) MCM2 and Ki-67 expression in human lung adenocarcinoma: prognostic implications. Pathobiology 71:193–200

Hassan R, Ho M (2008) Mesothelin targeted cancer immunotherapy. Eur J Cancer 44:46–53

Herrick SE, Mutsaers SE (2004) Mesothelial progenitor cells and their potential in tissue engineering. Int J Biochem Cell Biol 36:621–642

Hillegass JM, Shukla A, Lathrop SA et al (2010) Inflammation precedes the development of human malignant mesotheliomas in a SCID mouse xenograft model. Ann N Y Acad Sci 1203:7–14

Hillegass JM, Miller JM, MacPherson MB et al (2013) Asbestos and erionite prime and activate the NLRP3 inflammasome that stimulates autocrine cytokine release in human mesothelial cells. Part Fibre Toxicol 10:39

Hinescu ME, Gherghiceanu M, Suciu L et al (2011) Telocytes in pleura: two- and three-dimensional imaging by transmission electron microscopy. Cell Tissue Res 343:389–397

Hirano S, Kanno S, Furuyama A (2011) Macrophage receptor with collagenous structure (MARCO) is a dynamic adhesive molecule that enhances uptake of carbon nanotubes by CHO-KI cells. Toxicol Appl Pharmacol 259:96–103

Hoang CD, D'Cunha J, Kratzke MG et al (2004) Gene expression profiling identifies matriptase overexpression in malignant mesothelioma. Chest 125:1843–1852

Hodgson DC, Gilbert ES, Dores GM et al (2007) Long-term solid cancer risk among 5-year survivors of Hodgkin's lymphoma. J Clin Oncol 25:1489–1497

Hosako M, Muto T, Nakamura Y et al (2012) Proteomic study of malignant pleural mesothelioma by laser microdissection and two- dimensional difference gel electrophoresis identified cathepsin D as a novel candidate for a differential diagnosis biomarker. J Proteome 75:833–844

Huang H, Regan KM, Wang F et al (2005) Skp2 inhibits FOXO1 in tumor suppression through ubiquitin-mediated degradation. Proc Natl Acad Sci U S A 102:1649–1654

Iijima S, Ichihashi T (1993) Single-shell carbon nanotubes of 1 nm diameter. Nature 363:603–605

International Agency for Research on Cancer (2009) Asbestos (chrysolite, amosite, crocidolite, tremolite, actinolite, and anthophyllite). In: IARC Monographs. Arsenic, Metals, fibres and dusts. International Agency for Research on Cancer, Lyon, pp 147–167

Jackson DE (2003) The unfolding tale of PECAM-1. FEBS Lett 540:7–14

Jacquemont C, Taniguchi T (2007) Proteasome function is required for DNA damage response and fanconi anemia pathway activation. Cancer Res 67:7395–7405

Jagadeeswaran R, Ma PC, Seiwert TY et al (2006) Functional analysis of c-Met/hepatocyte growth factor pathway in malignant pleural mesothelioma. Cancer Res 66:352–361

Jaurand MC, Fleury-Feith J (2005) Pathogenesis of malignant pleural mesothelioma. Respirology 10:2–8

Jaurand MC, Kheuang L, Magne L et al (1986) Chromosomal changes induced by chrysotile fibres or benzo-3,4-pyrene in rat pleural mesothelial cells. Mutat Res 169:141–148

Jean D, Daubriac J, Le Pimpec-Barthes F et al (2011) Molecular changes in mesothelioma with an impact on prognosis and treatment. Arch Pathol Lab Med 136:277–293

Joshi TK, Bhuva UB, Katoch P (2006) Asbestos ban in India: challenges ahead. Ann N Y Acad Sci 1076:292–308

Jung BH, Beck SE, Cabral J et al (2007) Activin type 2 receptor restoration in MSI-H colon cancer suppresses growth and enhances migration withactivin. Gastroenterology 132:633–644

Kanehisa M, Araki M, Goto S et al (2008) KEGG for linking genomes to life and the environment. Nucleic Acids Res 36:D480–D484

Kato T, Totsuka Y, Ishino K et al (2013) Genotoxicity of multi-walled carbon nanotubes in both in vitro and in vivo assay systems. Nanotoxicology 7:452–461

Kauffmann A, Rosselli F, Lazar V et al (2008) High expression of DNA repair pathways is associated with metastasis in melanoma patients. Oncogene 27:565–573

Kennedy RD, D'Andrea AD (2006) DNA repair pathways in clinical practice: lessons from pediatric cancer susceptibility syndromes. J Clin Oncol 24:3799–3808

Kettunen E, Nissén AM, Ollikainen T et al (2001) Gene expression profiling of malignant mesothelioma cell lines: cDNA array study. Int J Cancer 91:492–496

Kettunen E, Nicholson AG, Nagy B et al (2005) L1CAM, INP10, P-cadherin, tPA and ITGB4 over-expression in malignant pleural mesotheliomas revealed by combined use of cDNA and tissue microarray. Carcinogenesis 26:17–25

Kim JC, Badano JL, Sibold S et al (2004) The Bardet-Biedl protein BBS4 targets cargo to the pericentriolar region and is required for microtubule anchoring and cell cycle progression. Nat Genet 36:462–470

Kim JS, Song KS, Yu IJ (2015) Evaluation of in vitro and in vivo genotoxicity of single-walled carbon nanotubes. Toxicol Ind Health 31:747–757

Kirschner MB, Cheng YY, Badrian B et al (2012) Increased circulating miR-625-3p: a potential biomarker for patients with malignant pleural mesothelioma. J Thorac Oncol 7:1184–1191

Kirschner MB, Cheng YY, Armstrong NJ et al (2015) MiR-score: a novel 6-microRNA signature that predicts survival outcomes in patients with malignant pleural mesothelioma. Mol Oncol 9:715–726

Kjærheim K, Røe OD, Waterboer T et al (2007) Absence of SV40 antibodies or DNA fragments in prediagnostic mesothelioma serum samples. Int J Cancer 120:2459–2465

Kothmaier H, Quehenberger F, Halbwedl I et al (2008) EGFR and PDGFR differentially promote growth in malignant epithelioid mesothelioma of short and long term survivors. Thorax 63:345–351

Kraemer S, Vaught JD, Bock C et al (2011) From SOMAmer-based biomarker discovery to diagnostic and clinical applications: a SOMAmer-based, streamlined multiplex proteomic assay. PLoS One 6:e26332

Krätschmer W, Lamb LD, Fostiropoulos K et al (1990) Solid C_{60}: a new form of carbon. Nature 347:354–358

Kwon YK, Tomanek D (1998) Electronic and structural properties of multiwall carbon nanotubes. Phys Rev B 16:001–004

Langhoff MD, Kragh-Thomsen MB, Stanislaus S et al (2014) Almost half of women with malignant mesothelioma were exposed to asbestos at home through their husbands or sons. Dan Med J 61:A4902

Levallet G, Vaisse-Lesteven M, Le Stang N et al (2012) Plasma cell membrane localization of c-MET predicts longer survival in patients with malignant mesothelioma: a series of 157 cases from the MESOPATH Group. J Thorac Oncol 7:599–606

Light RW, Lee YCG (eds) (2003) Textbook of pleural diseases, 1st edn. Arnold, London

Lindberg HK, Falck GC, Suhonen S et al (2009) Genotoxicity of nanomaterials: DNA damage and micronuclei induced by carbon nanotubes and graphite nanofibers in human bronchial epithelial cells in vitro. Toxicol Lett 186:166–173

Lippmann M (1994) Deposition and retention of inhaled fibres: effects on incidence of lung cancer and mesothelioma. Occup Environ Med 51:793–798

Lohcharoenkal W, Wang L, Stueckle TA et al (2013) Exposure to carbon nanotubes induces invasion of human mesothelial cells through matrix metalloproteinase-2. ACS Nano 7:7711–7723

Lopez-Rios F, Chuai S, Flores R et al (2006) Global gene expression profiling of pleural mesotheliomas: overexpression of aurora kinases and P16/CDKN2A deletion as prognostic factors and critical evaluation of microarray-based prognostic prediction. Cancer Res 66:2970–2979

Lu F, Lingrong G, Mohammed J et al (2009) Advances in bioapplications of carbon nanotubes. Adv Mater 21:139–152

Luo S, Liu X, Mu S et al (2003) Asbestos related diseases from environmental exposure to crocidolite in Da-yao, China. I. Review of exposure and epidemiological data. Occup Environ Med 60:35–41. discussion 41–42

Magnani C, Dalmasso P, Biggeri A et al (2001) Increased risk of malignant mesothelioma of the pleura after residential or domestic exposure to asbestos: a case-control study in Casale Monferrato, Italy. Environ Health Perspect 109:915–919

Mäki-Nevala S, Sarhadi VK, Knuuttila A et al (2016) Driver gene and novel mutations in asbestos-exposed lung adenocarcinoma and malignant mesothelioma detected by exome sequencing. Lung 194:125–135

Matullo G, Guarrera S, Betti M et al (2008) Genetic variants associated with increased risk of malignant pleural mesothelioma: a genome-wide association study. PLoS One 8:e61253

McDonald JC, Armstrong BG, Edwards CW et al (2001) Case-referent survey of young adults with mesothelioma: I. Lung fibre analyses. Ann Occup Hyg 45:513–518

Mehara NK, Jain NK (2013) Development, characterization and cancer targeting potential of surface engineered carbon nanotubes. J Drug Target 8:745–758

Metintas S, Metintas M, Ucgun I et al (2002) Malignant mesothelioma due to environmental exposure to asbestos: follow-up of a Turkish cohort living in a rural area. Chest 122:2224–2229

Mirabelli D, Cavone D, Merler E et al (2010) Non-occupational exposure to asbestos and malignant mesothelioma in the Italian National Registry of Mesotheliomas. Occup Environ Med 67:792–794

Morinaga K, Kishimoto T, Sakatani M et al (2001) Asbestos-related lung cancer and mesothelioma in Japan. Ind Health 39:65–74

Murthy SS, Testa JR (1999) Asbestos, chromosomal deletions, and tumor suppressor gene alterations in human malignant mesothelioma. J Cell Physiol 180:150–157

Musk AW, de Klerk NH (2004) Epidemiology of malignant mesothelioma in Australia. Lung Cancer 45(Suppl 1):S21–S23

Musti M, Pollice A, Cavone D et al (2009) The relationship between malignant mesothelioma and an asbestos cement plant environmental risk: a spatial case-control study in the city of Bari (Italy). Int Arch Occup Environ Health 82:489–497

Mutsaers SE (2004) The mesothelial cell. Int J Biochem Cell Biol 36:9–16

Neri M, Ugolini D, Dianzani I et al (2008) Genetic susceptibility to malignant pleural mesothelioma and other asbestos-associated diseases. Mutat Res 659:126–136

Ostroff RM, Mehan MR, Stewart A et al (2012) Early detection of malignant pleural mesothelioma in asbestos-exposed individuals with a noninvasive proteomics-based surveillance tool. PLoS One 7:e46091

Pacurari M (2008) Raw single-wall carbon nanotubes induce oxidative stress and activate MAPKs, AP-1, NKκB and Akt in normal and malignant human mesothelial cells. Environ Health Perspect 116:121

Pacurari M, Qian Y, Porter DW et al (2011) Multi-walled carbon nanotube-induced gene expression in the mouse lung: association with lung pathology. Toxicol Appl Pharmacol 255:18–31

Palomaki J, Valimaki E, Sund J (2011) Long, needle-like carbon nanotubes and asbestos activate the NLPR3 inflammasome sensing of asbestos and silica. ACS Nano 5:6861–6870

Panou V, Vyberg M, Weinreich UM et al (2015) The established and future biomarkers of malignant pleural mesothelioma. Cancer Treat Rev 41:486–495

Pass HI, Lott D, Lonardo F et al (2008) Asbestos exposure, pleural mesothelioma, and serum osteopontin levels. N Engl J Med 53:1564–1573

Pass HI, Levin SM, Harbut MR et al (2012) Fibulin-3 as a blood and effusion biomarker for pleural mesothelioma. N Engl J Med 367:1417–1427

Peto J, Decarli A, La Vecchia C et al (1999) The European mesothelioma epidemic. Br J Cancer 79:666–672

Porter DW, Hubbs AF, Mercer RR et al (2010) Mouse pulmonary dose- and time course-responses induced by exposure to multi-walled carbon nanotubes. Toxicology 269:136–147

Prato M, Kostarelos K, Bianco A (2008) Functionalized carbon nanotubes in drug design and discovery. Acc Chem Res 41:60–68

Program NT (2004) NTP 11th report on carcinogens. Rep Carcinog 11:A1–A32

Ramos-Nino ME, Timblin CR, Mossman BT (2002) Mesothelial cell transformation requires increased AP-1 binding activity and ERK-dependent Fra-1 expression. Cancer Res 62:6065–6069

Ramos-Nino ME, Blumen SR, Sabo-Attwood T et al (2008) HGF mediates cell proliferation of human mesothelioma cells through a PI3K/MEK5/Fra-1 pathway. Am J Respir Cell Mol Biol 38:209–217

Rapp GR (2009) Archaeomineralogy, vol XV. Springer, Berlin/London, 348 pp

Reid G (2015) MicroRNAs in mesothelioma: from tumour suppressors and biomarkers to therapeutic targets. J Thorac Dis 7:1031–1040

Ribak J, Lillis R, Suzuki Y et al (2008) Malignant mesothelioma in a cohort of asbestos insulation workers: clinical presentation, diagnosis, and causes of death. Br J Ind Med 45:182–187

Rinkcvich Y, Mori T, Sahoo D et al (2012) Identification and prospective isolation of a mesothelial precursor lineage giving rise to smooth muscle cells and fibroblasts for mammalian internal organs, and their vasculature. Nat Cell Biol 14:1251–1260

Robinson BW, Creaney J, Lake R et al (2003) Mesothelin-family proteins and diagnosis of mesothelioma. Lancet 362:1612–1616

Robinson BW, Musk AW, Lake RA (2005) Malignant mesothelioma. Lancet 366:397–408

Røe OD, Stella GM (2015) Malignant pleural mesothelioma: history, controversy and future of a manmade epidemic. Eur Respir Rev 24:115–131

Røe OD, Creaney J, Lundgren S et al (2008) Mesothelin-related predictive and prognostic factors in malignant mesothelioma: a nested case-control study. Lung Cancer 61:235–243

Røe OD, Anderssen E, Helge E et al (2009) Genome-wide profile of pleural mesothelioma versus parietal and visceral pleura: the emerging gene portrait of the mesothelioma phenotype. PLoS One 4:e6554

Røe OD, Anderssen E, Sandeck H et al (2010) Malignant pleural mesothelioma: genome-wide expression patterns reflecting general resistance mechanisms and a proposal of novel targets. Lung Cancer 67:57–68

Roushdy-Hammady I, Siegel J, Emri S et al (2001) Genetic-susceptibility factor and malignant mesothelioma in the Cappadocian region of Turkey. Lancet 357:444–445

Rump A, Morikawa Y, Tanaka M et al (2004) Binding of ovarian cancer antigen CA125/MUC16 to mesothelin mediates cell adhesion. J Biol Chem 279:9190–9198

Ryman-Rasmussen JP, Cesta MF, Brody AR et al (2009) Inhaled carbon nanotubes reach the subpleura tissue in mice. Nat Nanotechnol 4:747–751

Sakellariou K, Malamou-Mitsi V, Haritou A et al (1996) Malignant pleural mesothelioma from nonoccupational asbestos exposure in Metsovo (north-west Greece): slow end of an epidemic? Eur Respir J 9:1206–1210

Salvador-Morales C, Townsendb P, Flahautc E et al (2007) Binding of pulmonary surfactant proteins to carbon nanotubes; potential for damage to lung immune defense mechanisms. Carbon 45:607–617

Sartore-Bianchi A, Gasparri F, Galvani A et al (2007) Bortezomib inhibits nuclear factor-kappaB dependent survival and has potent in vivo activity in mesothelioma. Clin Cancer Res 13:5942–5951

Sebastien P, Janson X, Gaudichet A et al (1980) Asbestos retention in human respiratory tissues: comparative measurements in lung parenchyma and in parietal pleura. IARC Sci Publ 30:237–246

Shukla A, Hillegass JM, MacPherson MB et al (2011) ERK2 is essential for the growth of human epithelioid malignant mesotheliomas. Int J Cancer 129:1075–1086

Shulte PA, Kuempel ED, Zumwalde RD et al (2012) Focused actions to protect carbon nanotube workers focused actions to protect carbon nanotube workers. Am J Ind Med 55:395–411

Shvedova AA, Tkach AV, Kisin ER et al (2013) Carbon nanotubes enhance metastatic growth of lung carcinoma via up-regulation of myeloid-derived suppressor cells. Small 9:1691–1695

Stanton MF, Wrench C (1972) Mechanisms of mesothelioma induction with asbestos and fibrous glass. J Natl Cancer Inst 48:797–821

Stella GM (2011) Carbon nanotubes and pleural damage: perspectives of nanosafety in the light of asbestos experience. Biointerphases 6:P1–17

Sun X, Gulyás MM, Hjerpe A et al (2006) Proteasome inhibitor PSI induces apoptosis in human mesothelioma cells. Cancer Lett 232:161–169

Suzuki Y, Yuen SR, Ashley R (2005) Short, thin asbestos fibers contribute to the development of human malignant mesothelioma: pathological evidence. Int J Hyg Environ Health 208:201–210

Takagi A, Hirose A, Futakuchi M et al (2012) Dose-dependent mesothelioma induction by intraperitoneal administration of multi-wall carbon nanotubes in p53 heterozygous mice. Cancer Sci 103:1440–1444

Takahashi K, Karjalainen A (2003) A cross-country comparative overview of the asbestos situation in ten Asian countries. Int J Occup Environ Health 9:244–248

Taskinen E, Ahlamn K, Wukeri M (1973) A current hypothesis of the lymphatic transport of inspired dust to the parietal pleura. Chest 64:193–196

Testa JR, Cheung M, Pei J et al (2011) Germline BAP1 mutations predispose to malignant mesothelioma. Nat Genet 43:1022–1025

Thickett DR, Armstrong L, Millar AB (1999) Vascular endothelial growth factor (VEGF) in inflammatory and malignant pleural effusions. Thorax 54:707–710

Thiele C, Das R (2009) Carbon nanotubes and graphene for electronics applications: technologies, players and opportunities. IDTechEX, Santa Clara, CA

Tossavainen A (2004) Global use of asbestos and the incidence of mesothelioma. Int J Occup Environ Health 10:22–25

Travis LB, Fossa SD, Schonfeld SJ et al (2005) Second cancers among 40,576 testicular cancer patients: focus on long-term survivors. J Natl Cancer Inst 97:1354–1365

Ugolini D, Neri M, Ceppi M et al (2013) Genetic susceptibility to malignant mesothelioma and exposure to asbestos: the influence of the familial factor. Mutat Res 658:162–171

Ugurluer G, Chang K, Gamez ME et al (2016) Genome-based mutational analysis by next generation sequencing in patients with malignant pleural and peritoneal mesothelioma. Anticancer Res 36:2331–2338

Varga C, Szendi K (2010) Carbon nanotubes induce granulomas but not mesotheliomas. In Vivo 24:153–156

Wagner JC, Sleggs CA, Marchand P (1960) Diffuse pleural mesothelioma and asbestos exposure in the North Western Cape Province. Br J Ind Med 17:260–271

Wagner JC, Berry G, Skidmore JW et al (1974) The effects of the inhalation of asbestos in rats. Br J Cancer 29:252–269

Wilson SM, Barbone D, Yang TM et al (2012) mTOR mediates survival signals in malignant mesothelioma grown as tumor fragment spheroids. Am J Respir Cell Mol Biol 39:576–583

Xia T, Hamilton RF, Bonner JC et al (2013) Interlaborator evaluation of in vitro cytotoxicity and inflammatory responses to engineered nanomaterials: the NIEHS Nano GO Consortium. Environ Health Perspect 121:683–690

Xu J, Alexander DB, Futakuchi M et al (2014) Size- and shape-dependent pleural translocation, deposition, fibrogenesis, and mesothelial proliferation by multiwalled carbon nanotubes. Cancer Sci 105:763–769

Yang CT, You L, Yeh CC et al (2000) Adenovirus-mediated p14(ARF) gene transfer in human mesothelioma cells. J Natl Cancer Inst 92:636–641

Yang H, Bocchetta M, Bg K et al (2006) TNF-alpha inhibits asbestos-induced cytotoxicity via a NF-kappaB-dependent pathway, a possible mechanism for asbestos-induced oncogenesis. Proc Natl Acad Sci U S A 103:10397–10402

Yoshikawa Y, Sato A, Tsujimura T et al (2012) Frequent inactivation of the BAP1 gene in epithelioid-type malignant mesothelioma. Cancer Sci 103:868–874

Chapter 5
Communities at High Risk in the Third Wave of Mesothelioma

Edward A. Emmett and Brigid Cakouros

Abstract In this chapter, we describe and discuss communities that have a high incidence of mesothelioma. These communities are part of a third wave of asbestos exposures and consequent asbestos-related diseases (ARD). Many of the current paradigms applied to ARD arose to address the first and second waves associated with mining and the industrial use of asbestos, respectively. We examine the lessons from a number of communities where there is an elevated risk of mesothelioma not restricted to specific occupations: Wittenoom, Western Australia, where crocidolite was mined; Libby Montana where amphibole asbestos contaminated vermiculite was mined and processed; Broni Italy, and Ambler Pennsylvania where asbestos-cement products were manufactured; and Karain in Cappadocia Turkey where the asbestiform mineral erionite occurs naturally. In these communities, in addition to occupational exposures, paraoccupational, residential, and environmental lifestyle asbestos exposures appear to contribute to the mesothelioma burden. Finally, we discuss a number of issues germane to non-occupational community mesothelioma risk: age and gender distribution of non-occupational mesothelioma; prevention appropriate to the third wave; shortcomings of the regulatory definition of asbestos; vulnerable groups in the community, diffuse administrative responsibility; diverse community attitudes to risk and prevention; difficulties in quantifying exposures and justifying remediation actions; surveillance, diagnostic and care requirements in high-risk communities; legal responsibilities and compensation for nonoccupational ARD; the application of epidemiology to third wave high-risk communities; differing expressions of ARD from community exposures; and estimating the magnitude of the third mesothelioma wave.

Keywords Mesothelioma • Risk factors • Epidemiology • Waves of asbestos exposure/disease • High-risk communities • Remediation • Prevention • Asbestos definition • Asbestos-related diseases

E.A. Emmett (✉) • B. Cakouros
Superfund Research Program, Perelman School of Medicine, University of Pennsylvania, Philadelphia, PA 19104, USA
e-mail: emmetted@mail.med.upenn.edu

© Springer International Publishing AG 2017
J.R. Testa (ed.), *Asbestos and Mesothelioma*, Current Cancer Research,
DOI 10.1007/978-3-319-53560-9_5

5.1   Waves of Asbestos Exposure and Disease

As a result of the long latent period of 30 to 50 or more years between asbestos exposure and the occurrence of mesothelioma, the peak expression of adverse effects occurs long after the peak exposure. This characteristic delay underscores the importance of recognizing and eliminating or minimizing exposures long before clinical disease is apparent. Understanding this delay also allows us to define several waves of ARD.

The *first wave* was recognized in countries with significant asbestos mining operations in those occupationally exposed through mining, milling, and packaging asbestos. A *second wave,* also industrial and predominantly occupational, resulted from manufacturing various asbestos containing products and from the use of asbestos in construction. From small beginnings in the 1890s the use of asbestos in industrial fabrication, including asbestos cement products, structural insulation, shipbuilding and a multitude of miscellaneous uses, rapidly increased to reach a maximum in the mid-twentieth century (Henderson and Leigh 2012). This resulted in a wave of occupational asbestos-related disease, including lung cancer and mesothelioma whose effects continue to the present. During these first two waves it became apparent that ARD, particularly mesothelioma, were not confined to workers but could also be seen in family members who resided with asbestos workers and were exposed to asbestos bought home on the clothes, footwear, skin and hair of workers, and spread within the home through laundry, dusting and sweeping. These exposures have been variously described as familial, domestic, or "paraoccupational," we will use the latter in this chapter, since this effect is not necessarily confined to family members but could affect others who share a domicile with an asbestos worker. Mesothelioma was also described in connection with residing near an asbestos-manufacturing site (Newhouse and Thompson 1965). In many developed countries the exposures that bought on the first two waves were bought to a halt in the late twentieth century, initially by strict regulations controlling occupational and environmental exposures associated with mining, industrial use, and construction, and later by a total ban on the import or use of asbestos. However elsewhere asbestos use continues, greatest in the BRIC countries: Brazil, Russia, India, and China (Algrantia et al. 2015). For these countries, action to ban the use of asbestos appears imperative.

However, even where there is a ban on asbestos use we can still confront a *third wave* of asbestos exposure and ARD resulting from the previous dissemination of asbestos and asbestos-containing products or from exposure to naturally occurring asbestos. Initially the third wave concept was applied to what was termed asbestos-in-place, particularly asbestos in buildings (Landrigan 1991). Concern was particularly directed at exposures and ARD in groups of workers who had not customarily been considered as at risk from asbestos, such as railroad workers (Maltoni et al. 1991) and merchant seamen (Greenberg 1991). Wide dissemination of asbestos was also recognized. For example, asbestos bodies could be found in the lungs of children living in urban settings (Haque et al. 1991). More recently, there has been increased recognition that the third wave includes communities that are hotspots for ARD including mesothelioma. These include sites where asbestos was mined or used in manufacturing, where there is substantial asbestos-containing waste, where asbestos fibers or products using asbestos have been widely disseminated, and where asbestos fibers occur naturally. In Australia, third wave ARD has been found in non-professional do-it-yourself home renovators who cut and repair or demolish asbestos cement products in home renovation or maintenance. Family members present during these activities are at risk (Olsen et al. 2011; Gordon and Leigh 2011). These types of community third wave exposures raise new issues for which the existing prevention paradigms developed for industrial and occupational exposures are not always adequate, as will be discussed in the final section of this chapter.

Although asbestos use has been banned in many countries there is emerging concern that we may need further action to prevent a *fourth wave* of ARD. For regulatory purposes the term asbestos applies to six types of mineral fibers that were used in commerce at the time of the first and second waves of ARD. However there are other asbestiform minerals that have the same deleterious carcinogenic and other toxic properties that are not regulated because they were not used commercially when the current regulatory definition was developed. Consequently, these carcinogenic, but unregulated fibers, which share some of the useful properties that made asbestos use popular in the early twentieth century could legally be incorporated into materials that could legally be imported into countries where regulated asbestos fibers are banned, e.g., for use in construction. This creates a risk that legally acceptable exposure to such fibers could in turn inadvertently cause a *fourth wave* of exposure and ARD, despite a "ban" on asbestos. This issue will be discussed further in the final section of this chapter.

5.2   Lessons from Exposed Communities

The third wave of asbestos-related events has been recognized and studied most intensively in certain communities where exposure and effect are more concentrated. We will next address the lessons being learned in a number of these high-mesothelioma risk communities around the world.

5.2.1   Libby, Montana

Libby, MT is a small town (2010 census population: 2628) on the Kootenay River in a mountainous area of Western Montana, USA. On July 17, 2009, the U.S. Environmental Protection Agency (EPA) declared the first US Public Health Emergency, using the Comprehensive Environmental Response, Compensation, and Liability Act (CERCLA), in Libby as a result of documentation of hundreds of ARD over the past several years (USEPA 2009). The declaration also covered neighboring Troy, Montana (2010 census population: 938). About 10,000 people live in a 10-mile radius of Libby including many former workers at the Libby vermiculite mine and processing operations. In addition, the EPA estimated as many as 80,000 individuals were exposed during the life of the mine.

Citizens and workers of these communities had been exposed to high levels of asbestos from vermiculite mines. Vermiculite was discovered by gold miners in 1881. In the 1920s, the Zonolite Company began to mine, mill, screen, exfoliate, process, and ship the ore in Libby, transporting both milled and raw vermiculite from Libby by way of the Kootenay River. In 1963, the mine was purchased by WR Grace and production expanded greatly. Using regulations for asbestos introduced in the 1970s, EPA, NIOSH, and state inspections in the 1980s found that asbestos fiber counts in downtown Libby exceeded allowable limits. Additionally, WR Grace lost its largest customer, Scotts Company in Marysville, Ohio in the 1980s, when ARD were found in workers in their processing plant. Vermiculite production ceased in 1990. Two separate but parallel cohort studies showed excess mortality from lung cancer, mesothelioma, and non-malignant respiratory disease among Libby vermiculite miners (Amandus et al. 1987; Amandus and Wheeler 1987; McDonald et al. 1986). A cross sectional community study showed that radiologic pleural abnormalities related to asbestos were most common in former workers with vermiculite, but also occurred in household contactants (paraoccupational) and those with environmental exposures (Peipens et al. 2003). Libby was added to the National Priority List as a "superfund site" in 2002. It is estimated that the Libby mine was the source of over 70% of all vermiculite sold in the United States from 1919 to 1990 (USEPA 2009).

The presence of asbestiform fibers in the mined vermiculite was not acknowledged at first. The contaminant, a unique mixture of amphiboles now known as Libby Amphibole Asbestos (LAA), consists of winchite, richterite, lesser amounts of tremolite and trace amphiboles (Meeker et al. 2003). LAA could be present in high concentrations; in some locations, it comprised nearly 100% of the ore, and produced abundant, extremely fine fibers on gentle abrasion or crushing. Although winchite and richterite appear to have similar toxicologic and carcinogenic properties to tremolite, because of a legacy regulatory definition from the days of the first and second waves of asbestos disease, only tremolite was officially considered to be a health risk at the time of the plant closure.

Studies of LAA exposure illustrate the complexity of evaluating and reconstructing historic pathways of asbestos exposures in community settings. The most comprehensive analysis, by Noonan et al. (2015), evaluated four categories of exposure: occupational, sharing a household with a worker, residence in Libby or Troy, and environmental pathways.

5.2.1.1 Occupational Exposures

Occupational exposures occurred directly to employees or contracted workers for Zoolite or WR Grace. For this group, quantifiable cumulative exposures could often be reconstructed based on years worked, job categories, and when available, workplace air monitoring data. A second potential occupational exposure group had exposures from disturbing dust-containing vermiculite or LAA through local work at construction, demolition or excavation sites, the Montana railroad industry, work with commercial boilers or incinerators, agriculture or silviculture, cleaning residences or businesses, logging, plywood manufacturing, and other wood processing or finishing. A third potential occupational exposure group included those previously identified in the literature as having an increased risk of exposure to asbestos not necessarily mined at Libby (such as working with brake or clutch linings, high temperature gaskets, cement sheets, pipes or heat-resistant panels, insulation, electric cloth wrap or high-temperature wiring, fire-proofing materials, heat-protective clothing such as gloves, aprons or coats, joint compounds and sheetrock/drywall, heating and ventilation ducts or duct connecting materials, roofing materials, thermal taping compounds, and heat-resistant plastic parts such as Bakelite).

5.2.1.2 Household Contact (Paraoccupational) Exposure

These exposures occurred from sharing a household with Zonolite/WR Grace employees. Elements contributing to the extent of exposure included whether the worker wore visibly dusty clothes at home or in the household car, time spent by adults in the laundry/utility room, and the job classification of the worker. WR Grace had no formal industrial hygiene program to control take-home asbestos exposure.

5.2.1.3 Residential Exposure

Cumulative exposure estimates were developed for Libby and Troy residents using soil and dust sampling at various properties, and limited activity-based sampling to estimate air levels of LAA fibers associated with activities. Geospatial approaches were used to predict soil and dust concentrations at residences that had not been sampled; however, these did not provide useful additional predictive quantitative information to explain ARD phenomena and were not used further.

5.2.1.4 Environmental Exposure Pathways

Eleven potential pathways of environmental exposure were identified based on activity-based sampling and any other available data. Each pathway was categorized as having high (4), medium (3), or low (2) exposure potential. Table 5.1 lists the pathways identified for Libby and the assigned exposure potential. This methodology appears applicable to other communities with non-occupational exposures.

Using this array of exposure estimates for 3031 persons seen at the Center for Asbestos Related Diseases (CARD) clinic in Libby, MT, significant but small or modest correlations with ARD including pleural disease were seen for 22 of 28

Table 5.1 Example of environmental exposure pathway survey for Libby, MT[a]

Questionnaire language	Description of pathway impact	Weight factor
Shoveling and/or hauling vermiculite outside of work?	Ore piles were always available and local citizens were encouraged to take what they needed	4
Playing in or around the vermiculite piles?	Children played in the piles all of the time	4
Handling vermiculite insulation outside of any job?	Many people installed their own insulation because it was easy to get	4
Fishing on the Kootenai River near the mouth of Rainy Creek?	Near a poorly covered conveyor belt that leaked asbestos-containing dust	3
Heating vermiculite ore to make it expand or pop?	Raw ore was used during science lessons	3
Cutting or collecting firewood near Rainy Creek Road?	Common area to gather firewood but very close to the mine	3
Gardening in soil that was observed or known to contain vermiculite?	Vermiculite was free and readily available for gardening use	3
Using the Libby Middle School track beyond scheduled gym classes?	Historically, vermiculite ore was used to cover the track	2
Playing in or watching games at the downtown ballfields?	Plant was adjacent to the fields and they were highly contaminated	2
Recreational activities (hunting, hiking, etc.) along Rainy Creek Road?	Dusty public access road used by trucks containing uncovered vermiculite	2
Burning firewood in your home?	Wood is used as a primary heat source and much of the firewood was found to be contaminated	n/a

[a]Modified from Noonan et al. (2015), from a survey used at Libby, MT to help determine the extent to which residents near the mine and factory were exposed to asbestos from lifestyle environmental exposures. The weight factor helped estimate the impact of the exposure for a study participant

studied estimates, with three of the four higher correlations seen within the household contact exposure pathways. Overall, men had the highest estimates for occupational exposures, whereas women had the highest estimates for household contact exposure, being almost twice that of men. Estimates for environmental exposure pathways were not significantly different by age or gender. Such detailed community exposure analyses help elucidate the importance of specific exposure pathways and enhance risk assessments that can support rational decisions about this superfund site and other similar community exposure situations.

Work at WR Grace and/or residence in Libby has now been associated with mesothelioma (Dunning et al. 2012; Whitehouse et al. 2008), progressive pulmonary disease (Whitehouse 2004; Black et al. 2014), and asbestos-related mortality (Naik et al. 2016). There may be distinctive features of ARD from LAA, compared with ARD in populations occupationally exposed to chrysotile. LAA is associated with an increased frequency of antinuclear autoantibodies (ANA) (Pfau et al. 2005; Pfau et al. 2015), and an increased risk of systemic autoimmune disease (Noonan et al. 2006) not described to date in other asbestos-exposed groups. Furthermore, LAA induces mesothelial cell autoantibodies (MCAA), which induce collagen deposition by mesothelial cells both in vitro (Serve et al. 2013) and in vivo (Gilmer et al. 2016), and is associated with radiographic changes in the pleura (Marchand et al. 2012). In contrast, chrysotile does not induce autoantibodies in mice or humans, MCAA occur with less frequency, and is not associated with pleural disease (Pfau et al. 2011; Pfau et al. 2015).

Following a study showing greatly increased mortality from asbestosis (ATSDR 2002), the Libby community founded CARD in 2000 with a local Board of Directors to provide community health screening, patient care, and social service support and counseling to individuals and families. With significant U.S. Federal Government funding, CARD now operates out of a modern purpose-built facility in Libby. Since 2009, medical records have been electronic, and the population regularly followed now exceeds 5000. CARD activities have engendered remarkable community acceptance and local support.

5.2.2   Broni, Italy

Broni is a small town (approximately 10,000 inhabitants) in Lombardy, Italy. The second oldest and largest asbestos cement factory (Fibronit) in Italy is about 600 m west of the historic town center (Mirabelli et al. 2010). The factory produced asbestos cement pipes and sheets from 1932 to 1993, initially about 8000 ton (metric tons; each equivalent to ~2200 pounds) per year, but increasing in the 1960s up to 100,000 ton/year. Chrysotile, crocidolite, and smaller quantities of amosite were added to the cement in proportions of 10–15% in sheets and up to more than 30% in pipes (Mensi et al. 2015). About 2741 men and 714 women were employed overall at Fibronit. As of the 1970s, several tasks were performed manually, there were no ventilation systems, and work hygiene was generally poor without personal protection or change of clothes or showering after shifts. In the late 1970s, air filtration units were installed and automated processes introduced (Oddone et al. 2014). Asbestos use ceased by 1993 following Italian Law 257/1992 banning asbestos (Mensi et al. 2015). The factory continued cement production until 1997 without any remediation work, and closed in 2000. In 2002, Broni was included in a government list of environmentally contaminated sites (Siti di Interesse Nazionale, SIN) under Italian law 388/2000 (Pirastu et al. 2011).

Oddone et al. (2014) investigated 1296 workers (1254 men, 42 women) who had been working in the Broni factory in 1970 or were hired subsequently: the standardized mortality ratio (SMR) for pleural cancer was 18 in males (26 observed vs. 1.45 expected) and 69 in women (2 observed, 0.03 expected). Seven men (SMR 10) died from peritoneal or retroperitoneal cancers and asbestosis, and three deaths from asbestosis (SMR 130), with no deaths in women from these causes.

Mensi et al. (2015) were able to quantify the total impact of asbestos on meso-thelioma incidence in Broni for workers employed at the Broni factory (occupa-tional); familial exposure arising from fibers on the workers' clothes or hair (paraoccupational); and residential exposure in Broni and surrounding towns (envi-ronmental exposure arising from outdoor pollution related to the factory). Mesothelioma cases were obtained from the Lombardy Mesothelioma Registry, a component of the National Register of Malignant Mesotheliomas, in Italian "Registro Nazionale dei Mesoteliomi" (ReNaM), which collects information on all cases of mesothelioma of the pleura, peritoneum, pericardium, and tunica vaginalis of testis diagnosed either in Lombardy (currently almost 10 million inhabitants) and or from a hospital outside Lombardy (Mensi et al. 2007). The registry record includes information on occupational exposures, domestic cohabitants, residential history including proximity to asbestos sources, and lifestyle including domestic and leisure-time activities involving potential asbestos exposure, all collected from interviews of patients or next-of-kin by trained personnel using a standardized ques-tionnaire (Nesti et al. 2003). From 2000–2011, 147 mesothelioma cases (17.45 expected) were attributable to occupational, familial, or environmental asbestos exposure from the Broni factory. The absolute and relative mesothelioma excess was greater in women (87 cases; 7.6 expected) than in men (60 cases; 9.9 expected). There were 138 pleural and 9 peritoneal mesotheliomas but no mesothelioma of the pericardium or testicular tunica vaginalis.

Where individuals had experienced multiple types of exposures the cause was assigned using Italian national guidelines in the order: occupational > familial > certain environmental > potential environmental (Nesti et al. 2003). Applying this rubric, 38 cases were designated occupational (32 men, 6 women), 37 were paraoc-cupational (5 men, 32 women), and 72 were environmental, of which 48 were in Broni (20 men, 28 women) and 24 in surrounding towns within ~10 km. Among the occupationally exposed, and when both occupational and paraoccupational expo-sure groups were combined, the standardized incidence ratios for men and women were similar. Community epidemiologic studies based on registries recording the site of residence at the time of diagnosis may underestimate the true disease burden resulting from past exposures; however, the authors believed this effect would be modest for Broni because of limited outmigration.

Although there were some historical records of intermittent measurements of exposure within the Fibronit factory, there was no data on exposure levels sustained by workers families. Some airborne fiber counts were available for Broni from 1991–1993 (median fiber counts up to ~0.6 f/L); however, at that time production output was rapidly declining and measures to reduce fiber dispersion had been introduced, so that no useful information concerning community or residential exposures is available for the vast majority of the production period.

The Mensi et al. (2007) study of Broni underlines the importance of assessing the impact of asbestos exposure for the community at large. Overall, approximately half the mesothelioma cases in Broni and surrounding towns were attributable to envi-ronmental exposure, a quarter to occupational exposure, and a quarter to paraoccu-pational exposure.

5.2.3   Non-Occupational Asbestos Exposure and Disease Elsewhere in Italy

One of the earliest non-occupational cohort studies of mesothelioma was of wives of asbestos workers employed at the "Eternit" plant in Casale Monferrato (Italy) from 1950 to 1986, when the plant closed: published by Magnani et al. (1993) and later updated (Ferrante et al. 2007). Eternit, one of the largest asbestos cement manufacturing facilities in Italy, used chrysotile and crocidolite to make high-pressure pipes, plain and corrugated sheets, chimney tubes, and other products (Magnani et al. 1996). The factory had no laundry facilities, so work clothes were taken home for cleaning. Wives were tracked through Registrar's Office records, kept in every Italian town, of vital and marital status for each resident and allowed tracking movement to another town. Women who had worked at the plant, and who had no domestic exposure (e.g., married after worker's employment at the plant terminated) were excluded. The final cohort of 1740 women was followed until 2003, when 67% were still alive, 32.3% dead, and 0.7% lost to follow-up. Mortality from pleural mesothelioma over the period 1965 to 2002 was markedly increased (21 observed vs. 1.2 expected; SMR = 18.00; 95% CI 11.14–27.52), whereas mortality from lung cancer was not increased. Most of the mesothelioma was reported in more recent years with 12 cases over the period 1990–2001.

Marinaccio et al. (2015) used mesothelioma incidence data from ReNaM, which covers 98.5% of the Italian population, to examine non-occupational mesothelioma across Italy for the 1993–2008 period. Excluding occupational exposure, mesotheliomas were categorized as caused by familial (paraoccupational) exposures, environmental (residence near a source of asbestos pollution without occupational or familial exposure) and leisure activities (without occupational familial or environmental exposure). For the period 1993 to 2008, 15,845 cases of mesothelioma were identified, of which 93% were pleural, 6.4% peritoneal, and 0.3% pericardial or testicular. The male/female ratio was 2.6 for pleural mesothelioma, 1.4 for peritoneal, and 1.9 for pericardial. The mean age at diagnosis was 68.3 years (SD ±10.6) in men and 69.8 (SD ±11.6) in women. Age less than 45 was rare: 2.4% of all cases. The exposure source could be characterized in 12,065 instances: most were occupational, but 530 (4.4%) had familial (paraoccupational) exposure, 514 (4.3%) had environmental exposure through living near a source of asbestos pollution, and 188 (1.6%) were exposed through hobby-related or other leisure activities. For 2466 cases (20.4%), no asbestos exposure could be found. Females predominated in non-occupational cases overall (female to male ratio 2.3:1), and particularly for paraoccupational cases (5.9:1). The mean age at diagnosis was slightly, but statistically significantly, lower for nonoccupational cases at 67.2 vs. 68.1 years, $p < 0.01$).

Nonoccupational cases were not distributed uniformly across Italy. Distinct geographic clusters were observed in areas where asbestos-cement plants had operated (Broni, Casale Monferrato, and Bari), areas of shipbuilding and repair (Monfalcone, Trieste, La Spezia, Genova, Castellammare di Stabia, Livorno, and Taranto) and in Biancavilla, Sicily, where the asbestiform amphibole fluoroedenite was used in

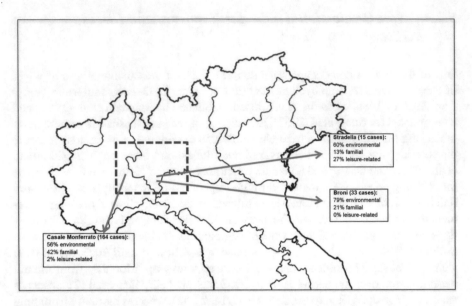

Fig. 5.1 Mesothelioma cases in three communities in Italy (2008–2013). Map highlighting the variation in community exposure within a small area of Italy. Mesothelioma cases were tracked in the Italian National Mesothelioma Register (ReNaM) between the years of 2008 and 2013. Modified from Marinaccio et al. (2015)

large amounts in construction and road paving. Different towns had quite different proportions for the categories of nonoccupational exposure, environmental (residential), familial (paraoccupational, and leisure-related (environmental pathways)). Figure 5.1 displays this variation for the three Northern Italian towns of Broni, Stradella, and Casale Monferrato. The authors commented on the need for a framework to deal with compensation rights for mesothelioma cases induced by nonoccupational asbestos exposure.

5.2.4 Wittenoom, Western Australia

Wittenoom is a remote inland community in Western Australia, approximately 1000 miles north of the state capital of Perth. Rocks exposed in Wittenoom Gorge are remarkable for narrow bands of crocidolite (blue asbestos), averaging about 2.5 in. in width about 25 ft apart. In the 1930s, the seams were worked by hand using primitive methods, and bags of asbestos were carried by donkey to outside the gorge. High prices for crocidolite in 1937–1938 bought a rush of prospectors to the area. Production increased from 1943 to 1966 when ABA (Australian Blue Asbestos) took over the leases and operated a mine and mill in the gorge. Milling was particularly problematic: it consisted of dry mechanical crushing, grinding, and aspiration with persistent problems with dust control, ventilation, fiber purity, and abrasive hard host rock (ironstone). All mining and milling areas were very extensively contaminated with asbestos dust; work conditions were very hot and dusty with almost no use of respirators. A new, somewhat improved, mill built in 1958 still had problems from dustiness. The only adequate industrial hygiene survey made during 1966, the final year of the plant's operation, found fiber levels above 100 f/ml in many areas of the plant (Musk et al. 1992), subsequent reevaluation suggests that these levels were underestimated possibly by several orders of magnitude (Rogers 1990). No asbestos standard was in place in Western Australia until 1978, long after the mine had closed, although standards were in place elsewhere in Australia. The entire operation was only profitable from 1955 to 1960 when there was an export contract to the USA (Musk et al. 1992).

Originally the town settlement was in the Gorge, about a mile from the mine; later a township was built at the entrance to the Gorge about 12 miles away by the state government with an agenda of developing the north subsidized housing and transport (Musk et al. 1992). In 1961, the population was 671 males and 309 females. Tailings from the mine were used in and around the town to pave roads and parking lots, reduce dust and mud in backyards and the school playground and also for the airport runway; tailing uses continued to the mid-1960s. Vehicle movement over the roads produced so much dust that airline pilots claimed to identify Wittenoom from considerable distances by a blue haze on the horizon (Reid et al. 2008). Cumpston (1978, 1979) reported on measured ambient environmental exposures with levels of 0.01–0.21 f/ml. No non-work indoor air exposure measurements from Wittenoom have been reported.

The sociologist Layman (1983) described the community. Wittenoom was a typical company-dominated mining town except for a high degree of both geographic and interpersonal isolation, and an apathetic rather than conflicted community with a high turnover. Although the maximum workforce at any time was about 500, approximately 6500 men and 500 women in total worked for ABA from 1943 from to 1966. Most employees were unskilled; many were migrants from Italy lured by 2-year contracts. Forty-four percent of workers stayed in the community less than 3 months, and only 22% stayed longer than 1 year. About 50% of the workers were in their 20s and only 16% were over 40 years of age. Most desired to make money and leave. Single males lived in particularly squalid conditions. Families were mostly young couples with small children; most women were dismayed by the isolation and primitive conditions with the hotel and alcohol too central to the way of life. The young demographic perversely provided residents with a long time period in which to experience mesothelioma, because of the long latency.

The Western Australian state government began decommissioning the town in the 1980s, by 1992 all government-owned buildings were demolished and new residents officially discouraged (Graham 1994). The town was virtually abandoned when it was degazetted by the state government in 2007, with 150,000 tons of raw, exposed asbestos fibers remaining at the site (Bennett 2016). As of 2015 three remaining residents of the town refused to leave (Daily Telegraph 2015). Cleanup is contemplated (Moulton 2015).

The first case of mesothelioma among ex-Wittenoom workers was detected in 1961 (McNulty 1962), and numerous cases were recognized by 1967 (Elder 1967). Mortality studies of workers (Hobbs et al. 1980; Armstrong et al. 1988) found excesses of many diseases, including cancers of the trachea, bronchus and lung, mesothelioma, pneumoconiosis, mental disorders and alcoholism, cirrhosis of the liver, and injuries and poisonings.

Hansen et al. (1993) examined the risks of non-occupational exposure to cro-cidolite in a cohort of 4890 residents of Wittenoom during the period 1943–1993, who had never worked for ABA but had lived at Wittenoom for at least 1 month. The cohort was assembled using a wide variety of records: electoral rolls, local school records, hospital and medical records, church records, birth certificates, employ-ment lists for employers other than ABA, answers to a 1979 questionnaire to work-ers, and participants in a Vitamin A cancer prevention trial, in all 18,553 individual sources of information. Comparison between records suggested that the cohort was complete. Mesothelioma was identified from State and Australia-wide Mesothelioma registries. Wittenoom residents included families of ABA workers, government employees (teachers, hospital staff, police, etc.), employees in agriculture or mining for other companies who used Wittenoom as a base camp, self-employed individu-als and families of those people. Almost all had little chance of exposure to asbestos elsewhere. Fifty-five percent were families of workers, 55% women, 50% children of whom 43% were first at Wittenoom when aged <10; 51% of the entire cohort lived at Wittenoom for less than 2 years. As of 1993 the whereabouts of 71.4% of the cohort was known (Hansen et al. 1998). Twenty-seven subjects had developed mesothelioma, the majority since 1989. There was an excess of females: 18 vs. 9 males. Paraoccupational exposures predominated: 12 wives, 11 children, and 1 brother. The mean duration of Wittenoom residence was 60 months (range 2 months to 17 years). Compared with the rest of the cohort, mesothelioma cases had stayed longer at Wittenoom (64.8 months vs. 32.8 months, p 0.001), had a higher esti-mated intensity of exposure (mean 0.8 f/ml vs. 0.5 f/ml; $p < 0.001$), and a higher estimated cumulative exposure to crocidolite (mean 16.3 f/mly vs. 5.4 f/mly; $p < 0.001$). Nine of the 27 subjects (33%) were younger than 40 at the time of diagnosis. However, there was no significant effect of age after adjustment for time since first exposure and duration of residence; the high number of early-age cases at Wittenoom was simply a result of larger proportions of exposed children compared with other populations. Reid et al. (2008) further examined the causes of death for women in the Wittenoom non-occupational cohort up to 2004 finding significantly increased mortality rates from all causes, all neoplasms, mesothelioma, lung cancer, and pneumoconiosis (asbestosis).

5.2.5   Karain, Turkey

Karain is a village in Cappadocia, Turkey, which had a population of around 2000 in 1950, but more recently less than 150. Residents of Karain and of the nearby vil-lages of Tuzkoy and Sarihidir have very to extremely high rates of mesothelioma

(Baris et al. 1978; Artvinli and Baris 1979). Mesothelioma is responsible for more than 50% of deaths in Karain. Significant numbers of villagers had also migrated to Stockholm, studies of 162 emigrants from Karain found 18 deaths, at least 14 of which were from mesothelioma (Metintas et al. 1999). Around Karain, erionite, a fibrous zeolite, occurs naturally in volcanic rocks in zeolite-rich layers. Stones containing zeolite with deposits of fibrous, whitish, soft and friable erionite were quarried from the nearby mountain and river and used to build houses in these three villages (Carbone et al. 2007). Erionite is found in the air of these villages (Baris et al. 1987) and in the lungs of residents (Sebastien et al. 1981). Experimentally, erionite is a highly potent cause of mesothelioma in rats (Wagner et al. 1985).

However, some villages nearby, including Karlik 3 km away did not experience epidemic proportions of mesothelioma, despite having similar stone in the houses. Pedigree studies of Karain residents found that mesothelioma was concentrated in some families but not others (Roushdy-Hammady et al. 2001). Moreover, members of high-risk families who were born and lived outside Cappadocia did not develop mesothelioma. Current evidence indicates that the extraordinary rates of mesothelioma in Karain, Tuzkoy, and Sarihidir are due to the interaction of genetic predisposition and environmental erionite exposure (Dogan et al. 2006).

Beginning around 2005, a new village has been constructed in Tuzkoy using erionite-free bricks and cement and with asphalt roads. Free radiology screening and medical treatment for mesothelioma are now available through the Turkish Directorate of Cancer Control. Free biomonitoring screening was made available, and approximately 50% of villagers accepted this opportunity; others believed that screening would be useless unless there was effective treatment to offer (Carbone et al. 2007).

5.2.6 Ambler, Pennsylvania

Ambler, located in the suburbs of greater Philadelphia, was at one time home to the world's largest asbestos cement manufacturing operation (Quattrone 2004). Asbestos-containing products were produced in Ambler from the late 1890s; activity peaked before the Great Depression and was very substantial in both World Wars. Mainly chrysotile was used; much imported from a Canadian mine the facility owned. The wide variety of products included piping, electrical insulation, millboard, brake linings, roofing shingles, cement siding, asbestos paper, conveyer belts, laboratory bench tops, and many others. Production was largely discontinued in the 1970s coinciding with stricter occupational health and environmental laws, with the last operations ceasing in 1988. A company town, Ambler was largely built for workers and their families who primarily came from Italy and Virginia. Many residents worked in the asbestos plant. Family members recall that workers would return home covered in so much white dust as to be barely recognizable. Workers houses extended up to the boundary of the plant. Particularly noticeable were the "White Mountains," which consisted of large piles of asbestos-containing waste

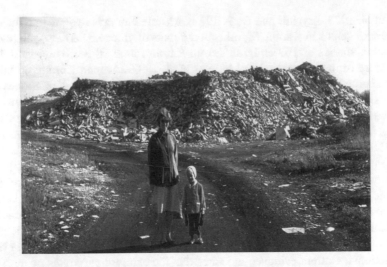

Fig. 5.2 Family photograph from around 1963, showing children in proximity to Ambler, PA asbestos-containing waste piles. Photographer: Joe Marincola with permission from Greg Marincola

material from the plants where children and adolescents played extensively. Figure 5.2 is a family photograph from around 1960 showing family members alongside some of these piles.

Initially very prosperous, Ambler underwent a period of unemployment and urban decay after the plants closed, but a renaissance starting in the 1990s resulted in a currently desirable place to live with substantial family-friendly amenities and a thriving restaurant scene. Since the plant closure, attention has focused on two large accumulations of asbestos-containing waste material, both adjoining residential areas. The first, a 24-acre, 30-foot high asbestos-containing waste area, was remediated by the EPA in the 1980s and 1990s by covering with soil and geotextile, grading, and erecting an 8-foot fence to eliminate access and use (USEPA 1988, 1989). The second site of approximately 28 acres known as Bo-Rit is currently designated as a superfund site: hazard reduction activities have been undertaken and a final decision on further remediation is imminent. Decisions on future access and use for the area are complex because of the many parties involved, as discussed later in this chapter.

Using data for 1992–2008 from the Pennsylvania Cancer Registry, the incidence of mesothelioma in residents of the Ambler zip code was found to be 2.7 times that of Pennsylvania as a whole for men and 4.5 times higher for women, both statistically significant, while there was no increase in surrounding zip codes (Pennsylvania Department of Health 2011). The previous manufacturing operations and the Bo-Rit site are both located within the Ambler zip code. Studies are continuing to help determine the excess attributable to past occupational, paraoccupational, residential, and environmental exposures.

To understand the views of Ambler community stakeholders about asbestos hazards, we conducted community surveys and semi-structured in-depth interviews with a purposive sample of diverse Ambler residents from different socio-economic and professional backgrounds (e.g., real estate agent, property developer, environmental scientist, local business owner, urban planner, and others) and officials from different governmental agencies. Attitudes and perceptions were grouped according to a number of themes including: time, space, activities resulting in asbestos exposure, community input and Community Advisory Group, attitudes toward asbestos and risk, choice of remediation remedy, lessons for other communities from Ambler, and research needs and information gaps. There was a high concordance of views amongst community members in most thematic areas. Interviewees were uniformly quite well informed about the hazards of asbestos and all could identify at least one individual who had died as a result of ARD. Community attitudes had changed dramatically from the earlier remediation in the 1980s when attitudes were characterized as "clean it up and get out, we don't want the stigma" to the 2010s "sustainability and future use are important," "it is no longer acceptable just to fence off about 65 acres in the center of town." Residents now question the long-term effectiveness of the 1980s remediation because whitish waste (presumably asbestos-containing) is visible on eroded slopes and near the roots of fallen trees and animal burrows. Despite the similarity of views on most topics, there are widely divergent views in the community and sometimes within the same family about the risk posed by asbestos and the preferred remediation remedy. Interviewees saw limitations in seemingly rigid EPA risk assessment processes in dealing with this complexity.

5.3 Distinctive Features of Third Wave Mesothelioma in Communities

As we address the issue of disease and exposure in communities, we need to think outside the prevailing exposure effect and prevention paradigms appropriate to the first and second waves associated with industrial and mining operations that resulted in occupational disease. In the *third wave*, we face more diffuse, complex and in many ways more difficult situations. To help address this novel situation we will discuss 12 distinctive aspects of non-occupational asbestos exposures and ARD in present-day communities.

5.3.1 Appropriate Prevention for the Third Wave, Banning Asbestos Use is Not Enough

The only known effective measure for preventing mesothelioma is to prevent asbestos exposure. Banning the import, export, and use of asbestos will end the first and second waves of asbestos-related disease. The ILO has called for national bans on asbestos: for example, the Resolution of the 95th Convention June 1, 2006 promotes the elimination of future use of all forms of asbestos and asbestos containing materials in all member states (ILO 2006). As of September 2015 at least 57 countries had instituted such bans (International Ban Secretariat 2015), mostly industrialized nations. There is an undeniable and urgent need for other countries to follow suit.

However, even effective bans on asbestos importation and use will not necessarily eliminate third wave exposures such as those from asbestos-containing products in building and construction, waste sites and communities contaminated with asbestos, exposure to "natural" asbestos fibers, and the like. Preventing these exposures requires additional actions and especially awareness.

5.3.2   Shortcomings of the Regulatory Definition for Asbestos

Preventing a fourth wave may also require an expanded regulatory definition of asbestos. Asbestos is a generic term describing a number of silicate minerals that produce thin, flexible fibers when crushed and which have high tensile strength and resistance to heat and chemicals. Six types of asbestos are regulated: the serpentine mineral chrysotile and five amphibole minerals, crocidolite (mineralogically fibrous riebeckite), amosite, tremolite, actinolite, and anthophyllite (USDOL 1975), the choice based on commercial use as of 1975. All are carcinogenic (International Agency for Research on Cancer 2012). For the purposes of U.S. EPA, U.S. OSHA and WHO, fibers of each of these types are regulated if they are longer than 5 µm and have a length to width (aspect ratio) of at least 3:1 (Case et al. 2011). There is no strict minerologic definition to correspond to this regulatory definition (Lowers and Meeker 2002).

Although this definition may have been appropriate for controlling occupational workplace exposures to asbestos in industrial operations, it is inappropriate to many community exposures as exemplified by exposures to erionite (fibrous zeolite) in Cappadocia, and exposures predominantly to winchite and richterite in LAA. For both erionite (Emri et al. 2002; Baris and Grandjean 2006; Carbone et al. 2007) and LAA, there is strong evidence of carcinogenicity from both laboratory animal and human epidemiologic studies.

Ideally regulations for both occupational and environmental health exposures should address all fibers capable of producing mesothelioma and other asbestos-related diseases. Revising the definition of asbestos for regulatory applications will involve toxicologic, minerologic, and analytic considerations and could require a protracted process. If this proves difficult, at the very least the regulatory definition should be extended to include winchite, richterite, and erionite.

5.3.3   Age and Gender Distribution of Nonoccupational
              Mesothelioma

As discussed with specific communities, third wave pleural mesothelioma from community exposure is characterized by a higher proportion of females, and sometimes by cases arising at a younger age than those from occupational exposures.

The younger age distribution appears to be a result of younger age at first exposure so that at any given age there has been greater opportunity to have accrued the characteristically long latent period. This effect is greatest where exposure started in very early childhood. However, mesothelioma risk still rises with age and the rate of mesothelioma still increases 50 years after exposure (Reid et al. 2013). Apart from this exposure-cohort effect, children have not been shown to be more vulnerable to mesothelioma than adults. Peritoneal mesothelioma is uncommon from most community exposures, as is asbestosis; both are more strongly associated with characteristically higher occupational exposures (Reid et al. 2014).

5.3.4 Vulnerable Groups in the Community

Familial clustering of cases of mesothelioma occurs as a direct consequence of paraoccupational exposures to those who are domiciled with asbestos workers, an effect that could be potentially related to shared residential neighborhood and lifestyle-dependent environmental exposures. There is also a strong possibility the familial clustering could reflect an additional or even primary genetic component. De Klerk et al. (2013) have estimated the additional genetically derived familial risk of mesothelioma in the Wittenoom cohort, after allowing for common exposures. This required fitting a statistical survival model to all the data, based on time from first exposure, duration and intensity of exposure and age, which allowed estimation of the expected number of mesotheliomas in family groupings. Of 369 families with at least one case of mesothelioma, 25 mesotheliomas were found in relatives vs. 12.9 expected. The risk ratio for blood relatives after this adjustment was 1.9 (95% CI 1.3 to 2.9, $p = 0.002$). This suggested an important though not dominant genetic component at Wittenoom. A larger genetic component was estimated by Roushdy-Hammady et al. (2001) for mesothelioma resulting from exposure to erionite in the Cappadocia region of Turkey.

An important social vulnerability occurs in those who are unknowingly exposed to asbestos by any pathway. This has been an important characteristic of residents of several high-risk communities in the past. Ignorance of asbestos exposure and effects appears more likely to be associated with non-occupational exposure at present, at least in developed countries, as asbestos awareness is generally high in employers, in the skilled trades, and amongst unionized employees. The role of socioeconomic factors in the risk of mesothelioma does not appear to have been studied even though there appear to be significant environmental justice concerns in the distribution of risk.

General population exposure can include exposures to groups of people who are not usually in the workforce such as those with serious diseases as well as the very young and aged. There is no convincing evidence that there is any increased predisposition to mesothelioma in any such group or amongst different ethnic groups, although it remains a possibility.

5.3.5   Diffuse Administrative Responsibility

For the first and second waves of exposure, the lines of administrative responsibility
to protect workers' health were clear, i.e., a responsible party, the employer, and a
single enforcing agency. In the USA, the general duty clause of the Occupational
Safety and Health Act of 1970, enforced by OSHA, states that "each employer (1)
shall furnish to each of his employees a place of employment which is free from
recognized hazards that are causing or are likely to cause death or serious physical
harm to his employees and (2) shall comply with occupational safety and health
standards promulgated under this Act." Asbestos has its own standard with detailed
requirements for permissible exposures, risk identification and assessment, engineering controls, work practices and respiratory protection, proper hazard communication, demarcation of areas where there are risks, separate decontamination and
luncheon areas, training requirements, medical surveillance, and record keeping.
Most other countries have similar regulations.

In contrast in many non-occupational exposure situations such as asbestos exposures in residences, asbestos encountered during lifestyle activities, or environmental exposures the chain of responsibility can be very complex. For example for the
Bo-Rit Superfund site in Ambler, PA is an area of approximately 25 acres with
much asbestos-containing material and potentially contaminated surrounding areas
including creeks and parkland. The U.S. EPA is responsible for the cleanup on the
site itself but does not even have automatic right of access to surrounding private
properties where additional contamination is possible. Present or future use and
control of access to potentially contaminated areas is, or will be, variously controlled by several different landowners, the Pennsylvania Department of
Environmental Protection, four different local municipalities, the County Planning
Department, other important stakeholders including neighborhood residents and
businesses, the State Health Department, and a federal health agency (Agency for
Toxic Substances and Disease Control). In other community sites, the parties
involved may vary but responsibility is likely equally diffuse. When there is a shared
common appreciation of risks and commitment to working with others, satisfactory
and sustainable control of long-term risks acceptable to at least a majority of stakeholders may be obtainable. Where there are sufficiently divergent views amongst
major stakeholders, achieving appropriate hazard control can be contentious,
prolonged, and potentially ineffective.

5.3.6   Diverse Community Attitudes to Risk and Prevention

The stakeholders we interviewed regarding Ambler's asbestos-containing waste
sites had wide divergence within a community expressed widely divergent views
about risk and the appropriate future use of potentially contaminated areas.
Interviewees also cited marked changes in community attitudes to asbestos risks

over recent decades with increasing importance now given to long-term sustainability. More research is needed to understand how these different views are generated. We need methodology to help communities develop consensus around acceptable solutions, especially in third wave exposure situations where collaborative efforts involving many different parties are necessary to reduce or remove risks in a sustainable manner.

5.3.7 Quantifying Nonoccupational Exposures, Justifying Remediation and Action

In general the data quantifying non-occupational community exposures is sparse and often sporadic or absent. This is true for paraoccupational exposures (Goswami et al. 2013), residential exposures and the various pathways for environmental and lifestyle exposures. Moreover, individuals often sustain multiple exposure pathways: those with occupational exposures may have additional non-occupational exposures. Thus it is difficult or impossible to study the outcomes from a single exposure pathway in isolation. Furthermore, the cumulative "dose" from non-occupational asbestos exposures is likely to be site-specific and not easily extrapolated from one community to another: for example, ambient exposures in a wet temperate climate may differ markedly from those from a dry dusty tropical climate, and all will be affected by the local culture, lifestyle, and activities. Much information about community exposures is based on subjective historical recollection and relates to exposures and practices many years ago that are not readily reconstructed; and past measurement may have had very serious methodologic limitations (Rogers 1990). These inherent limitations in the exposure database pose difficulties for the types of quantitative risk assessments preferred by the U.S. EPA and similar agencies to support decisions as to remediation and prioritization of hazards.

We should be cautious not to overly discount the potential for risk of mesothelioma given the apparent dose response relationship with no known threshold and, in contrast to other ARDs, demonstrable risk from very low exposures. Limitations in our ability to recognize potentially carcinogenic exposures are illustrated by the findings of Leigh and Driscoll (2003): 19% of subjects with mesothelioma in the Australian Mesothelioma Registry gave no known history of any asbestos exposure; however, when lung tissue was analyzed for fibers, 81% of this group had fiber counts >200,000 fibers/g dry lung, and 30% had more than 10^6 fibers/g >2 μm, including "long" (>10 μm) fibers, suggesting that nearly all had been exposed to asbestos but could not recall or had never recognized the exposure.

5.3.8 Surveillance/Early Diagnosis in High-Risk Communities

Any enthusiasm for surveillance of those with previous exposure to asbestos must be tempered by the dismal prognosis once the disease is recognized. Using national U.S. Surveillance, Epidemiology and End-Results (SEER) data from 1973 to 2009,

Taioli et al. (2015) found no significant improvement in the mean survival time for pleural mesothelioma over four decades. However, in Australia (Soeberg et al. 2016) and the Netherlands (Damhuis et al. 2012) modest improvements (in the order of a few months increased survival for pleural mesothelioma) have been noted during the last few years, largely corresponding with the introduction of new chemotherapeutic regimes. Furthermore, currently no evidence-based interventions are able to reduce the incidence or prognosis of cancers in those who have been exposed other than smoking cessation, which might help prevent lung cancer but does not influence mesothelioma outcomes. This grim picture emphasizes the need for primary prevention through elimination of exposure rather than secondary or tertiary prevention. Perhaps this situation will change. There is close surveillance of some high-risk community populations such as in Libby, MT, so that more data will become available on any benefits of close follow-up. Efforts to find biomarkers of early effects and to develop effective chemoprevention and treatments continue, so that more optimistic scenarios may emerge.

Importantly, high-risk communities need services to ensure prompt diagnosis and treatment of those ARD that do occur and to provide sociologic and psychologic support. Many high-risk communities contain a substantial number of former asbestos workers. In the USA, current Occupational Health and Safety Regulations are not particularly helpful for retired workers, as employers are required to provide periodic medical evaluations while working with asbestos, but no systematic surveillance or other follow-up after leaving that job. Yet, due to the long latent period for mesothelioma, the greatest risk occurs after work with asbestos has ceased.

Khatab et al. (2014) have developed a risk-based tool to predict which former asbestos workers would benefit most from participation in prospective surveillance for ARD. Risk factors include age, exposure duration, time since first exposure, age at first exposure, and job (partly as a proxy for degree of exposure). Since the primary target of their model is lung cancer where the benefit of early detection on mortality is demonstrated, smoking is included in the risk model. Should the prognosis of treated mesothelioma improve, a model specifically directed at mesothelioma risk might help identify both high-risk communities and individuals within a community who would have the greatest benefit from surveillance.

5.3.9   Legal Responsibility and Compensation for Non-Occupational ARD

The assignment of responsibility and legal recourse for compensation for mesothelioma and other "injury' suffered as a result of exposure was relatively straightforward during the first and second waves of ARD. As a base, Workers Compensation Insurance would apply, although in many countries including the USA, third-party suits against the supplier of asbestos were successful and resulted in much greater monetary settlements for plaintiffs. Community non-occupational exposures have the potential for new legal challenges, particularly where a single responsible party is difficult to identify. For example, in Italy, Marinaccio et al. (2015) have reported concern about insurance and welfare protection for mesothelioma sufferers and note that different pathways of non-occupational exposure to asbestos pose different concerns with respect to the welfare protection framework. They argue that a suitable framework needs to incorporate economic, ethical, and insurance points of view. Environmental exposure to natural asbestiform fibers may pose the greatest challenge.

Gordon and Leigh (2011) cite third wave risks to non-professionals who cut and fix asbestos cement products in home renovation or maintenance and other do-it-yourself activities. They maintain that manufacturers of asbestos-containing products have a continuing duty of care to inform such users about asbestos risks. They see major issues of controversy as the claimant's ability to prove that the manufacturer could, and should, have taken steps that would (before the time of exposure) have drawn the risk to the user's attention; and proving, more probably than not, that the exposure in such limited circumstances was the cause of, or made a contribution to, the mesothelioma manifesting many years later.

5.3.10 Epidemiology for Communities at High Risk for Mesothelioma

National Mesothelioma Registries have been invaluable for discovering trends in mesothelioma incidence and uncovering effects of third wave exposures. These registries overcome weaknesses in other systems that include underreporting of data, uncertain diagnosis, poor elucidation of occupational and environmental exposures, and less than comprehensive coverage (Ferguson et al. 1987). Mesothelioma Registries operate in Italy, France, and Australia. In Italy, ReNaM has recorded mesothelioma cases and collected information on asbestos exposure from 1993 to the present, although as of 2015 some regional data was still not available (Marinaccio et al. 2005; Marinaccio et al. 2015). A French National Registry has operated since 1998 (Goldberg et al. 2006; Galateau-Sallé et al. 2014). In Australia, national data on mesothelioma has been collected under two successive schemes: the Australian Mesothelioma Surveillance Program (1979–1985) and the Australian Mesothelioma Register (1986–2002), the latter operated by the National Occupational Health and Safety Commission (NOHSC) up to 2001 (Leigh and Driscoll 2003). As a consequence of funding cutbacks and interpretations of privacy legislation preventing comparisons with state cancer registries, data was incomplete from 2001 to 2010, when the registry was reconstituted. All Australians diagnosed with mesothelioma who consent to an asbestos exposure assessment complete questionnaires for the registry to record their residential and occupational history, any tasks outside paid work and other circumstances likely to have exposed them to asbestos (Australian Mesothelioma Registry 2014).

Mesothelioma registries have important characteristics for addressing third wave exposures including standardized diagnostic criteria, collection of exposure data that enables trends in the incidence attributable to different exposure types to be monitored, ability to track trends in different regions, and the ability to identify communities with clusters of mesothelioma.

The very long latency period between exposure and effect and the short median survival time after mesothelioma diagnosis pose methodological issues for conventional case-control and cohort studies of communities. In many modern communities, few people reside in the same location 40 or more years later, so that the studies of survivor populations may greatly underestimate the risk from past exposures. Short survival periods allow a brief window to question the patient about exposures, and next-of-kin may be ignorant of exposures many years ago. Occupational studies have used lists of past employees or in some cases union membership to identify cohorts of workers exposed to asbestos (Selikoff et al. 1965; Selikoff and Seidman 1991). Cohorts of children exposed to asbestos (Reid et al. 2013) and of spouses of asbestos workers (Ferrante et al. 2007; Reid et al. 2008) have contributed comprehensive information on long-term effects of exposure to those groups. Cohort studies following an entire community exposed to asbestos are rare; however, studies of former Wittenoom residents show they are possible through innovative methods and exhaustive follow-up.

5.3.11   Estimating the Magnitude and Timing of Third Wave Mesothelioma

Driscoll et al. (2005) estimated a global annual burden of 43,000 deaths and 564,000 disability-adjusted life years (DALYs) from mesothelioma assuming that virtually all mesothelioma is caused by exposure to asbestos. In some countries, mesothelioma incidence appears to have reached a plateau. Soeberg et al. (2016) analyzed the incidence and survival trends for pleural and peritoneal mesothelioma for Australia from 1982–2009. Very high asbestos consumption levels peaked from 1970–1979 and declined rapidly thereafter. Overall, mesothelioma incidence rates appeared to have reached maximum levels in the early 2000s, consistent with the earlier predictions based on consumption patterns (Leigh et al. 1997), but there were differences over time by age, gender, and tumor location. During 2003–2009, the incidence for men aged <65 was declining by about 5% per year, whereas for women and men aged >75 the incidence was increasing by about 5% per year. Although data for peritoneal mesothelioma were sparse, the incidence appeared to be slowly rising over the entire period studied.

Reid et al. (2014) pooled data from Italy and Australia using six cohort studies of exposed workers and two cohorts with residential exposure. Both the rate and risk of pleural mesothelioma increased until 45 years after first exposure and then appeared to increase at a slower rate. The authors commented that while the rate of increase appears to start to level out after 40–50 years, no one survives long enough for the excess risk to disappear. The rate of increase for peritoneal mesothelioma continued to increase over the entire 50 years of study. Women appeared to have a longer latent period than men and mostly obtained their asbestos exposure from paraoccupational, residential, or environmental sources which tend to be associated with lower exposures levels than occupational settings. Lower exposures appear associated with longer latency in other studies. Amongst Turkish emigrants to Sweden lower asbestos exposure was associated with a longer latency period (Metintas et al. 1999), and Wittenoom women who worked for the asbestos company had a shorter latency period than those with only residential exposure (Reid et al. 2008).

Predicting the magnitude of third wave ARD is difficult because of the paucity of good non-occupational exposure data. However, in countries with mesothelioma registries that record both exposure and diagnosis, we are already able to discern third wave mesothelioma from non-occupational exposures, including those in Italian communities with mesothelioma clusters (Marinaccio et al. 2015) and Australian home do-it-yourself renovators (Olsen et al. 2011) mentioned earlier in this chapter.

5.3.12 Varying Expressions of ARD in Different Communities

The pattern of ARD in an affected community can be influenced by amount of exposure, age at exposure, fiber type, and genetic predisposition. The highest exposures, seen predominantly in occupational groups, are associated with excess lung cancer and asbestosis and a higher proportion of peritoneal mesothelioma in addition to pleural mesothelioma; for the lower exposures experienced by non-occupational exposure groups, pleural mesothelioma predominates (Reid et al. 2014). Follow-up of the cohort of children (aged <15 years) exposed at Wittenoom found in addition to a very great excess of mesothelioma, excesses in other cancers including ovarian and brain cancers in women as well as leukemia, prostate, brain, and colorectal cancers, and mortality from "all causes" in men (Reid et al. 2013). With respect to fiber type: the association of LAA with more marked pleural changes and autoimmune manifestations is discussed in the section of this chapter dealing with Libby, MT.

5.4 Conclusion

Mesothelioma caused by asbestos has largely been considered and dealt with as an occupational disease. However recent research demonstrates an elevated incidence in a number of communities where there are important contributions not only from occupational exposures but also from non-occupational exposures. These include paraoccupational, residential, and lifestyle/behaviorally determined exposures. Although these exposures can be clearly identified, they are seldom accurately quantifiable. Genetic vulnerabilities may be important and can play a major role.

Each community cluster appears to have unique characteristics and a distinctive local history. Collectively prevention and attribution of ARD from non-occupational community exposures can be more complex and raise additional and different issues compared with prevention of occupational asbestos exposure. Their issues have been discussed in this chapter.

Acknowledgements Research reported in this publication was supported by National Institute Environmental Health Sciences of the National Institutes of Health under award number P42 ES023720 Penn Superfund Research Program Center Grant. The content is solely the responsibility of the authors and does not necessarily represent the official views of the National Institutes of Health.

Conflict of Interest The authors have no conflicts of interest to disclose.

References

Algrantia E, Saitob CA, Carneiroc APS et al (2015) The next mesothelioma wave: mortality trends and forecast to 2030 in Brazil. Cancer Epidemiol 39:687–692

Amandus HE, Wheeler R, Jankovic J et al (1987) The morbidity and mortality of vermiculite miners and millers exposed to tremolite-actinolite. Part I. Exposure estimates. Am J Ind Med 11:1–14

Amandus HE, Wheeler R (1987) The morbidity and mortality of vermiculite miners and millers exposed to tremolite-actinolite. Part II. Mortality. Am J Ind Med 11:15–26

AMR (Australian Mesothelioma Registry) (2014) Australian Mesothelioma Registry 3rd annual report: Mesothelioma in Australia 2013. Safe Work Australia, Canberra. Available at: http://www.mesothelioma-australia.com/publications-and-data/publications

Armstrong BK, de Klerk NH, Musk AW et al (1988) Mortality in miners and millers of crocidolite in Western Australia. Brit J Ind Med 45:5–13

Artvinli M, Baris YI (1979) Malignant mesotheliomas in a small village in the Anatolian region of Turkey: an epidemiologic study. J Natl Cancer Inst 63:17–22

ATSDR (2002) Health Consultation Libby Asbestos Site, Libby, Lincoln County Montana. Agency for Toxic Substances and Disease Registry, Atlanta, GA

Musk AW, de Klerk NH, Eccles JL et al (1992) Wittenoom, Western Australia: a modern industrial disaster. Am J Ind Med 21:735–747

Baris YI et al (1978) An outbreak of pleural mesothelioma and chronic fibrosing pleurisy in the village of Karain/Urgup in Anatolia. Thorax 33:181–192

Baris YI, Grandjean P (2006) Prospective study of mesothelioma mortality in Turkish villages with exposure to fibrous zeolite. J Natl Cancer Inst 98:414–417

Baris YI, Simonato L, Artvinli M et al (1987) Epidemiological and environmental evidence of health effects of exposure to erionite fibers: a four year study in the Cappodocian region in Turkey. Int J Cancer 39:10–17

Bennett C (2016) The Blue Ghosts of Wittenoom. Watoday.com. http://www.watoday.com.au/interactive/2015/blueGhosts/. Accessed 11 March 2016

Black B, Szeinuk J, Whitehouse AC et al (2014) Rapid progression of pleural disease due to exposure to Libby amphibole: "Not your grandfather's asbestos related disease.". Am J Ind Med 57:1197–1206

Case BW, Abraham JL, Meeker G et al (2011) Applying definitions of "asbestos" to environmental and "low-dose" exposure levels and health effects, particularly malignant mesothelioma. J Toxicol Environ Health B Crit Rev 14:3–39

Carbone M, Emri S, Dogan AU et al (2007) A mesothelioma epidemic in Cappadocia: scientific developments and unexpected social outcomes. Nat Rev Cancer 7:147–154

Cumpston AG (1978) The health hazard at Wittenoom. Public Health Department of Western Australia, Perth

Cumpston AG (1979) Exposure to crocidolite at Wittenoom. Public Health Department of Western Australia, Perth

Damhuis RAM, Schroten C, Burgers JA (2012) Population-based survival for malignant mesothelioma after introduction of novel chemotherapy. Eur Respir J 40:185–189

de Klerk N, Alfonso H, Olsen N et al (2013) Familial aggregation of malignant mesothelioma in former workers and residents of Wittenoom, Western Australia. Int J Cancer 136:1423–1428

Dogan AU, Baris YI, Dogan M et al (2006) Genetic predisposition to fiber carcinogenesis causes a mesothelioma epidemic in Turkey. Cancer Res 66:5063–5068

Driscoll T, Nelson DI, Steenland K et al (2005) The global burden of disease due to occupational carcinogens. Am J Ind Med 48:419–431

Dunning KK, Adjei S, Levin L et al (2012) Mesothelioma associated with commercial use of vermiculite containing Libby amphibole. J Occup Environ Med 54:1359–1363

Elder J (1967) Asbestosis in Western Australia. Med J Aust 2:579–583

Emri S, Demir A, Dogan M et al (2002) Lung diseases due to environmental exposures to erionite and asbestos in Turkey. Toxicol Lett 27:251–257

Ferguson DA, Berry G, Jelihovsky T et al (1987) The Australian Mesothelioma Surveillance Program 1979–1985. Med J Aust 147:166–172

Ferrante D, Bertolotti M, Todesco A et al (2007) Cancer mortality and incidence of mesothelioma in a cohort of wives of asbestos workers in Casale Monferrato, Italy. Environ Health Perspect 115:1401–1405

Galateau-Sallé F, Gilg Soit Ilg A, Le Stang N et al (2014) The French mesothelioma network from 1998 to 2013. Ann Pathol 34:51–63

Gilmer J, Serve KM, Davis C et al (2016) Libby amphibole-induced mesothelial cell autoantibodies promote collagen deposition in mice. Am J Physiol Lung Cell Mol Physiol 310.L1071–L1077

Goldberg M, Imbernon E, Rolland P et al (2006) The French National Mesothelioma Surveillance Program. Occup Environ Med 63:390–395

Gordon JRC, Leigh J (2011) Medicolegal aspects of the third wave of asbestos-related disease in Australia. Med J Aust 195:247–248

Goswami E, Craven V, Dahlstrom DL et al (2013) Domestic asbestos exposure: a review of epidemiologic and exposure data. Int J Environ Res Public Health 10:5629–5670

Graham L (1994) Report of the select committee appointed to inquire into Wittenoom. Legislative Assembly of the Parliament of Western Australia, Perth

Greenberg M (1991) Cancer mortality in merchant seamen. Ann N Y Acad Sci 643:321–332

Hansen J, de Klerk NH, Eccles J et al (1993) Malignant mesothelioma after environmental exposure to blue asbestos. Int J Cancer 54:578–581

Hansen J, de Klerk NH, Musk AW et al (1998) Environmental exposure to crocidolite and mesothelioma exposure-response relationships. Am J Respir Crit Care Med 157:69–75

Haque AK, Kanz MF, Mancuso MG et al (1991) Asbestos in the lungs of children. Ann N Y Acad Sci 643:419–429

Henderson DW, Leigh J (2012) The history of asbestos utilization and recognition of asbestos-induced disease. In: Dodson RF, Hammer SP (eds) Asbestos, risk assessment, epidemiology and health, 2nd edn. CRC Press, Boca Raton, FL, pp 1–22

Hobbs MST, Woodward SD, Murphy B et al (1980) The incidence of pneumoconiosis, mesothelioma and other respiratory cancers in men engaged in mining and milling crocidolite in Western Australia. In: Wagner JC (ed) Biological effects of mineral fibers. International Agency for Research on Cancer. IARC Scientific Publication No 30, Lyon

International Agency for Research on Cancer (2012) Asbestos (chrysotile, amosite, crocidolite, tremolite, actinolite, and anthophyllite). IARC Monogr Eval Carcinog Risks Chem Hum 100(Pt C):219–309

International Ban Asbestos Secretariat (2015) Chronology of National Asbestos Bans, Compiled by Laurie Kazan-Allen. http://www.ibasecretariat.org/chron_ban_list.php

International Labour Organization (2006) Resolution concerning asbestos. http://www.ilo.org/safework/info/standards-and-instruments/WCMS_108556/lang--en/index.htm

Khatab K, Felten M, Kandala NB et al (2014) Risk factors associated with asbestos-related diseases: results of the asbestos surveillance programme Aachen. Eur Med J Respir 1:1–9

Naik SL, Lewin M, Young R, et al. (2016) Mortality from asbestos-associated disease in Libby, Montana 1979–2011. J Expo Sci Environ Epidemiol 2 doi: 10.1038/jes.2016.18 [Epub ahead of print]

Landrigan PJ (1991) The third wave of asbestos disease: exposure to asbestos in place–Public health control. Introduction. Ann N Y Acad Sci 643:xv–xvi

Layman L (1983) Work and workers' response at Wittenoom 1943–1966. Community Health Stud 7:1–18

Leigh J, Driscoll T (2003) Malignant mesothelioma in Australia, 1945–2002. Int J Occup Environ Health 9:206–217

Leigh J, Hull B, Davidson P (1997) Malignant mesothelioma in Australia (1945–1995). Ann Occup Hyg 41:161–167

Lowers HA, Meeker GP (2002) Tabulation of asbestos-related terminology. U.S. Geological Survey open-file report 02–458, Version 1.0. USGS http://pubs.usgs.gov/of/2002/ofr-02-458/OFR-02-458-508

Magnani C, Terracini B, Ivaldi C et al (1993) A cohort study on mortality among wives of workers in the asbestos cement industry in Casale Monferrato, Italy. Br J Ind Med 50:779–784

Magnani C, Terracini B, Ivaldi C et al (1996) Mortalità per tumori e altre cause tra i lavoratori del cemento-amianto a Casale Monferrato. Uno studio di coorte storico. Med Lav 87:133–146

Maltoni C, Pinto C, Mobiglia A (1991) Mesothelioma due to asbestos used in railroads in Italy. Ann N Y Acad Sci 643:347–367

Marchand LS, St-Hilaire S, Putnam EA et al (2012) Mesothelial cell and anti-nuclear autoantibodies associated with pleural abnormalities in an asbestos exposed population of Libby MT. Toxicol Lett 208:168–173

Marinaccio A, Montanaro F, Mastrantonio M et al (2005) Predictions of mortality from pleural mesothelioma in Italy: a model based on asbestos consumption figures supports results from age-period-cohort models. Int J Cancer 115:142–147

Marinaccio A, Binazzi A, Bonafede M et al (2015) Malignant mesothelioma due to non-occupational asbestos exposure from the Italian national surveillance system (ReNaM): epidemiology and public health issues. Occup Environ Med 72:648–655

McDonald JC, McDonald AD, Armstrong B et al (1986) Cohort study of mortality of vermiculite miners exposed to tremolite. Br J Ind Med 43:436–444

McNulty JC (1962) Malignant pleural mesothelioma in an asbestos worker. Med J Aust 49:953–954

Meeker GP, Bern AM, Brownfield HA et al (2003) The composition and morphology of amphiboles from the rainy creek complex, near Libby, Montana. Am Mineral 88:1955–1969

Mensi C, Termine L, Canti Z et al (2007) The Lombardy Mesothelioma Register, Regional Operating Centre (ROC) of National Mesothelioma Register: organizational aspects. Epidemiol Prev 31:283–289

Mensi C, Riboldi L, DeMatteis S et al (2015) Impact of an asbestos cement factory on mesothelioma incidence: global assessment of effects of occupational, familial, and environmental exposure. Environ Int 74:191–199

Metintas M, Hillerdal G, Metintas S (1999) Malignant mesothelioma due to environmental exposure to erionite: follow-up of a Turkish emigrant cohort. Eur Respir J 13:523–526

Mirabelli D, Cavone D, Luberto F et al (2010) Il comparto della produzione di cemento-amianto. In: Marinaccio A et al (eds) Registro Nazionale Mesoteliomi Terzo Rapporto. ISPESL, Roma, pp 105–121

Moulton E (2015) Geotechnical work to begin in Wittenoom to determine how to clean up the contaminated site. News.com.au May 17. http://www.news.com.au/technology/environment/

geotechnical-work-to-begin-in-wittenoom-to-determine-how-to-clean-up-the-contaminated-site/news-story/2896d2221712698708836578829b83f7

Nesti M, Adamoli S, Ammirabile F et al (2003) Linee guida per la rilevazione e la definizione dei casi di mesotelioma maligno e la trasmissione delle informazioni all'ISPESL da parte dei Centri Operativi Regionali, Seconda edizione. ISPESL, Roma

Newhouse ML, Thompson H (1965) Mesothelioma of pleura and peritoneum following exposure to asbestos in the London area. Brit J Ind Med 22:262–269

Noonan CW, Pfau JC, Larson TC et al (2006) Nested case-control study of autoimmune disease in an asbestos-exposed population. Environ Health Perspect 114:1243–1247

Noonan CN, Conway K, Landguth EL et al (2015) Multiple pathway asbestos exposure assessment for a Superfund community. J Exposure Sci Environ Epidemiol 25:18–25

Oddone E, Ferrante D, Cena T et al (2014) Asbestos cement factory in Broni (Pavia, Italy): a mortality study. Med Lav 105:15–29

Olsen NJ, Franklin PJ, Reid A et al (2011) Increasing incidence of malignant mesothelioma after exposure to asbestos during home maintenance and renovation. Med J Aust 195:271–274

Peipens LA, Lewin M, Campolucci S et al (2003) Radiographic abnormalities and exposure to asbestos-contaminated vermiculite in the community of Libby, Montana, USA. Environ Health Perspect 111:1753–1759

Pennsylvania Department of Health 2011. Cancer evaluation, Ambler area, Montgomery County. July 11, 2011, Harrisburg, PA

Pfau JC, Sentissi JJ, Weller G et al (2005) Assessment of autoimmune responses associated with asbestos exposure in Libby, Montana, USA. Environ Health Perspect 113:25–30

Pfau JC, Li S, Holland S et al (2011) Alteration of fibroblast phenotype by asbestos-induced auto-antibodies. J Immunotoxicol 8:159–169

Pfau JC, Serve KM, Woods L et al (2015) Asbestos exposure and autoimmunity. In: Biological effects of fibrous and particulate substances. Current topics in environmental health and preventive medicine. Springer, Japan

Pirastu R, Zona A, Ancona C et al (2011) Mortality results in SENTIERI Project(Italian). Epidemiol Prev 35:29–152

Quattrone F (2004) Images of America: Ambler. Arcadia Publishing, Charleston, SC

Reid A, de Klerk NH, Magnani C et al (2014) Mesothelioma risk after 40 years since first exposure to asbestos: a pooled analysis. Thorax 69:843–850

Reid A, Hayworth J, de Klerk N et al (2008) The mortality of women exposed environmentally and domestically to blue asbestos at Wittenoom, Western Australia. Occup Environ Med 65:743–749

Reid A, Franklin P, Olsen N et al (2013) All-cause mortality and cancer incidence among adults exposed to blue asbestos during childhood. Am J Ind Med 56:133–145

Rogers A (1990) Cancer mortality and crocidolite. Brit J Ind Med 47:286

Roushdy-Hammady I, Siegel J, Emri S et al (2001) Genetic-susceptibility factor and malignant mesothelioma in the Cappadocian region of Turkey. Lancet 357:444–445

Sebastien P, Gaudichet A, Bignon J et al (1981) Zeolite bodies in human lungs from Turkey. Lab Invest 44:420–425

Selikoff IJ, Churg J, Hammond EC (1965) The occurrence of asbestosis among insulation workers in the United States. Ann N Y Acad Sci 132:139–155

Selikoff IJ, Seidman H (1991) Asbestos-associated deaths among insulation workers in the United States and Canada, 1967–1987. Ann N Y Acad Sci 643:1–14

Serve KM, Black B, Szeinuk J et al (2013) Asbestos-associated mesothelial cell autoantibodies promote collagen deposition in vitro. Inhalation Toxicol 25:774–784

Soeberg MJ, Leigh J, Driscoll T et al (2016) Incidence and survival trends for malignant pleural and peritoneal mesothelioma, Australia, 1982–2009. Occup Environ Med 73:187–194

Taioli E, Wolf AS, Camancho-Rivera M et al (2015) Determinants of survival in malignant pleural mesothelioma: a surveillance, epidemiology, and end results (SEER) study of 14,228 patients. PLoS One 10:e0145039

United States Department of Labor (1975) Occupational exposure to asbestos. Fed Regist 40:47652–47665

USEPA 2009. https://yosemite.epa.gov/opa/admpress.nsf. EPA announces Public Health Emergency in Libby Montana. 06/17/2009

USEPA Superfund, 1988. Record of Decision Ambler Asbestos Piles EPA ID: PAD000436436, OU 1. Ambler, PA; Washington DC. U.S. Environmental Protection Agency.

USEPA Superfund, 1989. Record of Decision Ambler Asbestos Piles EPA ID: PAD000436436, OU 2. Ambler, PA; Washington DC. U.S. Environmental Protection Agency.

Wagner JC, Skidmore JW, Hill RJ et al (1985) Erionite exposure and mesotheliomas in rats. Br J Cancer 51:727–730

Whitehouse AC (2004) Asbestos-related pleural disease due to tremolite associated with progressive loss of lung function: serial observations in 123 miners, family members and residents of Libby Montana. Am J Ind Med 46:219–225

Whitehouse AC, Black CB, Heppe MS et al (2008) Environmental exposure to Libby asbestos and mesotheliomas. Am J Ind Med 51:877–880

Wittenoom's asbestos history still looms large but some residents won't leave. The Daily Telegraph, May 11, 2015. http://www.dailytelegraph.com.au/news/wittenooms-asbestos-history-still-looms-large-but-some-residents-wont-leave/news-story/eec0f1fd82bf076ebe84c6e02fb5ac1f

Chapter 6
Mesothelioma Pathology

Elizabeth N. Pavlisko, John M. Carney, Thomas A. Sporn,
and Victor L. Roggli

Abstract Malignant mesothelioma can arise from pleura, peritoneum, pericardium, and the tunica vaginalis. It has the propensity to encase organs with rind-like growth over serosal surfaces and can demonstrate a variety of histomorphologic growth patterns ranging from epithelial to sarcomatoid. Given such, securing a diagnosis of malignant mesothelioma entails proper gross distribution of tumor in combination with histomorphology compatible with mesothelioma and exclusion of another primary source metastatic to the serosal cavity through immunohistochemistry. While employed less often, electron microscopy still holds value in distinguishing epithelioid malignancies from malignant epithelial mesothelioma. Recent studies have shown BAP1 immunohistochemistry in conjunction with fluorescence in-situ hybridization for homozygous loss of the gene encoding 16INK4A to be beneficial in separating benign/reactive from malignant mesothelial proliferations.

Keywords Mesothelioma • Histopathology • Immunohistochemical stains • Other mesothelioma markers • Immunohistochemical panels and differential diagnosis • Electron microscopy

6.1 Gross Morphology

Malignant mesotheliomas are typically diffuse neoplasms, whose characteristic growth pattern is that of thick and confluent involvement of the serosal membrane where it originates. This includes pleural (Fig. 6.1), peritoneal (Fig. 6.2), and pericardial (Fig. 6.3) cavities as well as the tunica vaginalis testis (Churg et al. 2006). Associated effusions involving these body cavities are usually symptomatic and precipitate clinical detection of the mesothelioma itself. With advanced disease, the combination of tumor and effusion leads to obliteration of pleural or peritoneal spaces and thick confluent growth of tumor invades and compresses regional structures extrinsically. Malignant mesothelioma most commonly originates in the pleura, with the ratio of pleural to peritoneal tumors being approximately 10:1

E.N. Pavlisko • J.M. Carney • T.A. Sporn • V.L. Roggli (✉)
Department of Pathology, Duke University Medical Center, Durham, NC 27710, USA
e-mail: Elizabeth.pavlisko@duke.edu; Roggl002@mc.duke.edu

© Springer International Publishing AG 2017
J.R. Testa (ed.), *Asbestos and Mesothelioma*, Current Cancer Research,
DOI 10.1007/978-3-319-53560-9_6

Fig. 6.1 Coronal slice of
the right lung in a patient
with malignant (diffuse)
pleural mesothelioma
demonstrating encasement
of the lung by a whitish
rind of tumor. There is
superficial invasion of
underlying parenchyma.
(Reprinted from Roggli
VL, Kolbeck J, Sanfilippo
F, Shelburn JD (1987)
Pathology of human
mesothelioma: etiologic
and diagnostic
considerations. Pathol
Annu 22(Part2):91–131,
Fig. 2, with permission)

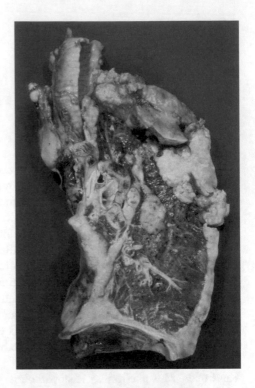

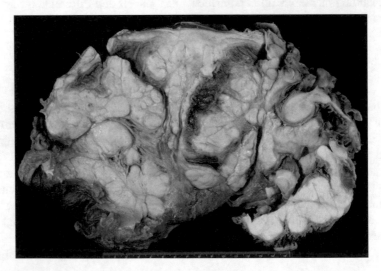

Fig. 6.2 Coronal slice of abdominal viscera in a patient with malignant (diffuse) peritoneal mesothelioma demonstrating encasement and compression of bowel (dark areas) by confluent tumor
nodules. (Reprinted from Pavlisko EN, Sporn TA (2014) Mesothelioma. Chapter 5. In: Pathology
of Asbestos-Associated Diseases, 3rd ed. Oury TD, Sporn TA, Roggli VL, eds. Springer, New York,
NY, Fig. 5.19, with permission)

Fig. 6.3 Transverse section of the heart, showing complete encasement by malignant pericardial mesothelioma. (Reprinted from Pavlisko EN, Sporn TA (2014) Mesothelioma. Chapter 5. In: Pathology of Asbestos-Associated Diseases, 3rd ed., Oury TD, Sporn TA, Roggli VL, eds. Springer: New York, NY, Fig. 5.23, with permission)

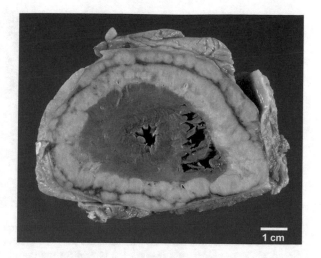

1 cm

(Hillerdal 1983). Pericardial mesotheliomas are quite rare, with approximately 200 cases reported to date in the literature (Gossinger et al. 1988; Pavlisko and Sporn 2014). Pericardial mesothelioma accounts for 2–3% of all cardiac/pericardial malignancies and 1% of all mesotheliomas (Burke et al. 1996).

6.1.1   Pleural Mesothelioma

As the list of differential diagnostic considerations of tumors involving the serosa is extensive, in order to make an accurate diagnosis the pathologist must use all available data (clinical, historical, and radiological) as well as have an understanding of the gross distribution of disease (Moran et al. 1992). Malignant pleural mesotheliomas typically begin as multiple small discrete nodules or macules originating on the surface of the parietal pleura and parallel the distribution of the lymphatics (Boutin et al. 1996; Corson 1997). Presenting complaints are often dyspnea and chest pain secondary to large pleural effusions, which can be viewed on chest radiographs (Fig. 6.4a). Plain film chest radiographs are limited in that a large effusion can obscure underlying tumor. Chest computerized tomography (CT) may assist in elucidating the underlying pathology (Fig. 6.4b). Due to ease of accessibility, effusion cytology is often employed as the first step towards a diagnosis.

With progression of disease, there is coalescence of individual tumor nodules culminating in fusion of visceral and parietal pleura, resulting in encasement of the lung by tumor and extension follows along pleura within fissures and into interlobular septa. Tumor may invade into adjacent structures including bone and soft tissues of the chest wall, diaphragm, pericardium, and other mediastinal structures. Tumor growth is typically thickest at the base of the pleural cavity. Some tumors elaborate abundant amounts of hyaluronic acid, leading to cyst-like accumulations of the

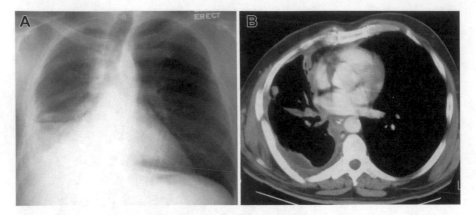

Fig. 6.4 (**a**) Posteroanterior chest X-ray shows a unilateral pleural effusion. (**b**) Computed tomography of the thorax from the same patient shows irregular pleural thickening with encasement of the lung. These radiographic features are typical for malignant (diffuse) pleural mesothelioma. (Courtesy of Dr. Caroline Chiles, Duke University Medical Center. Reprinted from Pavlisko EN, Sporn TA (2014) Mesothelioma. Chapter 5. In: Pathology of Asbestos-Associated Diseases, 3rd ed., Oury TD, Sporn TA, Roggli VL, eds. Springer: New York, NY, Fig. 5.4, with permission)

viscous material within the lung and pleura. At late stage, the contralateral pleural cavity and peritoneum may become involved. Parenchymal lung involvement in the form of tumor masses is not common, and the presence of a dominant intraparenchymal lung mass should raise the possibility of an alternative diagnosis. Similarly, it is the exceptional case of mesothelioma whose gross distribution is that of a large and localized mass, although these have been described (Allen et al. 2005; Crotty et al. 1994; Obers et al. 1988).

The pleurotropic gross distribution of pleural mesothelioma (Fig. 6.1), while distinctive, is not pathognomonic of the entity. There are other malignant neoplasms, both primary within the lung and metastatic to the lung and pleura, that may display such characteristic pleurotropic growth. The term "pseudomesotheliomatous adenocarcinoma" has been proposed for primary pulmonary adenocarcinomas originating in the extreme periphery of the lung and disseminating through the pleura (Hammar 1994; Koss et al. 1992). Attanoos and Gibbs described a series of pseudomesotheliomatous carcinomas, and they found that the majority of tumors represented pleurotropic growth of pulmonary adenocarcinomas. A small number of those cases represented metastasis from extrathoracic sites such as the genitourinary tract, pancreas, and salivary gland (Attanoos and Gibbs 2003). In addition to some carcinomas, angiosarcomas and the closely related epithelioid hemangioendotheliomas originating in the pleura may display pleurotropic growth (Sporn et al. 2002).

Pleural mesotheliomas most commonly metastasize via the lymphovasculature to hilar and mediastinal lymph node stations, yet spread may also be hematogenous. Clinically evident metastatic disease outside the thorax is not common at time of diagnosis, but is detected at autopsy in at least 50% of cases (Churg et al. 2006). Mesothelioma also shows a propensity for growth in subcutaneous tracks and surgical wounds following needle biopsy or ports for thoracoscopy, which necessitates the excision of such when surgical debulking of tumor takes place. Mesotheliomas are only rarely localized, and these tend to have a better prognosis as they lack the diffuse infiltrative pleurotropic growth (Nakas et al. 2008).

6.1.2   Peritoneal Mesothelioma

Peritoneal mesotheliomas grow in a similar manner (Fig. 6.2), tend to form bulky nodules invading omentum and can be distributed widely through the peritoneal cavity, often accompanied by ascites. As within the pleura, this growth pattern is not pathognomonic. By gross morphology alone, malignant mesothelioma cannot be distinguished from peritoneal carcinomatosis. With advanced disease, mesothelioma may encase the abdominal viscera and demonstrate extramural invasion into viscera, particularly in the bowel. Rarely, these tumors may be discovered microscopically (incidentally) at a very early stage during histologic examination of surgical specimens sampling colon, ovary, and uterus. In a series of 13 sarcomatoid peritoneal mesotheliomas, presenting symptoms in women mimicked acute cholecystitis while men presented with abdominal pain, increased abdominal girth and weight loss (Pavlisko and Roggli 2015). As one might expect, bowel obstruction from tumor may occur leading to clinical presentation.

Malignant peritoneal mesothelioma must be distinguished from other tumors that result in peritoneal carcinomatosis, particularly those serous papillary carcinomas arising from Müllerian epithelium and tumors of renal origin. As pleural mesotheliomas may also seed the peritoneal membranes and vice versa, knowledge of the gross distribution of disease on either side of the diaphragm is necessary in establishing site of origin. Similar to pleural mesotheliomas, distant metastases from peritoneal mesotheliomas are seldom of clinical significance, although they may be detected postmortem.

6.1.3   Other Mesothelioma

Mesothelioma rarely involves the vaginalis testis and pericardium. Mesotheliomas involving the tunica vaginalis testis, an outpouching of abdominal peritoneum, are usually focal abnormalities which may mimic the benign condition of inguinal hernia or hydrocele or present as a paratesticular mass. Despite focality, these uncommon tumors may behave aggressively and metastasize (Jones et al. 1995). Pericardial mesotheliomas have gross morphology similar to that of their pleural and peritoneal counterparts with eventual fusion of pericardium to epicardium and rind-like encasement of the heart (Fig. 6.3). Presenting symptomatology can include shortness of breath and dyspnea on exertion secondary to a pericardial effusion, mimicking constrictive pericarditis and congestive heart failure (Churg et al. 2006).

Well-differentiated papillary mesotheliomas (WDPM) more commonly involve the peritoneum of young women, often as incidental findings at abdominal or pelvic surgery, and are not generally related to an exposure to asbestos (Daya and McCaughey 1990). They may be unifocal or multifocal and importantly lack stromal invasion. WDPM rarely arises from the pleura, and may radiographically be observed as unilateral pleural effusions without nodularity. If numerous, WDPM may impart a granular or velvety gross appearance to the pleura. There is no sex predominance with pleural WDPM (Galateau-Salle et al. 2004). There are case reports of WDPM of the tunica vaginalis testis (Erdogan et al. 2014; Manganiello et al. 2014; Tan et al. 2016). WDPM is frequently asymptomatic and tends to pursue an indolent clinical course (Butnor et al. 2001; Galateau-Salle et al. 2004; Hoekstra et al. 2005).

6.2   Histopathology

Malignant mesothelioma is characterized by a broad range of microscopic appearances and features, both across the spectrum of the disease entity and within individual tumors. The World Health Organization recognizes three basic subtypes: epithelioid, sarcomatoid, and biphasic (Travis et al. 2015). The desmoplastic variant is considered a subtype of sarcomatoid mesothelioma. The "epithelioid" designation (as opposed to "epithelial") is not without controversy as mesotheliomas are most properly considered neoplasms originating in the epithelium of the serosal membrane.

Within the pleura the epithelial subtype of mesothelioma predominates, accounting for 50% of cases. The biphasic and sarcomatoid subtypes of pleural mesotheliomas account for 30 and 20%, respectively (Roggli et al. 1987). The representation of mesothelioma subtypes within the peritoneum differs from that of the pleura. Churg and Kannerstein reported 75% epithelioid, 24% biphasic, and 1% sarcomatoid subtype in a series of peritoneal mesotheliomas (Kannerstein and Churg 1977). The histomorphology of malignant mesothelioma subtypes is not significantly different in pleural, peritoneal, or pericardial locations.

6.2.1   Epithelial Mesothelioma

The epithelial variant may demonstrate a variety of histologic growth patterns including trabecular, tubulopapillary (Fig. 6.5a, b), and solid (Fig. 6.5c) (Churg et al. 2006; Travis et al. 2015). Epithelial mesotheliomas often demonstrate histomorphologic heterogeneity and may incorporate different combinations of trabecular, tubulopapillary, and solid patterns. Tubulopapillary consists of branching tubules (Fig. 6.5a) and short papillary structures (with true fibrovascular cores)

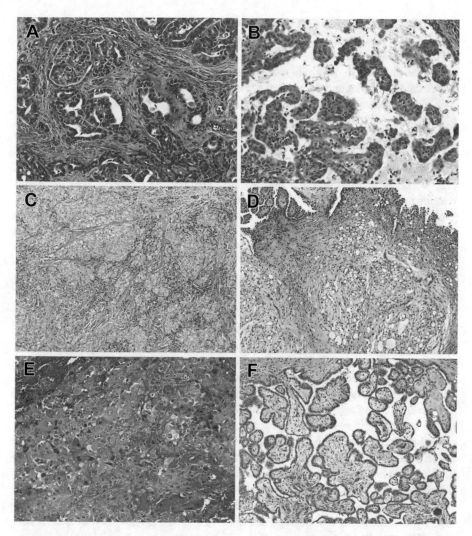

Fig. 6.5 Histologic patterns of the epithelial variant of malignant (diffuse) mesothelioma. (**a, b**) Tubulopapillary. (**c**) Solid. (**d**) Adenomatoid (microcystic) pattern. (**e**) Pleomorphic pattern of epithelial mesothelioma. (**f**) Well-differentiated papillary pattern. H&E: Parts (**a, c, e**): 20×; Parts (**b, d, f**): 10×

lined by flat or cuboidal tumor cells (Fig. 6.5b). Unlike papillary carcinomas arising from other organ systems, columnar tumor cells are not common. Psammoma bodies may be observed in some 5–10% of mesotheliomas with papillary morphology (Attanoos and Gibbs 1997). However, the existence of large numbers of psammoma bodies suggests papillary adenocarcinoma. This is especially the case in tumors involving the peritoneum, and immunohistochemical stains are necessary to confirm the tumor's tissue of origin. Micropapillary histomorphology consists of tufts of tumor cells lacking true fibrovascular cores.

The cytologic features of most epithelial mesotheliomas include cuboidal or polygonal shape with moderate to abundant cytoplasm and paracentric nuclei, bland vesicular chromatin, and occasional prominent nucleoli. Higher-grade mesotheliomas display prominent nucleoli, which along with atypical mitoses and elevated mitotic count were demonstrated by Kadota to correlate with survival (Kadota et al. 2012). While the pleomorphic pattern of epithelial mesothelioma is recognized, extreme cytologic atypia, with anaplastic or extremely pleomorphic cells, is not typical of epithelial mesothelioma. Multinucleate forms and occasional mitoses may be observed, but atypical mitoses are extremely uncommon. The epithelial variant most closely mimics adenocarcinoma, and this distinction becomes more problematic with the mesotheliomas that show higher degrees of cytologic atypia and pleomorphism. The diagnosis of malignant mesothelioma on cytologic grounds alone is controversial as reactive mesothelial proliferations can demonstrate considerable cytologic atypia.

Somewhat less common histomorphologic patterns of epithelial mesothelioma include the adenomatoid, deciduoid, and small cell variants. The adenomatoid variant, also termed microcystic, shows microglandular growth with lumina containing hyaluronic acid, closely mimicking adenomatoid tumors (Fig. 6.5d). The small cell variant superficially resembles small cell carcinoma, but generally lacks necrosis, elevated mitotic rate and other distinctive histomorphologic features of true small cell carcinoma. Deciduoid mesothelioma was originally described as aggressive peritoneal tumors of young women, unrelated to asbestos exposure (Ordonez 2012a, b). Features include sheets of large, round to polygonal cells with abundant cytoplasm superficially resembling the uterine decidual reaction. This variant has been described in men as well, involving both pleura and peritoneum, and has been reported in association with asbestos exposure in a number of cases (Nascimento et al. 1994; Shanks et al. 2000). Two subsets of deciduoid mesotheliomas have been described which differ in terms of survival. While both subsets demonstrate the typical deciduoid cytomorphology described above, pleomorphism, elevated mitotic activity, and loss of cell cohesion were observed by Ordonez to confer shorter survival (Ordonez 2012a).

Still other variants of epithelial mesothelioma include the pleomorphic, adenoid cystic, and clear cell forms. The pleomorphic variant is exceptional amongst the other epithelial histologies in view of its high cytologic grade, nuclear pleomorphism, and mitotic activity (Fig. 6.5e), and is apt to be confused with pleomorphic carcinomas of the lung or epithelioid sarcomas involving the pleura.

6.2.2   Well-Differentiated Papillary Mesothelioma

WDPM is classified separately by the WHO (Travis et al. 2015). Butnor et al. described a series of 14 cases of WDPM that included 7 pleural tumors and 1 from the tunica vaginalis testis. The histologic features of WDPM are those of prominent

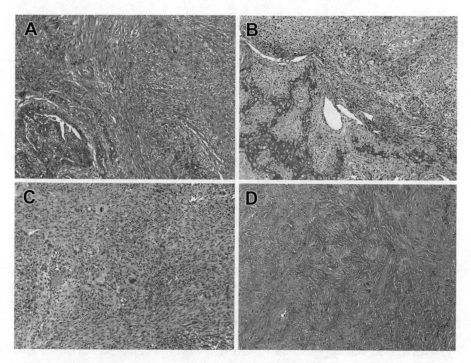

Fig. 6.6 Histologic patterns of biphasic and sarcomatoid variant of malignant (diffuse) mesothelioma. (**a**) Biphasic mesothelioma. (**b**) Mesothelioma with heterologous elements, including osetosarcomatous and chondrosarcomatous. (**c**) Pleomorphic variant of sarcomatoid mesothelioma. (**d**) Desmoplastic variant of sarcomatoid mesothelioma. H&E: All parts (**a–d**): 10×

fibrovascular cores lined by a single layer of relatively uniform cuboidal cells with minimal nuclear atypia, no mitoses, and no stromal invasion (Fig. 6.5f). Death from WDPM has been reported following demonstration of invasion, and such cases should be classified as true epithelial mesothelioma.

6.2.3   Biphasic Mesothelioma

The biphasic subtype of malignant mesothelioma, consisting of both epithelial and sarcomatoid subtypes is quite distinctive (Fig. 6.6a). Each pattern must account for at least 10% of the tumor (Travis et al. 2015). The distinction from a fibrosing serosal reaction to the presence of epithelial mesothelioma or epithelial mesothelioma invading pleural plaque makes the identification of a true sarcomatoid component challenging.

6.2.4   Sarcomatoid Mesothelioma

The least common histologic subtype of mesothelioma is sarcomatoid. Tumor cells are discohesive, elongate to spindled and may be bland or show considerable pleomorphism and mitotic activity. Similar to the epithelial subtype, sarcomatoid mesothelioma is heterogeneous and multiple patterns may be observed within an individual tumor. Growth patterns can consist of broad fascicles or storiform growth that mimics other typical soft tissue sarcomas such as osteogenic sarcoma, leiomyosarcoma, neurogenic sarcomas, and dedifferentiated chondrosarcoma. Mesotheliomas may show foci of osseous metaplasia, but true heterologous elements consisting of foci showing osteo- or chondrosarcomatous differentiation have also been described in otherwise typical malignant mesotheliomas (Fig. 6.6b). Klebe and colleagues described a series of malignant mesotheliomas with heterologous elements; only one case demonstrated epithelial histology, the remaining 26 being biphasic or sarcomatoid (Klebe et al. 2008).

There are several other morphologic subtypes within sarcomatoid mesothelioma that are recognized: pleomorphic, lymphohistiocytoid, transitional and desmoplastic mesothelioma. Pleomorphic sarcomatoid mesothelioma (Fig. 6.6c) has features otherwise typical of the sarcomatoid variant with discohesive, ovoid to spindled cells but the degree of cytologic atypia is greatly magnified. This pattern should be distinguished from its similarly named counterpart, pleomorphic epithelial mesothelioma.

The lymphohistiocytoid variant of sarcomatoid mesothelioma consists of large histiocytoid cells admixed with a dense lymphoplasmacellular infiltrate in a background of frankly sarcomatoid tumor. Transitional mesothelioma references those tumors whose plump spindle cells are cytologically bland, making their distinction from epithelial mesothelioma difficult. Clinically, their behavior is similar to that of other sarcomatoid mesothelioma variants.

A diagnostically challenging and rare pattern of sarcomatoid mesothelioma is the desmoplastic variant. While foci of desmoplastic growth may be seen in sarcomatoid mesotheliomas, true desmoplastic malignant mesothelioma (DMM), as described in detail below, constitutes approximately 10% of all malignant mesotheliomas. The deceptive nature of DMM lies in its mimic of benign and reactive processes, typically the fibrosing serositis that may occur in post-operative or post-inflammatory conditions. DMM is typically far less cellular than its sarcomatoid counterparts, and features largely hyalinized and collagenous stroma (Fig. 6.6d). DMM was originally described by Kannerstein and Churg (1980); specific diagnostic criteria were introduced by Mangano et al. (1998). The most striking feature of this paucicellular tumor is the whorled and twisted array of distinct collagen bundles, forming the "patternless pattern" of Stout (1965). The storiform pattern can be found at least focally as a component of a large percentage of malignant mesotheliomas, so the term is restricted to cases in which this pattern predominates (Adams and Unni 1984).

The diagnostic criteria for desmoplastic mesothelioma includes >50% of the tumor must consist of this dense collagen organized in a storiform or patternless pattern and at least one of the following four features. (1) Invasion of subpleural

Fig. 6.7 Sarcomatoid subtype of malignant mesothelioma. (**a**) Tumor with atypical spindled cells invading adipose tissue. (**b**) Cytokeratin cocktail (AE1/3, CAM5.2, MNF.116) demonstrating invasion of adipose tissue by spindled tumor cells. H&E and cytokeratin cocktail: 10×

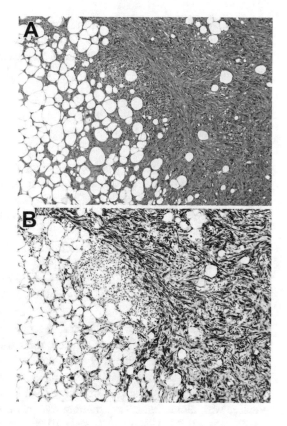

adipose tissue, chest wall, or lung by neoplastic spindle cells. This may be facilitated by cytokeratin immunostains (Fig. 6.7a, b), but mere expression of cytokeratins by the spindle cells within the lesion does not suffice to establish the diagnosis, as cytokeratin immunostaining may be observed in reactive processes as well. Cytokeratin staining must be present within subpleural tissue to be considered diagnostic, (2) "Bland" tumor necrosis. This is defined as foci of necrotic tumor with minimal associated inflammatory infiltrate. Necrosis may be detected by karyorrhexis and subtle changes in the tinctorial quality of the fibrosis, (3) Frankly sarcomatoid foci. This is evidenced by alternation of paucicellular zones with those of denser spindled cellularity. Areas of increased cytologic atypia may assist in the distinction of frankly sarcomatoid foci. The demonstration of mitoses is not particularly useful, as these are not numerous in either fibrosing pleuritis or desmoplastic mesothelioma and (4) Distant metastases with boney metastases being particularly common (Galateau-Salle et al. 2016; Husain et al. 2013; Mangano et al. 1998). In addition to these specific criteria, other helpful findings which favor a reactive process include (1) demonstration of a "top heavy" cellularity in benign reactions, where there is a crescendo of cellularity toward the luminal aspect of the pleura and (2) presence of numerous capillaries oriented perpendicularly with respect to pleura, diffusely through the thickness of the pleura (Churg et al. 2000). Tumors that have greater than 10% but less than 50% desmoplastic components may be classified as sarcomatoid mesothelioma with desmoplastic features, or sarcomatoid and desmoplastic variants.

6.3 Histochemistry

Approximately two thirds of pulmonary adenocarcinomas produce neutral mucin, and approximately one quarter of epithelial mesotheliomas produce hyaluronic acid, in quantities readily visible on hematoxylin and eosin (H&E)-stained sections. These observations provide the basis for the histochemical distinction between epithelial mesothelioma and pulmonary adenocarcinoma (Roggli et al. 1987). Neutral mucin stains positive with periodic acid-Schiff (PAS) and is distinguishable from cytoplasmic glycogen by predigestion of the section with diastase, which removes glycogen. Similarly, alcian blue stains a variety of acid mucopolysaccharides, and the staining is made specific for hyaluronic acid by prior treatment of the section with hyaluronidase.

In mucin-positive adenocarcinomas, the mucin secretions may be seen within glandular spaces, in the apex of tall columnar tumor cells, or as vacuoles within individual tumor cells. With PAS stain, the secretions typically stain dark red and often have a spidery appearance (Fig. 6.8a). Such adenocarcinomas also usually produce acid mucopolysaccharides other than hyaluronic acid, and therefore stain positive with alcian blue. This staining remains after treatment with hyaluronidase (McCaughey 1965; Aisner and Wiernik 1978; Craighead et al. 1982; Hillerdal 1983; Roggli et al. 1987; Hammar 1994; Attanoos and Gibbs 1997; Corson 1997; Churg 1998; Magnani et al. 2000).

The secretions visible on H&E in epithelial mesotheliomas may be present within tubular lumens, microcystic spaces or cytoplasmic vacuoles within individual tumor cells. They typically have a wispy basophilic appearance on H&E. These secretions stain positive with alcian blue (Fig. 6.8b), staining of which is abolished by pretreatment with hyaluronidase (Fig. 6.8c). They are negative with PAS following digestion with diastase (Fig. 6.8d) (McCaughey 1965; Aisner and Wiernik 1978; Craighead et al. 1982; Hillerdal 1983; Roggli et al. 1987; Hammar 1994; Attanoos and Gibbs 1997; Churg 1998).

As a practical matter, we only use histochemistry when there are obvious secretions on H&E. This is because the yield is extremely low when secretions are not visible on H&E. Histochemistry is especially useful when there are visible secretions and the results of immunohistochemistry (see below) are ambiguous. PAS with diastase is especially useful in the distinction between serous papillary carcinoma of the ovary or peritoneum and peritoneal mesothelioma. This is due to the fact that there is significant overlap in the immunohistochemical profile of these malignancies. Histochemistry is of no use in the diagnosis of sarcomatoid or desmoplastic mesothelioma.

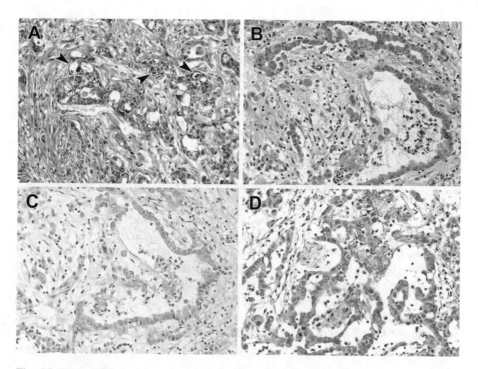

Fig. 6.8 Epithelial mesothelioma versus adenocarcinoma. (**a**) Adenocarcinoma shows positive staining with PAS following diastase digestion, with a spidery appearance within cytoplasmic vacuoles (*arrows*) indicative of neutral mucin. (**b**) Epithelial mesothelioma with microcystic pattern showing intense intraluminal staining for alcian blue. (**c**) Serial section treated with hyaluronidase showing abolished staining, indicating that the material is hyaluronic acid. (**d**) Serial section stained with PAS following diastase digestion shows no appreciable staining, indicating an absence of neutral mucin. Part (**a**): 10×; Parts (**b–d**): 20×

There are several pitfalls of which the reader should be aware. We do not use mucicarmine to make the histochemical distinction between mesothelioma and mucinous adenocarcinoma. This is because in some cases of mesothelioma, hyaluronic acid stains positive for mucicarmine, giving a false impression of neutral mucin production. In addition, one must use caution in interpreting PAS with diastase stains, since basal lamina material stains positive and hence may be confused with neutral mucin. This is especially the case for some papillary variants of mesothelioma where there is excess basal lamina material at the core of the papilla. Also, incomplete removal of glycogen by diastase may lead to a false positive interpretation. Hence controls should be run in parallel.

Finally, there have been a number of reports in the literature of mucin-positive mesotheliomas (MacDougall et al. 1992; Hammar 1994; Cook et al. 2000). In our experience, these are quite uncommon (less than 1% of cases). This unusual variant has been attributed to the production of crystallized proteoglycans which aberrantly stain for PAS following diastase (Hammar et al. 1996). The material is also resistant to hyaluronidase digestion and therefore alcian blue staining persists after treatment with this enzyme. One should only make a diagnosis of mucin-positive mesothelioma when all other diagnostic modalities (immunohistochemistry and/or ultrastructure) support the diagnosis of mesothelioma.

6.4 Immunohistochemistry

In addition to the gross distribution of tumor and histomorphology, securing the diagnosis of mesothelioma may necessitate the use of confirmatory immunohistochemical stains. These are often most helpful in tumors with epithelial morphology and become less helpful due to loss of antigen expression with progression of tumors to biphasic and sarcomatoid morphology. As there is no marker with complete sensitivity and specificity for mesothelioma, it is recommended that a panel of at least two positive (mesothelioma) markers and two negative markers be employed when distinguishing mesothelioma from other malignant neoplasms involving the thoracic cavity or peritoneum (Husain et al. 2013). Of course, the negative markers chosen should be reflective of the differential diagnosis based on histomorphology, gross distribution of tumor, and clinical history.

6.4.1 Cytokeratins

Cytokeratins form intermediate filaments found in the cytoplasm of benign, reactive, and malignant epithelial cells and mesothelium. Broad-spectrum cytokeratin (CK) cocktails, including those of both high and low molecular weights, are of great utility in determining if a tumor is of epithelial or mesothelial origin. Mesotheliomas have been described to express cytokeratins 4, 5, 6, 14, and 17 (Wick et al. 1990). From a practical perspective, we use an anticytokeratin cocktail consisting of AE1/AE3, CAM5.2, and MNF.116.

Cytokeratins 5/6 (Fig. 6.9a) can assist in the distinction between mesothelioma and pulmonary adenocarcinoma, but not squamous cell carcinoma or large cell carcinoma of lung (Miettinen and Sarlomo-Rikala 2003; Comin et al. 2014). Ordonez described positive immunoreactivity in 100% of 40 epithelial mesotheliomas, whereas 30 pulmonary adenocarcinomas were non-immunoreactive (Ordonez 1998). Later studies demonstrated slightly less sensitivity and specificity for CK5/6 in the distinction between two tumors (Cury et al. 2000; Chu and Weiss 2002). Cytokeratin 7 is expressed by pulmonary and mammary adenocarcinomas as well as mesotheliomas, and thus is not useful in the distinction between these tumors involving the pleura.

While cytokeratins do not distinguish benign from malignant epithelial or mesothelial cells, they are useful in that they can assist in demonstrating tissue invasion, a feature of malignancy. Our experience is that 100% of epithelial and biphasic

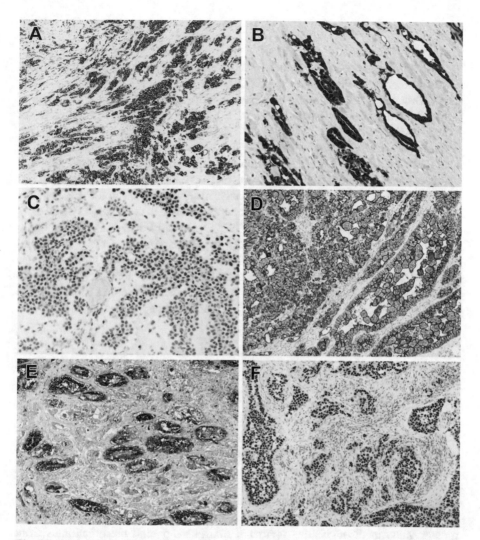

Fig. 6.9 Mesothelioma immunostaining. (**a**) Strong cytoplasmic staining of an epithelial mesothelioma for cytokeratins 5/6. (**b**) Strong nuclear and cytoplasmic staining of an epithelial mesothelioma for calretinin. (**c**) Nuclear staining of WT1 in same peritoneal mesothelioma. (**d**) Membranous staining of epithelial mesothelioma for D2-40. (**e**) Adenocarcinoma showing positive staining for carcinoembryonic antigen (CEA). (**f**) Adenocarcinoma showing strong nuclear staining for thyroid transcription factor-1 (TTF-1). Parts (**a, c–f**): 10×; Part (**b**): 20×

mesotheliomas of pleural and peritoneal locations stain positively for an anticytokeratin cocktail. This drops to 92% with sarcomatoid mesothelioma, pleural and peritoneal combined (Pavlisko and Sporn 2014). Immunoreactivity for cytokeratin is useful in excluding tumors such as melanoma, lymphoma, and epithelioid hemangioendothelioma. It should be remembered that there are some sarcomas, such as synovial sarcoma and epithelioid angiosarcoma, that can show patchy reactivity for cytokeratins.

6.4.2 Calretinin

Calretinin is a member of the cytoplasmic calcium-binding protein family, and is a useful marker in the diagnosis of mesothelioma (Doglioni et al. 1996; Mimura et al. 2007; Ordonez 2013a). In our experience, it is expressed in a high percentage of epithelial and biphasic mesotheliomas, 97% and 90%, respectively, and to a lesser extent in sarcomatoid mesotheliomas at 47% (Pavlisko and Sporn 2014). This corresponds to what has been reported in the literature (Ordonez 2013a, b, c, d). Calretinin's specificity for mesothelioma is better with nuclear staining, although concurrent cytoplasmic staining is also seen (Fig. 6.8b). Calretinin expression has been reported in a small subset of mammary carcinoma (higher grade, ER negative and basal type) as well as in 1/3 of thymic carcinomas (Pan et al. 2003; Powell et al. 2011), lung carcinoma (Doglioni et al. 1996; Oates and Edwards 2000; Miettinen and Sarlomo-Rikala 2003; Ordonez 2003), serous carcinoma (Cathro and Stoler 2005; Ordonez 2006a) and in a very small number of renal cell carcinomas (Osborn et al. 2002). One should use caution as metastatic breast carcinoma or thymic carcinoma may be misinterpreted as malignant mesothelioma if calretinin and CK5/6 are relied upon too heavily. Negative staining is evidence against the diagnosis of epithelial mesothelioma.

6.4.3 WT1

WT1, also known as Wilms Tumor suppressor gene protein, demonstrates positive nuclear staining (Fig. 6.8c) in approximately 43–100% of malignant epithelial mesotheliomas (Amin et al. 1995; Kumar-Singh et al. 1997; Ordonez 2002). Our experience is that WT1 positively stains 91% of epithelial pleural and peritoneal mesotheliomas as well as 80% and 50% of pleural and peritoneal biphasic malignant mesotheliomas, respectively (Pavlisko and Sporn 2014). As most ovarian serous carcinomas and some renal cell carcinomas stain positively, WT1 holds greater value in distinguishing epithelial malignant pleural mesotheliomas from lung adenocarcinomas and squamous cell carcinomas (Ordonez 2013a). In tumors of sarcomatoid morphology, we have found WT1 to be unhelpful in discriminating mesothelioma from other spindle cell tumors.

6.4.4 Podoplanin (D2-40)

Podoplanin or D2-40, an anti-podoplanin antibody, is a transmembrane glycoprotein of uncertain function (Ordonez 2006b). D2-40 demonstrates positive membranous cytoplasmic staining (Fig. 6.8d) in 72–96% of epithelial mesotheliomas (Chu et al. 2005; Ordonez 2005a, b; Pavlisko and Sporn 2014). We find it to be more useful than some of the other mesothelioma markers for mesotheliomas with sarco-matoid morphology with staining seen in 55% of our sarcomatoid mesothelioma cases (Pavlisko and Sporn 2014). In a series by Takeshima and colleagues, sarcoma-toid mesothelioma demonstrated immunoreactivity for D2-40 in 87% versus 26% of pulmonary sarcomatoid carcinomas (Takeshima et al. 2009). However, others have found D2-40 less helpful in making this distinction (Ordonez 2005a; Muller et al. 2006). Podoplanin is of value in distinguishing epithelial mesothelioma from lung adenocarcinoma. Other tumors with positive staining for podoplanin include lung squamous carcinoma and ovarian serous carcinomas.

6.4.5   Other Mesothelioma Markers

Mesothelin is a glycoprotein expressed on the cell surface of mesothelial cells. However, other tumors including non-mucinous ovarian, pancreatic, and extrahe-patic biliary tree carcinomas as well as transitional cell carcinoma, clear cell carci-noma and lung adenocarcinomas, also express mesothelin. Its rate of expression in triple-negative breast cancer was reported to be 56% and 3% in ER-positive breast cancer (Ordonez and Sahin 2014). As with calretinin, in tumors with epithelial mor-phology, negative staining for mesothelin should suggest another diagnosis.

Thrombomodulin is a cell surface glycoprotein that serves to abrogate the coagu-lation cascade. Thrombomodulin is expressed on vascular and lymphatic endothe-lial cells as well as on mesothelial cells, transitional cells, squamous cells, and syncytiotrophoblasts. A membranous pattern of staining is typically observed. Because there are other markers with higher sensitivity and specificity, we use thrombomodulin as a second line positive mesothelioma antibody if results of first line antibodies are equivocal. Caution should be use as angiosarcomas and epitheli-oid hemangioendotheliomas will stain positively for thrombomodulin.

HBME-1, a monoclonal antibody developed to well-differentiated epithelial mesothelioma, is not specific for mesothelium, as positive reactivity has been dem-onstrated in adenocarcinomas including thyroid papillary and follicular carcinomas and ovarian cystadenocarcinoma (Pan et al. 2003). Synovial sarcomas have also shown positive immunoreactivity for HBME-1 (Miettinen and Sarlomo-Rikala 2003). It holds limited utility, but some investigators continue to use HBME-1 at much higher dilutions (1:5000–15,000) than the manufacturer's recommendation (1:50) (Pavlisko and Sporn 2014). Negative staining for HBME-1 would argue against a diagnosis of epithelial mesothelioma.

6.4.6   Carcinoma Markers

Carcinoembryonic antigen (CEA), a glycoprotein, was one of the first antibodies used in the distinction of mesothelioma from other malignancies, as mesotheliomas are non-immunoreactive for CEA (Wang 1979). CEA (Fig. 6.9e) is expressed by a number of adenocarcinomas including those of lung (50–95%), gastrointestinal tract, breast, liver, and pancreas. It is not expressed by serous ovarian tumors, renal cell carcinoma, and carcinoma of the prostate limiting its utility in the peritoneum (Mezger et al. 1990; Garcia-Prats et al. 1998; Comin et al. 2001; Roberts et al. 2001; Abutaily et al. 2002; Ordonez 2003). While it has been reported that some mesotheliomas stain positively for CEA, newer and commercially available antibodies to CEA have improved specificity with some reduction in sensitivity (Sheibani et al. 1986a, b). We have not observed any false positive staining of mesotheliomas using a monoclonal antibody to CEA.

Ber-EP4, a monoclonal antibody derived from mice immunized with a cellular extract of breast cancer, has great utility in the ability to distinguish mesothelioma from adenocarcinoma. Ber-EP4 immunoreactivity has been reported in 100% of lung adenocarcinomas, 93% of non-lung adenocarcinomas, and only 26% of mesotheliomas (Ordonez 1989). We have observed occasional patchy staining for Ber-EP4 in 9% of our epithelial peritoneal mesotheliomas, but never strong/diffuse staining. This is consistent with results reported by others (Ordonez 1989). Of interest, renal cell carcinomas do not express Ber-EP4.

B72.3, a monoclonal antibody to tumor-associated glycoproteins derived from human breast cancer cells, will positively stain adenocarcinomas of lung as well as other adenocarcinomas. Positive immunoreactivity for B72.3 has been reported in 100% of lung adenocarcinomas and in 72–100% of serous ovarian tumors (Johnston et al. 1986; Johnston 1987; Rothacker and Mobius 1995; Bollinger et al. 1989; Gitsch et al. 1992). Renal cell carcinomas do not express B72.3 (Ordonez 2004). Focal immunoreactivity has been described in up to 5% of mesotheliomas, though most series observed no staining (Szpak et al. 1986; Bollinger et al. 1989; Ordonez 1989; Ordonez 2003). We observed no immunoreactivity in 48 peritoneal epithelial mesotheliomas and 3 peritoneal biphasic mesotheliomas (Pavlisko and Sporn 2014).

LeuM1 (CD15), a myelomonocytic antigen, was an early marker used in distinguishing carcinoma from mesothelioma. Immunoreactivity has been reported in 50–94% of lung adenocarcinomas and in 30–60% of non-lung adenocarcinomas with no immunoreactivity in mesotheliomas (Sheibani et al. 1986a, b; Ordonez 1989; Wick et al. 1990; Doglioni et al. 1996; Roberts et al. 2001; Ordonez 2003). Kao et al. report the benefit of non-immunoreactivity for LeuM1 in the distinction between malignant pleural mesotheliomas and carcinomas of other sites (Kao et al. 2011). In addition to carcinomas, such as renal cell carcinoma, both Hodgkin and non-Hodgkin lymphomas as well as leukemias have shown positive immunoreactivity (Sheibani et al. 1986a, b). Positive staining for LeuM1 would argue against the diagnosis of mesothelioma whereas negative staining is not as helpful.

MOC-31 is an antibody to EP-CAM formed using small cell lung carcinoma cells treated with neuraminidase (de Leij et al. 1984). MOC-31 has immunoreactivity in adenocarcinoma and squamous cell lung carcinomas with reported rates of 90–100% and 97%, respectively. Positive staining has also been demonstrated in 98% of serous ovarian/peritoneal tumors (Sosolik et al. 1997; Ordonez 2003; Ordonez 2006a). Of note, as with Ber-EP4, focal positive staining has been reported in 2–10% of mesotheliomas (Ruitenbeek et al. 1994; Riera et al. 1997; Ordonez

1998; Oates and Edwards 2000; Carella et al. 2001; Ordonez 2006a). Thus, diffuse (as opposed to focal) positive staining for this antibody would suggest a diagnosis other than mesothelioma.

6.5 Immunohistochemical Panels and Differential Diagnosis

As mentioned above, because there is no singular immunohistochemical stain with 100% specificity and sensitivity for malignant mesothelioma, a panel of antibodies is needed. We employ a panel of both positive and negative stains with a specificity of ≥80% as is recommended in the International Mesothelioma Interest Group guidelines for the diagnosis of mesothelioma (Husain et al. 2009; Husain et al. 2013). As the differential diagnosis varies by tumor morphology, location, gross distribution of tumor as well as the patient's clinical history, these panels should also vary by morphology and location reflecting common malignancies arising in each site (Table 6.1) (Pavlisko and Sporn 2014). The utility of BAP1 immunohisto-chemistry and fluorescence in situ hybridization (FISH) for the gene encoding 16INK4A is discussed below.

For pleurotropic epithelial tumors, malignant mesothelioma, pseudomesothelio-matous adenocarcinoma of lung and metastatic breast carcinoma are to be considered in the differential as well as other metastatic carcinomas. For peritoneal epithelial tumors, renal and genitourinary tumors enter the differential. In addition to markers typically positive in mesothelioma, we complete our panels with positive carcinoma markers including monoclonal CEA and TTF-1 (Fig. 6.9e, f) for pleural tumors and Ber-EP4 and B72.3 for peritoneal epithelial tumors.

Table 6.1 First and second line immunohistochemical panels for pleural and peritoneal locations with epithelial/biphasic or sarcomatoid morphology

	Epithelial and/or biphasic		Sarcomatoid
	Pleural	Peritoneal	
First line	Cytokeratin cocktail	Cytokeratin cocktail	Cytokeratin cocktail
	Cytokeratin 5/6	Cytokeratin 5/6	Vimentin
	Calretinin	Calretinin	Calretinin
	D2-40	D2-40	D2-40
	WT-1	WT-1	
	TTF-1	BerEP4	
	CEA	B72.3	
Second line	LeuM1	LeuM1	
	B72.3	Thrombomodulin	

Reprinted from Pavlisko EN, Sporn TA (2014) Mesothelioma. Chapter 5. In: Pathology of Asbestos-Associated Diseases, 3rd ed., Oury TD, Sporn TA, Roggli VL, eds. Springer: New York, NY. Table 5.3, with permission

If a renal or gynecologic primary is suspected, PAX8 and claudin-4 are helpful. Positive immunoreactivity for PAX 8 and claudin-4 were reported in 93% and 91% of metastatic renal cell carcinoma to pleura, respectively (Ordonez 2013d). For serous carcinomas of the peritoneum/ovary, 89 and 91% expressed PAX8 and claudin-4, whereas no immunoreactivity was seen for these two markers in epithelial mesotheliomas (Ordonez 2013c). Claudin-4 is also expressed by estrogen receptor (ER)-positive breast carcinomas as well as the triple-negative phenotype (Ordonez and Sahin 2014) and can assist in the differentiation of mesothelioma versus breast carcinoma. GATA3, a relatively newer antibody that has utility in identifying breast and renal/urinary tumors, has been reportedly positive in 28–58% of mesotheliomas, and thus is not of great utility in this arena (Miettinen et al. 2014; Ordonez and Sahin 2014). Ordonez investigated the value of ER and progesterone receptor (PR) in distinguishing peritoneal epithelial mesothelioma, WDPM, and adenomatoid tumor from serous carcinomas (metastatic and primary peritoneal). He observed that 86% of primary peritoneal carcinomas and 88% of metastatic serous carcinomas had positive immunoreactivity for ER with no staining of mesotheliomas or adenomatoid tumors. For PR, 56% of primary peritoneal serous carcinomas and 60% of metastatic serous carcinomas were immunoreactive with no staining observed in mesotheliomas and adenomatoid tumors (Ordonez 2005a, b). Thus, positive staining for ER and/or PR would assist in excluding mesothelioma while a negative stain is less helpful.

When biphasic morphology exists, biphasic synovial sarcoma and epithelioid angiosarcoma enter the differential diagnosis. Sarcomatoid morphology brings about a differential of both malignant and benign entities including fibrous pleurisy (fibrosing pleuritis), sarcomatoid variant of malignant mesothelioma, epithelioid hemangioendothelioma, solitary/localized fibrous tumor, monophasic synovial sarcoma, and other sarcomas. Most sarcomas tend to have negative or patchy reactivity for cytokeratins. It is our experience that an anticytokeratin cocktail in combination with vimentin performs best for sarcomatoid mesothelioma as the other markers tend to be lost. We observed positive immunoreactivity for D2-40 in 55% and calretinin in 47% of our sarcomatoid mesothelioma cases (Pavlisko and Sporn 2014).

6.6   Electron Microscopy

Mesothelial cells have long slender surface microvilli devoid of glycocalyx, a feature that is retained in many epithelial mesotheliomas. These microvilli tend to have a high aspect ratio (length to diameter), typically greater than 15. In contrast, pulmonary adenocarcinomas typically have short blunt microvilli, often associated with a fuzzy glycocalyx and intraluminal glycocalyceal bodies. The microvilli may also be associated with rootlets and typically have an aspect ratio that is less than 10. These observations form the basis for the ultrastructural diagnosis of malignant mesothelioma and its distinction from pulmonary adenocarcinoma (Wang 1973; Davis 1974; Warhol et al. 1982; Burns et al. 1985; Warhol and Corson 1985; Oury et al. 1998).

Table 6.2 Ultrastructure of mesothelioma versus adenocarcinoma

Mesothelioma	Adenocarcinoma
Long sinuous surface MV	Short stubby surface MV with glycocalyx
AR > 15	AR < 10
No glycocalyx	Glycocalyceal bodies
May abutt collagen fibers	May be associated with rootlets
Perinuclear tonofilaments	Tonofilaments not prominent but may be seen in AdSq Ca
Prominent macula adherens jcns	Prominent apical zona occludens (tight) jcns
Cytoplasmic crystalloid structures	Mucous granules, Clara cell granules

AdSq Ca adenosquamous carcinoma, *AR* aspect ratio, *jcns* junctions, *MV* microvilli

Other ultrastructural features commonly observed in epithelial mesotheliomas include perinuclear tonofilaments and well-formed macula-adherens (desmosomal) type intercellular junctions. Some epithelial mesotheliomas form long (greater than 1 μm in length) desmosomes, a feature which may be of diagnostic utility when present (Burns et al. 1988; Ghadially et al. 1995). In addition, some epithelial mesotheliomas have microvilli on the abluminal surface making direct contact with collagen fibers through defects in the basal lamina (Dewar et al. 1987). No single ultrastructural feature of mesothelioma is pathognomonic for the diagnosis. Rather, a constellation of ultrastructural findings tends to be supportive of the diagnosis (Table 6.2 and Fig. 6.10).

Certain ultrastructural features when present tend to detract from a diagnosis of mesothelioma. These include the finding of mucous granules, zymogen granules, Clara cell granules, premelanosomes, Weibel-Palade bodies, and dense core (neuroendocrine-type) granules. Mucous granules must be distinguished from crystalloids in the cytoplasm of some mesothelial cells associated with proteoglycan production (Hammar et al. 1996; Ordonez 2012b). Weibel-Palade bodies are indicative of endothelial differentiation and suggest a diagnosis of epithelioid hemangioendothelioma or angiosarcoma, whereas premelanosomes point towards a diagnosis of melanoma (Oury et al. 1998). Although the finding of dense core neurosecretory granules would favor a diagnosis of neuroendocrine carcinoma, it should be noted that we have identified such granules in the cytoplasm of tumor cells from one epithelial mesothelioma with small cell features (Fig. 6.11).

As epithelial mesotheliomas become more poorly differentiated, they may lose some of the distinctive ultrastructural features noted above. Thus, the absence of any or all of the typical fine structural details does not necessarily exclude a diagnosis of mesothelioma (Dardick et al. 1987). For sarcomatoid mesotheliomas, ultrastructural features are not usually helpful in coming to the correct diagnosis (Oury et al. 1998). Nonetheless, some sarcomatoid mesotheliomas may have intercellular junctions, occasional surface microvilli, partial or incomplete basal lamina, or even a few tonofilaments. These features, if present, would then support the diagnosis of mesothelioma (Klima and Bossart 1983).

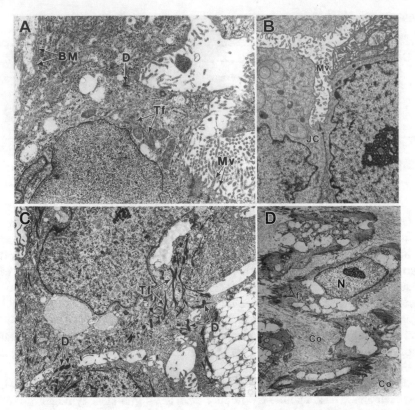

Fig. 6.10 Transmission electron microscopy of mesothelioma. (**a**) Epithelial mesothelioma with long sinuous surface microvilli (Mv), perinuclear tonofilaments (Tf), desmosomes (D), and basal lamina (BM). (**b**) Adenocarcinoma metastatic to the pleura shows blunt surface microvilli (Mv) and a junctional complex (JC). (**c**) Squamous cell carcinoma has prominent perinuclear tonofilaments (Tf) and prominent desmosomes (D). (**d**) Sarcomatoid mesothelioma consisting of spindle cells with cytoplasmic filaments (f) and abundant extracellular collagen (Co). N = nucleus. Transmission electron microscopy in (**a**): ×10,000, (**b, c**): ×6000, and (**d**): ×4000. (Reprinted from Pavlisko EN, Sporn TA (2014) Mesothelioma, Chapter 5. In: Pathology of Asbestos-Associated Diseases, 3rd ed., Oury TD, Sporn TA, Roggli VL, eds. Springer: New York, NY, Fig.5.14, with permission)

6.7 Molecular Analysis

The most frequent molecular alterations in mesothelioma include mutations of tumor suppressor genes encoding BRCA-associated protein-1 (BAP1), cyclin-dependent kinase inhibitor 2A (CDKN2A/p16INK4A) and neurofibromin 2 (NF2/Merlin) (Guo et al. 2015). *CDKN2A/p16INK4A* gene analysis via fluorescence in-situ hybridization (FISH) in conjunction with BAP1 staining via immunohistochemistry hold diagnostic utility, as recent studies have shown promise in distinguishing

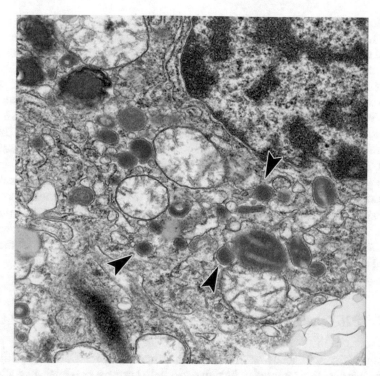

Fig. 6.11 Small cell variant of epithelial mesothelioma containing cytoplasmic structures consistent with dense core neurosecretory type granules (Ng). This tumor also stained positive for CD56 and TTF-1. Transmission electron microscopy: ×17,000

benign/reactive mesothelial processes from malignant mesothelioma (Sheffield et al. 2015; Hwang et al. 2016b). Studies have not explored NF2's utility for this purpose.

6.7.1 BAP1

BAP1, a nuclear deubiquitinase protein, is a tumor suppressor gene and has a number of functions including DNA double-strand break repair as well as gene expression and transcription. Pleural malignant mesotheliomas frequently have BAP1 loss, which can occur through point mutations, deletions, and insertions. Somatic point mutations are estimated to occur in up to about 65% of sporadic mesotheliomas and germline mutations in <5% (Nasu et al. 2015; Travis et al. 2015; Walts et al. 2016). Immunohistochemical staining holds strong utility as an accessible and reliable technique for the evaluation of BAP1 loss (McGregor et al. 2015; Nasu et al. 2015; Sheffield et al. 2015). When nuclear immunoreactivity for BAP1 is absent in a tumor, it is not possible to determine whether the mutation is of germline or somatic nature. However, immunohistochemistry is a useful screening tool for BAP1 loss in malignant mesothelioma, but gene sequencing on blood or other non-malignant tissue is necessary to determine if a germline mutation is present (Testa et al. 2011). Germline *BAP1* mutations occur in families with increased rates of various malignancies including malignant mesothelioma and melanocytic tumors (uveal melanoma, cutaneous melanoma and atypical Spitz tumors) (Testa et al. 2011; Wiesner et al. 2011; Abdel-Rahman et al. 2011; Wiesner et al. 2016; Ohar et al. 2016). This has been termed BAP1 cancer predisposition syndrome. Thus far, 67 families have been identified with 56 germline mutations described (Betti et al. 2016). The sensitivity for BAP1 loss via immunohistochemistry is approximately 50–70% for epithelial, 15–50% for biphasic, and 15–63% for sarcomatoid subtypes of mesothelioma (Churg et al. 2016a). The specificity has been reported at 100% (Cigognetti et al. 2015; McGregor et al. 2015; Sheffield et al. 2015). While a negative stain is helpful in distinguishing malignant mesothelioma from a benign/reactive mesothelial process, a positive stain does not exclude malignant mesothelioma (Churg et al. 2016a, b; Cigognetti et al. 2015).

6.7.2   P16 (Cyclin-Dependent Kinase Inhibitor 2A; CDKN2A)

Deletion of the 9p21 locus, where the tumor suppressor gene *CDKN2A/p16INK4A* resides, has not been reported in benign mesothelial processes (Galateau-Salle et al. 2016). Loss of *p16INK4A* is one of the most common genetic aberrations in malignant mesothelioma and has been reported in 33–100% of pleural mesotheliomas and in 14–51% of peritoneal mesotheliomas. The incidence is higher in malignant mesothelioma with sarcomatoid morphology (Churg et al. 2016b). Homozygous loss of *p16INK4A* detected through FISH holds value in separating benign/reactive from malignant mesothelial proliferations (Sheffield et al. 2015; Galateau-Salle et al. 2016; Hwang et al. 2016b; Walts et al. 2016). The reader should be cautioned that p16INK4A immunohistochemistry cannot be substituted for FISH and that the diagnostic finding is homozygous loss (not heterozygous loss of *p16INK4A*) (Galateau-Salle et al. 2016). As with a negative BAP1 test (retention of BAP1 nuclear staining), a negative *p16INK4A* test (heterozygous loss or wild type *p16INK4A*) does not help exclude malignant mesothelioma. In combination, BAP1 immunohistochemistry and FISH for homozygous loss of *p16INK4A* can be helpful in separating benign/reactive from malignant mesothelial proliferations.

Declaration of Interests Drs. V.L. Roggli and T.A. Sporn consult with both plaintiff and defense attorneys in asbestos litigation. The other authors have no conflicts of interest.

References

Abdel-Rahman MH, Pilarski R, Cebulla CM et al (2011) Germline bap1 mutation predisposes to uveal melanoma, lung adenocarcinoma, meningioma, and other cancers. J Med Genet 48: 856–859

Abutaily AS, Addis BJ, Roche WR (2002) Immunohistochemistry in the distinction between malignant mesothelioma and pulmonary adenocarcinoma: a critical evaluation of new antibodies. J Clin Pathol 55:662–668

Adams VI, Unni KK (1984) Diffuse malignant mesothelioma of pleura: diagnostic criteria based on an autopsy study. Am J Clin Pathol 82:15–23

Aisner J, Wiernik PH (1978) Malignant mesothelioma. Current status and future prospects. Chest 74:438–444

Allen TC, Cagle PT, Churg AM et al (2005) Localized malignant mesothelioma. Am J Surg Pathol 29:866–873

Amin KM, Litzky LA, Smythe WR et al (1995) Wilms' tumor 1 susceptibility (WT1) gene products are selectively expressed in malignant mesothelioma. Am J Pathol 146:344–356

Attanoos RL, Gibbs AR (1997) Pathology of malignant mesothelioma. Histopathology 30: 403–418

Attanoos RL, Gibbs AR (2003) 'Pseudomesotheliomatous' carcinomas of the pleura: a 10-year analysis of cases from the environmental lung disease research group, Cardiff. Histopathology 43:444–452

Betti M, Aspesi A, Biasi A et al (2016) CDKN2A and BAP1 germline mutations predispose to melanoma and mesothelioma. Cancer Lett 378:120–130

Bollinger DJ, Wick MR, Dehner LP et al (1989) Peritoneal malignant mesothelioma versus serous papillary adenocarcinoma. A histochemical and immunohistochemical comparison. Am J Surg Pathol 13:659–670

Boutin C, Dumortier P, Rey F et al (1996) Black spots concentrate oncogenic asbestos fibers in the parietal pleura. Thoracoscopic and mineralogic study. Am J Respir Crit Care Med 153: 444–449

Burke A, Virmani R, Armed Forces Institute of Pathology (U.S.), et al (1996) Tumors of the heart and great vessels. Washington, D.C., Bethesda, MD, Published by the Armed Forces Institute of Pathology under the auspices of the Universities Associated for Research and Education in Pathology

Burns TR, Greenberg SD, Mace ML et al (1985) Ultrastructural diagnosis of epithelial malignant mesothelioma. Cancer 56:2036–2040

Burns TR, Johnson EH, Cartwright J Jr et al (1988) Desmosomes of epithelial malignant mesothelioma. Ultrastruct Pathol 12:385–388

Butnor KJ, Sporn TA, Hammar SP et al (2001) Well-differentiated papillary mesothelioma. Am J Surg Pathol 25:1304–1309

Carella R, Deleonardi G, D'Errico A et al (2001) Immunohistochemical panels for differentiating epithelial malignant mesothelioma from lung adenocarcinoma: a study with logistic regression analysis. Am J Surg Pathol 25:43–50

Cathro HP, Stoler MH (2005) The utility of calretinin, inhibin, and wt1 immunohistochemical staining in the differential diagnosis of ovarian tumors. Hum Pathol 36:195–201

Chu AY, Litzky LA, Pasha TL et al (2005) Utility of d2-40, a novel mesothelial marker, in the diagnosis of malignant mesothelioma. Mod Pathol 18:105–110

Chu PG, Weiss LM (2002) Expression of cytokeratin 5/6 in epithelial neoplasms: an immunohistochemical study of 509 cases. Mod Pathol 15:6–10

Churg A (1998) Neoplastic asbestos-induced disease. In: Churg A, Green FHY (eds) Pathology of occupational lung disease, 2nd edn. Williams & Wilkins, Baltimore, pp 339–392

Churg A, Attanoos R, Borczuk AC et al (2016a) Dataset for reporting of malignant mesothelioma of the pleura or peritoneum: recommendations from the international collaboration on cancer reporting (iccr). Arch Pathol Lab Med 140:1104–1110

Churg A, Cagle PT, Roggli VL (2006) Tumors of the serosal membranes. In: AFIP atlas of tumor pathology, 4th edn. American Registry of Pathology, Washington, DC

Churg A, Colby TV, Cagle P et al (2000) The separation of benign and malignant mesothelial proliferations. Am J Surg Pathol 24:1183–1200

Churg A, Sheffield BS, Galateau-Salle F (2016b) New markers for separating benign from malignant mesothelial proliferations: are we there yet? Arch Pathol Lab Med 140:318–321

Cigognetti M, Lonardi S, Fisogni S et al (2015) BAP1 (BRCA1-associated protein 1) is a highly specific marker for differentiating mesothelioma from reactive mesothelial proliferations. Mod Pathol 28:1043–1057

Comin CE, Novelli L, Boddi V et al (2001) Calretinin, thrombomodulin, CEA, and CD15: a useful combination of immunohistochemical markers for differentiating pleural epithelial mesothelioma from peripheral pulmonary adenocarcinoma. Hum Pathol 32:529–536

Comin CE, Novelli L, Cavazza A et al (2014) Expression of thrombomodulin, calretinin, cytokeratin 5/6, D2-40 and WT-1 in a series of primary carcinomas of the lung: an immunohistochemical study in comparison with epithelioid pleural mesothelioma. Tumori 100:559–567

Cook DS, Attanoos RL, Jalloh SS et al (2000) 'Mucin-positive' epithelial mesothelioma of the peritoneum: an unusual diagnostic pitfall. Histopathology 37:33–36

Corson JM (1997) Pathology of diffuse malignant pleural mesothelioma. Semin Thorac Cardiovasc Surg 9:347–355

Craighead JE, Abraham JL, Churg A et al (1982) The pathology of asbestos-associated diseases of the lungs and pleural cavities: diagnostic criteria and proposed grading schema. Report of the pneumoconiosis committee of the College of American Pathologists and the National Institute for Occupational Safety and Health. Arch Pathol Lab Med 106:544–596

Crotty TB, Myers JL, Katzenstein AL et al (1994) Localized malignant mesothelioma. A clinicopathologic and flow cytometric study. Am J Surg Pathol 18:357–363

Cury PM, Butcher DN, Fisher C et al (2000) Value of the mesothelium-associated antibodies thrombomodulin, cytokeratin 5/6, calretinin, and CD44H in distinguishing epithelioid pleural mesothelioma from adenocarcinoma metastatic to the pleura. Mod Pathol 13:107–112

Dardick I, Jabi M, McCaughey WT et al (1987) Diffuse epithelial mesothelioma: a review of the ultrastructural spectrum. Ultrastruct Pathol 11:503–533

Davis JM (1974) Ultrastructure of human mesotheliomas. J Natl Cancer Inst 52:1715–1725

Daya D, McCaughey WT (1990) Well-differentiated papillary mesothelioma of the peritoneum. A clinicopathologic study of 22 cases. Cancer 65:292–296

de Leij L, Poppema S, Nulend JK et al (1984) Immunoperoxidase staining on frozen tissue sections as a first screening assay in the preparation of monoclonal antibodies directed against small cell carcinoma of the lung. Eur J Cancer Clin Oncol 20:123–128

Dewar A, Valente M, Ring NP et al (1987) Pleural mesothelioma of epithelial type and pulmonary adenocarcinoma: an ultrastructural and cytochemical comparison. J Pathol 152:309–316

Doglioni C, Dei Tos AP, Laurino L et al (1996) Calretinin: a novel immunocytochemical marker for mesothelioma. Am J Surg Pathol 20:1037–1046

Erdogan S, Acikalin A, Zeren H et al (2014) Well-differentiated papillary mesothelioma of the tunica vaginalis: a case study and review of the literature. Korean J Pathol 48:225–228

Galateau-Salle F, Churg A, Roggli V et al (2016) The 2015 world health organization classification of tumors of the pleura: advances since the 2004 classification. J Thorac Oncol 11:142–154

Galateau-Salle F, Vignaud JM, Burke L et al (2004) Well-differentiated papillary mesothelioma of the pleura: a series of 24 cases. Am J Surg Pathol 28:534–540

Garcia-Prats MD, Ballestin C, Sotelo T et al (1998) A comparative evaluation of immunohistochemical markers for the differential diagnosis of malignant pleural tumours. Histopathology 32:462–472

Ghadially FN, Rippstein PU, Cavell S et al (1995) Giant desmosomes in tumors. Ultrastruct Pathol 19:469–474

Gitsch G, Tabery U, Feigl W et al (1992) The differential diagnosis of primary peritoneal papillary tumors. Arch Gynecol Obstet 251:139–144

Gossinger HD, Siostrzonek P, Zangeneh M et al (1988) Magnetic resonance imaging findings in a patient with pericardial mesothelioma. Am Heart J 115:1321–1322

Guo G, Chmielecki J, Goparaju C et al (2015) Whole-exome sequencing reveals frequent genetic alterations in BAP1, NF2, CDKN2A, and CUL1 in malignant pleural mesothelioma. Cancer Res 75:264–269

Hammar SP (1994) The pathology of benign and malignant pleural disease. Chest Surg Clin North Am 4:405–430

Hammar SP, Bockus DE, Remington FL et al (1996) Mucin-positive epithelial mesotheliomas: a histochemical, immunohistochemical, and ultrastructural comparison with mucin-producing pulmonary adenocarcinomas. Ultrastruct Pathol 20:293–325

Hillerdal G (1983) Malignant mesothelioma 1982: review of 4710 published cases. Br J Dis Chest 77:321–343

Hoekstra AV, Riben MW, Frumovitz M et al (2005) Well-differentiated papillary mesothelioma of the peritoneum: a pathological analysis and review of the literature. Gynecol Oncol 98:161–167

Husain AN, Colby T, Ordonez N et al (2013) Guidelines for pathologic diagnosis of malignant mesothelioma: 2012 update of the consensus statement from the international mesothelioma interest group. Arch Pathol Lab Med 137:647–667

Husain AN, Colby TV, Ordonez NG et al (2009) Guidelines for pathologic diagnosis of malignant mesothelioma: a consensus statement from the international mesothelioma interest group. Arch Pathol Lab Med 133:1317–1331

Hwang HC, Pyott S, Rodriguez S et al (2016a) Bap1 immunohistochemistry and p16 FISH in the diagnosis of sarcomatous and desmoplastic mesotheliomas. Am J Surg Pathol 40:714–718

Hwang HC, Sheffield BS, Rodriguez S et al (2016b) Utility of BAP1 immunohistochemistry and p16 (CDKN2A) FISH in the diagnosis of malignant mesothelioma in effusion cytology specimens. Am J Surg Pathol 40:120–126

Johnston WW (1987) Applications of monoclonal antibodies in clinical cytology as exemplified by studies with monoclonal antibody B72.3. The George N. Papanicolaou Award Lecture. Acta Cytol 31:537–556

Johnston WW, Szpak CA, Thor A et al (1986) Phenotypic characterization of lung cancers in fine needle aspiration biopsies using monoclonal antibody B72.3. Cancer Res 46:6462–6470

Jones MA, Young RH, Scully RE (1995) Malignant mesothelioma of the tunica vaginalis. A clinicopathologic analysis of 11 cases with review of the literature. Am J Surg Pathol 19:815–825

Kadota K, Suzuki K, Colovos C et al (2012) A nuclear grading system is a strong predictor of survival in epithelioid diffuse malignant pleural mesothelioma. Mod Pathol 25:260–271

Kannerstein M, Churg J (1980) Desmoplastic diffuse mesothelioma. In: Fenoglio CM, Wolff M (eds) Progress in surgical pathology. Masson Pub, New York, pp 19–29

Kannerstein M, Churg J (1977) Peritoneal mesothelioma. Hum Pathol 8:83–94

Kao SC, Griggs K, Lee K et al (2011) Validation of a minimal panel of antibodies for the diagnosis of malignant pleural mesothelioma. Pathology 43:313–317

Klebe S, Mahar A, Henderson DW et al (2008) Malignant mesothelioma with heterologous elements: clinicopathological correlation of 27 cases and literature review. Mod Pathol 21:1084–1094

Klima M, Bossart MI (1983) Sarcomatous type of malignant mesothelioma. Ultrastruct Pathol 4:349–358

Koss M, Travis W, Moran C et al (1992) Pseudomesotheliomatous adenocarcinoma: a reappraisal. Semin Diagn Pathol 9:117–123

Kumar-Singh S, Segers K, Rodeck U et al (1997) WT1 mutation in malignant mesothelioma and WT1 immunoreactivity in relation to p53 and growth factor receptor expression, cell-type transition, and prognosis. J Pathol 181:67–74

MacDougall DB, Wang SE, Zidar BL (1992) Mucin-positive epithelial mesothelioma. Arch Pathol Lab Med 116:874–880

Magnani C, Agudo A, Gonzalez CA et al (2000) Multicentric study on malignant pleural mesothelioma and non-occupational exposure to asbestos. Br J Cancer 83:104–111

Manganiello M, Cassalman C, Dugan J et al (2014) Scrotal mesothelioma. Can J Urol 21:7163–7165

Mangano WE, Cagle PT, Churg A et al (1998) The diagnosis of desmoplastic malignant mesothelioma and its distinction from fibrous pleurisy: a histologic and immunohistochemical analysis of 31 cases including p53 immunostaining. Am J Clin Pathol 110:191–199

McCaughey W (1965) Criteria for the diagnosis of diffuse mesothelial tumors. Ann N Y Acad Sci 132:603–613

McGregor SM, Dunning R, Hyjek E et al (2015) Bap1 facilitates diagnostic objectivity, classification, and prognostication in malignant pleural mesothelioma. Hum Pathol 46:1670–1678

Mezger J, Lamerz R, Permanetter W (1990) Diagnostic significance of carcinoembryonic antigen in the differential diagnosis of malignant mesothelioma. J Thorac Cardiovasc Surg 100:860–866

Miettinen M, McCue PA, Sarlomo-Rikala M et al (2014) GATA3: a multispecific but potentially useful marker in surgical pathology: a systematic analysis of 2500 epithelial and nonepithelial tumors. Am J Surg Pathol 38:13–22

Miettinen M, Sarlomo-Rikala M (2003) Expression of calretinin, thrombomodulin, keratin 5, and mesothelin in lung carcinomas of different types: an immunohistochemical analysis of 596 tumors in comparison with epithelioid mesotheliomas of the pleura. Am J Surg Pathol 27:150–158

Mimura T, Ito A, Sakuma T et al (2007) Novel marker D2-40, combined with calretinin, CEA, and TTF-1: an optimal set of immunodiagnostic markers for pleural mesothelioma. Cancer 109:933–938

Moran CA, Suster S, Koss MN (1992) The spectrum of histologic growth patterns in benign and malignant fibrous tumors of the pleura. Semin Diagn Pathol 9:169–180

Muller AM, Franke FE, Muller KM (2006) D2-40: a reliable marker in the diagnosis of pleural mesothelioma. Pathobiology 73:50–54

Nakas A, Martin-Ucar AE, Edwards JG et al (2008) Localised malignant pleural mesothelioma: a separate clinical entity requiring aggressive local surgery. Eur J Cardiothorac Surg 33:303–306

Nascimento AG, Keeney GL, Fletcher CD (1994) Deciduoid peritoneal mesothelioma. An unusual phenotype affecting young females. Am J Surg Pathol 18:439–445

Nasu M, Emi M, Pastorino S et al (2015) High incidence of somatic bap1 alterations in sporadic malignant mesothelioma. J Thorac Oncol 10:565–576

Oates J, Edwards C (2000) HBME-1, MOC-31, WT1 and calretinin: an assessment of recently described markers for mesothelioma and adenocarcinoma. Histopathology 36:341–347

Obers VJ, Leiman G, Girdwood RW et al (1988) Primary malignant pleural tumors (mesotheliomas) presenting as localized masses. Fine needle aspiration cytologic findings, clinical and radiologic features and review of the literature. Acta Cytol 32:567–575

Ohar JA, Cheung M, Talarchek J et al (2016) Germline BAP1 mutational landscape of asbestos-exposed malignant mesothelioma patients with family history of cancer. Cancer Res 76:206–215

Ordonez NG (1989) The immunohistochemical diagnosis of mesothelioma. Differentiation of mesothelioma and lung adenocarcinoma. Am J Surg Pathol 13:276–291

Ordonez NG (1998) Role of immunohistochemistry in distinguishing epithelial peritoneal mesotheliomas from peritoneal and ovarian serous carcinomas. Am J Surg Pathol 22:1203–1214

Ordonez NG (2002) Immunohistochemical diagnosis of epithelioid mesotheliomas: a critical review of old markers, new markers. Hum Pathol 33:953–967

Ordonez NG (2003) The immunohistochemical diagnosis of mesothelioma: a comparative study of epithelioid mesothelioma and lung adenocarcinoma. Am J Surg Pathol 27:1031–1051

Ordonez NG (2004) The diagnostic utility of immunohistochemistry in distinguishing between mesothelioma and renal cell carcinoma: a comparative study. Hum Pathol 35:697–710

Ordonez NG (2005a) D2-40 and podoplanin are highly specific and sensitive immunohistochemical markers of epithelioid malignant mesothelioma. Hum Pathol 36:372–380

Ordonez NG (2005b) Value of estrogen and progesterone receptor immunostaining in distinguishing between peritoneal mesotheliomas and serous carcinomas. Hum Pathol 36:1163–1167

Ordonez NG (2006a) The diagnostic utility of immunohistochemistry and electron microscopy in distinguishing between peritoneal mesotheliomas and serous carcinomas: a comparative study. Mod Pathol 19:34–48

Ordonez NG (2006b) Podoplanin: a novel diagnostic immunohistochemical marker. Adv Anat Pathol 13:83–88

Ordonez NG (2012a) Deciduoid mesothelioma: report of 21 cases with review of the literature. Mod Pathol 25:1481–1495

Ordonez NG (2012b) Mesotheliomas with crystalloid structures: report of nine cases, including one with oncocytic features. Mod Pathol 25:272–281

Ordonez NG (2013a) Application of immunohistochemistry in the diagnosis of epithelioid mesothelioma: a review and update. Hum Pathol 44:1–19

Ordonez NG (2013b) Value of claudin-4 immunostaining in the diagnosis of mesothelioma. Am J Clin Pathol 139:611–619

Ordonez NG (2013c) Value of PAX8, PAX2, claudin-4, and h-caldesmon immunostaining in distinguishing peritoneal epithelioid mesotheliomas from serous carcinomas. Mod Pathol 26:553–562

Ordonez NG (2013d) Value of PAX8, PAX2, napsin A, carbonic anhydrase IX, and claudin-4 immunostaining in distinguishing pleural epithelioid mesothelioma from metastatic renal cell carcinoma. Mod Pathol 26:1132–1143

Ordonez NG, Sahin AA (2014) Diagnostic utility of immunohistochemistry in distinguishing between epithelioid pleural mesotheliomas and breast carcinomas: a comparative study. Hum Pathol 45:1529–1540

Osborn M, Pelling N, Walker MM et al (2002) The value of 'mesothelium-associated' antibodies in distinguishing between metastatic renal cell carcinomas and mesotheliomas. Histopathology 41:301–307

Oury TD, Hammar SP, Roggli VL (1998) Ultrastructural features of diffuse malignant mesotheliomas. Hum Pathol 29:1382–1392

Pan CC, Chen PC, Chou TY et al (2003) Expression of calretinin and other mesothelioma-related markers in thymic carcinoma and thymoma. Hum Pathol 34:1155–1162

Pavlisko EN, Roggli VL (2015) Sarcomatoid peritoneal mesothelioma: clinicopathologic correlation of 13 cases. Am J Surg Pathol 39:1568–1575

Pavlisko EN, Sporn TA (2014) Mesothelioma. In: Oury TD, Sporn TA, Roggli VL (eds) Pathology of asbestos-associated diseases, 3rd edn. Springer, Berlin Heidelberg, pp 81–140

Powell G, Roche H, Roche WR (2011) Expression of calretinin by breast carcinoma and the potential for misdiagnosis of mesothelioma. Histopathology 59:950–956

Riera JR, Astengo-Osuna C, Longmate JA et al (1997) The immunohistochemical diagnostic panel for epithelial mesothelioma: a reevaluation after heat-induced epitope retrieval. Am J Surg Pathol 21:1409–1419

Roberts F, Harper CM, Downie I et al (2001) Immunohistochemical analysis still has a limited role in the diagnosis of malignant mesothelioma. A study of thirteen antibodies. Am J Clin Pathol 116:253–262

Roggli VL, Kolbeck J, Sanfilippo F et al (1987) Pathology of human mesothelioma. Etiologic and diagnostic considerations. Pathol Annu 22(Pt 2):91–131

Rothacker D, Mobius G (1995) Varieties of serous surface papillary carcinoma of the peritoneum in northern germany: a thirty-year autopsy study. Int J Gynecol Pathol 14:310–318

Ruitenbeek T, Gouw AS, Poppema S (1994) Immunocytology of body cavity fluids. MOC-31, a monoclonal antibody discriminating between mesothelial and epithelial cells. Arch Pathol Lab Med 118:265–269

Shanks JH, Harris M, Banerjee SS et al (2000) Mesotheliomas with deciduoid morphology: a morphologic spectrum and a variant not confined to young females. Am J Surg Pathol 24:285–294

Sheffield BS, Hwang HC, Lee AF et al (2015) Bap1 immunohistochemistry and p16 FISH to separate benign from malignant mesothelial proliferations. Am J Surg Pathol 39:977–982

Sheibani K, Battifora H, Burke JS (1986a) Antigenic phenotype of malignant mesotheliomas and pulmonary adenocarcinomas. An immunohistologic analysis demonstrating the value of Leu M1 antigen. Am J Pathol 123:212–219

Sheibani K, Battifora H, Burke JS et al (1986b) Leu-M1 antigen in human neoplasms. An immunohistologic study of 400 cases. Am J Surg Pathol 10:227–236

Sosolik RC, McGaughy VR, De Young BR (1997) Anti-MOC-31: a potential addition to the pulmonary adenocarcinoma versus mesothelioma immunohistochemistry panel. Mod Pathol 10:716–719

Sporn TA, Butnor KJ, Roggli VL (2002) Epithelioid hemangioendothelioma of the pleura: an aggressive vascular malignancy and clinical mimic of malignant mesothelioma. Histopathology 41:173–177

Stout A (1965) Biological effects of asbestos. Ann NY Acad Sci 130:680–682

Szpak CA, Johnston WW, Roggli V et al (1986) The diagnostic distinction between malignant mesothelioma of the pleura and adenocarcinoma of the lung as defined by a monoclonal antibody (B72.3). Am J Pathol 122:252–260

Takeshima Y, Amatya VJ, Kushitani K et al (2009) Value of immunohistochemistry in the differential diagnosis of pleural sarcomatoid mesothelioma from lung sarcomatoid carcinoma. Histopathology 54:667–676

Tan WK, Tan MY, Tan WS et al (2016) Well-differentiated papillary mesothelioma of the tunica vaginalis: case report and systematic review of literature. Clin Genitourin Cancer 14: e435–e439

Testa JR, Cheung M, Pei J et al (2011) Germline BAP1 mutations predispose to malignant mesothelioma. Nat Genet 43:1022–1025

Travis WD, Brambilla E, Burke A et al (2015) Who classification of tumours of the lung, pleura, thymus and heart. In: Bosman FT, Jaffe ES, Lakjani SR, Ohgaki H (eds) World Health Organization classification of tumours, 4th edn. International Agency for Research on Cancer, Lyon. p. 412

Walts AE, Hiroshima K, McGregor SM et al (2016) BAP1 immunostain and CDKN2A (p16) FISH analysis: clinical applicability for the diagnosis of malignant mesothelioma in effusions. Diagn Cytopathol 44:599–606

Wang NS (1973) Electron microscopy in the diagnosis of pleural mesotheliomas. Cancer 31:1046–1054

Wang NS, Huang SN, Gold P (1979) Absence of carcinoembryonic antigen material in mesothelioma. Cancer 44:937–943.

Warhol MJ, Corson JM (1985) An ultrastructural comparison of mesotheliomas with adenocarcinomas of the lung and breast. Hum Pathol 16:50–55

Warhol MJ, Hickey WF, Corson JM (1982) Malignant mesothelioma: ultrastructural distinction from adenocarcinoma. Am J Surg Pathol 6:307–314

Wick MR, Loy T, Mills SE et al (1990) Malignant epithelioid pleural mesothelioma versus peripheral pulmonary adenocarcinoma: a histochemical, ultrastructural, and immunohistologic study of 103 cases. Hum Pathol 21:759–766

Wiesner T, Obenauf AC, Murali R et al (2011) Germline mutations in BAP1 predispose to melanocytic tumors. Nat Genet 43:1018–1021

Wiesner T, Kutzner H, Cerroni L et al (2016) Genomic aberrations in spitzoid melanocytic tumours and their implications for diagnosis, prognosis and therapy. Pathology 48:113–131

Chapter 7
Asbestos-Induced Inflammation in Malignant Mesothelioma and Other Lung Diseases

Joyce K. Thompson and Arti Shukla

Abstract Asbestos exposure can lead to many lung and mesothelial cell diseases, including fibrosis and malignant mesothelioma. These are devastating diseases that are difficult to treat due to the long latency period and lack of predictive markers. Available literature shows that there is consensus among researchers that inflammation plays a significant role in the development of these diseases. Furthermore, there is a potential that early inflammatory signatures could be exploited as biomarkers for diagnosis and targets for treatment. This chapter reviews recent information, ranging from experimental disease models to asbestos-exposed individuals, that suggests a critical role for asbestos-induced inflammation in disease causation; this information has implications for the identification of novel predictive biomarkers and therapeutic targets to aid in early diagnosis and treatment of asbestos-associated diseases.

Keywords Asbestos • Mesothelioma • Lung cancer • Fibrosis • Inflammation • Predictive biomarkers • Molecular therapeutic targets

7.1 Introduction

The group of hydrated silica fibers, collectively referred to as asbestos fibers, was used extensively during the industrial age due to their high tensile strength, thermal and fire resistance. As such, they were employed in construction work for insulation and fireproofing as well as in shipbuilding. Any endeavor that required insulation from high temperatures and provided great fire risks relied on asbestos. Now that asbestos use has been reduced and banned in the construction industry, we are left with large numbers of buildings and ships that contain copious amounts of asbestos. Members of the workforce that were involved in the mining, weaving into textile,

J.K. Thompson • A. Shukla (✉)
Department of Pathology and Laboratory Medicine, College of Medicine,
University of Vermont, Burlington, VT 05405, USA
e-mail: arti.shukla@med.uvm.edu

© Springer International Publishing AG 2017
J.R. Testa (ed.), *Asbestos and Mesothelioma*, Current Cancer Research,
DOI 10.1007/978-3-319-53560-9_7

application of and plumbing with asbestos fibers were exposed to asbestos fibers from their work environment. Unfortunately, these workers also carried the fibers home with them in the form of the dust on their work clothes, which were handled and laundered by family members, exposing them to asbestos fibers in the process (Rom and Palmer 1974). Towns that surrounded asbestos mines and textile mills were not spared this exposure either, as their air was filled with dust from these activities (Lemen et al. 1980). So long as asbestos sheets and other products are intact, they are relatively safe. Should they break or fracture in any way, however, they then pose a health risk to those exposed. One might ask, why is this the case? The answer lies in the friable nature of the asbestos fiber. Once broken, the fiber and any product made from it continues to break into ever-smaller pieces like fabric that is unraveling and fraying. This produces fiber particles that are small enough to become airborne and, thus, respirable. It was noted well before the twentieth century that people who worked with asbestos died earlier than others and presented with symptoms that were in one case referred to as pneumoconiosis. The only common thread between these cases was the occupation of the individuals and the role asbestos played in those occupations.

Reports indicate that miners of asbestos who happened to smoke have a 95% increase in their risk of developing lung cancer (Norbet et al. 2015). Cases referred to as pneumoconiosis, and later on determined to be asbestos-induced lung or pleural fibrosis, seemed to be most common in individuals with a history of occupational exposure (Manning et al. 2002). In some cases, individuals developed pleural plaques with and without pleural effusions, which were sometimes termed malignant. However, the deadliest disease ascribed to asbestos exposure is malignant mesothelioma (MM), which affects only a small subset of exposed individuals (Norbet et al. 2015; Neumann et al. 2013; Broaddus et al. 2011). An underlying thread found in these asbestos-related diseases is their latency period, which ranged in duration from 10–60 years after initial exposure. The level of exposure and time span of exposure also plays a role in the latency period of these diseases. Asbestos fibers, especially the amphiboles such as crocidolite, are non-degradable and persist in parts of the body where they are eventually deposited (typically the pleural cavity). Macrophages and other phagocytic cells attempt to clear the asbestos fibers, but they only succeed in removing short fibers. Long asbestos fibers, because of their high aspect ratio, pose a problem for these cells, as they are not able to engulf the fibers fully (Moolgavkar et al. 2001; Sanchez et al. 2009). As a result, there are repeated attempts to phagocytose the fibers, which results in frustrated phagocytosis, the accompanying release of superoxide, and the eventual death of the cells involved (Sanchez et al. 2009; Murphy et al. 2013). This process of frustrated phagocytosis and cell death leads to the establishment of a vicious cycle in which inflammatory cells are repeatedly recruited to sites of asbestos fiber deposition accompanied by the secretion of inflammatory factors and chemokines that facilitate an inflammatory environment/niche (Mossman et al. 2013). In this chapter, we cover some of the ways in which asbestos promotes chronic inflammation and how such an environment can engender the development of asbestos-related diseases.

7.2   Asbestos-Related Diseases

The commonest asbestos-related diseases are pleural in nature and range from benign pleural plaques and benign (or sometimes malignant) pleural effusions to pleural fibrosis, asbestosis, and lung cancer (Manning et al. 2002; Prazakova et al. 2014; Norbet et al. 2015). The less common diseases include the fatal disease MM (primarily pleural and peritoneal, and to lesser extent, pericardial mesothelioma) (Mossman et al. 2013), the rare asbestos-induced IgG-related disease (Onishi et al. 2016), as well as autoimmune diseases that affect the joints (Pfau et al. 2014). The presentation and outcomes of these diseases vary. At times, the disease goes undiagnosed and is only observed post-mortem upon autopsy after death from an unrelated cause.

7.2.1   Pleural Plaques

Pleural plaques, the commonest asbestos-related disease, arises predominantly on the parietal pleura (O'Reilly et al. 2007). These plaques are distinct areas of fibrosis that can be found classically on the dome of the diaphragm, on the back wall of the chest between the seventh and tenth ribs, as well as laterally between the sixth and ninth ribs (Peacock et al. 2000; Becklake et al. 2007; Norbet et al. 2015). Pleural plaques can be diagnosed with a chest X-ray depending on the position of the plaque (Peacock et al. 2000). In addition, examination of such plaques can reveal the presence of asbestos fibers. The plaques are believed to develop as part of an inflammatory response to asbestos fibers (Manning et al. 2002). Although calcification of asbestos-induced pleural plaques is uncommon, there are reports of some calcification in about 10–15% of pleural plaques (Norbet et al. 2015). Pleural plaques are generally presumed to be benign but some patients experience a small reduction in lung function as well as neuropathic pain (Becklake et al. 2007; Norbet et al. 2015).

7.2.2   Pleural Effusion

The accumulation of fluid in the pleural space of individuals with a history of asbestos exposure may be a benign or malignant manifestation of asbestos-related disease (Prazakova et al. 2014; Manning et al. 2002). As with all asbestos-related diseases, there is a long latency period. Pleural effusions are typically observed within 10–20 years after initial asbestos exposure (Myers 2012; O'Reilly et al. 2007). However, since other conditions can lead to the development of pleural effusions, diagnosis depends heavily on the exclusion of all other potential causes (O'Reilly et al. 2007). Due to the association of MM with pleural manifestation, a waiting period of 3 years without the manifestation of a neoplasm is required before a pleural effusion incident is deemed benign (Peacock et al. 2000). As such, thoracoscopic examination of the pleural space and cytological analysis of the effusion is performed to ascertain the presence of malignant cells and asbestos fibers (Peacock et al. 2000). Like many other diseases, the level of morbidity associated with pleural effusions depends on the amount of the effusion and the time it takes to resolve.

7.2.3 Asbestosis

Asbestosis, also known as asbestos-induced pulmonary fibrosis, is an interstitial lung disease that causes fibrosis of the lung parenchyma and honeycombing (Norbet et al. 2015; Manning et al. 2002). In some cases, there are calcifications of the lung interstitia. Asbestosis shares characteristics with idiopathic pulmonary fibrosis and severely compromises lung function, leading to dyspnea and drastic reduction in lung flow volume (Manning et al. 2002; Prazakova et al. 2014). Asbestosis generally occurs within 10–30 years after asbestos exposure as a result of unresolved inflammation in response to the presence of long thin asbestos fibers in the small airways and alveoli (Manning et al. 2002). The inflammation causes scarring and thickening of the interstitia and subsequent loss of elasticity of the type II alveoli epithelium, thereby compromising lung function (Norbet et al. 2015).

7.2.4 Lung Cancer

Inhalation of asbestos can also lead to the development of lung cancer. While the majority of lung cancers are related to smoking, asbestos exposure accounts for about 3–8% of all lung cancer cases (Prazakova et al. 2014). Asbestos exposure is believed to increase the risk of developing lung cancer in smokers by as much as 4- to 9-fold (Ngamwong et al. 2015; Swiatkowska et al. 2015). Like other asbestos-associated diseases, asbestos-related lung cancer has a long latency period (20–40 years after asbestos exposure) (Manning et al. 2002; Ngamwong et al. 2015; Swiatkowska et al. 2015). For a diagnosis of lung cancer to be attributed to asbestos exposure, however, the patient has usually been heavily exposed to asbestos with an exposure rate of about 25 fibers/mL per year or more (Prazakova et al. 2014). In addition to the presence of asbestos fibers in the lung interstitium, presentation with lung cancer must be found to occur more than 10 years after exposure in order to establish causality (Norbet et al. 2015). In a number of cases of asbestos-related lung cancer, there is concurrent asbestosis. Asbestos-related lung cancer cannot be differentiated phenotypically from lung cancer in non-asbestos exposed individuals, but there appears to be a propensity for this type of lung cancer to develop in the lower lung compared to non-asbestos related lung cancer (Inamura et al. 2014;

Manning et al. 2002). Studies have shown that cumulative asbestos exposure is proportionally related to the development of asbestos-related lung cancer (Inamura et al. 2014).

7.2.5   Malignant Mesothelioma

The deadliest disease attributed to asbestos exposure is MM, which arises in the serosal lining (mesothelium) of the pleura, peritoneum, and sometimes the pericardium (Manning et al. 2002; Mossman et al. 2013). Even rarer is the occasional incidence of MM in the tunica vaginalis of the testis (Jankovichova et al. 2015; Trpkov et al. 2011; Chekol and Sun 2012). As with all asbestos-related diseases, MM has a long latency period (10–40 years) (Mossman et al. 2013). MM is considered an occult cancer that is difficult to detect until it is advanced enough to cause appreciable symptoms. Symptoms usually include chest pain, coughing, dyspnea, pleural effusions (in the case of pleural MM), pain, and discomfort with distention of the abdomen due to ascites build up, and night sweats/fever (in peritoneal MM) (Moore et al. 2008; Prazakova et al. 2014). Thin and long asbestos fibers are believed to translocate to the mesothelium outside of the lung, by mechanisms that are still poorly understood, ultimately causing MM in the pleura or peritoneum (Mossman et al. 2013; Murphy et al. 2013). In addition to asbestos fibers, erionite—a non-asbestos fiber—has been shown to be more mesotheliomagenic and is responsible for an MM epidemic in the Cappadocia region in Turkey (Heintz et al. 2010; Dikensoy 2008). Erionite has been found in different areas here in the United States and has the potential to cause cases of MM because of environmental exposure.

7.3   Asbestos, Inflammation, and Asbestos-Related Diseases

All types of asbestos elicit an immune response in the cells they come into contact with either directly or indirectly through the release of danger associated molecular pattern molecules from cells they encounter (Ballan et al. 2014; Donaldson et al. 2010; Haegens et al. 2007). The amphibole asbestos fibers are bio-persistent compared to the serpentine asbestiform, chrysotile, which can be degraded by bodily fluids and cells due to its more compressible fibril nature and the leaching of magnesium from the fibers (chemical composition: $Mg_3Si_2O_5(OH)_4$) (Manning et al. 2002). A recent review by Acencio et al. (2015) clearly summarized the role of inflammatory cytokines in chrysotile- and crocidolite-induced mesothelial cell injury leading to diseases. Studies from our group have also demonstrated that asbestos can cause increased gene expression and protein levels of various inflammatory cytokines (IL-13, bFGF, VEGF, GSF) from mesothelial cells (Shukla et al.

2009) and that many of these cytokines are required for MM development in mice (Hillegass et al. 2010). Chrysotile asbestos has been shown to elicit an acute immune response 3 and 9 days post inhalation of this fiber type (Haegens et al. 2007). In an examination of mice exposed to chrysotile asbestos for 6 h a day, an increase in the number of immune cells retrieved from the lungs through bronchoalveolar lavage showed an increase in infiltrating cells in the asbestos-exposed mice when compared to sham-exposed mice (Haegens et al. 2007). Increases in the number of infiltrating eosinophils and neutrophils were observed, and the number of lymphocytes increased after 9 days of exposure (Haegens et al. 2007).

Amphibole asbestos fibers are generally regarded as the main culprits behind MM, although chrysotile asbestos has also been shown to cause the disease. Among the amphiboles, crocidolite asbestos is classified as the most carcinogenic (Dopp et al. 2005; Ballan et al. 2014), and studies into reactive oxygen species (ROS) production, cell signaling, and genotoxicity have generally been carried out using crocidolite or amosite (Dopp et al. 2005). Crocidolite asbestos elicits an acute immune response, and because of its biopersistence can cause chronic inflammation by recruiting inflammatory cells which then die in the process of attempting to clear the asbestos fibers (Moolgavkar et al. 2001). The death of such immune cells then elicits a new wave of inflammatory cell influx, thus leading to a never-ending cycle of inflammation in response to the presence of the fibers. Amphiboles such as amosite and crocidolite also contain iron in their crystal structures ($[(Mg, Fe)_7Si_8O_{22}(OH)_2]_n$ and $[NaFe_3^{2+}Fe_2^{3+}Si_8O_{22}(OH)_2]_n$, respectively), and the valency state of these iron moieties determines their ability to participate in Fenton reactions (Dopp et al. 2005). These Fenton reactions promote the production of reactive species such as the hydroxyl ion (Dopp et al. 2005; Mossman et al. 2011). Regulators of expression of various cytokines (transcription factors, e.g., NFκB and AP-1) are affected by the redox state of the cell (Shukla et al. 2003). Raising the oxidation state or altering the redox balance of the cell can thereby lead to their aberrant activation or inhibition, resulting in the production of more inflammatory cytokines in response to asbestos exposure. Exposure to crocidolite/amosite has been shown to increase the production and secretion of a number of inflammatory cytokines, including but not limited to IL-1β, IL-5, IL-6, IL-8, and IL-18 (Haegens et al. 2007; Hillegass et al. 2013).

While tracheal instillation of asbestos into mice has been shown to result in death of epithelial and mesothelial cells as well as alveolar macrophages, some of these cells appear to escape such death and survive longer than cells from control animals or cells unexposed to asbestos (Nishimura et al. 2013). Alveolar macrophages that survive chrysotile asbestos exposure have been reported to live longer and secrete increased amounts of the fibrogenic factor TGFβ, leading to the conclusion that such alterations contribute directly to the fibrosis observed in response to asbestos exposure (Nishimura et al. 2013). These inflammatory responses to asbestos have been observed both in vitro and in vivo. Recent studies of patients with history of asbestos exposure have shown that these patients have elevated levels of IL-8 and other cytokines, as well as their respective receptors (Comar et al. 2016; Comar et al. 2014). Levels of vascular endothelial growth factor (VEGF), platelet derived growth factor b (PDGFb), and basic fibroblast growth factor (bFGF) were also significantly increased upon exposure to asbestos and further increased in some cases with disease (Comar et al. 2016). VEGF and bFGF are both angiogenic factors that stimulate proliferation of mesothelial cells (Comar et al. 2016; Strizzi et al. 2001; Van et al. 2012) and alter the permeability of the mesothelium (VEGF) (Hillegass et al. 2013; Strizzi et al. 2001). PDGFb has been shown to promote the growth of fibroblasts and the progression of fibrosis in lung disease (Safi et al. 1992).

Asbestos fibers can cause systemic changes in inflammatory cytokines (Gavett et al. 2016; Fukagawa et al. 2008; Dragon et al. 2015), and these changes can lead to the creation of a pro-tumorigenic environment (Okada 2014). The initial site of contact for inhaled fibers is the lung, where alveolar macrophages and epithelial cells encounter the inhaled asbestos. In as early as 3 days after asbestos exposure, the inflammatory profile in the lung changes. An increase in the number of infiltrating eosinophils and neutrophils is observed (Haegens et al. 2007). As cells attempt to clear the foreign objects, the high aspect ratio of the asbestos fibers leads to frustrated phagocytic events that promote death of the phagocytic cells. Consequently, greater numbers of inflammatory cells are recruited to the site of injury. An overproduction of collagen by fibroblasts recruited to these sites of injury promotes parenchymal fibrosis, because the injury is not resolved due to the continued presence of the asbestos fibers. As cells attempt to clear asbestos fibers and resolve the injury, more and more extracellular matrix will be deposited and stromal cells will be recruited. These may be the underlying contributing factors to the development of asbestosis and potentially lung cancer (Heintz et al. 2010).

Asbestos fibers have been found to translocate to the interpleural space by mechanisms that are still incompletely understood. Studies indicate that asbestos or carbon nanotubes 10 μm or greater in length cause acute inflammation and fibrosis on the parietal surface of the pleural mesothelium in a length dependent manner due to an inhibition of clearance through the pleural stomata (Fig. 7.1) (Murphy et al. 2011; Schinwald et al. 2012). It has been proposed that the length of a fraction of the asbestos fibers interferes with their clearance through the lymphatic drainage, as they cannot go through the pleural stomata. As a result, fibers within a particular length range accumulate on the parietal pleura, leading to the formation of pleural plaques and pleural fibrosis by propagating chronic inflammation and injury to the mesothelium (Donaldson et al. 2010). Recent studies have shown that asbestos-like fibers such as carbon nanotubes are capable of eliciting the same kind of inflammatory and fibrotic responses in the pleural mesothelium as does asbestos (Murphy et al. 2011; Murphy et al. 2012; Nagai and Toyokuni 2010). Asbestos bodies are not always associated with pleural plaques, suggesting that an intermediate inflammatory mediator may be involved. Macrophages, mesothelial cells, and other phagocytic cells undergo frustrated phagocytosis while attempting to clear these high aspect ratio fibers and secrete a host of inflammatory mediators. Thus, pleural macrophages secreting a number of inflammatory cytokines may also play a role in facilitating inflammation-induced injury and repair in the pleura that could promote asbestos-related disease formation (Mossman et al. 2011). One study has shown that supernatants from macrophages exposed to long carbon nanotubes serve as

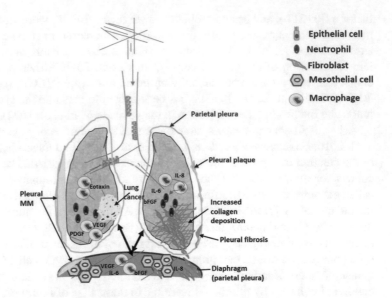

bFGF- basic FGF; VEGF- vascular endothelial growth factor and PDGF- platelet derived growth factor

Fig. 7.1 Inflammation plays a role in asbestos-related diseases. Asbestos fibers first encounter bronchial epithelial cells when inhaled, and long fibers may become lodged at bifurcations in the bronchi and lead to chronic inflammation at those sites that recruits inflammatory cells. Such chronic inflammation can lead to the development of bronchogenic diseases at those sites. In the lung parenchyma, long and thin asbestos fibers can travel deeper and interact with alveolar macrophages, which will attempt to clear these fibers. While fibers that are short enough to be completely engulfed and cleared, longer fibers will cause frustrated attempts of clearing, leading to more inflammation. The production of various signaling and inflammatory molecules in response to this assault over time contributes to the interstitial lung diseases observed in response to asbestos. Longer asbestos fibers have been found to accumulate on the parietal pleura and are also believed to become lodged in the stomata of the mesothelium at those points where they may potentiate chronic inflammation that contribute to pleural asbestos diseases. It also appears that events occurring in the lung may influence or affect disease in the parietal pleura and vice versa

potent activators of mesothelial cells and significantly increase their secretion of inflammatory cytokines such as IL-1β and eotaxin (Murphy et al. 2012). This same phenomenon has been demonstrated for asbestos as well. Studies indicate that one of the inflammatory cascades activated by asbestos in macrophages and mesothelial cells is the activation of the inflammasome (Dostert et al. 2008; Hillegass et al. 2013). The inflammasome is a special component of inflammation, where nod like receptor containing pyrin domain 3 (NLRP3), a cytoplasmic protein complex, senses fibers. This results in caspase-1 activation and secretion of the pro-inflammatory cytokines IL-1β and IL-18. There are several nod like receptors reported in literature; however, only activation of the NLRP3 inflammasome in macrophages and mesothelial cells by asbestos has been demonstrated to increase secretion of IL-1β, IL-18, and other pro-inflammatory cytokines as a result of IL-1β signaling (Dostert et al. 2008; Hillegass et al. 2013). Additionally, asbestos-induced inflammasome activation can lead to the release of a pro-inflammatory danger-associated molecule, high mobility group box 1 (HMGB1), from mesothelial cells, which is also a potent inducer of inflammation (Hillegass et al. 2013; Yang et al. 2010; Carbone and Yang 2012).

Inflammasome activation induced by asbestos plays an important role in the development of MM when coupled with genetic predisposition and cumulative exposure to asbestos (Kadariya et al. 2016; Hillegass et al. 2010). In contrast, a recent study of MM tumor cells and tissue arrays showed attenuated levels of the NLRP3 inflammasome and caspase-1 activation (Westbom et al. 2015). Treatment of these tumors with cisplatin caused increased NLRP3 priming and activation. To the contrary, treatment of tumors with a combination of cisplatin and an IL-1 receptor antagonist resulted in better tumor reduction as compared to cisplatin alone. These findings again point towards a tumor promoting role of IL-1β, a pro-inflammatory cytokine (Westbom et al. 2015). Although there are various ways through which the inflammasome is activated by asbestos, NADPH oxidase and thioredoxin interacting protein (TXNIP) appear to play prominent roles (Thompson et al. 2014; Dostert et al. 2008). This attests to the role of ROS in inflammasome regulation. The inflammatory profile of patients with MM has been recently suggested to offer insights into the interactions between a tumor and its microenvironment, which promote tumorigenesis (Judge et al. 2016). Analysis of sera and peritoneal ascites fluid from patients with peritoneal MM showed localized elevation in a number of pro-inflammatory cytokines (IL-6, IL-8, MCP-1, MIP-1β, MIP1α, IL-10, VEGF and TNFα) when compared to control sera (Judge et al. 2016). In vivo and in vitro studies of the growth of MM from our group have also demonstrated that inflammation is an active component of MM growth in SCID mice (Hillegass et al. 2010; Westbom et al. 2014). The risk of developing MM has been shown to rise with increased exposure to asbestos (Mossman et al. 2013; Landrigan and Collegium 2016). In a small fraction of patients, germline mutations of the BRCA1 associated protein 1 gene (*BAP1*) have been shown to increase the risk of developing MM even at lower levels of asbestos exposure (Testa et al. 2011; Napolitano et al. 2016; Ohar et al. 2016). It is, however, interesting to note that in a heterozygous *Bap1*-mutant murine model, exposure to low doses of asbestos led to a stronger inflammatory response and higher incidence of MM when compared to their wild type littermates (Napolitano et al. 2016). This suggests that the higher inflammatory response may play a crucial role in the development of MM in patients with *BAP1* mutations as well, indicating a putative link between the function of BAP1 and inflammatory responses (Napolitano et al. 2016).

With the postulated hypothesis of how a fraction of longer asbestos fibers are deposited on the parietal pleura over time, the observation that MM originates from the parietal pleura before spreading to the visceral pleura is somewhat explained (Donaldson et al. 2010; Murphy et al. 2011). Asbestos activates a number of signaling cascades that are involved in the regulation of inflammatory responses, and this may play a large role in the sustained inflammatory response to asbestos fibers that eventually lead to the development of the various asbestos-related diseases (Shukla et al.

2003; Haegens et al. 2007; Heintz et al. 2010; Nishimura et al. 2013). In fact, our next-generation sequencing studies of primary mesothelial cells indicate that asbestos exposure predominantly upregulates inflammatory networks (Dragon et al. 2015). Such chronic inflammation eventually leads to DNA damage and may be responsible for the many deletions and mutations observed in MM (see Chapters Asbestos-Induced Inflammation in Malignant Mesothelioma and Other Lung Diseases and Germline and Somatic Mutations in Human Mesothelioma and Lessons from Asbestos-Exposed Genetically Engineered Mouse Models of this volume). Inflammation induced by asbestos has been shown to promote the formation of 8-oxoguanine adducts in nuclear and mitochondrial DNA (Fung et al. 1997; Okada 2007). The formation of a number of nitrosylation products, including 8-nitroguanine, also results from the generation of ROS as a combined result of Fenton reactions facilitated by asbestos fibers and the induction of the nitric oxide synthase enzyme by inflammatory cells (Fung et al. 1997; Okada 2007; Hiraku et al. 2010). Thus, not only does asbestos cause mechanical injury to the mesothelium that can lead to aberrant repair, but its chemical composition also promotes inflammation via the recruitment of inflammatory cells (Shukla et al. 2003; Shukla et al. 2007; Okada 2007). Asbestos exposure also leads to the activation of cellular pathways that are sensitive to the redox state of the cell and involved in the regulation of inflammation (Thompson et al. 2014; Shukla et al. 2003).

A recent study of asbestos-exposed workers from an Italian coastal area showed the presence of elevated chemokines and pro-inflammatory cytokines in serum of asbestos-exposed workers as compared to healthy controls (Comar et al. 2016). Inflammatory parameters have been suggested to have prognostic significance in MM. For example, lymphocyte-to-monocyte (LMR) ratio (Yamagishi et al. 2015) or neutrophil-to-lymphocyte (NLR) ratio along with red cell distribution width (RDW) (Abakay et al. 2014) could be projected as predictive factors for MM prognosis. Furthermore, inhibition of inflammation by natural compounds (Benvenuto et al. 2016; Pietrofesa et al. 2016) has also been shown to inhibit asbestos-induced inflammation and carcinogenesis in animal models, confirming the role of inflammation in asbestos-induced diseases.

7.4   Conclusions

Asbestos-related diseases have a long latency period and are end result of aberrant wound healing responses, chronic inflammation, and (in the case of lung cancer and MM) inflammation-related genetic mutation and deviant gene expression or silencing. The inflammasome and its products, IL-1β and IL-18, may play an important role in promoting a myofibroblastic transition in mesothelial cells as well as in activating fibroblasts to create a microenvironment in which damaged cells survive and go on to acquire mutations and activate gene programs that enable them to become malignant and clonally expand. More studies are needed to help uncover the mechanisms involved in the development of these diseases, as this would lead to discovery of potential biomarkers and therapeutic targets to aid in early diagnosis and treatment.

Acknowledgements This work is supported by a grant from NIEHS (RO1ES021110) and a Pathology and Laboratory Medicine fellowship.

Conflict of Interest The authors have no conflicts of interest to disclose.

References

Abakay O, Tanrikulu AC, Palanci Y et al (2014) The value of inflammatory parameters in the prognosis of malignant mesothelioma. J Int Med Res 42:554–565

Acencio MM, Soares B, Marchi E et al (2015) Inflammatory cytokines contribute to asbestos-induced injury of mesothelial cells. Lung 193:831–837

Ballan G, Del Brocco A, Loizzo S et al (2014) Mode of action of fibrous amphiboles: the case of Biancavilla (Sicily, Italy). Ann Ist Super Sanita 50:133–138

Becklake MR, Bagatin E, Neder JA (2007) Asbestos-related diseases of the lungs and pleura: uses, trends and management over the last century. Int J Tuberc Lung Dis 11:356–369

Benvenuto M, Mattera R, Taffera G et al (2016) The potential protective effects of polyphenols in asbestos-mediated inflammation and carcinogenesis of mesothelium. Nutrients 8:275

Broaddus VC, Everitt JI, Black B et al (2011) Non-neoplastic and neoplastic pleural endpoints following fiber exposure. J Toxicol Environ Health B Crit Rev 14:153–178

Carbone M, Yang H (2012) Molecular pathways: targeting mechanisms of asbestos and erionite carcinogenesis in mesothelioma. Clin Cancer Res 18:598–604

Chekol SS, Sun CC (2012) Malignant mesothelioma of the tunica vaginalis testis: diagnostic studies and differential diagnosis. Arch Pathol Lab Med 136:113–137

Comar M, Zanotta N, Bonotti A et al (2014) Increased levels of C-C chemokine RANTES in asbestos exposed workers and in malignant mesothelioma patients from an hyperendemic area. PLoS One 9:e104848

Comar M, Zanotta N, Zanconati F et al (2016) Chemokines involved in the early inflammatory response and in pro-tumoral activity in asbestos-exposed workers from an Italian coastal area with territorial clusters of pleural malignant mesothelioma. Lung Cancer 94:61–67

Dikensoy O (2008) Mesothelioma due to environmental exposure to erionite in Turkey. Curr Opin Pulm Med 14:322–325

Donaldson K, Murphy FA, Duffin R et al (2010) Asbestos, carbon nanotubes and the pleural mesothelium: a review of the hypothesis regarding the role of long fibre retention in the parietal pleura, inflammation and mesothelioma. Part Fibre Toxicol 7:5

Dopp E, Yadav S, Ansari FA et al (2005) ROS-mediated genotoxicity of asbestos-cement in mammalian lung cells in vitro. Part Fibre Toxicol 2:9

Dostert C, Petrilli V, Van Bruggen R et al (2008) Innate immune activation through Nalp3 inflammasome sensing of asbestos and silica. Science 320:674–677

Dragon J, Thompson J, MacPherson M et al (2015) Differential susceptibility of human pleural and peritoneal mesothelial cells to asbestos exposure. J Cell Biochem 116:1540–1552

Fukagawa NK, Li M, Sabo-Attwood T et al (2008) Inhaled asbestos exacerbates atherosclerosis in apolipoprotein E-deficient mice via CD4+ T cells. Environ Health Perspect 116:1218–1225

Fung H, Kow YW, Van Houten B et al (1997) Patterns of 8-hydroxydeoxyguanosine formation in DNA and indications of oxidative stress in rat and human pleural mesothelial cells after exposure to crocidolite asbestos. Carcinogenesis 18:825–832

Gavett SH, Parkinson CU, Willson GA et al (2016) Persistent effects of Libby amphibole and amosite asbestos following subchronic inhalation in rats. Part Fibre Toxicol 13:17

Haegens A, Barrett TF, Gell J et al (2007) Airway epithelial NF-kappaB activation modulates asbestos-induced inflammation and mucin production in vivo. J Immunol 178:1800–1808

Heintz NH, Janssen-Heininger YM, Mossman BT (2010) Asbestos, lung cancers, and mesotheliomas: from molecular approaches to targeting tumor survival pathways. Am J Respir Cell Mol Biol 42:133–139

Hillegass JM, Miller JM, MacPherson MB et al (2013) Asbestos and erionite prime and activate the NLRP3 inflammasome that stimulates autocrine cytokine release in human mesothelial cells. Part Fibre Toxicol 10:39

Hillegass JM, Shukla A, Lathrop SA et al (2010) Inflammation precedes the development of human malignant mesotheliomas in a SCID mouse xenograft model. Ann N Y Acad Sci 1203:7–14

Hiraku Y, Kawanishi S, Ichinose T et al (2010) The role of iNOS-mediated DNA damage in infection- and asbestos-induced carcinogenesis. Ann N Y Acad Sci 1203:15–22

Inamura K, Ninomiya H, Nomura K et al (2014) Combined effects of asbestos and cigarette smoke on the development of lung adenocarcinoma: different carcinogens may cause different genomic changes. Oncol Rep 32:475–482

Jankovichova T, Jankovich M, Ondrus D et al (2015) Extremely rare tumour--malignant mesothelioma of tunica vaginalis testis. Bratisl Lek Listy 116:574–576

Judge S, Thomas P, Govindarajan V et al (2016) Malignant peritoneal mesothelioma: characterization of the inflammatory response in the tumor microenvironment. Ann Surg Oncol 23:1496–1500

Kadariya Y, Menges CW, Talarchek J et al (2016) Inflammation-related IL1β/IL1R signaling promotes the development of asbestos-induced malignant mesothelioma. Cancer Prev Res 9:406–414

Landrigan PJ, Collegium R (2016) Comments on the causation of malignant mesothelioma: rebutting the false concept that recent exposures to asbestos do not contribute to causation of mesothelioma. Ann Glob Health 82:214–216

Lemen RA, Dement JM, Wagoner JK (1980) Epidemiology of asbestos-related diseases. Environ Health Perspect 34:1–11

Manning CB, Vallyathan V, Mossman BT (2002) Diseases caused by asbestos: mechanisms of injury and disease development. Int Immunopharmacol 2:191–200

Moolgavkar SH, Brown RC, Turim J (2001) Biopersistence, fiber length, and cancer risk assessment for inhaled fibers. Inhal Toxicol 13:755–772

Moore AJ, Parker RJ, Wiggins J (2008) Malignant mesothelioma. Orphanet J Rare Dis 3:34

Mossman BT, Lippmann M, Hesterberg TW et al (2011) Pulmonary endpoints (lung carcinomas and asbestosis) following inhalation exposure to asbestos. J Toxicol Environ Health B Crit Rev 14:76–121

Mossman BT, Shukla A, Heintz NH et al (2013) New insights into understanding the mechanisms, pathogenesis, and management of malignant mesotheliomas. Am J Pathol 182:1065–1077

Murphy FA, Poland CA, Duffin R et al (2011) Length-dependent retention of carbon nanotubes in the pleural space of mice initiates sustained inflammation and progressive fibrosis on the parietal pleura. Am J Pathol 178:2587–2600

Murphy FA, Poland CA, Duffin R et al (2013) Length-dependent pleural inflammation and parietal pleural responses after deposition of carbon nanotubes in the pulmonary airspaces of mice. Nanotoxicology 7:1157–1167

Murphy FA, Schinwald A, Poland CA et al (2012) The mechanism of pleural inflammation by long carbon nanotubes: interaction of long fibres with macrophages stimulates them to amplify proinflammatory responses in mesothelial cells. Part Fibre Toxicol 9:8

Myers R (2012) Asbestos-related pleural disease. Curr Opin Pulm Med 18:377–381

Nagai H, Toyokuni S (2010) Biopersistent fiber-induced inflammation and carcinogenesis: lessons learned from asbestos toward safety of fibrous nanomaterials. Arch Biochem Biophys 502:1–7

Napolitano A, Pellegrini L, Dey A et al (2016) Minimal asbestos exposure in germline BAP1 heterozygous mice is associated with deregulated inflammatory response and increased risk of mesothelioma. Oncogene 35:1996–2002

Neumann V, Loseke S, Nowak D et al (2013) Malignant pleural mesothelioma: incidence, etiology, diagnosis, treatment, and occupational health. Dtsch Arztebl Int 110:319–326

Ngamwong Y, Tangamornsuksan W, Lohitnavy O et al (2015) Additive synergism between asbestos and smoking in lung cancer risk: a systematic review and meta-analysis. PLoS One 10:e0135798

Nishimura Y, Maeda M, Kumagai-Takei N et al (2013) Altered functions of alveolar macrophages and NK cells involved in asbestos-related diseases. Environ Health Prev Med 18:198–204

Norbet C, Joseph A, Rossi SS et al (2015) Asbestos-related lung disease: a pictorial review. Curr Probl Diagn Radiol 44:371–382

O'Reilly KM, McLaughlin AM, Beckett WS et al (2007) Asbestos-related lung disease. Am Fam Physician 75:683–688

Ohar JA, Cheung M, Talarchek J et al (2016) Germline BAP1 mutational landscape of asbestos-exposed malignant mesothelioma patients with family history of cancer. Cancer Res 76:206–215

Okada F (2007) Beyond foreign-body-induced carcinogenesis: impact of reactive oxygen species derived from inflammatory cells in tumorigenic conversion and tumor progression. Int J Cancer 121:2364–2372

Okada F (2014) Inflammation-related carcinogenesis: current findings in epidemiological trends, causes and mechanisms. Yonago Acta Med 57:65–72

Onishi Y, Nakahara Y, Hirano K et al (2016) IgG4-related disease in asbestos-related pleural disease. Respirol Case Rep 4:22–24

Peacock C, Copley SJ, Hansell DM et al (2000) Asbestos-related benign pleural disease. Clin Radiol 55:422–432

Pfau JC, Serve KM, Noonan CW et al (2014) Autoimmunity and asbestos exposure. Autoimmune Dis 2014:782045

Pietrofesa RA, Velalopoulou A, Arguiri E et al (2016) Flaxseed lignans enriched in secoisolarici-resinol diglucoside prevent acute asbestos-induced peritoneal inflammation in mice. Carcinogenesis 37:177–187

Prazakova S, Thomas PS, Sandrini A et al (2014) Asbestos and the lung in the 21st century: an update. Clin Respir J 8:1–10

Rom WN, Palmer PE (1974) The spectrum of asbestos-related diseases. West J Med 121:10–21

Safi A, Sadmi M, Martinet N et al (1992) Presence of elevated levels of platelet-derived growth factor (PDGF) in lung adenocarcinoma pleural effusions. Chest 102:204–207

Sanchez VC, Pietruska JR, Miselis NR et al (2009) Biopersistence and potential adverse health impacts of fibrous nanomaterials: what have we learned from asbestos? Wiley Interdiscip Rev Nanomed Nanobiotechnol 1:511–529

Schinwald A, Murphy FA, Prina-Mello A et al (2012) The threshold length for fiber-induced acute pleural inflammation: shedding light on the early events in asbestos-induced mesothelioma. Toxicol Sci 128:461–470

Shukla A, Lounsbury KM, Barrett TF et al (2007) Asbestos-induced peribronchiolar cell proliferation and cytokine production are attenuated in lungs of protein kinase C-delta knockout mice. Am J Pathol 170:140–151

Shukla A, MacPherson MB, Hillegass J et al (2009) Alterations in gene expression in human mesothelial cells correlate with mineral pathogenicity. Am J Respir Cell Mol Biol 41:114–123

Shukla A, Ramos-Nino M, Mossman BT (2003) Cell signaling and transcription factor activation by asbestos in lung injury and disease. Int J Biochem Cell Biol 35:1198–1209

Strizzi L, Catalano A, Vianale G et al (2001) Vascular endothelial growth factor is an autocrine growth factor in human malignant mesothelioma. J Pathol 193:468–475

Swiatkowska B, Szubert Z, Sobala W et al (2015) Predictors of lung cancer among former asbestos-exposed workers. Lung Cancer 89:243–248

Testa JR, Cheung M, Pei J et al (2011) Germline BAP1 mutations predispose to malignant mesothelioma. Nat Genet 43:1022–1025

Thompson JK, Westbom CM, MacPherson MB et al (2014) Asbestos modulates thioredoxin-thioredoxin interacting protein interaction to regulate inflammasome activation. Part Fibre Toxicol 11:24

Trpkov K, Barr R, Kulaga A et al (2011) Mesothelioma of tunica vaginalis of "uncertain malignant potential" – an evolving concept: case report and review of the literature. Diagn Pathol 6:78

Van TT, Hanibuchi M, Goto H et al (2012) SU6668, a multiple tyrosine kinase inhibitor, inhibits progression of human malignant pleural mesothelioma in an orthotopic model. Respirology 17:984–990

Westbom C, Thompson JK, Leggett A et al (2015) Inflammasome modulation by chemotherapeutics in malignant mesothelioma. PLoS One 10:e0145404

Westbom CM, Shukla A, MacPherson MB et al (2014) CREB-induced inflammation is important for malignant mesothelioma growth. Am J Pathol 184:2816–2827

Yamagishi T, Fujimoto N, Nishi H et al (2015) Prognostic significance of the lymphocyte-to-monocyte ratio in patients with malignant pleural mesothelioma. Lung Cancer 90:111–117

Yang H, Rivera Z, Jube S et al (2010) Programmed necrosis induced by asbestos in human mesothelial cells causes high-mobility group box 1 protein release and resultant inflammation. Proc Natl Acad Sci U S A 107:12611–12616

Chapter 8
Germline and Somatic Mutations in Human Mesothelioma and Lessons from Asbestos-Exposed Genetically Engineered Mouse Models

Mitchell Cheung, Craig W. Menges, and Joseph R. Testa

Abstract Like cancer generally, malignant mesothelioma is a genetic disease at the cellular level. Specific genes most frequently linked to mesothelioma include the tumor suppressor genes *BAP1*, *CDKN2A*, and *NF2*. Somatic (acquired) mutations of these and other tumor suppressor genes often occur in combination in a given mesothelioma, suggesting that a cascade of genomic alterations is involved in the pathogenesis of this deadly disease. Overall, only a small fraction of individuals exposed to asbestos fibers develop the disorder, suggesting that inherited genetic factors may play a role in predisposing to mesothelioma. A person who is genetically predisposed to mesothelioma carries a DNA variant in one or possibly more genes, but the disease may not be triggered unless there is exposure to asbestos—perhaps even minimally—or some other relevant carcinogenic environmental factor. For example, clustering of mesothelioma cases has been documented in some, but not all, families with a germline inactivating mutation of *BAP1*. People without a genetic predisposition also develop the disease when exposed to asbestos, but studies in humans and genetically engineered mouse models indicate that the risk is likely to be much lower. In this review, we highlight the current understanding of the role of both hereditary and somatic mutations in human malignant mesothelioma, as well as what has been learned from experimental studies of asbestos-exposed rodent models of mesothelioma.

Keywords Mesothelioma • Genetics • Tumor suppressor genes • Somatic and germline mutations • BAP1 syndrome • Mouse models of mesothelioma

Mitchell Cheung and Craig W. Menges have contributed equally to this review.

M. Cheung • C.W. Menges • J.R. Testa (✉)
Cancer Biology Program, Fox Chase Cancer Center, Philadelphia, PA 19111, USA
e-mail: joseph.testa@fccc.edu

© Springer International Publishing AG 2017
J.R. Testa (ed.), *Asbestos and Mesothelioma*, Current Cancer Research,
DOI 10.1007/978-3-319-53560-9_8

8.1 Somatic Mutations in Malignant Mesothelioma

Several prominent sites of somatic (non-germline) chromosomal loss have been identified in human mesothelioma, including recurring deletions of chromosomes 3, 9, and 22, specifically at genomic locations ("bands") 3p21, 9p21, and 22q12, respectively. These acquired chromosome abnormalities often occur in combination in a given tumor, suggesting a multi-step pathogenetic process (Murthy and Testa 1999). Work performed in the 1990s implicated tumor suppressor loci at two of these chromosomal sites: *CDKN2A* (Cheng et al. 1994; Xio et al. 1995; Altomare et al. 2005), located at 9p21, and *NF2* (Bianchi et al. 1995; Sekido et al. 1995), residing at 22q12. The identity of the critical 3p21 gene in mesothelioma had remained a mystery until 2011, when somatic point mutations of the BRCA1 associated protein-1 gene, *BAP1*, located at 3p21.3, were identified in 20–25% of sporadic mesotheliomas (Bott et al. 2011; Testa et al. 2011). In 2012, Yoshikawa and colleagues uncovered biallelic alterations of *BAP1*, including homozygous deletions of part or all of this tumor suppressor gene as well as sequence-level mutations, in 61% of sporadic mesotheliomas (Yoshikawa et al. 2012). Subsequent studies with newer next generation and multiplex ligation-dependent probe amplification platforms confirmed a similarly high incidence of *BAP1* mutations in this disease (Lo Iacono et al. 2015; Nasu et al. 2015).

In vivo work has demonstrated that the BAP1 protein is a bona fide tumor suppressor (Kadariya et al. 2016a). Functionally, BAP1 and its *Drosophila* homolog Calypso are nuclear-localized deubiquitinating enzymes and members of the polycomb-group of highly conserved transcriptional repressors, which are required for long-term silencing of genes that regulate stem cell pluripotency, cell fate determination, and other developmental processes (Gaytan de Ayala Alonso et al. 2007). BAP1 has also been shown to play an important role in double-strand break repair by homologous recombination, thereby suggesting a potential mechanism by which *BAP1* mutations might contribute to genomic instability and tumor formation (Ismail et al. 2014). Further functional implications of *BAP1* mutations in mesothelioma are described in the following section.

The *CDKN2A* locus encodes two important tumor suppressors, p16INK4A and p14ARF, which are known to regulate the critical Rb and p53 cell cycle regulatory pathways, respectively. Deletions of *CDKN2A* have been reported in 75–90% of mesothelioma samples and tumor-derived cell lines (Cheng et al. 1994; Xio et al. 1995; Altomare et al. 2005). Re-expression of p16INK4A in p16INK4A-null mesothelioma cells has been shown to cause cell cycle arrest and tumor suppression or regression (Frizelle et al. 1998), while re-expression of p14ARF in mesothelioma cells induced G1-phase cell cycle arrest and apoptosis (Yang et al. 2000). As noted above, p14ARF is an integral component of the p53 pathway, and mutations of the p53 gene, *TP53*, have also been reported in a subset of mesotheliomas (Cote et al. 1991; Altomare et al. 2005). For example, we identified *TP53* mutations in 3 of 20 (15%) malignant mesotheliomas we tested. Notably, two of these three tumor samples with *TP53* mutations did not show homozygous loss of *p14(ARF)*, indicating that alterations of the p53 pathway in mesothelioma can occur in connection with defects in either gene, thereby providing further support for a critical role of this pathway in mesothelioma pathogenesis.

Mutations of *NF2* have been reported in 20–55% of mesothelioma specimens and tumor-derived cell lines (Bianchi et al. 1995; Sekido et al. 1995; Cheng et al. 1999; Bott et al. 2011). Interestingly, mesotheliomas have been reported in several individuals with neurofibromatosis type 2 (Baser et al. 2002; Baser et al. 2005), an autosomal dominant disorder caused by germline mutation of *NF2*. In genetically engineered mouse models, there is ample evidence demonstrating that germline mutations of *Nf2*, like mutations of *Cdkn2a* or *Bap1*, contribute significantly to mesothelioma development (see below). The *NF2* product, merlin, is known to repress cyclin D1 expression, and merlin loss in mesothelioma cells leads to cell cycle progression via up regulation of cyclin D1 (Xiao et al. 2005). In our studies, adenovirus-mediated re-expression of merlin in *NF2*-deficient mesothelioma cells resulted in decreased expression of cyclin D1 mRNA (Xiao et al. 2005). Merlin has also been proposed to regulate cyclin D1 post-transcriptionally through the activation of mTORC1 (James et al. 2009; Lopez-Lago et al. 2009). Merlin also inhibits Rac/Pak and FAK signaling, which are implicated in cell migration and spreading, respectively, and inactivation of *NF2* in mesothelioma cells was found to promote invasiveness and spreading (Xiao et al. 2002; Poulikakos et al. 2006). More recently, deregulation of the Hippo signaling pathway, one of the downstream cascades regulated by merlin, has been implicated in mesothelioma. Notably, in addition to *NF2*, alterations of genes encoding several other components in the Hippo pathway have been reported in mesothelioma. These include somatic mutations of the tumor suppressor genes *LATS1* and *LATS2*, and upregulation of the transcriptional coactivator YAP, the main downstream effector of the pathway and a putative oncogene (Bott et al. 2011; Murakami et al. 2011). Given their frequent involvement in human mesothelioma, alterations of *CDKN2A*, *NF2*, and *BAP1* appear to be primary drivers in this malignancy.

Recently, investigators have begun to use massively parallel next-generation sequencing for comprehensive genomic analysis of malignant mesotheliomas, which has confirmed and extended earlier single gene studies on mesothelioma. In one report, Guo and colleagues performed whole-exome sequencing on 22 pleural malignant mesotheliomas and matched blood, which revealed frequent alterations in *BAP1*, *NF2*, *CDKN2A*, and *CUL1* (Guo et al. 2015). In a much larger study, Bueno and colleagues analyzed transcriptomes, whole exomes and targeted exomes from a total of 216 pleural mesotheliomas (Bueno et al. 2016). Using exome analysis, they found *BAP1*, *NF2*, *TP53*, *SETD2*, *DDX3X*, *ULK2*, *RYR2*, *CFAP45*, *SETDB1*, and *DDX51* to be significantly mutated. Besides the more commonly mutated genes, i.e., *BAP1*, *NF2*, and *TP53*, mutation of *SETD2* (8%) was the most frequently mutated of the remaining seven genes newly implicated in this disease. The remaining six newer genes were mutated in 4% of less of cases. Whole-genome sequencing revealed additional structural variations that resulted in loss of gene function or copy number loss. For example, of the 20 samples analyzed using whole-genome sequencing, chromosomal rearrangements within *BAP1*, *NF2*, or

CDKN2A were identified in 9 (45%) cases, and recurrent gene fusions and splice alterations appeared to be common mechanisms for the inactivation of *NF2, BAP1,* and *SETD2* (Bueno et al. 2016).

While most mesotheliomas investigated genetically have involved the pleura, a recent report by Borczuk and colleagues included a series of peritoneal mesotheliomas (Borczuk et al. 2016). The group compared DNA array-based findings from 48 epithelioid peritoneal mesotheliomas and 41 epithelioid pleural mesotheliomas to identify similarities and differences in DNA copy number alterations. Recurrent losses in 3p (including *BAP1*), 9p (*CDKN2A*), and 22q (*NF2*) were seen in mesotheliomas from both tumor sites, although losses of *CDKN2A* and *NF2* occurred more frequently in pleural disease. Interestingly, whereas DNA copy number losses were more frequent in pleural mesotheliomas, copy number gains were more common in the peritoneal tumors, with regions of gain encompassing genes encoding receptor tyrosine kinase pathway members. Also noteworthy, among the peritoneal tumors, deletions in chromosome arms 6q, 14q, 17p, and 22q, and gain of 17q were observed in asbestos-associated cases but not in cases in which the disease was linked to radiation exposure. The investigators concluded that the pattern of genomic imbalances suggests both overlapping and distinct molecular genetic pathways in mesothelioma of the pleura and peritoneum, and that differences in causation—i.e., asbestos versus radiation—may explain some of the site-dependent genomic differences observed (Borczuk et al. 2016).

8.2 Germline Mutations in Malignant Mesothelioma

Since only a small percentage of asbestos-exposed individuals develop mesothelioma, and because familial clustering of the disease occurs in some families, it was proposed that genetic factors are likely to play a role in the etiology of mesothelioma (Roushdy-Hammady et al. 2001). The following section provides compelling evidence in support of this idea.

8.2.1 Early Evidence for the Possible Involvement of Germline Mutations in Mesothelioma

An early report suggesting that genetic susceptibility may play a role in mesothelioma development was published in the late 1970s (Li et al. 1978). The paper described the presence of mesothelioma in the wife and daughter of a man who was a pipe insulator at a shipyard. The man developed asbestosis and died from metastatic lung adenocarcinoma, possibly linked to heavy smoking. Family members reported that this individual frequently came home from work with his clothes covered with white dust, possibly asbestos, and the authors suggested "… the dosage of asbestos to induce mesothelioma in susceptible persons may be low and hardly noticed." In another report, a statistically significant number of families of female mesothelioma patients with non-occupational asbestos exposure were found to have parents with gastric or intestinal carcinomas (Vianna and Polan 1978). Since the authors did not find any evidence of asbestos exposure in this group of parents, they proposed that these individuals were from cancer-prone families. On a much larger scale, genetic susceptibility to mesothelioma has been proposed to explain the high incidence of mesothelioma in certain villages in Cappadocia, Turkey, where a meso-thelioma epidemic was first reported by Baris and colleagues in 1978 (Baris et al. 1978). The authors later proposed the possibility that an asbestos-like mineral fiber, erionite, may be the cause of this epidemic (Baris et al. 1981). A role for genetic susceptibility to mesothelioma was later proposed when investigators found a high incidence of the disease in some homes but not in other adjacent homes made with the same type of erionite-containing building blocks (Roushdy-Hammady et al. 2001; Carbone et al. 2007). However, to date a candidate gene(s) involved in this epidemic has not been discovered.

8.2.2   Clues Incriminating the BAP1 Gene in Mesothelioma

Carbone, Testa and colleagues initiated studies to identify a mesothelioma predispo-sition gene(s) using linkage analysis and/or a candidate gene approach in families from Cappadocia, Turkey, as well as in two unrelated families residing in two dif-ferent states, Wisconsin and Louisiana (W and L families, respectively), in the USA (Testa et al. 2011). Chromosome microarray analysis on tumor samples from the W and L families, and later linkage analysis on germline DNA, led to the implication of a candidate gene at chromosome band 3p21 (Testa et al. 2011). Notably, Harbour, Bowcock, and colleagues had previously uncovered inactivating somatic mutations of *BAP1* in 26 of 31 (84%) metastasizing uveal melanomas, and one of their patients had a germline mutation in *BAP1*, suggesting the existence of a tumor susceptibility allele in this individual (Harbour et al. 2010). This finding piqued our interest for three reasons: (1) our chromosome microarray analysis on two mesothelioma sam-ples from the W and L families had uncovered genomic alterations that either encompassed *BAP1* (homozygous deletion) or involved a chromosomal break within the *BAP1* locus; (2) our group's L family had two individuals with uveal melanomas (including one with metastasis to the liver); and (3) the *BAP1* gene is located at 3p21, a chromosomal site previously implicated in our extensive earlier cytogenetic and loss of heterozygosity (LOH) studies of sporadic mesotheliomas (Flejter et al. 1989; Lu et al. 1994). Spurred by these clues, we took a candidate approach which led to the discovery of germline inactivating mutations of *BAP1* in both the W and the L families (Testa et al. 2011). Interestingly, none of the members in these two families reported any occupational exposure to asbestos, and only trace amounts of asbestos were found in their homes. In family W, a germline splice site mutation in intron 6 was discovered in five family members with mesothelioma and three members with kidney, breast, or ovarian carcinomas. This mutation was shown to result in an aberrantly spliced mRNA leading to nonsense-mediated mRNA decay or a truncated protein due to a frameshift and premature stop codon. In the L family, a different germline *BAP1* alteration, a nonsense mutation, was found in seven family members with mesothelioma, one individual with a uveal melanoma, and one other with both a mesothelioma and a uveal melanoma. Immunohistochemistry performed on mesothelioma specimens from these families revealed loss of BAP1 nuclear expression and only weak cytoplasmic staining (Testa et al. 2011). Interestingly, germline *BAP1* mutations were also discovered in 2 of 26 sporadic mesotheliomas tested, and both of these mutation carriers were previously diagnosed with uveal melanoma.

Intriguingly, in the same issue of *Nature Genetics* as our report (Testa et al. 2011), Wiesner, Speicher, and colleagues reported two families in which germline inactivating mutations of *BAP1* were connected with predisposition to melanocytic tumors (Wiesner et al. 2011). Both of their families were characterized by high incidence of benign melanocytic tumors with some overlapping features common to cutaneous melanoma. A frameshift germline *BAP1* mutation was found to co-segregate with affected individuals in family 1, including one person who also developed UM. The second family had multiple relatives with benign melanocytic lesions as well as the co-occurrence of cutaneous melanoma in three family members, and a uveal melanoma in a fourth individual. Affected members of this family had a germline acceptor splice site mutation in *BAP1*, which leads to a predicted frameshift and truncation of the protein. Also notable, at the time of publication, there were no mesotheliomas reported in these two families. After the simultaneous publications by Testa et al. and Wiesner et al. in the same journal issue, communication between the two groups was initiated. This led to the reexamination and discovery of one member (previously known to have benign melanocytic lesions and cutaneous melanoma) of family 2 who was later found to have peritoneal mesothelioma with no known asbestos exposure (Wiesner et al. 2012). One month after the initial reports of BAP1 families, a report was released online by Abdel-Rahman and colleagues, who provided further evidence for a novel hereditary cancer syndrome caused by germline *BAP1* mutation (Abdel-Rahman et al. 2011). They reported a family with predisposition to uveal melanoma, lung carcinoma, meningioma, and possibly other cancers in connection with a germline *BAP1* nonsense mutation. Although not emphasized in this report, it is very noteworthy that one mutation carrier in this family had a mesothelioma, and that individual's son and a nephew both had mesothelioma and second tumors, although *BAP1* sequencing results were not available in these two cases. As in other studies (Testa et al. 2011; Wiesner et al. 2011), DNA analysis and immunohistochemical studies revealed loss of the wild type *BAP1* allele in tumor specimens from the germline mutation carriers.

8.3 BAP1 Cancer Predisposition Syndrome

Since the time of these initial reports, many other studies have uncovered germline *BAP1* mutations in familial mesothelioma and other cancers (Wiesner et al. 2012; Njauw et al. 2012; Wadt et al. 2012; Cheung et al. 2013; Hoiom et al. 2013; Popova et al. 2013; Wadt et al. 2014; Carbone et al. 2015; Cheung et al. 2015a; de la Fouchardiere et al. 2015; Ohar et al. 2016). Collectively, these findings suggest a single BAP1-related tumor predisposition syndrome in which affected families are predisposed to mesothelioma, uveal and cutaneous melanoma, benign melanocytic tumors, renal cell carcinoma, meningioma, basal cell carcinoma, cholangiocarcinomas, and potentially other less common cancers. In Table 8.1, we summarize the frequency of each tumor type reported to date in connection with germline *BAP1* mutations. The numbers in parentheses represent additional individuals with the indicated type of malignancy in the same families as the probands, but whose germline DNA was not directly sequenced. To date, the two most common types of cancers observed among *BAP1* mutation carriers are mesothelioma and uveal melanoma (Table 8.1). The fact that biallelic inactivation of *BAP1* has been documented in multiple tumors from these high-risk families implies that *BAP1* acts as a classical tumor suppressor gene. Consistent with these exciting genetic discoveries, BAP1 has also been found to exhibit tumor suppressor activity in cell-based transfection assays, and such tumor suppression requires both nuclear localization and BAP1 deubiquitinase activity (reviewed in Fang et al. 2010).

Over the past 5 years, a number of remarkable clinical features have been reported with regard to mesotheliomas seen in *BAP1* mutation carriers. While approximately 20% of all sporadic mesotheliomas are found in the peritoneum (Faig et al. 2015), a higher proportion of peritoneal mesothelioma has been observed in *BAP1* mutation carriers (Baumann et al. 2015; Cheung et al. 2015a; Ohar et al. 2016). Second, our large-scale study of 150 mesothelioma patients revealed a 10-year younger age of mesothelioma diagnosis among germline *BAP1* mutation

Table 8.1 Summary of tumors reported in connection with germline BAP1 mutations

Tumor type	Number of cases[a]
Malignant mesothelioma	55 (+42) = 97 total
Uveal melanoma	57 (+36) = 93 total
Cutaneous melanoma	32 (+28) = 60 total
Renal cell carcinoma	18 (+26) = 44 total
Melanocytic tumor	34 (+3) = 37 total
Breast carcinoma	12 (+16) = 28 total
Basal cell carcinoma	16 (+9) = 25 total
Lung carcinoma	7 (+15) = 22 total

[a]Numbers in parentheses represent individuals with the indicated tumor type in the same families as the probands, but whose germline DNA was not directly sequenced

carriers when compared to mesothelioma patients without a germline mutation (Ohar et al. 2016). This early age of cancer onset phenotype is typical of other cancer predisposition syndromes such as Li-Fraumeni syndrome (Li et al. 1988; Malkin et al. 1990), hereditary breast and ovarian cancer syndrome (Lynch et al. 2013), familial adenomatous polyposis (Tezcan et al. 2016), and Lynch syndrome (Tezcan et al. 2016). Third, *BAP1* mutation carriers who develop mesothelioma have a 3.5- to 7-fold improved survival rate after tumor diagnosis compared to non-carriers (Baumann et al. 2015; Ohar et al. 2016). The reason(s) for the improved survival among *BAP1* mutation carriers may be connected with the younger age and/or higher proportion of the more treatable peritoneal tumor in this group (Cheung et al. 2015a; Ohar et al. 2016). Sporadic mesotheliomas also appear to have a better prognosis when there is loss of BAP1 immunohistochemical staining (Farzin et al. 2015). This is in stark contrast to the situation in sporadic uveal melanomas (Harbour et al. 2010) and clear cell renal cell carcinomas (Minardi et al. 2016; Pena-Llopis et al. 2012), where BAP1 loss is associated with a poor prognosis. Finally, we and others have observed a high number of mutation carriers having more than one type of primary cancer (Cheung et al. 2015a; Ohar et al. 2016), a phenomenon that mirrors what is seen in individuals with Li-Fraumeni syndrome (Hisada et al. 1998). An example is depicted in Fig. 8.1, showing a family in which five *BAP1* mutation carriers with mesothelioma had at least one other primary cancer. This is particularly pronounced in individual III-09 who has three different types of cancers: mesothelioma, basal cell carcinoma, and meningioma.

Despite the multiple studies implicating *BAP1* as an important player in familial mesothelioma, there are likely other genes that when mutated in the germline can lead to a similar cancer syndrome. In our study involving Sanger sequencing of *BAP1* in germline DNA from 150 mesothelioma patients with a family history of cancer, we uncovered 9 (6%) individuals who were *BAP1* mutation carriers (Ohar et al. 2016). Whether families of the remaining 141 patients harbor germline mutation of some other cancer predisposition gene is not known. Similarly, we reported a large family with eight mesotheliomas in which no *BAP1* germline mutation was identified (Cheung et al. 2015b). One recent paper described a family in which both mesothelioma and cutaneous melanoma cases were found to have a deleterious germline missense mutation in the *CDKN2A* gene (c.301G > T; p.Gly101Trp) (Betti et al. 2016). The proband with this mutation, a female who developed cutaneous melanoma at the age of 42, has a mother who also carried the mutation and developed cutaneous melanoma at age 62 and mesothelioma at 65 (Betti et al. 2016). The exposure level for the mother was determined to be of the "low exposure" category, which was defined as non-occupational exposure. This missense mutation has been previously reported in other familial cutaneous melanoma cases (reviewed in Goldstein 2004). Considering that the *CDKN2A* locus at 9p21 is the most frequently site of somatic deletions in sporadic mesotheliomas (Cheng et al. 1994; Murthy and Testa 1999), it is plausible that germline mutations in the *CDKN2A* gene could also lead to increased risk for developing mesothelioma. Germline mutations in the *TP53* tumor suppressor gene have also been reported in mesothelioma. A germline missense mutation (p.Arg213Gln) was reported in a large family characterized by a

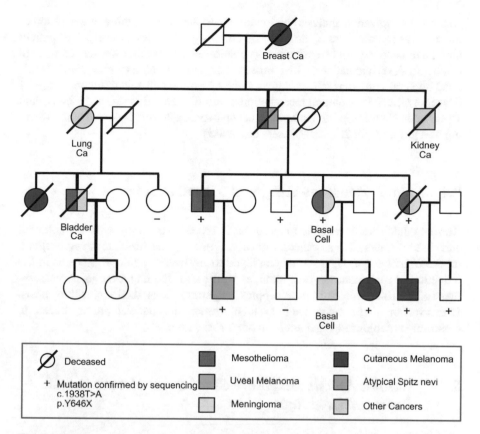

Fig. 8.1 Pedigree of BAP1 syndrome family with high incidence of multiple primary cancers. Affected family members have germline nonsense mutation in *BAP1* exon 15 (c.1938T>A). The family exhibits many neoplasms, including six family members with two or more primary tumors. Predominant cancers include mesothelioma and cutaneous melanoma, each observed in five family members. Modified from Cheung et al. (2015a); Cancer Lett 369:261–265. Copyright (2015), with permission from Elsevier

number of cancers, including breast and colon cancers (Ruijs et al. 2006). One mutation carrier in this family developed mesothelioma at the age of 55, with no asbestos exposure history described by the authors. Furthermore, a peritoneal mesothelioma was reported in an unrelated 60-year-old patient with Li-Fraumeni syndrome, in which a germline *TP53* missense mutation (p.R158H) was found (Ceelen et al. 2011). No known exposure to asbestos was reported for this individual. Finally, germline mutations in *NF2* have been reported in two studies. In the earlier report, an individual with NF2 disorder developed bilateral vestibular schwannomas and numerous spinal tumors in his 20s, and he later developed peritoneal mesothelioma at the age of 40 (Baser et al. 2002). Single-strand conformational polymorphism analysis did not reveal a germline mutation in the *NF2* gene; however, comparative genomic hybridization analysis and immunohistochemistry staining of the mesothelioma tissue revealed loss of the gene and protein product, respectively. This patient may have been exposed to asbestos occupationally, as he had worked as an auto mechanic. A second patient, with a missense mutation in *NF2* (p.Phe62Ser), developed bilateral vestibular schwannomas at the age of 66 and spinal tumors at age 74 (Baser et al. 2005). A pleural mesothelioma was discovered in this same individual 1 year later. He was reported to have an occupational asbestos exposure while working as a gas fitter for 25 years (Baser et al. 2005).

8.4 Animal Models of Malignant Mesothelioma

Animal models are invaluable tools for basic research on embryonic development and disease states such as cancer. Rodents, especially rat (*Rattus norvegicus*) and mouse (*Mus musculus*), are often employed to evaluate the role of asbestos in the induction of malignant mesothelioma, as well as for the unbiased genetic assessment of the role of mutant tumor suppressor genes in mesothelioma pathogenesis. In this section of our review, we focus on murine models but also provide a historic perspective of knowledge gained from other rodent models.

8.4.1 Chronic Asbestos Exposure Studies and Mesothelioma Pathogenesis in Rats

A strong epidemiological link between risk of mesothelioma and exposure to asbestos dust was established in the 1960s (reviewed in Gilson 1966). During the same decade, researchers began to formally test this hypothesis experimentally in laboratory rats by evaluating the carcinogenicity of both amphibole and serpentine mineral fibers (Wagner and Berry 1969). In 1962, Wagner and colleagues initiated a comprehensive study, in which 600 standard and 600 specific pathogen-free rats were inoculated intrapleurally with either amosite, chrysotile, crocidolite, extracted crocidolite (where oils were removed from the fibers with cyclohexane), silica or saline (~100 animals/arm/rat strain) and then followed until death (Wagner and Berry 1969). All carcinogenic mineral fibers tested were found to cause mesothelioma in a significant percentage of the animals irrespective of rat strain, thereby providing compelling experimental evidence for a causal relationship between asbestos and mesothelioma formation. This initial study was performed using a single inoculation of mineral fibers into the pleural space. However, in the occupational setting, humans typically inhale asbestos dust over a protracted time frame, different than what had been formally tested in rats. To address this discrepancy experimentally, in a subsequent investigation rats were chronically exposed to amphiboles and serpentine fibers using inhalation chambers. Animals were exposed to asbestos for 5, 8, and 10 weeks, as well as over longer time periods of 3, 6, 12, and 24 months, and then monitored for asbestos deposition in the lung and for disease onset (Wagner et al. 1974). In this study, a marked difference in lung deposition was observed between amphibole and serpentine fibers, with little to no deposition found in the lungs of chrysotile-exposed animals (Wagner et al. 1974). This observation led some to speculate that the serpentine shape of the chrysotile fibers makes it easier to expel in sputum from the lung (Bernstein et al. 2013). In the inhalation studies, a smaller percentage of mesotheliomas was observed compared to the previous study where asbestos was inoculated into the pleura, with Rhodesian chrysotile causing no mesotheliomas at all (Wagner et al. 1974). Asbestosis was a predominant disease observed in all exposed rats, although the authors also concluded that there was a positive correlation between asbestos exposure and mesothelioma development. Erionite, a zeolite mineral fiber implicated in the mesothelioma epidemic seen in several villages in Cappadocia, Turkey (Baris et al. 1978; Baris et al. 1981), was demonstrated to cause a very high rate of mesothelioma in rats when intrapleurally inoculated and was more carcinogenic than any amphibole or serpentine fiber tested in chronic inhalation experiments (Wagner et al. 1985).

These early studies in rats provided compelling evidence for the causal role of mineral fiber exposure in mesothelioma pathogenesis, a risk association previously identified in humans occupationally exposed to asbestos (Gilson 1966). Thus, rodents were established as an important tool for studies on the carcinogenicity of various types of mineral fibers.

8.4.2 Chronic Asbestos Exposure Studies and Mesothelioma Pathogenesis in Laboratory Mice

Initial rodent studies modeling asbestos-induced mesothelioma pathogenesis favored the rat over the mouse, due to the rat's larger pleural space for asbestos inoculation and lung capacity for mineral fiber inhalation studies. In some of the early investigations that did use mice, intrapleural inoculation of amphiboles and serpentine mineral fibers only caused granulomas and fibrosis (Davis 1970). Long-term asbestos inhalation studies in mice mainly caused fibrosis with occasional papillary carcinomas (Reeves et al. 1974). It was also demonstrated that very small amounts of asbestos deposition occur in the lung of mice via inhalation, presumably due to the mouse's smaller, more contorted nasal passages, such that asbestos fibers were less likely to enter the lung.

The first comprehensive mouse study testing the carcinogenicity of intraperitoneally inoculated asbestos and zeolite fibers was reported in the mid-1980s; in this investigation, more than 700 mice were injected with various concentrations and types of mineral fibers (Suzuki and Kohyama 1984). Malignant mesotheliomas were observed in 23.6% of the mice. This was a significantly higher incidence of mesothelioma than observed in mice either injected intrapleurally with mineral fibers or exposed to asbestos via inhalation (Davis 1970; Reeves et al. 1974; Suzuki and Kohyama 1984). Moreover, different laboratories have reported differing mesothelioma incidence and disease-free survival rates in wild type mice inoculated intraperitoneally with asbestos, due at least in part to differing types, amounts and fiber dimensions, variability of injection schedules, as well as differences in the genetic background of the strains of animals used (Marsella et al. 1997; Vaslet et al. 2002; Fleury-Feith et al. 2003; Altomare et al. 2005; Robinson et al. 2006; Altomare et al. 2009; Altomare et al. 2011; Chow et al. 2012; Xu et al. 2014; Menges et al. 2014; Kadariya et al. 2016a; Kadariya et al. 2016b; Pietrofesa et al. 2016). For example, laboratories that perform multiple injections of asbestos over time may observe a higher incidence of mesothelioma and shorter tumor-free survival than laboratories that inject mice with a single bolus of mineral fibers. Injection of asbestos into the peritoneal space induces an acute inflammation. This inflammatory response appears to contribute to mesothelioma pathogenesis via the repeated release of chemokines such as IL-1β, IL-6, and TNFα (Kadariya et al. 2016b; Pietrofesa et al. 2016). The acute inflammatory reaction to intraperitoneal injection of asbestos fibers declines after 21 days (Macdonald and Kane 1997). They found that a 3-week recovery period decreased the extent of fibrosis induced following repeated injections that can cause premature death in exposed mice before mesotheliomas have time to develop. Pilot studies using doses of 100, 200, or 500 μg revealed a dose-dependent increase in the acute inflammatory response (Macdonald and Kane 1997), and for most of our publications we selected repeated injections at a dose of 400 μg, which induced mesotheliomas in about 50% of wild-type mice (Altomare et al. 2005).

8.4.3 Chronic Asbestos Exposure Studies and Mesothelioma Pathogenesis in Genetically Engineered Mouse (GEM) Models

GEM models are mice that have had their genome altered through the use of genetic engineering, including gene knock-out and knock-in techniques, and have been used in science to understand embryonic development and to model disease states such as cancer. Genes frequently activated or inactivated in human cancers can be mutated or deleted in mice to unravel genetically the role of oncogenes and tumor suppressor genes, respectively, in development or tumorigenesis (Gopinathan and Tuveson 2008). Cytogenetic and molecular genetic analysis of human mesotheliomas by many different laboratories have revealed recurrent losses at chromosomal sites harboring known or suspected tumor suppressor loci (Tiainen et al. 1988; Flejter et al. 1989; Cheng et al. 1993; Taguchi et al. 1993; Lu et al. 1994; Lee et al. 1996; Bell et al. 1997; Bjorkqvist et al. 1997), and as noted above, mutations of several different tumor suppressor genes, especially *CDKN2A, BAP1,* and *NF2*, are considered to be driving events in this disease (Bianchi et al. 1995; Sekido et al. 1995; Cheng et al. 1999; Illei et al. 2003; Bott et al. 2011; Testa et al. 2011).

To determine if loss/inactivation of these tumor suppressor genes accelerates asbestos-induced mesothelioma development, various groups have conducted asbestos carcinogenicity studies with GEM models carrying germline mutations of these genes, along with wild type littermates that serve as controls. The first such studies involved a mouse model deficient for the *Tp53* gene, which encodes the tumor suppressor p53 (Marsella et al. 1997; Vaslet et al. 2002). Mice (129/Sv strain) with heterozygous (+/−) or homozygous (−/−) mutation of *Tp53*, along with wild type (+/+) littermates, were injected intraperitoneally with crocidolite every week. After 22 weekly injections, 76% of asbestos-exposed $Tp53^{+/-}$ mice developed mesothelioma (median latency: 44 weeks) compared to 32% of asbestos-exposed genetically normal ($Tp53^{+/+}$) mice (median latency: 67 weeks). Only 1 of 8 (12.5%) $Tp53^{-/-}$ mice developed a mesothelioma, with the remainder of this cohort dying of thymic lymphomas or hemangiosarcomas, which are known to arise spontaneously in such mice (Donehower et al. 1995).

The tumor suppressor gene *NF2* is mutated in up to 55% of mesotheliomas (Cheng et al. 1999). Two groups evaluated whether mice heterozygously deficient for Nf2 ($Nf2^{+/-}$) have increased susceptibility to asbestos-induced carcinogenesis (Fleury-Feith et al. 2003; Altomare et al. 2005). Both studies found that asbestos-injected $Nf2^{+/-}$ mice developed a higher incidence of peritoneal mesotheliomas and a shorter latency compared to mineral fiber-exposed wild-type cohorts. Interestingly, the second, wild-type copy of *Nf2* was lost in a high percentage of mesotheliomas from asbestos-exposed *Nf2*-deficient mice, a finding that mirrors what is observed in many human mesotheliomas (Altomare et al. 2005). Mesothelioma cell lines from asbestos-exposed $Nf2^{+/-}$ mice exhibited somatic genetic and cell signaling alterations recapitulating those of the human disease counterpart. Together, these data demonstrated that *Nf2* is a bona fide tumor suppressor gene and that, upon exposure to asbestos, *Nf2* inactivation can act as a primary driver in mesothelioma pathogenesis.

The next GEM model that was used to investigate mesothelioma formation was a transgenic model (C57/Bl 6 J background) expressing SV40 large T antigen (TAg) in the mesothelial lining (Robinson et al. 2006). Transgenic mice expressing a single copy or multiple copies of SV40 TAg, as well as non-transgenic littermates, were exposed to asbestos and followed for development of mesothelioma. TAg transgenic mice developed mesothelioma with a shorter latency than did wild type mice, with a direct relationship found between transgene copy number and survival after exposure to asbestos. This study demonstrated that SV40 TAg, presumably through its disruption of Rb and p53 pathways, can contribute to asbestos-induced mesothelioma pathogenesis, although this model has limited relevance to human disease, given that the proposed link between SV40 infection and human mesothelioma now appears unlikely (Lopez-Rios et al. 2004).

As mentioned earlier, the *CDKN2A* locus encodes two tumor suppressors, p16INK4A and p14ARF (p19Arf in mice), and deletion of this locus occurs in most mesotheliomas (Cheng et al. 1994; Xio et al. 1995; Altomare et al. 2005). Because that the genes encoding p16INK4A and p14/p19ARF share exon 2, the exon most often lost in mesotheliomas, deletions of *CDKN2A* usually inactivate both tumor suppressors. It was not clear until recently that both tumor suppressors contribute significantly to mesothelioma tumorigenesis. To address the potential role of p14/p19ARF loss in mesothelioma development, we used mice harboring a mutation in exon 1β of the *Cdkn2a* locus, which specifically inactivates p19Arf but not p16Ink4a (Altomare et al. 2009). Asbestos-exposed *p19Arf*[+/−] mice showed a higher incidence, and shorter latency, of mesothelioma formation compared to asbestos-exposed wild-type littermates. Mesotheliomas from *p19Arf*[+/−] mice showed recurrent genomic losses of chromosome 4, band C6, encompassing the Fas associated factor 1 gene, *Faf1*, which is known to play a role in apoptosis and cell death (Altomare et al. 2009; Menges et al. 2009). Additionally, its homolog, *FAF1*, is down-regulated in many human mesothelioma specimens and tumor-derived cell lines that were tested (Altomare et al. 2009). We also found that Faf1 regulates TNF-α-mediated NF-κB signaling, a signaling node that has been implicated in asbestos-induced carcinogenesis (Yang et al. 2006).

We next tested the relative contributions of both p16Ink4a and p19Arf to mesothelioma pathogenesis using mice with heterozygous deletions of one or the other genes (loss of exons 1α or 1β of *Cdkn2a*, respectively), or with a deletion knocking out both genes (loss of *Cdkn2a* exon 2) (Altomare et al. 2011). Asbestos-treated *p16Ink4a*[+/−] and *p19Arf*[+/−] mice each showed increased incidence and shorter latency of mesothelioma formation relative to wild type littermates. Mice deficient for both p16Ink4a and p19Arf showed accelerated asbestos-induced mesothelioma formation relative to mice deficient for *p16Ink4a* or *p19Arf* alone, and the resulting tumors exhibited biallelic loss of both tumor suppressor genes. Thus, these findings provided in vivo evidence indicating that both *Cdkn2a* gene products suppress asbestos carcinogenicity. Moreover, simultaneous inactivation of both genes appeared to cooperate to accelerate asbestos-induced tumor development and progression.

As stated above, human mesotheliomas frequently harbor alterations of both *NF2* and *CDKN2A*, suggesting cooperativity between losses of these two tumor suppressor genes. Tumorigenic cooperativity between these genes in mesothelioma pathogenesis was recently demonstrated in asbestos-exposed mice with germline mutation of one allele of each of these genes. These *Nf2*[+/−];*Cdkn2a*[+/−] mice showed markedly accelerated onset and progression of asbestos-induced mesothelioma compared to asbestos-exposed *Nf2*[+/−] or wild-type mice (Menges et al. 2014). Interestingly, ascites from the doubly mutant mice sometimes harbored large tumor spheroids, and tail vein injections of tumor-derived cell lines established from *Nf2*[+/−];*Cdkn2a*[+/−] mice, but not from *Nf2*[+/−] or wild type mice, produced numerous tumors in the lung, suggesting an increased metastatic potential. Additionally, these mesothelioma cell lines had increased markers of cancer stem cells (CSC) and formed CSC spheroids in vitro more efficiently than tumor cells from wild type or *Nf2*[+/−] mice. The mesothelioma cells from *Nf2*[+/−];*Cdkn2a*[+/−] mice had elevated levels of c-Met expression and activation, which was partly dependent on p53-mediated regulation of the microRNA miR-34a. This signaling axis appeared to be required for tumor migration, invasiveness and maintenance of the CSC population in the tumor cells from $Nf2^{+/-};Cdkn2a^{+/-}$ mice. Collectively, these studies implicate in vivo cooperativity between $Nf2$ and $Cdkn2a$ losses in the development of aggressive mesotheliomas that exhibit enhanced metastatic potential and an increased CSC population in connection with p53/miR-34a-dependent activation of c-Met (Menges et al. 2014). Thus, we proposed that cooperativity between losses of $Nf2$ and $Cdkn2a$ plays a fundamental role in driving the highly aggressive tumorigenic phenotype considered to be a hallmark of malignant mesothelioma.

At the time of the initial studies of germline $BAP1$ mutations in high-risk cancer families (Testa et al. 2011; Wiesner et al. 2011), it was unclear why mesothelioma was the main malignancy seen in some of these families (Testa et al. 2011), whereas melanocytic tumors predominated in other families (Wiesner et al. 2011). To address these questions experimentally, we generated GEM mice harboring a $Bap1$ deletion (designated $Bap1^{+/-}$ from here on) to assess whether $Bap1$ heterozygosity in the germline predisposes to asbestos-induced mesothelioma. $Bap1^{+/-}$ mice exhibited a significantly higher incidence of asbestos-induced mesotheliomas than wild type littermates (73% vs. 32%, respectively), and tumors arose at an accelerated rate in $Bap1^{+/-}$ mice as compared to wild type animals (median survival, 43 weeks vs. 55 weeks after initial exposure, respectively) (Xu et al. 2014). Mesothelioma cells from the $Bap1^{+/-}$ mice demonstrated biallelic inactivation of $Bap1$, consistent with the gene's proposed role as a recessive cancer susceptibility gene. Unlike the situation in wild type mice, mesothelioma cells from $Bap1^{+/-}$ mice did not require homozygous loss of $Cdkn2a$. Interestingly, normal mesothelial cells and mesothelioma cells from $Bap1^{+/-}$ mice showed down-regulation of Rb through a p16Ink4a-independent mechanism, suggesting that predisposition of $Bap1^{+/-}$ mice to mesothelioma may be facilitated, in part, by cooperation between Bap1 and Rb (Xu et al. 2014). In a subsequent study, a significantly higher incidence of mesothelioma was reported in $Bap1^{+/-}$ mice upon exposure to minimal doses of asbestos that rarely caused the disease in wild type mice, potentially connected with a deregulated inflammatory response (Napolitano et al. 2015). In another study (Fig. 8.2), we reported that knock-in mice harboring point mutations identical to those found in our first two BAP1 syndrome families (Testa et al. 2011) also demonstrated accelerated asbestos-induced mesothelioma development as compared to identically exposed wild-type littermates (Kadariya et al. 2016a). Taken together, these findings suggest that $BAP1$ carriers have markedly enhanced susceptibility to the carcinogenic effects of asbestos, even minimal doses (Napolitano et al. 2015), in comparison to the general population.

Finally, we should point out that BAP1's putative role in cancer has been somewhat perplexing, because $BAP1$ knockdown has been reported to inhibit cell proliferation and/or tumorigenicity. For example, Bott and colleagues reported that mesothelioma cell lines containing wild-type BAP1 showed decreased proliferation upon $BAP1$ knockdown, and that the reintroduction of wild-type $BAP1$ in $BAP1$-null mesothelioma cells resulted in an *increase* in cell proliferation, enigmatic findings for a putative tumor suppressor gene (Bott et al. 2011). Similarly, knockdown of $BAP1$ in breast cancer was shown to *inhibit* cell proliferation, tumorigenicity, and

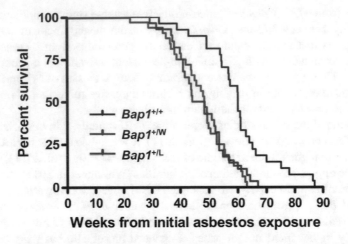

	Bap1 +/+	Bap1 +/W	Bap1 +/L	Significance
Median % disease-free (weeks)	60	48	46	p < 0.01 for Bap1+/+ mice vs. either Bap1+/W or Bap1+/L mice
Mesothelioma	35%	74%	71%	p < 0.01 for Bap1+/+ mice vs. either Bap1+/W or Bap1+/L mice

Fig. 8.2 GEM mice with clinically relevant germline mutations of *Bap1* show increased susceptibility to the carcinogenic effects of asbestos. *Top panel,* Kaplan-Meier survival curves showing markedly decreased survival (all deaths) in asbestos-exposed *Bap1*-mutant mice than in asbestos-exposed wild type (*Bap1+/+*) littermates. *Bap1+/W* mice have germline knock-in mutation identical to that of a BAP1 syndrome family from Wisconsin (W family), whereas *Bap1+/L* mice have the same germline mutation seen in a BAP1 syndrome family from Louisiana (L). *Lower panel,* Table summarizing statistically significant differences in disease-free time duration and mesothelioma incidence between *Bap1+/+* mice and *Bap1*-mutant cohorts. Modified from Kadariya et al. (2016a); Cancer Res 2016; 76:2836–2844. Copyright (2016), with permission from the American Association for Cancer Research (AACR)

metastasis (Qin et al. 2015). To examine experimentally whether germline *Bap1* mutations act as potent cancer susceptibility alleles, we monitored spontaneous tumor formation in three different heterozygous *Bap1*-mutant mouse models, including two with knock-in mutations identical to those reported in human BAP1 cancer syndrome families (Kadariya et al. 2016a). Spontaneous malignant tumors were observed in 54 of 93 (58%) *Bap1*-mutant mice versus only 4 of 43 (9%) wild-type littermates. The three *Bap1*-mutant models had a high incidence and similar spectrum of cancers, predominantly ovarian sex cord stromal tumors, lung and mammary carcinomas, as well as spindle cell tumors. Intriguingly, malignant mesotheliomas were seen in two *Bap1*-mutant mice but not in any wild-type mice, although this difference was not statistically significant. Together, these findings provided unbiased genetic evidence that *Bap1* is indeed a bona fide tumor suppressor gene, which when mutated in the germline predisposes to a wide spectrum of tumors, including occasional mesotheliomas, although high penetrance of mesothelioma was shown to require exposure to carcinogenic fibers (Kadariya et al. 2016a).

Declaration of Interests J.R.T. has served as a genetics consultant, and in one instance, as an expert witness for the plaintiff in a case involving the role of germline mutations of *BAP1* in mesothelioma. C.W.M. and M.C. declare no potential conflict of interest.

References

Abdel-Rahman MH, Pilarski R, Cebulla CM et al (2011) Germline BAP1 mutation predisposes to uveal melanoma, lung adenocarcinoma, meningioma, and other cancers. J Med Genet 48:856–859

Altomare DA, Vaslet CA, Skele KL et al (2005) A mouse model recapitulating molecular features of human mesothelioma. Cancer Res 65:8090–8095

Altomare DA, Menges CW, Pei J et al (2009) Activated TNF-alpha/NF-kappaB signaling via down-regulation of Fas-associated factor 1 in asbestos-induced mesotheliomas from Arf knockout mice. Proc Natl Acad Sci U S A 106:3430–3435

Altomare DA, Menges CW, Xu J et al (2011) Losses of both products of the Cdkn2a/Arf locus contribute to asbestos-induced mesothelioma development and cooperate to accelerate tumorigenesis. PLoS One 6:e18828

Baris YI, Sahin AA, Ozesmi M et al (1978) An outbreak of pleural mesothelioma and chronic fibrosing pleurisy in the village of Karain/Urgup in Anatolia. Thorax 33:181–192

Baris YI, Saracci R, Simonato L et al (1981) Malignant mesothelioma and radiological chest abnormalities in two villages in Central Turkey. An epidemiological and environmental investigation. Lancet 1:984–987

Baser ME, De Rienzo A, Altomare D et al (2002) Neurofibromatosis 2 and malignant mesothelioma. Neurology 59:290–291

Baser ME, Rai H, Wallace AJ et al (2005) Neurofibromatosis 2 (NF2) and malignant mesothelioma in a man with a constitutional NF2 missense mutation. Familial Cancer 4:321–322

Baumann F, Flores E, Napolitano A et al (2015) Mesothelioma patients with germline BAP1 mutations have 7-fold improved long-term survival. Carcinogenesis 36:76–81

Bell DW, Jhanwar SC, Testa JR (1997) Multiple regions of allelic loss from chromosome arm 6q in malignant mesothelioma. Cancer Res 57:4057–4062

Bernstein D, Dunnigan J, Hesterberg T et al (2013) Health risk of chrysotile revisited. Crit Rev Toxicol 43:154–183

Betti M, Aspesi A, Biasi A et al (2016) CDKN2A and BAP1 germline mutations predispose to melanoma and mesothelioma. Cancer Lett 378:120–130

Bianchi AB, Mitsunaga S-I, Cheng JQ et al (1995) High frequency of inactivating mutations in the neurofibromatosis type 2 gene (*NF2*) in primary malignant mesotheliomas. Proc Natl Acad Sci U S A 92:10854–10858

Bjorkqvist AM, Tammilehto L, Anttila S et al (1997) Recurrent DNA copy number changes in 1q, 4q, 6q, 9p, 13q, 14q and 22q detected by comparative genomic hybridization in malignant mesothelioma. Br J Cancer 75:523–527

Borczuk AC, Pei J, Taub RN et al (2016) Genome-wide analysis of abdominal and pleural malignant mesothelioma with DNA arrays reveals both common and distinct regions of copy number alteration. Cancer Biol Ther 17:328–335

Bott M, Brevet M, Taylor BS et al (2011) The nuclear deubiquitinase BAP1 is commonly inactivated by somatic mutations and 3p21.1 losses in malignant pleural mesothelioma. Nat Genet 43:668–672

Bueno R, Stawiski EW, Goldstein LD et al (2016) Comprehensive genomic analysis of malignant pleural mesothelioma identifies recurrent mutations, gene fusions and splicing alterations. Nat Genet 48:407–416

Carbone M, Emri S, Dogan AU et al (2007) A mesothelioma epidemic in Cappadocia: scientific developments and unexpected social outcomes. Nat Rev Cancer 7:147–154

Carbone M, Flores EG, Emi M et al (2015) Combined genetic and genealogic studies uncover a large BAP1 cancer syndrome kindred tracing back nine generations to a common ancestor from the 1700s. PLoS Genet 11:e1005633

Ceelen WP, Van Dalen T, Van Bockstal M et al (2011) Malignant peritoneal mesothelioma in a patient with Li-Fraumeni syndrome. J Clin Oncol 29:e503–e505

Cheng JQ, Jhanwar SC, Lu YY et al (1993) Homozygous deletions within 9p21-p22 identify a small critical region of chromosomal loss in human malignant mesothelioma. Cancer Res 53:4761–4763

Cheng JQ, Jhanwar SC, Klein WM et al (1994) *p16* alterations and deletion mapping of 9p21-p22 in malignant mesothelioma. Cancer Res 54:5547–5551

Cheng JQ, Lee WC, Klein MA et al (1999) Frequent mutations of NF2 and allelic loss from chromosome band 22q12 in malignant mesothelioma: evidence for a two-hit mechanism of NF2 inactivation. Genes Chromosomes Cancer 24:238–242

Cheung M, Talarchek J, Schindeler K et al (2013) Further evidence for germline BAP1 mutations predisposing to melanoma and malignant mesothelioma. Cancer Genet 206:206–210

Cheung M, Kadariya Y, Talarchek J et al (2015a) Germline BAP1 mutation in a family with high incidence of multiple primary cancers and a potential gene-environment interaction. Cancer Lett 369:261–265

Cheung M, Kadariya Y, Pei J, Talarchek J, Facciolo F, Visca P, Righi L, Cozzi I, Testa JR, Ascoli V (2015b) An asbestos-exposed family with multiple cases of pleural malignant mesothelioma without inheritance of a predisposing BAP1 mutation. Cancer Genet 208:502–507

Chow MT, Tschopp J, Möller A et al (2012) NLRP3 promotes inflammation-induced skin cancer but is dispensable for asbestos-induced mesothelioma. Immunol Cell Biol 90:983–986

Cote RJ, Jhanwar SC, Novick S et al (1991) Genetic alterations of the p53 gene are a feature of malignant mesothelioma. Cancer Res 51:5410–5416

Davis JM (1970) The long term fibrogenic effects of chrysotile and crocidolite asbestos dust injected into the pleural cavity of experimental animals. Br J Exp Pathol 51:617–627

de la Fouchardiere A, Cabaret O, Savin L et al (2015) Germline BAP1 mutations predispose also to multiple basal cell carcinomas. Clin Genet 88:273–277

Donehower LA, Harvey M, Vogel H et al (1995) Effects of genetic background on tumorigenesis in p53-deficient mice. Mol Carcinog 14:16–22

Faig J, Howard S, Levine EA et al (2015) Changing pattern in malignant mesothelioma survival. Transl Oncol 8:35–39

Fang Y, Fu D, Shen XZ (2010) The potential role of ubiquitin c-terminal hydrolases in oncogenesis. Biochim Biophys Acta 1806:1–6

Farzin M, Toon CW, Clarkson A et al (2015) Loss of expression of BAP1 predicts longer survival in mesothelioma. Pathology 47:302–307

Flejter WL, Li FP, Antman KH et al (1989) Recurring loss involving chromosomes 1, 3, and 22 in malignant mesothelioma: possible sites of tumor suppressor genes. Genes Chromosomes Cancer 1:148–154

Fleury-Feith J, Lecomte C, Renier A et al (2003) Hemizygosity of Nf2 is associated with increased susceptibility to asbestos-induced peritoneal tumours. Oncogene 22:3799–3805

Frizelle SP, Grim J, Zhou J et al (1998) Re-expression of p16INK4a in mesothelioma cells results in cell cycle arrest, cell death, tumor suppression and tumor regression. Oncogene 16:3087–3095

Gaytan de Ayala Alonso A, Gutierrez L, Fritsch C et al (2007) A genetic screen identifies novel polycomb group genes in *Drosophila*. Genetics 176:2099–2108

Gilson JC (1966) Health hazards of asbestos. Recent studies on its biological effects. Trans Soc Occup Med 16:62–74

Goldstein AM (2004) Familial melanoma, pancreatic cancer and germline CDKN2A mutations. Hum Mutat 23:630

Gopinathan A, Tuveson DA (2008) The use of GEM models for experimental cancer therapeutics. Dis Model Mech 1:83–86

Guo G, Chmielecki J, Goparaju C et al (2015) Whole-exome sequencing reveals frequent genetic alterations in BAP1, NF2, CDKN2A, and CUL1 in malignant pleural mesothelioma. Cancer Res 75:264–269

Harbour JW, Onken MD, Roberson ED et al (2010) Frequent mutation of BAP1 in metastasizing uveal melanomas. Science 330:1410–1413

Hisada M, Garber JE, Fung CY et al (1998) Multiple primary cancers in families with Li-Fraumeni syndrome. J Natl Cancer Inst 90:606–611

Hoiom V, Edsgard D, Helgadottir H et al (2013) Hereditary uveal melanoma: a report of a germline mutation in BAP1. Genes Chromosomes Cancer 52:378–384

Illei PB, Ladanyi M, Rusch VW et al (2003) The use of CDKN2A deletion as a diagnostic marker for malignant mesothelioma in body cavity effusions. Cancer Cytopathol 99:51–56

Ismail IH, Davidson R, Gagne JP et al (2014) Germline mutations in BAP1 impair its function in DNA double-strand break repair. Cancer Res 74:4282–4294

James MF, Han S, Polizzano C et al (2009) NF2/merlin is a novel negative regulator of mTOR complex 1, and activation of mTORC1 is associated with meningioma and schwannoma growth. Mol Cell Biol 29:4250–4261

Kadariya Y, Cheung M, Xu J et al (2016a) Bap1 is a bona fide tumor suppressor: genetic evidence from mouse models carrying heterozygous germline Bap1 mutations. Cancer Res 76:2836–2844

Kadariya Y, Menges CW, Talarchek J et al (2016b) Inflammation-related IL1beta/IL1R signaling promotes the development of asbestos-induced malignant mesothelioma. Cancer Prev Res 9:406–414

Lee WC, Balsara B, Liu Z et al (1996) Loss of heterozygosity analysis defines a critical region in chromosome 1p22 commonly deleted in human malignant mesothelioma. Cancer Res 56:4297–4301

Li FP, Lokich J, Lapey J et al (1978) Familial mesothelioma after intense asbestos exposure at home. JAMA 240:467

Li FP, Fraumeni JF Jr, Mulvihill JJ et al (1988) A cancer family syndrome in twenty-four kindreds. Cancer Res 48:5358–5362

Lo Iacono M, Monica V, Righi L et al (2015) Targeted next-generation sequencing of cancer genes in advanced stage malignant pleural mesothelioma: a retrospective study. J Thorac Oncol 10:492–499

Lopez-Lago MA, Okada T, Murillo MM et al (2009) Loss of the tumor suppressor gene NF2, encoding merlin, constitutively activates integrin-dependent mTORC1 signaling. Mol Cell Biol 29:4235–4249

Lopez-Rios F, Illei PB, Rusch V et al (2004) Evidence against a role for SV40 infection in human mesotheliomas and high risk of false-positive PCR results owing to presence of SV40 sequences in common laboratory plasmids. Lancet 364:1157–1166

Lu YY, Jhanwar SC, Cheng JQ et al (1994) Deletion mapping of the short arm of chromosome 3 in human malignant mesothelioma. Genes Chromosomes Cancer 9:76–80

Lynch HT, Snyder C, Casey MJ (2013) Hereditary ovarian and breast cancer: what have we learned? Ann Oncol 24(Suppl 8):viii83–viii95

Macdonald JL, Kane AB (1997) Mesothelial cell proliferation and biopersistence of wollastonite and crocidolite asbestos fibers. Fundam Appl Toxicol 38:173–183

Malkin D, Li FP, Strong LC et al (1990) Germ line p53 mutations in a familial syndrome of breast cancer, sarcomas, and other neoplasms. Science 250:1233–1238

Marsella JM, Liu BL, Vaslet CA et al (1997) Susceptibility of *p53*-deficient mice to induction of mesothelioma by crocidolite asbestos fibers. Environ Health Perspect 105:1069–1072

Menges CW, Altomare DA, Testa JR (2009) FAS-associated factor 1 (FAF1): diverse functions and implications for oncogenesis. Cell Cycle 8:2528–2534

Menges CW, Kadariya Y, Altomare D et al (2014) Tumor suppressor alterations cooperate to drive aggressive mesotheliomas with enriched cancer stem cells via a p53-miR-34a-c-Met axis. Cancer Res 74:1261–1271

Minardi D, Lucarini G, Milanese G et al (2016) Loss of nuclear BAP1 protein expression is a marker of poor prognosis in patients with clear cell renal cell carcinoma. Urol Oncol 34:338. e11–338.e18

Murakami H, Mizuno T, Taniguchi T et al (2011) LATS2 is a tumor suppressor gene of malignant mesothelioma. Cancer Res 71:873–883

Murthy SS, Testa JR (1999) Asbestos, chromosomal deletions, and tumor suppressor gene alterations in human malignant mesothelioma. J Cell Physiol 180:150–157

Napolitano A, Pellegrini L, Dey A et al (2015) Minimal asbestos exposure in germline BAP1 heterozygous mice is associated with deregulated inflammatory response and increased risk of mesothelioma. Oncogene 35:1996–2002

Nasu M, Emi M, Pastorino S et al (2015) High incidence of somatic BAP1 alterations in sporadic malignant mesothelioma. J Thorac Oncol 10:565–576

Njauw CN, Kim I, Piris A et al (2012) Germline BAP1 inactivation is preferentially associated with metastatic ocular melanoma and cutaneous-ocular melanoma families. PLoS One 7:e35295

Ohar JA, Cheung M, Talarchek J et al (2016) Germline BAP1 mutational landscape of asbestos-exposed malignant mesothelioma patients with family history of cancer. Cancer Res 76:206–215

Pena-Llopis S, Vega-Rubin-de-Celis S, Liao A et al (2012) BAP1 loss defines a new class of renal cell carcinoma. Nat Genet 44:751–759

Pietrofesa RA, Velalopoulou A, Arguiri E et al (2016) Flaxseed lignans enriched in secoisolariciresinol diglucoside prevent acute asbestos-induced peritoneal inflammation in mice. Carcinogenesis 37:177–187

Popova T, Hebert L, Jacquemin V et al (2013) Germline BAP1 mutations predispose to renal cell carcinomas. Am J Hum Genet 92:974–980

Poulikakos PI, Xiao GH, Gallagher R et al (2006) Re-expression of the tumor suppressor NF2/merlin inhibits invasiveness in mesothelioma cells and negatively regulates FAK. Oncogene 25:5960–5968

Qin J, Zhou Z, Chen W et al (2015) BAP1 promotes breast cancer cell proliferation and metastasis by deubiquitinating KLF5. Nat Commun 6:8471

Reeves AL, Puro HE, Smith RG (1974) Inhalation carcinogenesis from various forms of asbestos. Environ Res 8:178–202

Robinson C, van Bruggen I, Segal A et al (2006) A novel SV40 TAg transgenic model of asbestos-induced mesothelioma: malignant transformation is dose dependent. Cancer Res 66:10786–10794

Roushdy-Hammady I, Siegel J, Emri S et al (2001) Genetic-susceptibility factor and malignant mesothelioma in the Cappadocian region of Turkey. Lancet 357:444–445

Ruijs MW, Verhoef S, Wigbout G et al (2006) Late-onset common cancers in a kindred with an Arg213Gln TP53 germline mutation. Familial Cancer 5:169–174

Sekido Y, Pass HI, Bader S et al (1995) Neurofibromatosis type 2 (*NF2*) gene is somatically mutated in mesothelioma but not in lung cancer. Cancer Res 55:1227–1231

Suzuki Y, Kohyama N (1984) Malignant mesothelioma induced by asbestos and zeolite in the mouse peritoneal cavity. Environ Res 35:277–292

Taguchi T, Jhanwar SC, Siegfried JM et al (1993) Recurrent deletions of specific chromosomal sites in 1p, 3p, 6q, and 9p in human malignant mesothelioma. Cancer Res 53:4349–4355

Testa JR, Cheung M, Pei J et al (2011) Germline BAP1 mutations predispose to malignant mesothelioma. Nat Genet 43:1022–1025

Tezcan G, Tunca B, Ak S et al (2016) Molecular approach to genetic and epigenetic pathogenesis of early-onset colorectal cancer. World J Gastrointest Oncol 8:83–98

Tiainen M, Tammilehto L, Mattson K et al (1988) Non-random chromosomal abnormalities in malignant pleural mesothelioma. Cancer Genet Cytogenet 33:251–274

Vaslet CA, Messier NJ, Kane AB (2002) Accelerated progression of asbestos-induced mesotheliomas in heterozygous p53(+/−) mice. Toxicol Sci 68:331–338

Vianna NJ, Polan AK (1978) Non-occupational exposure to asbestos and malignant mesothelioma in females. Lancet 1:1061–1063

Wadt K, Choi J, Chung JY et al (2012) A cryptic BAP1 splice mutation in a family with uveal and cutaneous melanoma, and paraganglioma. Pigment Cell Melanoma Res 25:815–818

Wadt KA, Aoude LG, Johansson P et al (2014) A recurrent germline BAP1 mutation and extension of the BAP1 tumor predisposition spectrum to include basal cell carcinoma. Clin Genet 88:267–272

Wagner JC, Berry G (1969) Mesotheliomas in rats following inoculation with asbestos. Br J Cancer 23:567–581

Wagner JC, Berry G, Skidmore JW et al (1974) The effects of the inhalation of asbestos in rats. Br J Cancer 29:252–269

Wagner JC, Skidmore JW, Hill RJ et al (1985) Erionite exposure and mesotheliomas in rats. Br J Cancer 51:727–730

Wiesner T, Obenauf AC, Murali R et al (2011) Germline mutations in BAP1 predispose to melanocytic tumors. Nat Genet 43:1018–1021

Wiesner T, Fried I, Ulz P et al (2012) Toward an improved definition of the tumor spectrum associated with BAP1 germline mutations. J Clin Oncol 30:e337–e340

Xiao GH, Beeser A, Chernoff J et al (2002) p21-activated kinase links Rac/Cdc42 signaling to merlin. J Biol Chem 277:883–886

Xiao G, Gallagher R, Shetler J et al (2005) The NF2 tumor suppressor gene product, merlin, inhibits cell proliferation and cell cycle progression by repressing cyclin D1 expression. Mol Cell Biol 25:2384–2394

Xio S, Li D, Vijg J et al (1995) Codeletion of p15 and p16 in primary malignant mesothelioma. Oncogene 11:511–515

Xu J, Kadariya Y, Cheung M et al (2014) Germline mutation of Bap1 accelerates development of asbestos-induced malignant mesothelioma. Cancer Res 74:4388–4397

Yang CT, You L, Yeh CC et al (2000) Adenovirus-mediated p14(ARF) gene transfer in human mesothelioma cells. J Natl Cancer Inst 92:636–641

Yang H, Bocchetta M, Kroczynska B et al (2006) TNF-alpha inhibits asbestos-induced cytotoxicity via a NF-kappaB-dependent pathway, a possible mechanism for asbestos-induced oncogenesis. Proc Natl Acad Sci U S A 103:10397–10402

Yoshikawa Y, Sato A, Tsujimura T et al (2012) Frequent inactivation of the BAP1 gene in epithelioid-type malignant mesothelioma. Cancer Sci 103:868–874

Chapter 9
Gene Signature of Malignant Pleural Mesothelioma

Assunta De Rienzo, William G. Richards, and Raphael Bueno

Abstract Malignant pleural mesothelioma (MPM) is a rare deadly disease with limited therapeutic options. The application of tailored treatments may increase the efficacy of therapies. The promise of precision medicine is to improve human health by combining biomarkers with clinical data. Therefore, the discovery of gene signatures correlated to clinical characteristics is fundamental to identify patients that can benefit from a specific treatment. Although the "omics"-based analyses have become affordable and enabled a rapid identification of potential biomarkers, the application of gene signatures to personalized clinical decisions in order to improve patient outcome has not been delivered yet. Several attempts have been made using many different technologies such as sequencing, expression, and methylation arrays, and different signatures potentially specific to MPM have been generated. However, the lack of statistical power due to the absence of validation in large cohorts of samples has limited the implementation of these gene signatures in clinical practice. Large-scale validations in prospective cohorts are needed to bring the most promising gene signatures into the clinic.

Keywords Mesothelioma • Genetic signature • Profiling • Diagnosis • Prognosis

9.1 Introduction

Since the sequencing of the human genome was completed in 2003, one of the major focuses of medical science has been to characterize the molecular basis of cancer. *Omics*-based analyses have become an essential tool for the genetic profiling of biological samples due to their ability to study thousands of genes simultaneously (Broadhead et al. 2010; Shibata 2015). Often, such studies identify specific

A. De Rienzo (✉) • W.G. Richards • R. Bueno
The Thoracic Surgery Oncology Laboratory and the International Mesothelioma Program, Division of Thoracic Surgery, Brigham and Women's Hospital, and Harvard Medical School, Boston, MA 02115, USA
e-mail: aderienzo@partners.org

© Springer International Publishing AG 2017
J.R. Testa (ed.), *Asbestos and Mesothelioma*, Current Cancer Research,
DOI 10.1007/978-3-319-53560-9_9

patterns of mutation or gene expression associated with biological phenotypes and, if their specificity can be validated, may form the basis of new clinical tools to augment diagnosis, prognosis, or prediction of therapeutic response. Molecular signatures may also provide insights into biological processes associated with tumorigenesis, disease progression, and metastatic behavior [reviewed in (Chibon 2013)]. Increasing availability and diminishing cost of these novel technologies has led to a proliferation of putative signatures representing multiple malignancies; however, few of these have been properly validated and developed to the level of practical, widespread use to impact clinical decision making, and improve patient outcome. Several factors have contributed to the lagging clinical translation of gene signatures. During the discovery phase, the selection of the specimens is often not based on defined criteria for inclusion and exclusion of samples and the controls are not accurately chosen to reduce false discovery, reducing the likelihood of successive validation (Goossens et al. 2015). In the validation phase, lack of standardized methodology, the requirement for large, high-quality and well-annotated cohorts of samples along with the time, sample size, and resources needed for clinical adaptation and prospective validation of the signatures have inhibited progress. In general, the methods for identifying signatures have become accessible and relatively easy to accomplish, but appropriate validation and clinical translation remain extremely challenging [reviewed in (Poste 2011)]. Furthermore, functional studies of biomarkers and pathways identified by the signatures that could be informative of tumor biology and/or identify novel targets have been lacking.

Malignant pleural mesothelioma (MPM) is a highly lethal pleura-based malignancy associated with asbestos exposure. Despite abatement efforts, the incidence of MPM is estimated to increase in the next two decades (Henley et al. 2013). There are approximately 3200 new cases diagnosed yearly in the USA (Henley et al. 2013). Treatment with first-line combination chemotherapy (cisplatin and pemetrexed) is associated with median survival of between 10 and 12 months (Vogelzang et al. 2003). Only a small group of patients with early MPM who undergo multimodality therapy, including surgical resection and chemotherapy, benefit from longer-term survival of up to 20% at 5 years (Richards 2009). Therefore, there is a critical need for molecular tools that can enhance or replace existing methods of diagnosis, prognosis, clinical staging, and treatment design. Development of such tools for MPM is assisted by its relatively short natural history, but impeded by the rarity of the disease.

In this chapter, we review molecular studies on biological fluids and tumor tissue from MPM patients that have identified signatures representing patterns of gene expression, chromatin modification or mutation with potential diagnostic, prognostic or predictive value. Although many are currently too preliminary to be brought into daily clinical practice and have a widespread impact [reviewed in (Greillier et al. 2008)], we consider here the stage of each in the validation/development process and the potential impact on diagnosis, prognosis, treatment and ability to improve patients' outcome.

9.2   Signatures Reflecting Patterns of Gene Expression

9.2.1   RNA Expression Data

In the last few years, high-throughput gene expression has been widely used to understand tumor biology, and predict progression and treatments to which the tumor will respond. To overcome the difficulty to validate large gene signatures, our group has introduced the gene ratio-based method to translate expression profiles into simple tests with clinical relevancy (Gordon et al. 2002). This molecular algorithm is based on the expression levels of a relatively small number of genes. Initially, the gene expression array from a group of tissues is compared with the expression array of a second group of tissues that differs from the first group by a single condition (e.g., histology or outcome). Genes with significantly different expression between the two groups are selected and used to generate ratios of gene expression able to predict the clinical parameter for an individual patient (Gordon 2005). This method was applied to generate a 6-gene, 3-ratios test to distinguish MPM from adenocarcinoma, since these two malignancies are often difficult to differentiate without biopsy because such patients can show similar symptoms. We also generated a preoperative prognostic test able to identify patients likely to benefit from tumor resection using a 4-gene, 3-ratios signature (Gordon et al. 2002; Gordon et al. 2009; Gordon et al. 2003). Additional analyses showed that the prognostic test performed well in diverse cohorts of patients from different institutes and using different methods of analysis (e.g., SyBrGreen vs. TaqMan) (De Rienzo et al. 2017). Finally, this method was also applied to generate a test capable of discerning the epithelioid and sarcomatoid subtypes of MPM using a 4-gene 3-ratios signature (De Rienzo et al. 2013).

The ratio-based method presents several advantages: only a small number of genes are necessary to generate a test, it is independent from the microarray platform that is used to develop the test, it can be applied to primary tissues as well as biopsies, and it performs well in several types of cancers (De Rienzo et al. 2011; De Rienzo et al. 2014; Dong et al. 2009). One disadvantage is that the gene ratio test is able to discriminate only between two conditions. To overcome this limitation, a sequential combination of binary ratio tests was developed by our group to distinguish MPM from other thoracic malignancies included in the differential diagnosis of MPM as proof of principle. The aim of this work was to mimic the clinical diagnostic practice that pathologists use for the diagnosis of MPM. Thirty genes were selected to generate six different combinations of ratio tests. This algorithm showed high specificity and sensitivity, indicating that combinations of gene ratio tests can be used in clinical practice (De Rienzo et al. 2013).

A different study used expression arrays to investigate the biologic diversity of MPM samples (de Reynies et al. 2014). The aim was to discover pathways specifically deregulated in subgroups of MPM patients that could be targeted with specific therapies. Expression data were able to separate the samples in two clusters (1 and 2), partly related to histologic subtype. Epithelioid samples were distributed in both clusters, whereas sarcomatoid-desmoplastic samples were classified only in Cluster 2. Additional analyses identified three genes: periplakin (*PPL*), uroplakin 3B (*UPK3B*), and tissue factor pathway inhibitor (*TFPI*), able to predict the molecular cluster where a sample belongs. Interestingly, patients in Cluster 1 had a longer overall survival and high *BAP1* mutation rate compared to patients in Cluster 2, indicating that the epithelioid MPM tumors in Cluster 1 are molecularly different from the epithelioid samples present in Cluster 2. Furthermore, it was found that markers of epithelial to mesenchymal transition were differentially expressed in the two clusters, suggesting that the epithelioid tumors in Cluster 2 presented evidence of mesenchymal differentiation while retaining some epithelioid features (de Reynies et al. 2014).

9.2.2   microRNA Expression Data

MicroRNA (miRNA) are small (generally around 19–25 nucleotides), non-coding RNA that participate in the post-transcriptional regulation of gene expression regulating both pathological and physiological processes in the cell [reviewed in (Sethi et al. 2014)]. In general, the main function of miRNAs is to repress gene expression by binding to specific complementary regions in the 3′-untranslated regions (UTR) of their target mRNAs. This binding leads to degradation or inhibition of translation of the complementary RNA. To date, more than 2500 miRNA sequences have been identified in humans. The expression of many of them is altered in human cancers where they can act as oncogenes or tumor suppressor genes (Sethi et al. 2014). Since each cancer has a specific combination of miRNAs, it is possible that miRNA signatures may be used for patient stratification, prediction of prognosis, and personalized therapy (Goto et al. 2009; Shin and Chu 2014; Chandra et al. 2016; Guo et al. 2009; Guo et al. 2008). In the last few years, growing evidence indicates that MPM is characterized by significant alterations in microRNA expression; therefore, the understanding of the role of specific miRNA in this disease may lead to the discovery of novel molecular biomarkers [reviewed in (Reid 2015)].

One study of a large series of MPM tumors identified hsa-miR-29c* (now named miR-29c-5p) as an independent prognostic factor (Pass et al. 2010). In particular, longer survival was associated with increased expression of hsa-miR-29c*. When this miRNA was overexpressed in MPM cell lines, invasion, migration and proliferation decreased. Additional study of 15 MPM plasma samples confirmed the potential role of miR-29c* as candidate marker.

In 2010, Busacca and collaborators reported the first microRNA signature associated with prognosis (Busacca et al. 2010). Sixty-five microRNAs were found dysregulated in MPM cell lines based on miRNA expression profiles. The expression data were integrated by bioinformatic algorithms based on target predictions to identify potential candidates of the miRNA regulatory activities. Through this analysis, several potential target genes such as *CDKN1B*, which encodes cyclin-dependent kinase inhibitor 1B, and the B cell translocation gene 1 (*BTG1*) were identified. Finally, the expression of selected miRNAs was investigated in 24 MPM tumors. Markers miR-17-5p, miR-21, miR-29a, miR-30c, miR-30e-5p, miR-106a, and miR-143 were significantly associated with histology, whereas miR-17-5p and miR-30c correlated with longer overall survival in patients with sarcomatoid MPM (Busacca et al. 2010).

A different approach was used in a subsequent report in which 16 MPM specimens from long and short-term survivors following extrapleural pneumonectomy (EPP) were analyzed using expression arrays (Kirschner et al. 2015). Selected miRNAs were further validated in 48 additional EPP tumors by real-time PCR, and Kaplan-Meier analysis was used to investigate the correlation between overall survival of MPM patients and microRNA expression. A signature of six microRNAs (miR-21-5p, -23a-3p, -30e-5p, -221-3p, -222-3p, and -31-5p), named the "miR-Score," was found to predict with high accuracy the outcome of MPM patients (Kirschner et al. 2015).

Signatures of circulating microRNA have been also explored in the serum of MPM patients (Reid 2015). However, one of the most important limitations of these studies is the small number of samples analyzed and, in most of the cases, the absence of validation in large prospective cohorts (Kirschner et al. 2012; Santarelli et al. 2011; Weber et al. 2012). A study aimed to discover miRNA biomarkers in the serum of 14 MPM patients and ten controls identified two different miRNA signatures able to predict histological subtype and overall survival of the MPM patients (Lamberti et al. 2015). A recent comprehensive systematic review of miRNA expression signatures has been conducted to identify a set of circulating and tissue miRNAs with altered expression related to asbestos exposure and MPM (Micolucci et al. 2016). Qualitative meta-analysis of the collected data showed that the circulating miR-126-3p, miR-103a-3p, and miR-625-3p in combination with mesothelin were potential candidates to distinguish MPM patients from both the general population and asbestos-exposed subjects. In addition, nine miRNAs (miR-16-5p, miR-126-3p, miR-143-3p, miR-145-5p, miR-192-5p, miR-193a-3p, miR-200b-3p, miR-203a-3p, and miR-652-3p) were the most commonly identified miRNAs in MPM samples in relation to diagnosis (Micolucci et al. 2016).

9.2.3   RNA-Seq Data

Recently, our comprehensive genomic analysis of 216 MPM samples revealed novel molecular insights in MPM tumorigenesis (Bueno et al. 2016). In particular, four distinct molecular MPM subtypes were identified using unsupervised consensus clustering of RNA-seq–derived expression data. Interestingly, the samples were distributed in four clusters that were only partially associated with the pathological histologic subtype. Of the two most different clusters, one (Cluster 1) included all epithelioid and one biphasic sample, and the other (Cluster 4) contained all of the sarcomatoid-desmoplastic samples in addition to biphasic and epithelioid samples. The remaining biphasic and epithelioid samples were distributed in the other two clusters (2 and 3). Interestingly, the distribution of the samples in the four clusters was associated with the percentage of sarcomatoid content in the tumor. Consequently, Cluster 2 contained biphasic samples with predominantly epithelioid cells, and Cluster 3 included biphasic samples with high sarcomatoid cell content. Moreover, the histologically epithelioid samples, classified in Clusters 2, 3, and 4 were associated with shorter overall survival of MPM patients compared to the epithelioid samples in Cluster 1. Kaplan–Meier analysis illustrated that patients included in Cluster 1 had longer overall survival compared to patients present in the other three clusters (Bueno et al. 2016).

Although this classification appears powerful for identifying patients with longer overall survival, the use of extensive RNA-seq expression data is impractical (Poste 2011). Additional analyses using the same data set identified the log2 ratio of *CLDN15/VIM* (C/V) expression as significantly different among clusters, and the ability of this signature to discriminate MPM samples with different prognosis was further validated using published microarray data set (Bueno et al. 2016). *CLDN15* and *VIM* have been previously associated with MPM. CLDN15 was reported to be overexpressed in epithelioid MPM and absent in human airway epithelium (Chaouche-Mazouni et al. 2015). Vimentin staining was found to be a useful marker for the pathological diagnosis of sarcomatoid MPM (Husain et al. 2013). Although this signature is appealing in that expression of only two genes need be measured, further validation is necessary to confirm the correlation among the *CLDN15/VIM* expression signature, MPM phenotypes and patient prognosis. Differential expression analysis of the RNA-seq expression data revealed that several genes differentially expressed between consensus Clusters 1 and 4 are involved in the epithelial to mesenchymal transition, a finding consistent with previous investigations (de Reynies et al. 2014).

9.3   Signatures Reflecting Patterns of Chromatin Methylation

Although the difference between euchromatin (characteristic of gene activity) and heterochromatin (characteristic of gene repression) has been known for many years, only in the last 20 years the discovery of enzymes able to modify the chromatin and of the molecular mechanisms that change the chromatin status in response to cellular signals has transformed the field of epigenetics [reviewed in (Allis and Jenuwein 2016)]. Gene methylation is a highly controlled cellular process occurring during normal development. In cancer, DNA methylation is abnormal, and the causes of these alterations are unknown (Klutstein et al. 2016). In cancer cells, there are two major alterations in DNA methylation: hypomethylation, which occurs more commonly within the broad late-replicating Lamin-associated domains, areas of the DNA rich in repetitive sequences (Kulis et al. 2015); and hypermethylation, which is found at many CpG islands generally unmethylated in normal tissues

(Klutstein et al. 2016). Several factors seem to contribute to such molecular DNA alteration, e.g., it has been suggested that the transient silencing of tumor suppressor genes in stem cells may leave these genes susceptible to abnormal DNA hypermethylation during tumor progression (Ohm et al. 2007). On the other hand, it has been proposed that in tumors, de novo methylation may be a pre-programmed process mediated by an epigenetic system that usually represses genes during embryogenesis (Schlesinger et al. 2007). In addition to these major epigenetic mechanisms, several other posttranslational modifications (e.g., phosphorylation, ADP-ribosylation, biotinylation, ubiquitination) can regulate gene expression by altering the normal chromosomal condensation [reviewed in (Vandermeers et al. 2013)].

Several studies indicate that alteration of gene expression due to aberrant methylation is a common event in MPM (Vandermeers et al. 2013). Christensen and collaborators performed a comprehensive study of 1505 CpG dinucleotides associated with 803 cancer genes in 158 MPM tumors (Christensen et al. 2009). Unsupervised hierarchical clustering showed significant differences between the epigenetic profiles of MPM and those of the 18 normal pleurae included in the study. In addition, the tumors were stratified into seven classes according to their epigenetic profile. The methylation classes were significantly associated with lung asbestos body count, and were independent predictors of patient survival ($P < 0.01$) suggesting that abnormal methylation may be associated with disease progression. Another study investigated the epigenetic profiles of MPM and lung adenocarcinoma (Goto et al. 2009). Hierarchical cluster analysis showed that the methylation pattern was different between the two malignancies, most likely as the result of diverse pathologic events. Integrated analysis showed that methylation and/or tri-methylation of H3 lysine 27 (*H3K27me3*) affected ~11% of the genes where one allele was lost. A histone deacetylase inhibitor was able to reactivate a subset of genes silenced by H3K27me3. Furthermore, in a small subset of MPMs, low levels of DNA methylation were correlated to longer survival, potentially indicating that the progression of the disease may be related to the methylation levels. Finally, three genes, encoding the transmembrane protein 30B (*TMEM30B*), the Kazal type serine peptidase inhibitor domain 1 (*KAZALD1*), and the mitogen-activated protein kinase 13 (*MAPK13*) were found to be specific markers for methylation in MPM specimens compared to adenocarcinoma samples. It was suggested that these genes could be of diagnostic interest in MPM tumorigenesis (Goto et al. 2009).

Since the genetic landscape of MPM is mostly characterized by chromosomal rearrangement, bioinformatics studies were conducted to investigate how the measurements of DNA methylation vary in relation to the allelic copy number variation (Houseman et al. 2009). It was shown that copy number gain may introduce little bias in the methylation measurements, whereas, allelic lost may determine a small bias. On the other hand, homozygous losses seemed to introduce substantial bias in the measurements of the methylation status of the tumor. Therefore, a subsequent study investigated the relationship between copy number variation and methylation in 23 MPM tumors (Christensen et al. 2010). Interestingly, the results showed no significant correlation between copy number and methylation when a single locus was investigated. However, when the analysis was extended to the entire genome, a strong correlation between the two molecular mechanisms of inactivation was observed, suggesting that there is a significant relationship between epigenetic and genetic alterations in MPM.

Since alteration of gene expression due to promoter methylation is a common event in MPM, the use of pharmacological compounds able to interfere with DNA methylation is currently being tested in clinical trials (Vandermeers et al. 2013).

9.4 Signatures Reflecting Patterns of DNA Mutations

Recently, an iron signature has been identified in MPM samples (Crovella et al. 2016). Based on the observation that the asbestos pulmonary toxicity can be mediated by redox cycling of fiber-bound and iron (Fe) (Chew and Toyokuni 2015; Liu et al. 2013), 86 single nucleotide polymorphisms (SPNs) were investigated in ten Fe-metabolism genes in 77 MPM specimens. Results showed that three SNPs located in the genes encoding transferrin, hephaestin and ferritin heavy polypeptide were significantly related to MPM susceptibility.

Furthermore, next-generation sequencing analysis has identified gene signatures correlated to gender and histology (De Rienzo et al. 2016). In particular, epithelioid MPM showed higher mutation rates of *BAP1* single-nucleotide variants ($p < 0.001$), and more frequent loss of chromosome 22q ($p = 0.037$). The non-epithelioid subtypes displayed more frequent *CDKN2A* deletions among men ($p = 0.021$). Loss of *CDKN2A* was also correlated with shorter survival for the entire cohort ($p = 0.002$) and for men ($p = 0.012$). *TP53* was mutated more frequently in women ($p = 0.004$).

In our recent work, we have investigated recurrent gene alterations in the four MPM clusters identified by RNA-seq expression data to determine gene signature characteristics of each cluster (Bueno et al. 2016). Notably, four (*SETD2, TP53, NF2,* and *ULK2*) of the most significantly mutated genes showed mutation rates (including single nucleotide mutation, deletion, and amplification) significantly different between Cluster 1 and Clusters 2–4 (Table 9.1), indicating that the difference in the overall survival observed in Cluster 1 may be related to different combinations of mutations in these tumors.

In recent years, many investigations based on next-generation sequencing have highlighted the importance of BRCA1-associated protein (*BAP1*) in MPM (Bott et al. 2011; Testa et al. 2011). Although the role of *BAP1* in MPM is not fully described in this chapter, it is important to highlight that several studies have described the importance of *BAP1* in the diagnosis of MPM (Andrici et al. 2015; Henderson et al. 2013; Hwang et al. 2016). In particular, it has been described that BAP1 immunohistochemistry is able to distinguish mutated from wild-type *BAP1*, and therefore may be sufficient to diagnose MPM when all the other clinical, imaging, and cytological results strongly support the diagnosis of MPM (Panou et al. 2015; Walts et al. 2016). A more detailed discussion of the role of *BAP1* in MPM

Table 9.1 Number of mutations of the key mutated genes in Cluster 1 vs. Clusters 2–4 in 211 MPM samples (data from Bueno et al. 2016)

Gene name	Cluster C1 (%)	Clusters C2-4 (%)	p-value[a]
BAP1	14 (26)	45 (29)	0.8606
CCDC19	6 (11)	31 (20)	0.2125
DDX3X	1 (2)	6 (4)	0.6807
DDX51	6 (11)	27 (17)	0.386
NF2	7 (13)	50 (32)	0.0074
RYR2	6 (11)	34 (22)	0.1081
SETD2	17 (31)	27 (17)	0.0328
SETD5	5 (9)	28 (18)	0.1916
SETDB1	5 (9)	29 (18)	0.1354
TP53	3 (6)	33 (21)	0.0107
ULK2	2 (4)	23 (15)	0.028

[a]Significance based on analysis with Fisher's exact test

is presented in Chapter Germline and Somatic Mutations in Human Mesothelioma and Lessons from Asbestos-Exposed Genetically Engineered Mouse Models of this volume.

9.4.1   Future Directions

Recently, the basic concepts of cancer therapies have been revolutionized by the discovery that the blockade of immune checkpoints or the use of immune therapies, such as dendritic cell activation of T cells and adoptive T cell transfer, represents a valid treatment for a subset of cancer patients (Battaglia and Muhitch 2016). Therefore, the success in manipulating the human immune system to attack cancer cells has directed scientific efforts to further investigate changes in the tumor micro-environment and immune surveillance of human cancers (Li et al. 2016). Several immune gene signatures have been reported in several cancers based on expression data (Cheng et al. 2016; Clancy and Hovig 2016; Maglietta et al. 2016), and novel specific immune panels have been created to investigate immune-related genes. Although a specific immune gene signature has not been identified in MPM yet, the number of gene expression profiles associated with intratumoral immune response is expected to increase in the next few years. Recently, to investigate the immune profile of MPM, we used bioinformatic algorithms to determine the relative abundance of tumor-infiltrating lymphocytes (TILs) and macrophages by the analysis of RNA-seq data (Bueno et al. 2016). Sarcomatoid samples showed higher levels of T cells and M2 macrophages, as well as significantly higher PD-L1 expression compared to the other histological subtypes. In addition, the M2 macrophage to T cell ratio was found to be predictive of reduced overall survival.

9.5   Conclusions

MPM is a rare tumor with high morbidity and mortality rates. Although cytogenetic studies have revealed that chromosomal rearrangement events are common in MPM (Carbone et al. 2002), in the last few years, several studies have uncovered the genetic landscape of MPM (Bott et al. 2011; Bueno et al. 2016; Testa et al. 2011). The omics-based technologies allow rapid identification of gene signature based on patterns of expression, chromatin methylation, or sequencing data. The use of gene signatures is essential for precision medicine to classify patients with the same type of cancer in groups based on molecular characteristics or prognosis (Vargas and Harris 2016). However, most of the biomarkers identified cannot be used in a clinical setting, because they have not been properly validated [reviewed in (Chibon 2013; Poste 2011)]. Improvements in computational technologies will permit faster integration of multiple datasets; therefore, the identification of novel biomarkers is expected to rapidly increase. Consequently, it is desirable that large international consortiums participate in prospective studies to assure rapid validation of the most promising signatures and direct efficient functional studies of potential biomarkers.

Conflict of Interest Dr. R. Bueno receives funding through Brigham and Women's Hospital's *International Mesothelioma Program*, which receives support from plaintiff law firms. He is also supported by funds from NCI, Verastem, Genentech, Merck, Castle Biosciences, and Roche. The remaining authors have no potential conflicts of interest.

References

Allis CD, Jenuwein T (2016) The molecular hallmarks of epigenetic control. Nat Rev Genet 17:487–500

Andrici JA, Sheen L, Sioson K et al (2015) Loss of expression of BAP1 is a useful adjunct, which strongly supports the diagnosis of mesothelioma in effusion cytology. Mod Pathol 28:1360–1368

Battaglia S, Muhitch JB (2016) Unmasking targets of antitumor immunity via high-throughput antigen profiling. Curr Opin Biotechnol 42:92–97

Bott M, Brevet M, Taylor BS et al (2011) The nuclear deubiquitinase BAP1 is commonly inactivated by somatic mutations and 3p21.1 losses in malignant pleural mesothelioma. Nat Genet 43:668–672

Broadhead ML, Clark JC, Dass CR et al (2010) Microarray: an instrument for cancer surgeons of the future? ANZ J Surg 80:531–536

Bueno R, Stawiski EW, Goldstein LD et al (2016) Comprehensive genomic analysis of malignant pleural mesothelioma identifies recurrent mutations, gene fusions and splicing alterations. Nat Genet 48:407–416

Busacca S, Germano S, De Cecco L et al (2010) MicroRNA signature of malignant mesothelioma with potential diagnostic and prognostic implications. Am J Respir Cell Mol Biol 42:312–319

Carbone M, Kratzke RA, Testa JR (2002) The pathogenesis of mesothelioma. Semin Oncol 29:2–17

Chandra V, Kim JJ, Mittal B et al (2016) MicroRNA aberrations: an emerging field for gallbladder cancer management. World J Gastroenterol 22:1787–1799

Chaouche-Mazouni S, Scherpereel A, Zaamoum R et al (2015) Claudin 3, 4, and 15 expression in solid tumors of lung adenocarcinoma versus malignant pleural mesothelioma. Ann Diagn Pathol 19:193–197

Cheng W, Ren X, Zhang C et al (2016) Bioinformatic profiling identifies an immune-related risk signature for glioblastoma. Neurology 86:2226–2234

Chew SH, Toyokuni S (2015) Malignant mesothelioma as an oxidative stress-induced cancer: an update. Free Radic Biol Med 86:166–178

Chibon F (2013) Cancer gene expression signatures - the rise and fall? Eur J Cancer 49:2000–2009

Christensen BC, Houseman EA, Godleski JJ et al (2009) Epigenetic profiles distinguish pleural mesothelioma from normal pleura and predict lung asbestos burden and clinical outcome. Cancer Res 69(1):227–234

Christensen BC, Houseman EA, Poage GM et al (2010) Integrated profiling reveals a global correlation between epigenetic and genetic alterations in mesothelioma. Cancer Res 70:5686–5694

Clancy T, Hovig E (2016) Profiling networks of distinct immune-cells in tumors. BMC Bioinformatics 17:263

Crovella S, Bianco AM, Vuch J et al (2016) Iron signature in asbestos-induced malignant pleural mesothelioma: a population-based autopsy study. J Toxicol Environ Health A 79:129–141

de Reynies A, Jaurand MC, Renier A et al (2014) Molecular classification of malignant pleural mesothelioma: identification of a poor prognosis subgroup linked to the epithelial-to-mesenchymal transition. Clin Cancer Res 20:1323–1334

De Rienzo A, Archer MA, Yeap BY et al (2016) Gender-specific molecular and clinical features underlie malignant pleural mesothelioma. Cancer Res 76:319–328

De Rienzo A, Cook RW, Wilkinson J, Gustafson CE, Amin W, Johnson CE, Oelschlager KM, Maetzold DJ, Stone JF, Feldman MD, Becich MJ, Yeap BY, Richards WG, Bueno R (2017) Validation of a gene expression test for mesothelioma prognosis in formalin-fixed paraffin-embedded tissues. J Mol Diagn 19:65–71

De Rienzo A, Dong L, Yeap BY et al (2011) Fine-needle aspiration biopsies for gene expression ratio-based diagnostic and prognostic tests in malignant pleural mesothelioma. Clin Cancer Res 17:310–316

De Rienzo A, Richards WG, Yeap BY et al (2013) Sequential binary gene ratio tests define a novel molecular diagnostic strategy for malignant pleural mesothelioma. Clin Cancer Res 19:2493–2502

De Rienzo A, Yeap BY, Cibas ES et al (2014) Gene expression ratio test distinguishes normal lung from lung tumors in solid tissue and FNA biopsies. J Mol Diagn 16:267–272

Dong L, Bard AJ, Richards WG et al (2009) A gene expression ratio-based diagnostic test for bladder cancer. Adv Appl Bioinforma Chem 2:17–22

Goossens N, Nakagawa S, Sun X et al (2015) Cancer biomarker discovery and validation. Transl Cancer Res 4:256–269

Gordon GJ (2005) Transcriptional profiling of mesothelioma using microarrays. Lung Cancer 49(Suppl 1):S99–S103

Gordon GJ, Dong L, Yeap BY et al (2009) Four-gene expression ratio test for survival in patients undergoing surgery for mesothelioma. J Natl Cancer Inst 101:678–686

Gordon GJ, Jensen RV, Hsiao LL et al (2002) Translation of microarray data into clinically relevant cancer diagnostic tests using gene expression ratios in lung cancer and mesothelioma. Cancer Res 62:4963–4967

Gordon GJ, Jensen RV, Hsiao LL et al (2003) Using gene expression ratios to predict outcome among patients with mesothelioma. J Natl Cancer Inst 95:598–605

Goto Y, Shinjo K, Kondo Y et al (2009) Epigenetic profiles distinguish malignant pleural mesothelioma from lung adenocarcinoma. Cancer Res 69:9073–9082

Greillier L, Baas P, Welch JJ et al (2008) Biomarkers for malignant pleural mesothelioma: current status. Mol Diagn Ther 12:375–390

Guo J, Miao Y, Xiao B et al (2009) Differential expression of microRNA species in human gastric cancer versus non-tumorous tissues. J Gastroenterol Hepatol 24:652–657

Guo Y, Chen Z, Zhang L et al (2008) Distinctive microRNA profiles relating to patient survival in esophageal squamous cell carcinoma. Cancer Res 68(1):26–33

Henderson DW, Reid G, Kao SC et al (2013) Challenges and controversies in the diagnosis of malignant mesothelioma: Part 2. Malignant mesothelioma subtypes, pleural synovial sarcoma, molecular and prognostic aspects of mesothelioma, BAP1, aquaporin-1 and microRNA. J Clin Pathol 66:854–861

Henley SJ, Larson TC, Wu M et al (2013) Mesothelioma incidence in 50 states and the District of Columbia, United States, 2003–2008. Int J Occup Environ Health 19:1–10

Houseman EA, Christensen BC, Karagas MR et al (2009) Copy number variation has little impact on bead-array-based measures of DNA methylation. Bioinformatics 25:1999–2005

Husain AN, Colby T, Ordonez N et al (2013) Guidelines for pathologic diagnosis of malignant mesothelioma: 2012 update of the consensus statement from the International Mesothelioma Interest Group. Arch Pathol Lab Med 137:647–667

Hwang HC, Sheffield BS, Rodriguez S et al (2016) Utility of BAP1 Immunohistochemistry and p16 (CDKN2A) FISH in the Diagnosis of Malignant Mesothelioma in Effusion Cytology Specimens. Am J Surg Pathol 40:120–126

Kirschner MB, Cheng YY, Armstrong NJ et al (2015) MiR-score: a novel 6-microRNA signature that predicts survival outcomes in patients with malignant pleural mesothelioma. Mol Oncol 9:715–726

Kirschner MB, Cheng YY, Badrian B et al (2012) Increased circulating miR-625-3p: a potential biomarker for patients with malignant pleural mesothelioma. J Thorac Oncol 7:1184–1191

Klutstein M, Nejman D, Greenfield R et al (2016) DNA methylation in cancer and aging. Cancer Res 76:3446–3450

Kulis M, Merkel A, Heath S et al (2015) Whole-genome fingerprint of the DNA methylome during human B cell differentiation. Nat Genet 47:746–756

Lamberti M, Capasso R, Lombardi A et al (2015) Two different serum miRNA signatures correlate with the clinical outcome and histological subtype in pleural malignant mesothelioma patients. PLoS One 10:e0135331

Li Y, Li F, Jiang F et al (2016) A mini-review for cancer immunotherapy: molecular understanding of PD-1/PD-L1 pathway & translational blockade of immune checkpoints. Int J Mol Sci 17:1151

Liu G, Cheresh P, Kamp DW (2013) Molecular basis of asbestos-induced lung disease. Annu Rev Pathol 8:161–187

Maglietta A, Maglietta R, Staiano T et al (2016) The immune landscapes of polypoid and nonpolypoid precancerous colorectal lesions. PLoS One 11:e0159373

Micolucci L, Akhtar MM, Olivieri F et al (2016) Diagnostic value of microRNAs in asbestos exposure and malignant mesothelioma: systematic review and qualitative meta-analysis. Oncotarget 7(36):58606–58637

Ohm JE, McGarvey KM, Yu X et al (2007) A stem cell-like chromatin pattern may predispose tumor suppressor genes to DNA hypermethylation and heritable silencing. Nat Genet 39:237–242

Panou V, Vyberg M, Weinreich UM et al (2015) The established and future biomarkers of malignant pleural mesothelioma. Cancer Treat Rev 41:486–495

Pass HI, Goparaju C, Ivanov S et al (2010) hsa-miR-29c* is linked to the prognosis of malignant pleural mesothelioma. Cancer Res 70:1916–1924

Poste G (2011) Bring on the biomarkers. Nature 469:156–157

Reid G (2015) MicroRNAs in mesothelioma: from tumour suppressors and biomarkers to therapeutic targets. J Thorac Dis 7:1031–1040

Richards WG (2009) Recent advances in mesothelioma staging. Semin Thorac Cardiovasc Surg 21:105–110

Santarelli L, Strafella E, Staffolani S et al (2011) Association of MiR-126 with soluble mesothelin-related peptides, a marker for malignant mesothelioma. PLoS One 6:e18232

Schlesinger Y, Straussman R, Keshet I et al (2007) Polycomb-mediated methylation on Lys27 of histone H3 pre-marks genes for de novo methylation in cancer. Nat Genet 39:232–236

Sethi S, Ali S, Sethi S et al (2014) MicroRNAs in personalized cancer therapy. Clin Genet 86:68–73

Shibata T (2015) Current and future molecular profiling of cancer by next-generation sequencing. Jpn J Clin Oncol 45:895–899

Shin VY, Chu KM (2014) MiRNA as potential biomarkers and therapeutic targets for gastric cancer. World J Gastroenterol 20:10432–10439

Testa JR, Cheung M, Pei J et al (2011) Germline BAP1 mutations predispose to malignant mesothelioma. Nat Genet 43(10):1022–1025

Vandermeers F, Neelature Sriramareddy S, Costa C et al (2013) The role of epigenetics in malignant pleural mesothelioma. Lung Cancer 81:311–318

Vargas AJ, Harris CC (2016) Biomarker development in the precision medicine era: lung cancer as a case study. Nat Rev Cancer 16:525–537

Vogelzang NJ, Rusthoven JJ, Symanowski J et al (2003) Phase III study of pemetrexed in combination with cisplatin versus cisplatin alone in patients with malignant pleural mesothelioma. J Clin Oncol 21:2636–2644

Walts AE, Hiroshima K, McGregor SM et al (2016) BAP1 immunostain and CDKN2A (p16) FISH analysis: clinical applicability for the diagnosis of malignant mesothelioma in effusions. Diagn Cytopathol 44:599–606

Weber DG, Johnen G, Bryk O et al (2012) Identification of miRNA-103 in the cellular fraction of human peripheral blood as a potential biomarker for malignant mesothelioma–a pilot study. PLoS One 7:e30221

Chapter 10
Cell Signaling and Epigenetic Mechanisms in Mesothelioma

Brooke T. Mossman

Abstract Malignant mesotheliomas are a histologically diverse, polyclonal group of tumors arising most commonly in the pleura and to a lesser extent in the peritoneum, pericardium, and tunica vaginalis testis. They are primarily associated with exposures to naturally occurring mineral fibers including asbestos, erionite, and fluoro-edenite, although radiation- and chronic inflammation-associated as well as idiopathic mesotheliomas occur. Integrated analyses of pleural mesotheliomas have shown heterogeneous mutations in tumor suppressor genes, stimulation of multiple signaling cascades and transcription factors, and, most recently, epigenetic alterations that are defined as heritable and/or reversible changes in gene expression without changes in the DNA sequence. This review focuses on the epigenetic mechanisms reported in studies on mesotheliomas and mesothelial cells, emphasizing research that has linked these changes to critical survival and proliferative pathways in the development of mesotheliomas. This information is critical to understanding how key epigenetic effects modulate the carcinogenic process and will allow new strategies to prevent and treat mesotheliomas.

Keywords Mesothelioma • Epigenetics • Cell signaling • miRNAs • Histones • Methylation • Noncoding RNAs • Chromatin remodeling

10.1 Introduction

The pathogenesis of malignant mesotheliomas (MMs) is largely unexplained and may be different in individual tumors, which may be primarily epithelioid, sarcomatoid, biphasic, desmoplastic, or mixed in pathology (Husain et al. 2013). Phenotypic heterogeneity may reflect differences in genetic or epigenetic makeup of tumors, the stability or reversibility of these changes, and whether tumors arise from a single cell precursor or different subsets of dedifferentiating

B.T. Mossman (✉)
University of Vermont College of Medicine, Burlington, VT 05405, USA
e-mail: Brooke.Mossman@uvm.edu

© Springer International Publishing AG 2017
J.R. Testa (ed.), *Asbestos and Mesothelioma*, Current Cancer Research,
DOI 10.1007/978-3-319-53560-9_10

cells in the mesothelium. Because of difficulties in diagnosis of MMs, treatment of late-stage tumors has been discouraging. Unlike several cancers, few genomic abnormalities in MMs were revealed by comparative genomic hybridization analyses, DNA cytometry, and whole transcriptome sequencing approaches (Krismann et al. 2002; Sugarbaker et al. 2008). Moreover, there do not appear to be specific driver mutations in oncogenes that are signatures of asbestos exposures or are crucial to the development of MMs (Sugarbaker et al. 2008; Christensen et al. 2009a; Christensen et al. 2009b; Reid 2015; IARC 2012). For these reasons, discovery of diagnostic approaches and biomarkers based on epigenetic profiles of MMs vs. normal mesothelium or other tumor types has been the focus of several studies and reviews (Tsou et al. 2005; Tsou et al. 2007; Christensen et al. 2009a; Christensen et al. 2009b; Goto et al. 2009; Nelson et al. 2011; Zhang et al. 2015). Others have studied whether the epigenomic profiles of MMs can be used to indicate the prognosis of MM patients (Fischer et al. 2006; Tsou et al. 2007; Christensen et al. 2009b; Laszlo et al. 2015). More recently, epigenetic data on MM patients have been used to determine the efficacy of responsiveness to chemotherapeutic agents, chemoresistance, and other treatment options (Bowman et al. 2009; Vandermeers et al. 2013; LaFave et al. 2015; Zhang et al. 2015). Although searches for epigenetic biomarkers or diagnostic markers have not yielded global indicators of disease as yet, results have fostered promising novel approaches for treatment of MMs (reviewed in Vandermeers et al. 2013; Reid et al. 2016).

The goals of this chapter are to educate both basic and clinical scientists on the principles of epigenetics, the different types of epigenetic markers with an emphasis on histone modifications and DNA methylation, and interactions between epigenetic changes and cell signaling pathways that are critical to the pathogenesis of MMs. Information from functional studies that have used epigenetics to study the mechanisms of MM development is emphasized.

10.2   Basic Concepts of Epigenomics

"Epigenetics" is defined as the study of "changes in gene function that cannot be explained by changes in the DNA sequence" (Felsenfeld 2014). In eukaryotic cells, DNA is compactly wrapped around histones to form "nucleosomes," the basic repeating units of chromatin. The complex structural organization of chromosomes and chromatids is shown in Fig. 10.1. Chemical modifications catalyzed by specific enzymes or other processes to either histones, DNA, or chromatin remodeling affect both chromatin structure and gene/protein. Thus, chromatin structure is dynamically regulated by numerous epigenetic modifications that are elicited by the processes listed in Table 10.1. These processes do not entail a change in the DNA sequence but involve posttranscriptional and posttranslational modifications to histone proteins, DNA methylation, and noncoding RNAs

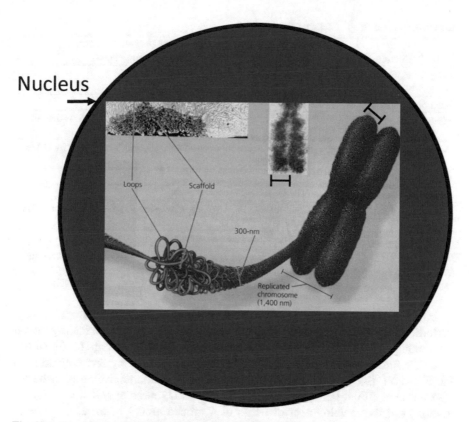

Fig. 10.1 Diagram showing intense chromatin packing in a chromosome. Histone proteins have a central role in organization of the DNA and DNA packing. More than 20% of the amino acids (lysine or arginine) of histones have a positive charge that allows their tight binding to negatively charged DNA. A nucleosome, consisting of DNA wound twice around a protein octamer core of histones, is formed in a bead-like structure that is strung together by linker DNA. The left of this figure shows the looped domain of 30-nm fibers, which then attach to a thick protein chromosome scaffold (300-nm fiber). During mitosis, the loops coil further to form a metaphase chromosome shown on the right. These are comprised of chromatids as indicated by the bars on the electron micrograph (inset) and diagram. Chemical modification (e.g., acetylation and methylation) of histones plays critical roles in the regulation of gene transcription and posttranscriptional events as the amino acids in the N-terminal tails of histones protrude outward in the nucleosome and are accessible to enzymes causing methylation and deacetylation (Modified from Campbell et al. Biology, 8th Edition, Pearson Benjamin Cummings, San Francisco, CA, 2008)

(microRNAs, i.e., miRNAs, and long noncoding mRNAs, i.e., lncRNAs). Inflammation and oxidant-dependent responses appear to be probable contributory factors to epigenetic processes (Peden 2011; Horsburgh et al. 2015; Vento-Tormo et al. 2017), concepts that may be of importance to the development of chronic inflammation, a predisposing factor to MMs both in animal models (Hillegass et al. 2013) and man (Pinato et al. 2012).

Table 10.1 Types of epigenetic mechanisms

MicroRNAs (miRNAs)	Family of noncoding small RNAs (~18–25 nucleotides) that silence gene expression by targeting mRNA
Long noncoding RNAs (lncRNAs)	Precise mechanisms unknown
Histone modifications	
Methylation	Addition of methyl groups on histidine, arginine, or lysine of histone tails by HMTs and HDMs
Acetylation	Occurs in lysine residues of histones and is catalyzed by HATs and HDACs
Other covalent	
Other modifications	
DNA methylation	Covalent attachment of a methyl group to the fifth carbon (C^5) in cytosine by DNMTs
Chromatin remodeling	ATP-dependent events altering histone-DNA complexes

DMNTs DNA methyltransferases, *HATs* histone acetyltransferases, *HDACs* histone deacetylases, *HDMs* histone demethylases, *HMTs* histone methyltransferases

Inflammation is associated with activation of multiple signaling pathways including inflammasome activation, a process associated with oxidant-generating, pathogenic asbestos fibers (reviewed in Sayan and Mossman 2016). In this regard, a fundamental component of inflammation is priming and activation of the NLRP3 (also known as cryopyrin and NALP3) inflammasome by asbestos (Dostert et al. 2008; Hillegass et al. 2013), which is linked to cell stress, inflammation, and the development of MMs in a mouse model of asbestos-induced MM (Kadariya et al. 2016). NLRP3 and its platform of proteins initiate cell signaling events in the cytoplasm of mesothelial cells and macrophages/monocytes to produce the mature form of the potent inflammatory cytokine, interleukin-1β (IL-1β). In the latter studies, mice deficient in Asc, a critical component of the NLRP3 inflammasome, and wild-type littermates were exposed to crocidolite asbestos and monitored for MM onset and incidence. Asc-deficient mice showed a significantly delayed onset and reduced numbers of MMs compared to wild-type mice. These studies were bolstered by administration of anakinra, an IL-1 receptor-antagonist, to crocidolite-exposed mice deficient in the tumor suppressors Nf2 and Cdkn2a, i.e., *Nf2$^{+/−}$;Cdkn2a$^{+/−}$* mice. Mice treated with anakinra showed a marked delay in the median time of MM onset compared to vehicle-control mice, again suggesting a critical role of IL-1β and IL-R signaling in development of MMs.

In recent studies, epigenetic control of inflammasome-associated genes has been shown in patients with autoinflammatory syndromes (Vento-Tormo et al. 2017). In brief, the role of DNA demethylation in activating inflammasome genes during macrophage differentiation and monocyte activation was investigated in both healthy subjects and patients with cryopyrin-associated periodic syndromes (CAPs) or familial Mediterranean fever. Inflammasome-related genes were rapidly demethylated during differentiation of monocytes to macrophages and during monocyte activation. Moreover, demethylation was associated with increased gene expression when either Tet methylcytosine dioxygenase 2 (TET2) or the transcription factor, nuclear factor-kappa B (NF-κB), was downregulated using siRNA interference or pharmacologic inhibition. Patients with CAPs administered anti-IL-1 drugs that displayed methylation levels similar to levels in healthy controls, suggesting a crucial link between epigenetic control of the inflammasome and novel clinical approaches to inflammasome-related diseases.

Although normally involved in developmental processes and balanced in normal cells, reprogramming or aberrations in epigenetic programs also result in cell transformation and/or malignant phenotypes during the development of cancers. Obesity-related chronic inflammation is implicated at the epigenetic level in the development of some forms of cancer (Lund et al. 2011), and chronic inflammation in general plays an essential role in tumorigenesis in a number of models (Wu et al. 2014).

Inflammatory mediators in the tumor microenvironment include cytokines, chemokines, and reactive oxygen and nitrogen species (ROS/RNS) that participate in host defense at low levels of injury or as chemoattractants recruiting leukocytes and other cells to sites of injury, leading to chronic inflammation and cancers at high levels of exposures. For example, NADPH oxidases (Nox family proteins) are upregulated in both cells of the immune system and in epithelial cells forming carcinomas (Wu et al. 2014). The ROS generated by Nox family proteins can then induce epigenetic changes and/or activate cell signaling cascades regulating cell proliferation, genetic instability, angiogenesis, and metastases. It should be noted that ROS are generated by long asbestos fibers (>5 μm) that are associated with the development of MMs (reviewed by Donaldson et al. 2010; Lippmann 2014; Roggli 2015). ROS are produced by an NADPH-dependent process (Dostert et al. 2008) or generated as the result of surface iron availability from the amphibole asbestos fibers, crocidolite, or amosite (reviewed in Shukla et al. 2003a; Shukla et al. 2003b).

Epigenetic changes can also result in regulation or deregulation of epithelial-mesenchymal transition (EMT) where epithelial cells or epithelioid MMs lose their epithelial properties and acquire properties of mesenchymal cells or sarcomatoid tumors exhibiting increased migratory or invasive properties (Sun and Fang 2016).

10.3   A Primer of Epigenetic Markers

10.3.1   Noncoding RNAs, Including microRNAs (miRNAs) and Long Noncoding RNAs (lncRNAs)

MiRNAs, small single-stranded RNA molecules, are the most studied class of epigenetic markers in MMs (Reid 2015) and in cancer in general (Zhang et al. 2007). Approximately 30% of protein-coding human genes are regulated by miRNAs. An estimated 1000 or more human miRNAs exist and may have originally evolved as part of a gamut of host defense mechanisms against foreign genetic materials such as DNA or RNA tumor viruses (Zhang et al. 2007). For example, viruses such as SV40 that are putative cofactors in MMs also encode miRNAs that may regulate their replication and pathogenesis (Toyooka et al. 2001).

Transcription of miRNA genes as primary transcripts (pri-miRNAs) occurs in the nucleus. After posttranscriptional processing, nucleotide precursors called pre-miRNAs are transported into the cytoplasm where they are further processed by Dicer, an RNA endonuclease, to generate a mature, double-stranded duplex (miRNA/miRNA) that binds to a protein (Argonaut 2) as part of an RNA-induced silencing complex (RISC). RISC and its miRNA complex then bind to a number of target mRNAs, specifically targeting sites in the 3′UTR region, to cause cleavage or translational repression. Thus, miRNAs are gene regulators mainly via mRNA degradation or translational repression of mRNA. There are two major groups of miRNAs: intergenic miRNAs that are found in the noncoding regions of chromosomes and intronic miRNAs that are expressed from a host gene promoter by RNA polymerase II and require RNA splicing.

The same molecular machinery may regulate both miRNAs and small interfering, double-stranded RNA (siRNA) molecules turning off expression of genes with the same sequence in a process known as RNA interference (RNAi). RNAi has been used by us and others to link gene expression to many functional changes in MMs. Although miRNAs and siRNAs can bind to the same proteins, miRNAs are formed from a single hairpin in precursor RNA, whereas siRNAs are formed from longer double-stranded RNAs.

The relevance of miRNA loss and dysregulation to development of cancers has been noted in a number of tumor types where tumors frequently exhibit global downregulation of miRNAs. Since a recent review highlights the changes observed in miRNA expression and function in MMs (Reid 2015), this chapter will focus primarily on other epigenetic signatures.

In contrast to miRNAs, lncRNAs have not been studied in MMs but are differentially transcribed in metastatic tumors and may act via many mechanisms to encourage EMT and tumor progression (Schmitz et al. 2016). LncRNAs can act as chromatin modulators in that they target histone-modifying enzymes to repress homeobox transcription factor (HOX) genes aberrantly expressed in human T cell and acute lymphomas and leukemias (Homminga et al. 2012). Many of these studies suggest cross talk between lncRNAs and miRNAs.

10.3.2 Histone Modifications

As illustrated in Fig. 10.1, chromatin structure consists of complex arrangements of DNA packaged by histone proteins. The five families of histones include H1, H2A, H2B, H3, and H4. All but H1, a linker histone, are core histones in which a pair of each forms a histone octamer that wraps around 146 bp of DNA. Initially, nucleosomes resemble "beads" that are connected to each other by linker DNA, forming a compact 30-nm fiber structure that subsequently undergoes thickening to a 300-nm fiber structure as metaphase approaches. DNA in the nucleosome is partially blocked from access to DNA polymerases and other regulatory proteins by histones, but the N-amino terminus of each histone that protrudes from the nucleosome can undergo posttranslational modifications including phosphorylation, ADP-ribosylation, sumoylation, ubiquitination, methylation, and acetylation, among other processes (Kouzarides 2007). Of these processes, histone acetylation (addition of –COCH$_3$) and removal, i.e., via deacetylation and methylation, have been primarily studied as modifications in histones that lead to alterations in nucleosome-DNA interactions and result in altered gene expression. In general, acetylation has been linked to a process where DNA becomes accessible as euchromatin and methylation (addition of –CH3 to histone tails) renders condensation of chromatin (heterochromatin) inaccessible for transcription.

As summarized in Table 10.1, two broad groups of enzymes, histone methyltransferases (HMTs) and histone demethylases (HDMs), participate in histone methylation. Methylation of histones catalyzed by HMTs can initiate either transcription or repression, depending upon the locus. An example is the tri-methylation of lysine residue 4 of histone 3 (H3K4me3) that causes gene transcription vs. the tri-methylation of lysine 9 (H3K9me3) or 27 (H3K27me3), which results in gene silencing. Histone modifications can also be mediated by SUV39H1 and G9a, which catalyze the mono-, di-, and tri-methylation of histone H3K9 (Martin and Zhang 2005; Shi and Whetstine 2007). G9a expression has been correlated with poor prognosis in lung cancer patients presumably by repressing the cell adhesion molecule, EPCAM, which is linked to catalyzing H3K9mc2 on its promoter. This then causes EMT and cancer metastasis (Chen et al. 2010). This mechanism has also been suggested in the development of human breast cancers (Dong et al. 2012) as well as head and neck carcinomas (Liu et al. 2015).

Another repressive histone modification, H3K27, is catalyzed by the embryonic ectoderm development protein of polycomb repressive complex 2 (EZH2) and its homolog, EZH1-containing polycomb repressive complex 2 (PRC2), which are important in both embryonic development and stem cell differentiation. Overexpression of EZH2 is a signature of poor prognosis in prostate and breast cancers (Margueron and Reinberg 2011), and PRC2/EZH2 expression is linked to reduction of E-cadherin expression, indicating a promoting role of this complex in EMT (Yu et al. 2012).

Histone acetylation, a process generally leading to transcriptional activation, occurs in the lysine regions of histone tails (Sterner and Berger 2000; Cress and Seto 2000). In brief, acetylation is regulated by histone acetyltransferases (HATs) and histone deacetylases (HDACs), which cause either decondensation or condensation of chromatin structure, respectively. Whereas HATs transfer acetyl groups to specific lysine side chains in the histone N-terminal tail, HDACs remove acetyl groups from lysine residues. There are several families of HATs including hMOF, TIP60, PCAF, and p300/CBT that act by neutralizing the negative charges of histones, weaken histone-DNA nucleosome interactions, and increase transcription. In addition, the attachment of acetyl groups via HATs creates an attachment site for other proteins that recruit chromatin remodeling constructs. As a result, chromatin is less tightly bound, and transcription factor binding can occur, resulting in gene activation. Several HATs are linked to Wnt and B-catenin-dependent EMT (Sun and Fang 2016), dissociation of ZEB1 from the miR-200c/141 promoter (Mizuguchi et al. 2012), and upregulation of TGF-β signaling that is known to occur in MMs.

Lysine acetylation is counteracted by HDACs that restore its positive charge, stabilize chromatin structure, and function primarily as corepressors of transcription. At least 18 mammalian HDACs occur in four classes. Inhibiting enzymatic activities of class I/II/III HDACs increases H3/H4 acetylation and derepresses gene expression in many types of cancer cells. Inhibition of class I HDACs using different approaches causes decreased cancer cell growth and metastases and abrogates EMT in many models (Takai et al. 2004; Srivastava et al. 2010; Ye et al. 2010; Shah et al. 2014). Data were initially encouraging in preclinical studies, resulting in the development of a number of small molecule inhibitors for clinical trials (West and Johnstone 2014). However, these compounds have had limited effects on solid tumors (Tam and Weinberg 2013) including MMs (Krug et al. 2015). Demonstration that inhibition of class I HDACs sensitizes melanoma cells to apoptosis after treatment with temozolomide has prompted co-therapeutic approaches using HDAC inhibitors with chemotherapy (Krumm et al. 2016; Kristensen et al. 2009) or immunotherapy (Hamaidia et al. 2016).

10.3.3   DNA Methylation

DNA methylation occurs via a different set of enzymes that methylate certain bases in DNA. The most frequently studied epigenetic marker is DNA methylation, a process catalyzed by DNA methyltransferases (DNMT) and resulting in covalent attachment of a methyl group to the fifth carbon of cytosine, i.e., 5-methylcytosine (5mC). This process occurs at sites of CpG dinucleotides that are located at promoter regions, i.e., transcription start sites of genes, and results in transcriptional silencing of gene expression by inhibition of transcription factor binding and/or recruitment of methyl-CpG binding proteins (MBPs). A number of DNMTs exist. For example, DNMT1 maintains methylation patterns during cell division, whereas DNMT3A and DNMT3B cause de novo DNA methylation, showing preference toward unmethylated CpG dinucleotides (Okano et al. 1999). Aberrant DNA methylation often occurs in cancers in which hypermethylation of CpG islands and hypomethylation of other regions are observed. These changes lead to tumor suppressor gene silencing and genomic instability (Sandoval and Esteller 2012). Overall, human tumors of a variety of types have been associated with global hypomethylation and hypermethylation of CpG islands in the promoter regions of tumor suppressor genes that lead to their inactivation.

DNA methylation-linked transcriptional silencing is connected with the recruitment of various methyl-DNA binding domain (MBD) proteins including MeCP2, MBD1-4, and Kaiso (Sansom et al. 2007). MBD proteins interact with different chromatin-modifying proteins to form compact chromatin, thus encouraging repression of transcription. Different CpG island methylation patterns recruit different sets of MBD proteins that may assume unique functions. For example, MeCP2 and MBD1/MBD2 bind to methylated CpG islands on the E-cadherin promoter and are associated with gene silencing in several types of tumor cells, whereas Kaiso also binds to the E-cadherin promoter as well as a methylated sequence in the miR-31 promoter to encourage EMT via unique signaling pathways (Jones et al. 2014; Wang et al. 2016).

The involvement of DNMTs in tumor growth and progression has also been indicated in knockdown studies using mice depleted of DNMT3a in a lung cancer model—these mice exhibit, in comparison to wild-type mice, significantly increased promotion of tumor cell growth and progression (Gao et al. 2011). Genome-wide DNA hypomethylation induced by DNMT1 deficiency also increases chromosome instability and tumor incidence in mice (Eden et al. 2003; Gaudet et al. 2003).

DNA demethylation changes may also be important in epithelial cell gene silencing and the development of EMT and cancers (Sun and Fang 2016). Passive DNA methylation occurs during replication, and active demethylation can be mediated by three ten-eleven translocation (TET1-3) proteins. These oxygenases convert 5mC to oxidatively modified derivatives. In particular, TET1 interacts with hypoxia-inducible factors (HIF-1α and HIF-1β) to enhance their transactivation, processes contributing to hypoxia-induced EMT.

10.3.4 Chromatin Remodeling and Interactions

ATP-dependent chromatin remodeling allows both compaction and decompaction of DNA in processes such as DNA replication, DNA repair, and regulation of gene expression (Sun and Fang 2016). The four major families of chromatin remodeling complexes are SWI/SNF, ISWI, CHD, and INO80. Most importantly, they commonly contain a catalytic ATPase subunit that undergoes ATP hydrolysis and alters histone-DNA interactions to restructure nucleosomes; however, they also have non-catalytic components that contribute to their complex targeting processes.

It is important to realize that there is cross talk between the different categories of epigenetic changes listed in Table 10.1. For example, often the expression of miRNAs is due to other epigenetic modifications on their promoter regions. Several examples are relevant to the development of cancers. First, during the development of EMT, the promoters of miR-200a/200b/429 and miR-200c/141 are embellished by repressive histone modifications, suggesting that several chromatin-modifying enzymes and DNMTs are important in miRNA regulation (Vrba et al. 2010). Silencing of miR-205 requires both DNA methylation and H3K27me3. These data suggest that different chromatin-modifying proteins and their catalyzed modifications, as well as miRNAs, regulate the same set of genes or act in concert.

An exciting recent report by Bintu and colleagues indicates how various individual chromatin regulators (CRs) acting on chromatin in diverse ways are temporally regulated and operative in a unifying model of epigenetic regulation (Bintu et al. 2016; Keung and Khalil 2016). In brief, in order to determine the kinetics of gene regulation and reporter protein levels, these investigators tracked the reporter activity of four repressive CRs (H3K27 methylation, H39L9 methylation, DNMT3B, and HDAC4) and silencing events in individual cells during CR recruitment. Reactivation events upon release of CRs by time-lapse microcopy were also studied. The data showed that all of the CRs silenced and reactivated reporter genes in an all-or-none fashion. These processes were characterized by stochastic transitions between active, reversibly silent, and irreversibly silent states with different timescales. For example, DNMT3B caused slow and complete commitment of cells to an irreversibly silent state, whereas HDAC4 initiated rapid silencing and reactivation. These observations may explain, in part, why DNA methylation is widely associated with heritable gene repression as opposed to histone acetylation, which is typically transient. The data also may have relevance to silencing of a number of tumor suppressor or other genes in MMs. Different fractions of cell populations may exhibit distinctive dynamics of epigenetic regulation due to the different timescales of activity and "memory" of CR-induced gene expression.

10.4 Involvement of Epigenetics in Molecular Changes and Cell Signaling Pathways Related to Proliferation and Survival in Mesothelioma

10.4.1 Cell Signaling Pathways

MMs display many alterations in mitogenic signaling pathways that are linked to increased survival, proliferation, and disruption of cell cycle control. Persistent activations of receptor tyrosine kinases (RTKs), mitogen activated protein kinases (MAPKs or Ras/extracellular signal regulated kinases (ERK1/ERK2)), and phosphatidylinositol 3 (PI3)-kinase/AKT pathways are common features of MM cells (Altomare et al. 2005; Opitz et al. 2008; Wang et al. 2011; Shukla et al. 2011; Ramos-Nino et al. 2005). These signaling pathways can be altered by (1) aberrant activity of RTKs or receptors for other kinases, (2) alterations in signaling adaptor proteins, (3) constitutive activation of GTPases such as Ras and Raf, (4) overexpression of target transcription factors, and (5) inactivation of negative regulators. Mitogenic signaling pathways and loss of cell cycle checkpoints can also be regulated cooperatively with cross talk between signaling pathways to favor cell proliferation and survival. For example, MM cells show phosphorylation of multiple RTKs, with phosphorylation of epidermal growth factor receptor (EGFR) and MET, the most prominent among 42 RTKs studied (Sekido 2010). Inhibition of both these receptors decreased MM cell proliferation in a synergistic fashion (Sekido 2010) as did dual inhibition of PI3K and the MET pathway in MM cells in another mouse model of MM (Kanteti et al. 2016). In a recent study, 60 human MMs were examined for expression of the *MET* gene, which was rarely amplified (1.7% of total cases) or displayed polysomy (6.7%) using in situ hybridization approaches (Varesano et al. 2016). However, this pathway may be governed by multiple epigenetic mechanisms (Menges et al. 2014).

Mesothelial cells also exhibit a number of cytokine receptors that trigger cell proliferation. Thus, they respond to a broad array of growth factors, including epidermal growth factor (EGF), keratinocyte growth factor (KGF), hepatocyte growth factor (HGF), tumor necrosis factor α (TNF-α), interleukin 8 (IL-8), fibroblast growth factors (FGFs), transforming growth factor β (TGF-β), and insulin-like growth factor 1 (IGF-1) (reviewed in Heintz et al. 2010; Sekido 2010).

In mesothelial cells, asbestos fibers cause dose-dependent proliferation and cell death by necrosis, apoptosis, and pyroptosis, a type of death linked to inflammasome activation (Miller et al. 2014). These responses are dependent on fiber type, size, duration of exposure, and the biodurability of fibers (reviewed in Mossman et al. 2013). At low exposures, asbestos induces some production of ROS/RNS, increases in expression of antioxidants, and elevations in cell proliferation, whereas cytotoxic doses cause striking increases in oxidant release, depletion of glutathione (Janssen et al. 1995), mitochondrial dysfunction (Shukla et al. 2003a), and cell death (Goldberg et al. 1997). Asbestos fibers dimerize and activate EGFR (Zanella et al. 1996; Pache et al. 1998), and both EGFR and β1-integrin may upregulate activation of AKT and MAPK/ERK1,2 cascades (Berken et al. 2003; Wilson et al. 2008).

Activation of ERKs results in induction of AP-1, a heterodimeric transcription factor composed of members of the c-Fos and c-Jun proto-oncogene families. The c-Fos family member, Fra-1, is the primary component of AP-1 required for MM cell growth (Ramos-Nino et al. 2002). Moreover, *JUN* and other transcription factor genes are amplified in some human MMs (Taniguchi et al. 2007). The strength and duration of ERK1/ERK2 phosphorylation may be important in determining cell proliferation or death, as persistent activation and of ERK1/ERK2 by crocidolite asbestos results in downregulation of cyclin D1 and apoptotic cell death (Yuan et al. 2004). Individual members of the ERK family have also been implicated in chemoresistance and development of MMs (Shukla et al. 2010).

The sensitivity of mesothelial cells in response to asbestos and erionite fibers, oxidants, and a wide array of growth factors that induce alterations in mitogenic signaling of MMs as well as loss of function of tumor suppressor proteins may govern the transformation and pathogenesis of MMs. As illustrated in Fig. 10.2, a number of signaling pathways may be interactive in the transformation of MM cells. For example, cell surface receptors may be activated directly by mineral fibers or indirectly by the generation of oxidants. These interactions lead to phosphorylation of serine-threonine (MAPK) or RTKs and other growth promoting kinase cascades. In addition, antiapoptotic or survival pathways can be initiated by cytokines such as TNF-alpha (TNF-α) produced by inflammatory cell types or mesothelial cells. Several of these cascades also depend upon pathways that stimulate chronic inflammation and S-phase entry of mesothelial cells via formation and nuclear translocation of transcription factors. Redox-regulated transcription factors, i.e., FOXM1 (Newick et al. 2012); redox-sensitive proteins, i.e., thioredoxins

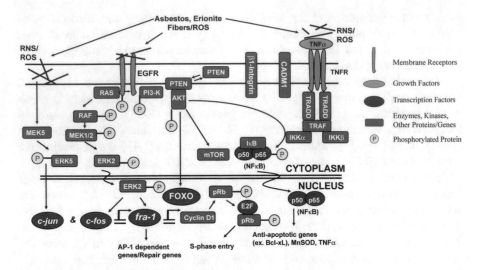

Fig. 10.2 Diagram illustrating the main cell signaling pathways in mesothelial cell transformation by carcinogenic mineral fibers and oxidants. Asbestos fibers may act directly at the cell membrane to cause activation of integrins or dimerization of surface receptors such as EGFR. Receptor-dependent and nonreceptor-activated pathways may also be stimulated indirectly via generation of oxidants such as ROS or RNS from asbestos fibers or cells of the immune system. Fiber-induced oxidant generation may occur both extracellularly due to bioavailable or adsorbed iron on the surfaces of fibers or intracellularly after uptake of fibers. Long asbestos fibers also cause frustrated phagocytosis in mesothelial cells and macrophages, a protracted source of oxidant generation. Mitogenic and other signaling pathways that are activated by growth factors and cytokines or chemokines then converge upon transcription factors that lead to loss of cell cycle control and the promotion of chronic cell inflammation, proliferation, and survival, key events in mesothelial cell transformation. Figure reproduced from Mossman et al. (2013)

(Tabata et al. 2013); and antioxidants (Stapelberg et al. 2005) have been suggested as biomarkers (Tabata et al. 2013), targets (Newick et al. 2012), and inhibitors (Stapelberg et al. 2005) of MM.

10.4.2   Alterations in Tumor Suppressor Genes/Proteins Linked to Cell Cycle Regulation

Loss of tumor suppressor gene and protein functions that negatively regulate cyclin D1, a requirement for cell proliferation, is also observed in MMs. For example, inactivation of the tumor suppressor neurofibromatosis type 2 gene (*NF2*), either by homozygous deletion or mutation, is observed in 40–50% of mesotheliomas (Bianchi et al. 1995). *NF2* encodes Merlin, a membrane-cytoskeleton protein that suppresses mitogenic signaling by sequestering growth factor receptors (Curto and McClatchey 2008). In cancer cells in general, Merlin also stops cell cycle progression by repressing expression of cyclin D1 (Xiao et al. 2005), which controls S-phase entry by phosphorylation of the retinoblastoma tumor suppressor protein (pRB) and activation of the transcription factor E2F1. A second regulator of cyclin D1 kinase activity, the tumor suppressor p16INK4A, is also deleted with high frequency in MMs, and inactivation of both p16Ink4a and p19Arf cooperates to accelerate asbestos-induced MMs in a mouse model of asbestos carcinogenesis (Altomare et al. 2011). Mice heterozygous (+/−) for *Nf2* also develop peritoneal MMs more quickly with a higher frequency than observed in wild-type littermates (Altomare et al. 2005). Interestingly, tumors from heterozygous *Nf2* mice also exhibit homozygous deletion of the *Cdkn2a* (p16Ink4a/p19Arf) locus frequently. Consistent with these observations, global gene expression studies indicate that regulation of E2F1 may represent a central control mechanism in MM cell proliferation (Gordon et al. 2005).

As emphasized above, there is a low frequency of consistent and global genetic abnormalities in MMs that are regarded as cancers primarily associated with loss of function of tumor suppressor genes (TSGs). A number of these negatively regulate the cyclin D1 regulatory axis. A frequent molecular change is deletion or hypermethylation at the *CDKN2A* (p16INK4A/p14ARF) and *CDKN2B* (encoding the tumor suppressor p15INK4B) loci in chromosome 9p21 (Murthy and Testa 1999). Frequent 16INK4A inactivation by homozygous deletion or methylation leads to the inactivation of 16INK4A in Japanese MM patients. Moreover, loss of expression of 16INK4A was associated with a poor prognosis (Kobayashi et al. 2008).

Hypermethylation and silencing of the *RASSFIA* and *GPC3* tumor suppressor genes has also been demonstrated in MMs (Murthy et al. 2000), and most recently, inactivation of the BRCA-associated protein 1 gene (*BAP1*) by germline mutations has been shown, suggesting a role in causation of familial MMs (Testa et al. 2011). A recent report shows that there are independent mutational and epigenetic control mechanisms in the loss of BAP1 function. In these studies, conditional *Bap1* loss in mice has multiple effects including elevations in H3K27me3 and increases in expression of enhancer of zeste 2 polycomb repressive complex 2 subunit (Ezh2) (LaFave et al. 2015). Conditional deletion of *Bap1* also resulted in a marked decrease in histone H4K20 monomethylation that has been shown to be important in the transcriptional regulation of EZH2. Moreover, MM cells that lacked BAP1 were more sensitive to EZH2 pharmacologic inhibition of cell proliferation.

BAP1 has been regarded as an epigenetic regulatory gene, as its loss of function as a deubiquitylase alters levels of HDAC1 and HDAC2 in lung cancers and MM cells in an opposite manner (Sacco et al. 2015). Whereas coordinated transcription of HDAC1 and HDAC2 occurs in lung cancer cell lines with genetic *BAP1* inactivation, *BAP1*-depleted MM cells show a reduction in HDAC2, but increased HDAC1 expression. This imbalance sensitizes some human MM cell lines to HDAC inhibitors, but other lines with low endogenous HDAC2 adapt to become resistant to HDAC inhibition.

Genomic profiling patterns of peritoneal MMs from 13 patients showed that recurrent alterations in *BAP1* and other epigenetic regulatory genes, including *SETD2* and *DDX3X*, are different from patterns observed in pleural MMs with nearly all of the peritoneal MMs (11/13) showing *BAP1* alterations as opposed to only 20–30% of pleural tumors (Joseph et al. 2016). In concert, studies summarized above and elsewhere (Guo et al. 2015; Alakus et al. 2015; Cigognetti et al. 2015; Chirac et al. 2016; Bueno et al. 2016) support the hypothesis that *BAP1* and other TSGs documented in MM to date are both important as epigenetic regulators and also are regulated themselves by multiple genetic and epigenetic control mechanisms.

10.4.3 Epigenetic Pathways in Responses to Asbestos and the Development of MMs

The terms "epigenetic" and "genotoxic" have been used historically to classify carcinogens. In the 1970s and 1980s, chemical carcinogens were generally classified as genotoxic because they interacted with DNA before or during their metabolism, whereas agents such as asbestos fibers were regarded as epigenetic in their effects and classified as tumor promoters or cocarcinogens as they did not interact directly with DNA nor form adducts with DNA (Williams 1979; Mossman et al. 1983; Eastman et al. 1983; Shelby 1988). Alternatively, many studies have shown that short asbestos fibers are phagocytized by mesothelial and lung epithelial cells and incorporated into membrane-bound phagolysosomes, which accumulate in the perinuclear region of the cell after size-dependent active transport along cytoplasmic microtubules (Cole et al. 1991). Long fibers then attach to the nuclear envelope and may sterically block cytokinesis (Jensen et al. 1996; Jensen and Watson 1999). Since some studies indicated possible physical interactions of asbestos fibers with chromosomes in rodent cells (Yegles et al. 1993), and large chromosomal deletions occurred at lethal concentrations of asbestos (Hei et al. 1992), the behavior of crocidolite asbestos fibers was studied using high-resolution time-lapse video-enhanced microscopy in living lung epithelial cells during mitosis (Ault et al. 1995). These studies showed that physical interactions between crocidolite fibers and chromosomes occurred randomly within the spindle. Moreover, crocidolite fibers showed no affinity toward chromatin, an observation that may be related to its lack of DNA accessibility due to compact and complex histone protein interactions. However, the more pathogenic types of asbestos, crocidolite, and amosite may generate epigenetic changes by oxidant-related mechanisms.

After inhalation and transport to the pleura, asbestos fibers first encounter the outer cell membrane of mesothelial cells where many signaling pathways can be initiated via a wide array of receptor-dependent or -independent pathways (reviewed in Mossman et al. 2013). As detailed above, these signaling cascades include activation of RTKs (Menges et al. 2010), Ras/ERK1/ERK2 pathways (reviewed in Mossman et al. 2013), and PI3K/Akt pathways (Altomare et al. 2005; Kanteti et al. 2016) that are also common features of MM cells. Upregulation of these pathways, which may be co-activated by various mechanisms, has been causally linked to proliferation and dysregulation of mesothelial cells after asbestos exposure.

In recent studies, alterations in the Wnt signaling pathway, which targets β-catenin expression (Kohno et al. 2010; Fox et al. 2013) and the Hippo pathway that is linked to inactivation of *NF2*, have been documented in MM cells and tissues

(Sekido 2010; Jaurand and Jean 2016; Bueno et al. 2016). The β-catenin pathway may be governed by methylation of a number of genes that may prove to be more important than genetic control, as examination of both MM cells and tissues showed no mutations in exon 3 of β-catenin, a signature of the canonical Wnt signaling pathway (Kohno et al. 2010). In contrast, the Hippo pathway has not been characterized functionally in the pathogenesis of MMs although alterations in regulation of this pathway by LATS1, LATS2, and SAV1 and overexpression of the transcription cofactor YAP have been observed in some MMs (Jaurand and Jean 2016).

10.5 Links Between Epigenetic Changes and Functional Alterations in the Development of Mesotheliomas

As described above, epigenetic alterations characterized by DNA methylation changes (Toyooka et al. 2001; Tsou et al. 2005) have been described in human MMs, but few studies have examined functional endpoints central to the development of these tumors. As miRNA findings in MMs have been recently reviewed (Reid 2015), studies in Table 10.2 emphasize methylation-related epigenetic changes and their functional effects on MMs, in chronological order.

Table 10.2 Types of methylation-related epigenetic changes and functional changes in malignant mesothelioma cells and tissues

Epigenetic change	Functional outcome	References
Silencing of SFRP by hypermethylation	Induction of apoptosis in β-catenin-deficient MM cells	Lee et al. (2004), He et al. (2005)
Depletion of *DNMT1/3b* using antisense oligonucleotides	Selective growth inhibition of MM vs. normal mesothelial cells	Kassis et al. (2006)
Hypermethylation of promoter regions of six TSGs (*APC, CCDN2, CDKN2A, CDKN2B, HPPBP1, RASSF1*) linked to cell cycle control	Increased asbestos (ferruginous) bodies in lung tissues	Christensen et al. (2008)
Silencing of *DNMT1*	Decreased cell survival	Amatori et al. (2009)
Hypermethylation of promoters of *WIF-1* and *SFRP*	Increased Wnt signaling	Kohno et al. (2010)
Inhibition of *miR-34b/c* expression by methylation	Induction of apoptosis by overexpression of *miR-34bc*	Kubo et al. (2011)
Hypermethylation of tumor suppressor mitogen α7 (*IGTA7*) promoter	Overexpression of ITGA7 in MM cells with low ITGA7 inhibited cell motility	Laszlo et al. (2015)
Reduced H3K27 tri-methylation by increased KDM6B histone demethylase	KDM6B regulated expression of estrogen receptor β, a putative TSG product in MM	Manente et al. (2016)

DNMT DNA methylation; *SFRP* secreted frizzled-related protein; *TSG* tumor suppressor gene

The first indication that DNMTs were important in cell growth and survival of MMs was work showing that expression of DNMT1, DNMT3a, and DNMT3b was upregulated in MMs, with DNMT1 being the most expressed DNA methyltransferase (>85% of total DNMTs). Silencing of DNMT1 or DNMT3b using antisense oligonucleotides resulted in inhibition of survival of MM cells, but not normal mesothelial cells, and resulted in caspase-dependent but p53-independent apoptosis (Kassis et al. 2006). The importance of silencing DNMT1 in MM cell survival was confirmed subsequently by another group (Amatori et al. 2009).

Others have focused on transcriptional downregulation of WIF-1, a negative regulator of the Wnt signaling pathway, or secreted frizzled-related protein (SFRP), which induces apoptosis in β-catenin-deficient MM cells (He et al. 2005). The promoters of these genes are hypermethylated in human MM cells and tissues (Lee et al. 2004; Kohno et al. 2010). Whereas WIF-1 promoter methylation was observed in 34 of 36 MMs (94%) and in each of eight MM lines tested, SFRP1, 2, and 4 methylation was seen in approximately 50 to 60% of MMs (Kohno et al. 2010). Treatment of MM cell lines with 5-aza-deoxycytidine showed WIF-1 promoter methylation recovery and restoration of WIF-1 expression.

Hypermethylation of the promoter regions of six TSGs (*APC, CCD2, CDKN2A, CDNKN2B, HPPBP1,* and *RASSF1*), all of which are linked to cell cycle control, was assessed in 70 human MM tissues (Christensen et al. 2008). These studies also evaluated lung content of asbestos (ferruginous) bodies as an indicator of patient exposure to asbestos. Significantly increased numbers of asbestos bodies were observed if any of these TSGs were methylated after controlling for age, gender, and tumor histology. By trend analysis, asbestos bodies increased as numbers of methylated genes increased, suggesting links between these TSGs and responses to asbestos. In addition, methylation of any one or more of the six TSGs was significantly associated with increased age. These data support the hypothesis that epigenetic gene silencing via promoter methylation of TSGs plays a role in asbestos carcinogenesis. Since hypermethylation of cell cycle regulatory genes, inflammation-associated genes, and apoptosis-related genes occurred in MMs, these authors hypothesized that hypermethylation and gene silencing play a role in selective survival of MMs during tumor development in an environment of persistent inflammation, tissue injury, and oxidative stress. Subsequent work by this group showed that methylation profiles also differentiated pleural MMs from normal pleural tissue. Moreover, methylation profiles and asbestos burden were independent predictors of MM patient survival (Christensen et al. 2009a). DNA methylation profiles also distinguished MMs from lung adenocarcinomas and nonmalignant lung tissues (Christensen et al. 2009b). The frequency of genetic and epigenetic alterations was then examined in a case series of 23 pleural MMs using comparisons between gene copy number alterations and DNA methylation profiles. Data showed prevalent allele loss at the DNMT1 gene locus and a strong association between global genetic and epigenetic alterations in MMs (Christensen et al. 2010).

Epigenetic profiles have been recently studied in heterogeneous side populations (SP) and non-SP populations isolated from a human MM line (Kim et al. 2016). Using integrated analyses of methylated DNA immunoprecipitation combined with high-throughput sequencing (MeDIP-sequencing) and RNA-sequencing to show concomitant changes in mRNA expression, changes in DNA methylation and mRNA expression were found in 122 genes, of which 118 were downregulated with hypermethylation and 4 were upregulated with hypomethylation. Genes functionally were related primarily to stem cell maintenance and development as well as negative regulation of developmental processes. The genes *BNC1*, *RPS6KA3*, *DUSP1*, and *TWSG1* most commonly showed aberrant methylation in the CpG islands of their promoter regions in a distinct population of MM cells. Thus, DNA methylation changes might predict different MM phenotypes and contribute to heterogeneity of MMs.

The aberrant promoter methylation of bone morphogenic proteins (BMPs), i.e., members of the TGF-β superfamily, has also been studied in human MM lines and tissues (Kimura et al. 2008). These studies showed that methylation status and expression of BMP3b and BMP6 were suppressed in two of seven cell lines. Significant changes in frequency of BMP3b were observed in MM cases from Japan (9 of 17 cases, 53%) vs. cases from the USA (3 of 40 cases, 8%), suggesting that methylation of this gene may have ethnic differences.

Hypermethylation of two other putative TSGs has recently been identified and characterized functionally in human MM cells (Table 10.2). Using MM cell lines exhibiting different cell motilities, researchers identified a set of 139 genes that were differentially expressed in MMs with high vs. low migration rates (Laszlo et al. 2015). When compared to normal mesothelial cells with low motility, MM cells showed hypermethylation of the promoter region of the integrin α7 promoter gene (*ITGA7*), which correlated with patterns of reduced expression of *ITGA7* mRNA and protein in highly motile cells. Overexpression of *ITGA7* in MM cells with low endogenous ITGA and high motility inhibited their migration, showing a functional regulatory role of ITGA7, a novel TSG, in MM cell motility. Normal human pleura robustly expressed ITGA7 protein that varied in a panel of 200 MMs; however, patients with high ITGA7 expression had an increased median overall survival compared to low- or no-expression groups. Thus, these data not only demonstrate the importance of epigenetic modulation of ITGA7 in a functional context but also suggest that its expression may be used in diagnosis or therapy of MMs.

Estrogen receptor β (ERβ), a positive prognostic marker and tumor suppressor, is maintained by selective ligand activation in human MMs (Pinton et al. 2009; Manente et al. 2013; Manente et al. 2015; Manente et al. 2016). To determine whether expression of ERβ is governed by epigenetic mechanisms, the expression of KDM6B, which reduces histone H3K27 tri-methylation, was studied in human MM cell spheroids under hypoxic conditions that promote ERβ expression in ERβ-negative MM cells (Manente et al. 2016). In hypoxia, HIF2α-KDM6B interactions induced ERβ expression and epithelioid morphology in biphasic MMs with an estrogen receptor-negative phenotype. MM cells exposed to the selective ERβ agonist, KB9520, during reoxygenation maintained ERβ expression, and their epithelioid phenotype related to less aggressive functional characteristics. These approaches illustrate the importance of epigenetic mechanisms in regulation of ERβ expression and cell phenotype.

Methylation of miRNA genes also occurs in MMs, indicating multiple mechanisms of epigenetic control. In studies by Kubo and colleagues, inhibition of miR-34a and miR-34b/c by methylation was observed in MM cells and tissues (Kubo et al. 2011). Overexpression of miR-34b/c resulted in decreased cell proliferation and apoptosis.

10.6 Conclusions and Clinical Relevance of Findings

In contrast to genetic alterations, epigenetic changes in MMs have been explored only recently. Although epigenetic signatures such as DNA methylation and histone modifications are linked to suppression of TSGs, the complexity of these processes are confounding. Responses may be different in subpopulations of MM cells and are further complicated by interactions between enzymes that facilitate these responses and cross talk, i.e., methylation of miRNAs. However, epigenomics is likely to play an important role in defining patient responsiveness to chemotherapy and in diagnosis and prognosis of MMs, although multiple epigenetic signatures may be required. An illustration of how epigenetic candidates, such as certain miRNAs, may be important as therapeutic targets is described briefly below.

Restoring miRNA levels that are frequently decreased in a number of cancers, most notably non-small cell lung cancer (NSCLC), has shown inhibition of tumor growth in several preclinical models. Based on the hypothesis that miRNA replacement therapy will be beneficial in the treatment of MM patients, a novel delivery system for miRNA mimetics, i.e., TargomiRs, which are delivered by targeted bacterial minicells, has been developed (Reid et al. 2016). This approach is bolstered by preliminary data in human MMs showing that downregulation of miR-16 and the entire miR-15/107 group (Reid et al. 2016) occurs commonly in MM tumors and cell lines. Thus synthetic miRNA mimics were created with novel sequences based on a consensus sequence derived from the miR-15/107 group. Use of this approach in a mouse xenograft model using human MM cells resulted in 60–80% growth inhibition, a greater inhibition than the use of native miR-16. A bacterially derived delivery system using nanocells, i.e., nonviable minicells (EDVs) that are coated with a bi-specific antibody with one arm binding to a target surface receptor on tumor cells, causes endocytosis. This novel delivery system has led to the development of a phase I trial, the MesomiR-1 trial, for MM patients that were initiated in December of 2014 in Australia and is near completion. Most exciting thus far are observations that TargomiR treatment is well tolerated and safe in patients and has achieved disease control in five of six MM patients after 8 weeks of treatment. Further studies are planned to evaluate this approach using miRNAs targeting the immune checkpoint protein, PD-L1, or in combination therapies with radiation or chemotherapeutic drugs. This is an encouraging example of how the focus on epigenetic targets has been translated into clinical use.

Acknowledgments Research on cell signaling in the Mossman laboratory has been supported by grants from NHLBI (P01 HL67004), NCI (P01 CA11407, M. Carbone, PI), and NIEHS (T32 ES00712). Jennifer Díaz (UVM) provided secretarial support for this chapter, and Maximilian MacPherson (UVM) assisted with figure preparation.

Dedication This chapter is dedicated to all patients with malignant mesotheliomas with the hope that new information here will be translated to the design of novel treatments.

Declaration of Interests The author has consulted with both plaintiff and defense lawyers and has been an expert witness in cosmetic talc litigation.

References

Alakus H, Yost SE, Woo B et al (2015) BAP1 mutation is a frequent somatic event in peritoneal malignant mesothelioma. J Transl Med 13:122

Altomare DA, You H, Xiao GH et al (2005) Human and mouse mesotheliomas exhibit elevated AKT/PKB activity, which can be targeted pharmacologically to inhibit tumor cell growth. Oncogene 24(40):6080–6089

Altomare DA, Menges CW, Xu J et al (2011) Losses of both products of the Cdkn2a/Arf locus contribute to asbestos-induced mesothelioma development and cooperate to accelerate tumorigenesis. PLoS One 6:e18828

Amatori S, Papalini F, Lazzarini R et al (2009) Decitabine, differently from DNMT1 silencing, exerts its antiproliferative activity through p21 upregulation in malignant pleural mesothelioma (MPM) cells. Lung Cancer 66:184–190

Ault JG, Cole RW, Jensen CG et al (1995) Behavior of crocidolite asbestos during mitosis in living vertebrate lung epithelial cells. Cancer Res 55:792–798

Berken A, Abel J, Unfried K (2003) B1-integrin mediates asbestos-induced phosphorylation of AKT and ERK1/2 in a rat pleural mesothelial cell line. Oncogene 22:8524–8528

Bianchi AB, Mitsunaga SI, Cheng JQ et al (1995) High frequency of inactivating mutations in the neurofibromatosis type 2 gene (NF2) in primary malignant mesotheliomas. Proc Natl Acad Sci U S A 92:10854–10858

Bintu L, Yong J, Antebi YE et al (2016) Dynamics of epigenetic regulation at the single-cell level. Science 351:720–724

Bowman RV, Wright CM, Davidson MR et al (2009) Epigenomic targets for the treatment of respiratory disease. Expert Opin Ther Targets 13:625–640

Bueno R, Stawiski EW, Goldstein LD et al (2016) Comprehensive genomic analysis of malignant pleural mesothelioma identifies recurrent mutations, gene fusions and splicing alterations. Nat Genet 48:407–416

Chen MW, Hua KT, Kao HJ et al (2010) H3K9 histone methyltransferase G9a promotes lung cancer invasion and metastasis by silencing the cell adhesion molecule Ep-CAM. Cancer Res 70:7830–7840

Chirac P, Maillet D, Lepretre F et al (2016) Genomic copy number alterations in 33 malignant peritoneal mesothelioma analyzed by comparative genomic hybridization array. Hum Pathol 55:72–82

Christensen BC, Godleski JJ, Marsit CJ et al (2008) Asbestos exposure predicts cell cycle control gene promoter methylation in pleural mesothelioma. Carcinogenesis 29:1555–1559

Christensen BC, Houseman EA, Godleski JJ et al (2009a) Epigenetic profiles distinguish pleural mesothelioma from normal pleura and predict lung asbestos burden and clinical outcome. Cancer Res 69:227–234

Christensen BC, Marsit CJ, Houseman EA et al (2009b) Differentiation of lung adenocarcinoma, pleural mesothelioma, and nonmalignant pulmonary tissues using DNA methylation profiles. Cancer Res 69:6315–6321

Christensen BC, Houseman EA, Poage GM et al (2010) Integrated profiling reveals a global correlation between epigenetic and genetic alterations in mesothelioma. Cancer Res 70:5686–5694

Cigognetti M, Lonardi S, Fisogni S et al (2015) BAP1 (BRCA1-associated protein 1) is a highly specific marker for differentiating mesothelioma from reactive mesothelial proliferations. Mod Pathol 28:1043–1057

Cole RW, Ault JG, Hayden JH et al (1991) Crocidolite asbestos fibers undergo size-dependent microtubule-mediated transport after endocytosis in vertebrate lung epithelial cells. Cancer Res 51:4942–4947

Cress WD, Seto E (2000) Histone deacetylases, transcriptional control, and cancer. J Cell Physiol 184:1–16

Curto M, McClatchey AI (2008) Nf2/Merlin: a coordinator of receptor signalling and intercellular contact. Br J Cancer 98:256–262

Donaldson K, Murphy FA, Duffin R et al (2010) Asbestos, carbon nanotubes and the pleural mesothelium: a review of the hypothesis regarding the role of long fibre retention in the parietal pleura, inflammation and mesothelioma. Part Fibre Toxicol 7:5

Dong C, Wu Y, Yao J et al (2012) G9a interacts with Snail and is critical for Snail-mediated E-cadherin repression in human breast cancer. J Clin Invest 122:1469–1486

Dostert C, Petrilli V, Van Bruggen R et al (2008) Innate immune activation through Nalp3 inflammasome sensing of asbestos and silica. Science 320:674–677

Eastman A, Mossman BT, Bresnick E (1983) Influence of asbestos on the uptake of benzo(a) pyrene and DNA alkylation in hamster tracheal epithelial cells. Cancer Res 43:1251–1255

Eden A, Gaudet F, Waghmare A et al (2003) Chromosomal instability and tumors promoted by DNA hypomethylation. Science 300:455

Felsenfeld G (2014) A brief history of epigenetics. Cold Spring Harb Perspect Biol 6:a018200

Fischer JR, Ohnmacht U, Rieger N et al (2006) Promoter methylation of RASSF1A, RARbeta and DAPK predict poor prognosis of patients with malignant mesothelioma. Lung Cancer 54:109–116

Fox SA, Richards AK, Kusumah I et al (2013) Expression profile and function of Wnt signaling mechanisms in malignant mesothelioma cells. Biochem Biophys Res Commun 440:82–87

Gao Q, Steine EJ, Barrasa MI et al (2011) Deletion of the de novo DNA methyltransferase Dnmt3a promotes lung tumor progression. Proc Natl Acad Sci U S A 108:18061–18066

Gaudet F, Hodgson JG, Eden A et al (2003) Induction of tumors in mice by genomic hypomethylation. Science 300:489–492

Goldberg JL, Zanella CL, Janssen YM et al (1997) Novel cell imaging techniques show induction of apoptosis and proliferation in mesothelial cells by asbestos. Am J Respir Cell Mol Biol 17:265–271

Gordon GJ, Rockwell GN, Jensen RV et al (2005) Identification of novel candidate oncogenes and tumor suppressors in malignant pleural mesothelioma using large-scale transcriptional profiling. Am J Pathol 166:1827–1840

Goto Y, Shinjo K, Kondo Y et al (2009) Epigenetic profiles distinguish malignant pleural mesothelioma from lung adenocarcinoma. Cancer Res 69:9073–9082

Guo G, Chmielecki J, Goparaju C et al (2015) Whole-exome sequencing reveals frequent genetic alterations in BAP1, NF2, CDKN2A, and CUL1 in malignant pleural mesothelioma. Cancer Res 75:264–269

Hamaidia M, Staumont B, Duysinx B et al (2016) Improvement of malignant pleural mesothelioma immunotherapy by epigenetic modulators. Curr Top Med Chem 16:777–787

He B, Lee AY, Dadfarmay S et al (2005) Secreted frizzled-related protein 4 is silenced by hypermethylation and induces apoptosis in beta-catenin-deficient human mesothelioma cells. Cancer Res 65:743–748

Hei TK, Piao CQ, He ZY et al (1992) Chrysotile fiber is a strong mutagen in mammalian cells. Cancer Res 52:6305–6309

Heintz NH, Janssen-Heininger YM, Mossman BT (2010) Asbestos, lung cancers, and mesotheliomas: from molecular approaches to targeting tumor survival pathways. Am J Respir Cell Mol Biol 42:133–139

Hillegass JM, Miller JM, MacPherson MB et al (2013) Asbestos and erionite prime and activate the NLRP3 inflammasome that stimulates autocrine cytokine release in human mesothelial cells. Part Fibre Toxicol 10:39

Homminga I, Pieters R, Meijerink JP (2012) NKL homeobox genes in leukemia. Leukemia 26(4):572–581

Horsburgh S, Robson-Ansley P, Adams R et al (2015) Exercise and inflammation-related epigenetic modifications: focus on DNA methylation. Exerc Immunol Rev 21:26–41

Husain AN, Colby T, Ordonez N et al (2013) Guidelines for pathologic diagnosis of malignant mesothelioma: 2012 update of the consensus statement from the International Mesothelioma Interest Group. Arch Pathol Lab Med 137:647–667

IARC (2012). 501 pp Arsenic Metals, fibres and dusts: a review of human carcinogens. In: IARC working group on the evaluation of carcinogenic risks to humans. International Agency for Research on Cancer, Lyon

Janssen YM, Heintz NH, Mossman BT (1995) Induction of c-fos and c-jun proto-oncogene expression by asbestos is ameliorated by N-acetyl-L-cysteine in mesothelial cells. Cancer Res 55:2085–2089

Jaurand MC, Jean D (2016) Biomolecular pathways and malignant pleural mesothelioma. In: Mineo TC (ed) Malignant pleural mesothelioma: present status and future directions. Bentham Science Publishers, Sharjah, pp 173–196

Jensen CG, Watson M (1999) Inhibition of cytokinesis by asbestos and synthetic fibres. Cell Biol Int 23:829–840

Jensen CG, Jensen LC, Rieder CL et al (1996) Long crocidolite asbestos fibers cause polyploidy by sterically blocking cytokinesis. Carcinogenesis 17:2013–2021

Jones J, Wang H, Karanam B et al (2014) Nuclear localization of Kaiso promotes the poorly differentiated phenotype and EMT in infiltrating ductal carcinomas. Clin Exp Metastasis 31:497–510

Joseph NM, Chen YY, Nasr A et al (2016) Genomic profiling of malignant peritoneal mesothelioma reveals recurrent alterations in epigenetic regulatory genes BAP1, SETD2, and DDX3X. Mod Pathol. doi:10.1038/modpathol.2016.188. [Epub ahead of print]

Kadariya Y, Menges CW, Talarchek J et al (2016) Inflammation-related IL1beta/IL1R signaling promotes the development of asbestos-induced malignant mesothelioma. Cancer Prev Res 9:406–414

Kanteti R, Riehm JJ, Dhanasingh I et al (2016) PI3 kinase pathway and MET inhibition is efficacious in malignant pleural mesothelioma. Sci Rep 6:32992

Kassis ES, Zhao M, Hong JA et al (2006) Depletion of DNA methyltransferase 1 and/or DNA methyltransferase 3b mediates growth arrest and apoptosis in lung and esophageal cancer and malignant pleural mesothelioma cells. J Thorac Cardiovasc Surg 131:298–306

Keung AJ, Khalil AS (2016) Molecular biology. A unifying model of epigenetic regulation. Science 351:661–662

Kim MC, Kim NY, Seo YR et al (2016) An integrated analysis of the genome-wide profiles of DNA methylation and mRNA expression defining the side population of a human malignant mesothelioma cell line. J Cancer 7:1668–1679

Kimura K, Toyooka S, Tsukuda K et al (2008) The aberrant promoter methylation of BMP3b and BMP6 in malignant pleural mesotheliomas. Oncol Rep 20(5):1265–1268

Kobayashi N, Toyooka S, Yanai H et al (2008) Frequent p16 inactivation by homozygous deletion or methylation is associated with a poor prognosis in Japanese patients with pleural mesothelioma. Lung Cancer 62:120–125

Kohno H, Amatya VJ, Takeshima Y et al (2010) Aberrant promoter methylation of WIF-1 and SFRP1, 2, 4 genes in mesothelioma. Oncol Rep 24:423–431

Kouzarides T (2007) Chromatin modifications and their function. Cell 128:693–705

Krismann M, Muller KM, Jaworska M et al (2002) Molecular cytogenetic differences between histological subtypes of malignant mesotheliomas: DNA cytometry and comparative genomic hybridization of 90 cases. J Pathol 197:363–371

Kristensen LS, Nielsen HM, Hansen LL (2009) Epigenetics and cancer treatment. Eur J Pharmacol 625:131–142

Krug LM, Kindler HL, Calvert H et al (2015) Vorinostat in patients with advanced malignant pleural mesothelioma who have progressed on previous chemotherapy (VANTAGE-014): a phase 3, double-blind, randomised, placebo-controlled trial. Lancet Oncol 16:447–456

Krumm A, Barckhausen C, Kucuk P et al (2016) Enhanced histone deacetylase activity in malignant melanoma provokes RAD51 and FANCD2-triggered drug resistance. Cancer Res 76:3067–3077

Kubo T, Toyooka S, Tsukuda K et al (2011) Epigenetic silencing of microRNA-34b/c plays an important role in the pathogenesis of malignant pleural mesothelioma. Clin Cancer Res 17:4965–4974

LaFave LM, Beguelin W, Koche R et al (2015) Loss of BAP1 function leads to EZH2-dependent transformation. Nat Med 21(11):1344–1349

Laszlo V, Hoda MA, Garay T et al (2015) Epigenetic down-regulation of integrin alpha7 increases migratory potential and confers poor prognosis in malignant pleural mesothelioma. J Pathol 237:203–214

Lee AY, He B, You L et al (2004) Expression of the secreted frizzled-related protein gene family is downregulated in human mesothelioma. Oncogene 23:6672–6676

Lippmann M (2014) Toxicological and epidemiological studies on effects of airborne fibers: coherence and public [corrected] health implications. Crit Rev Toxicol 44:643–695

Liu S, Ye D, Guo W et al (2015) G9a is essential for EMT-mediated metastasis and maintenance of cancer stem cell-like characters in head and neck squamous cell carcinoma. Oncotarget 6:6887–6901

Lund EK, Belshaw NJ, Elliott GO et al (2011) Recent advances in understanding the role of diet and obesity in the development of colorectal cancer. Proc Nutr Soc 70:194–204

Manente AG, Valenti D, Pinton G et al (2013) Estrogen receptor beta activation impairs mitochondrial oxidative metabolism and affects malignant mesothelioma cell growth in vitro and in vivo. Oncogenesis 2:e72

Manente AG, Pinton G, Zonca S et al (2015) Intracellular lactate-mediated induction of estrogen receptor beta (ERbeta) in biphasic malignant pleural mesothelioma cells. Oncotarget 6:25121–25134

Manente AG, Pinton G, Zonca S et al (2016) KDM6B histone demethylase is an epigenetic regulator of estrogen receptor beta expression in human pleural mesothelioma. Epigenomics 8:1227–1238

Margueron R, Reinberg D (2011) The Polycomb complex PRC2 and its mark in life. Nature 469:343–349

Martin C, Zhang Y (2005) The diverse functions of histone lysine methylation. Nat Rev Mol Cell Biol 6:838–849

Menges CW, Chen Y, Mossman BT et al (2010) A phosphotyrosine proteomic screen identifies multiple tyrosine kinase signaling pathways aberrantly activated in malignant mesothelioma. Genes Cancer 1:493–505

Menges CW, Kadariya Y, Altomare D et al (2014) Tumor suppressor alterations cooperate to drive aggressive mesotheliomas with enriched cancer stem cells via a p53-miR-34a-c-Met axis. Cancer Res 74:1261–1271

Miller JM, Thompson JK, MacPherson MB et al (2014) Curcumin: a double hit on malignant mesothelioma. Cancer Prev Res 7:330–340

Mizuguchi Y, Specht S, Lunz JG 3rd et al (2012) Cooperation of p300 and PCAF in the control of microRNA 200c/141 transcription and epithelial characteristics. PLoS One 7:e32449

Mossman BT, Eastman A, Landesman JM et al (1983) Effects of crocidolite and chrysotile asbestos on cellular uptake and metabolism of benzo(a)pyrene in hamster tracheal epithelial cells. Environ Health Perspect 51:331–335

Mossman BT, Shukla A, Heintz NH et al (2013) New insights into understanding the mechanisms, pathogenesis, and management of malignant mesotheliomas. Am J Pathol 182:1065–1077

Murthy SS, Testa JR (1999) Asbestos, chromosomal deletions, and tumor suppressor gene alterations in human malignant mesothelioma. J Cell Physiol 180:150–157

Murthy SS, Shen T, De Rienzo A et al (2000) Expression of GPC3, an X-linked recessive overgrowth gene, is silenced in malignant mesothelioma. Oncogene 19:410–416

Nelson HH, Almquist LM, LaRocca JL et al (2011) The relationship between tumor MSLN methylation and serum mesothelin (SMRP) in mesothelioma. Epigenetics 6:1029–1034

Newick K, Cunniff B, Preston K et al (2012) Peroxiredoxin 3 is a redox-dependent target of thiostrepton in malignant mesothelioma cells. PLoS One 7:e39404

Okano M, Bell DW, Haber DA et al (1999) DNA methyltransferases Dnmt3a and Dnmt3b are essential for de novo methylation and mammalian development. Cell 99:247–257

Opitz I, Soltermann A, Abaecherli M et al (2008) PTEN expression is a strong predictor of survival in mesothelioma patients. Eur J Cardiothorac Surg 33:502–506

Pache JC, Janssen YM, Walsh ES et al (1998) Increased epidermal growth factor-receptor protein in a human mesothelial cell line in response to long asbestos fibers. Am J Pathol 152:333–340

Peden DB (2011) The role of oxidative stress and innate immunity in O(3) and endotoxin-induced human allergic airway disease. Immunol Rev 242:91–105

Pinato DJ, Mauri FA, Ramakrishnan R et al (2012) Inflammation-based prognostic indices in malignant pleural mesothelioma. J Thorac Oncol 7:587–594

Pinton G, Brunelli E, Murer B et al (2009) Estrogen receptor-beta affects the prognosis of human malignant mesothelioma. Cancer Res 69:4598–4604

Ramos-Nino ME, Timblin CR, Mossman BT (2002) Mesothelial cell transformation requires increased AP-1 binding activity and ERK-dependent Fra-1 expression. Cancer Res 62:6065–6069

Ramos-Nino ME, Vianale G, Sabo-Attwood T et al (2005) Human mesothelioma cells exhibit tumor cell-specific differences in phosphatidylinositol 3-kinase/AKT activity that predict the efficacy of Onconase. Mol Cancer Ther 4:835–842

Reid G (2015) MicroRNAs in mesothelioma: from tumour suppressors and biomarkers to therapeutic targets. J Thorac Dis 7:1031–1040

Reid G, Kao SC, Pavlakis N et al (2016) Clinical development of TargomiRs, a miRNA mimic-based treatment for patients with recurrent thoracic cancer. Epigenomics 8:1079–1085

Roggli VL (2015) The so-called short-fiber controversy: literature review and critical analysis. Arch Pathol Lab Med 139:1052–1057

Sacco JJ, Kenyani J, Butt Z et al (2015) Loss of the deubiquitylase BAP1 alters class I histone deacetylase expression and sensitivity of mesothelioma cells to HDAC inhibitors. Oncotarget 6:13757–13771

Sandoval J, Esteller M (2012) Cancer epigenomics: beyond genomics. Curr Opin Genet Dev 22:50–55

Sansom OJ, Maddison K, Clarke AR (2007) Mechanisms of disease: methyl-binding domain proteins as potential therapeutic targets in cancer. Nat Clin Pract Oncol 4:305–315

Sayan M, Mossman BT (2016) The NLRP3 inflammasome in pathogenic particle and fibre-associated lung inflammation and diseases. Part Fibre Toxicol 13:51

Schmitz SU, Grote P, Herrmann BG (2016) Mechanisms of long noncoding RNA function in development and disease. Cell Mol Life Sci 73:2491–2509

Sekido Y (2010) Genomic abnormalities and signal transduction dysregulation in malignant mesothelioma cells. Cancer Sci 101:1–6

Shah P, Gau Y, Sabnis G (2014) Histone deacetylase inhibitor entinostat reverses epithelial to mesenchymal transition of breast cancer cells by reversing the repression of E-cadherin. Breast Cancer Res Treat 143:99–111

Shelby MD (1988) The genetic toxicity of human carcinogens and its implications. Mutat Res 204:3–15

Shi Y, Whetstine JR (2007) Dynamic regulation of histone lysine methylation by demethylases. Mol Cell 25:1–14

Shukla A, Jung M, Stern M et al (2003a) Asbestos induces mitochondrial DNA damage and dysfunction linked to the development of apoptosis. Am J Physiol Lung Cell Mol Physiol 285:L1018–L1025

Shukla A, Gulumian M, Hei TK et al (2003b) Multiple roles of oxidants in the pathogenesis of asbestos-induced diseases. Free Radic Biol Med 34:1117–1129

Shukla A, Hillegass JM, MacPherson MB et al (2010) Blocking of ERK1 and ERK2 sensitizes human mesothelioma cells to doxorubicin. Mol Cancer 9:314

Shukla A, Hillegass JM, MacPherson MB et al (2011) ERK2 is essential for the growth of human epithelioid malignant mesotheliomas. Int J Cancer 129:1075–1086

Srivastava RK, Kurzrock R, Shankar S (2010) MS-275 sensitizes TRAIL-resistant breast cancer cells, inhibits angiogenesis and metastasis, and reverses epithelial-mesenchymal transition in vivo. Mol Cancer Ther 9:3254–3266

Stapelberg M, Gellert N, Swettenham E et al (2005) Alpha-tocopheryl succinate inhibits malignant mesothelioma by disrupting the fibroblast growth factor autocrine loop: mechanism and the role of oxidative stress. J Biol Chem 280:25369–25376

Sterner DE, Berger SL (2000) Acetylation of histones and transcription-related factors. Microbiol Mol Biol Rev 64:435–459

Sugarbaker DJ, Richards WG, Gordon GJ et al (2008) Transcriptome sequencing of malignant pleural mesothelioma tumors. Proc Natl Acad Sci U S A 105:3521–3526

Sun L, Fang J (2016) Epigenetic regulation of epithelial-mesenchymal transition. Cell Mol Life Sci 73:4493–4515

Tabata C, Terada T, Tabata R et al (2013) Serum thioredoxin-1 as a diagnostic marker for malignant peritoneal mesothelioma. J Clin Gastroenterol 47:e7–e11

Takai N, Desmond JC, Kumagai T et al (2004) Histone deacetylase inhibitors have a profound antigrowth activity in endometrial cancer cells. Clin Cancer Res 10:1141–1149

Tam WL, Weinberg RA (2013) The epigenetics of epithelial-mesenchymal plasticity in cancer. Nat Med 19:1438–1449

Taniguchi T, Karnan S, Fukui T et al (2007) Genomic profiling of malignant pleural mesothelioma with array-based comparative genomic hybridization shows frequent non-random chromosomal alteration regions including JUN amplification on 1p32. Cancer Sci 98:438–446

Testa JR, Cheung M, Pei J et al (2011) Germline BAP1 mutations predispose to malignant mesothelioma. Nat Genet 43:1022–1025

Toyooka S, Pass HI, Shivapurkar N et al (2001) Aberrant methylation and simian virus 40 tag sequences in malignant mesothelioma. Cancer Res 61:5727–5730

Tsou JA, Shen LY, Siegmund KD et al (2005) Distinct DNA methylation profiles in malignant mesothelioma, lung adenocarcinoma, and non-tumor lung. Lung Cancer 47:193–204

Tsou JA, Galler JS, Wali A et al (2007) DNA methylation profile of 28 potential marker loci in malignant mesothelioma. Lung Cancer 58:220–230

Vandermeers F, Neelature Sriramareddy S, Costa C et al (2013) The role of epigenetics in malignant pleural mesothelioma. Lung Cancer 81:311–318

Varesano S, Salvi S, Boccardo S et al (2016) MET gene status in malignant mesothelioma using fluorescent in situ hybridization. J Thorac Oncol 11:e28–e30

Vento-Tormo R, Alvarez-Errico D, Garcia-Gomez A et al (2017) DNA demethylation of inflammasome-associated genes is enhanced in patients with cryopyrin-associated periodic syndromes. J Allergy Clin Immunol 139(1):202–211.e6

Vrba L, Jensen TJ, Garbe JC et al (2010) Role for DNA methylation in the regulation of miR-200c and miR-141 expression in normal and cancer cells. PLoS One 5:e8697

Wang H, Gillis A, Zhao C et al (2011) Crocidolite asbestos-induced signal pathway dysregulation in mesothelial cells. Mutat Res 723:171–176

Wang H, Liu W, Black S et al (2016) Kaiso, a transcriptional repressor, promotes cell migration and invasion of prostate cancer cells through regulation of miR-31 expression. Oncotarget 7:5677–5689

West AC, Johnstone RW (2014) New and emerging HDAC inhibitors for cancer treatment. J Clin Invest 124:30–39

Williams GM (1979) Review of in vitro test systems using DNA damage and repair for screening of chemical carcinogens. J Assoc Off Anal Chem 62:857–863

Wilson SM, Barbone D, Yang TM et al (2008) mTOR mediates survival signals in malignant mesothelioma grown as tumor fragment spheroids. Am J Respir Cell Mol Biol 39:576–583

Wu Y, Antony S, Meitzler JL et al (2014) Molecular mechanisms underlying chronic inflammation-associated cancers. Cancer Lett 345:164–173

Xiao GH, Gallagher R, Shetler J et al (2005) The NF2 tumor suppressor gene product, merlin, inhibits cell proliferation and cell cycle progression by repressing cyclin D1 expression. Mol Cell Biol 25:2384–2394

Ye Y, Xiao Y, Wang W et al (2010) ERalpha signaling through slug regulates E-cadherin and EMT. Oncogene 29:1451–1462

Yegles M, Saint-Etienne L, Renier A et al (1993) Induction of metaphase and anaphase/telophase abnormalities by asbestos fibers in rat pleural mesothelial cells in vitro. Am J Respir Cell Mol Biol 9:186–191

Yu H, Simons DL, Segall I et al (2012) PRC2/EED-EZH2 complex is up-regulated in breast cancer lymph node metastasis compared to primary tumor and correlates with tumor proliferation in situ. PLoS One 7:e51239

Yuan Z, Taatjes DJ, Mossman BT et al (2004) The duration of nuclear extracellular signal-regulated kinase 1 and 2 signaling during cell cycle reentry distinguishes proliferation from apoptosis in response to asbestos. Cancer Res 64:6530–6536

Zanella CL, Posada J, Tritton TR et al (1996) Asbestos causes stimulation of the extracellular signal-regulated kinase 1 mitogen-activated protein kinase cascade after phosphorylation of the epidermal growth factor receptor. Cancer Res 56:5334–5338

Zhang W, Dahlberg JE, Tam W (2007) MicroRNAs in tumorigenesis: a primer. Am J Pathol 171:728–738

Zhang X, Tang N, Rishi AK et al (2015) Methylation profile landscape in mesothelioma: possible implications in early detection, disease progression, and therapeutic options. Methods Mol Biol 1238:235–247

Chapter 11
3D Models of Mesothelioma in the Study of Mechanisms of Cell Survival

V. Courtney Broaddus, Carlo Follo, and Dario Barbone

Abstract Three-dimensional models can provide another experimental system for investigating many aspects of tumor biology, particularly of cell death and survival. These models, both in vitro and ex vivo, may be ideally suited for studying mesothelioma. Here we discuss the reports that are currently available on this subject and highlight areas in which 3D biology may provide insights into the mechanisms of cell death and survival in mesothelioma. It has long been known that single cells or monolayers are more sensitive to cell death than 3D aggregates or spheroids, which acquire resistance called "multicellular resistance." Possible survival mechanisms that have been studied using multicellular spheroids (in vitro) and tumor fragment spheroids (ex vivo) include growth factor pathways, calcium-dependent cell-cell adhesion, resistance to drug penetrance, gene expression, epigenetics, Bcl-2 antiapoptotic family expression, and autophagy. In general, cells in a 3D setting show many differences compared to the same cells in a 2D monolayer. Many of these differences appear to contribute to cell survival. In many cases, these features can be shown to be more similar to those in the actual tumor. Thus, whereas 3D studies offer more challenges for study, they offer the opportunity for new insights not possible in 2D studies. They may thus offer an intermediate model between the monolayer and in vivo studies and hopefully lead to discoveries that can be tested in clinical trials to benefit patients.

Keywords Mesothelioma • Chemoresistance • Aggregates • Spheroid • Matrix • Apoptosis • Autophagy • Epigenetics • Vorinostat

V. Courtney Broaddus (✉) • C. Follo • D. Barbone
Division of Pulmonary and Critical Care Medicine, Zuckerberg San Francisco General Hospital and Trauma Center, San Francisco, CA 94110-3518, USA
e-mail: Courtney.broaddus@ucsf.edu

© Springer International Publishing AG 2017
J.R. Testa (ed.), *Asbestos and Mesothelioma*, Current Cancer Research,
DOI 10.1007/978-3-319-53560-9_11

11.1   Introduction

Mesothelioma is currently incurable, thought to be due to its resistance to cell death. Mesothelioma is highly resistant to single agents, with less than a 20% response rate (Kindler 2008). With a two-chemotherapeutic regimen consisting of cisplatin plus pemetrexed, mesothelioma has a 41% response and patients can have an increased lifespan (from 9 to 12 months) (Vogelzang et al. 2003). Since this landmark study in 2003, there have been many clinical trials but no major breakthroughs. Mesothelioma represents a difficult challenge, an intractable tumor without an obvious vulnerability.

There are certain challenges in studying mesothelioma (Kindler 2008). It is difficult to study due to its relatively low frequency (~3000 annually in the USA) compared to other tumors and to its international distribution. Animal models have proved to have value in understanding mesothelioma, especially its genetic predispositions, but the long latency of the process to create the mesothelioma has limited their usefulness. Thus, three-dimensional (3D) models offer another avenue of study. They have many advantages compared to 2D models, especially in the study of mechanisms of cell death (Desoize and Jardillier 2000; Weiswald et al. 2015). In vitro 3D models can be used as a more realistic model of the tumor, and ex vivo 3D models can extend the study of the actual tumor in testing hypotheses worked out in the in vitro 3D setting, in finding biomarkers, and in screening for response to a variety of therapies.

11.2   Spheroids in the Study of Cancer

Multicellular 3D spheroids have been studied in cancer for more than 40 years (Sutherland et al. 1971; Kobayashi et al. 1993). Initially, 3D models were used for radiation studies of cell death because of their hypoxic core, which could represent the hypoxia known to be important in tumors (Leek et al. 2016). Over the subsequent decades, their use has expanded to the study of proliferation, metabolism, gene expression, and antibody and drug penetrance (Weiswald et al. 2015).

One of the theoretical advantages of the spheroid is its resemblance to the avascular region of tumors that lies between capillaries (Minchinton and Tannock 2006). Similar to the spheroid, the tumor that lies between capillaries relies on diffusion for survival. Both nutrients and oxygen must diffuse toward the center. In addition, therapeutic drugs and antibodies will need to diffuse to the center of the avascular regions to reach all the tumor cells. The nutrient and oxygen deficiencies in the interior may activate processes such as heat shock, the unfolded protein response, the hypoxic response, and autophagy that support cell survival. Other advantages of the 3D spheroid are that the cells assume more realistic cell shapes, cell-cell interactions, cell-matrix attachment, and stresses within and upon the cell (Weiswald et al. 2015; Nath and Devi 2016).

From the vantage point of 3D models, the traditional 2D monolayer model can be seen as a more artificial system. Although 2D has remained the standard model, cancer cells grown on plastic are stretched flat; have exposure to uniform and high, non-physiologic concentrations of nutrients and oxygen; and have limited cell-cell attachments. They are in a shape and environment quite different from the same cells in a 3D setting or in a tumor. Given that, it is not surprising that findings often differ between the monolayer and the spheroid.

Disadvantages of the 3D system today include the extra steps necessary to produce them and the different techniques sometimes needed to study them. Another disadvantage can be something of an advantage—namely, that there is less known about the response of cells in 3D and, thus, new and surprising findings can provide insights into tumor biology.

The study of ex vivo tumor as 3D spheroids has been less well accepted and less standardized as a model for investigation, presumably because of the complexity and the lack of availability of fresh tumor. Of course, the advantage to studying human tumor tissue ex vivo is that the model can exhibit the complexity of the actual tumor. The ex vivo tumor contains the variety of cells in the actual tumor, both malignant and nonmalignant. Unlike cell lines, the malignant cells are not clonal but instead represent the heterogeneous malignant cells of the actual tumor, including stem-like cells. The nonmalignant cells include immune and inflammatory cells, which are known to be important components in tumor biology, as well as the fibroblasts, endothelial cells, and other benign tissue cell types. The cell shape and arrangement of the cell types are as in the tumor, and the stroma constituents and structure are present as in the tumor. In the laboratory, the tumor can be studied ex vivo to test hypotheses worked out in the 3D multicellular spheroid model, as well as to test the value of prognostic biomarkers or screen for response to various therapies. The disadvantages of studying ex vivo tumor are also substantial given the complexity of the original tumor. There will be variation among the fragments taken from different parts of the tumor. With all the different cell types present, the identity of the mesothelioma cell or other cell types must be identified and distinguished from others. The study of such ex vivo tumor has challenges, but there is also great promise in studying the "real thing."

11.3   Production of Two Major Types of Spheroids

11.3.1   Multicellular Spheroids (MCS)

Multicellular spheroids (MCS) are most often generated from cancer cell lines. There are several techniques described in the literature including liquid overlay, hanging drop, matrix embedding, microfluidic devices, and spinner flask (Weiswald et al. 2015; Katt et al. 2016; Nath and Devi 2016). Among the various methods, features of the spheroids can be altered. The range of spheroid size, the numbers of spheroids produced, the use of a matrix, and the convenience of recovering the spheroids vary among the different methods. Interestingly, most mesothelioma studies including those from our laboratory use the liquid overlay method.

Spheroids can also be allowed to form spontaneously from cells plated on nonadherent surfaces and are thought to arise from single cells that have stem-like properties (Pastrana et al. 2011). Several groups have studied the factors that influence spheroid formation, e.g., spheroid formation has been shown to be associated with mesothelioma cell expression of CD9+ and CD24+ (Ghani et al. 2011), mTOR signaling (Hoda et al. 2011), mesothelioma (peritoneal) expression of stem cell markers (Myc, NES, and VEGFR2) (Varghese et al. 2012), cisplatin resistance (Cortes-Dericks et al. 2014), mesothelin expression (Melaiu et al. 2014), HGF (Deng et al. 2015), NF-κB (Nishikawa et al. 2014), c-Met (Menges et al. 2014), FGF (Schelch et al. 2014), Src family kinases (Eguchi et al. 2015), or aquaporin 1 (Jagirdar et al. 2016) and to be inhibited by mesenchymal stem cell-conditioned medium (Cortes-Dericks et al. 2016). A few of these groups have also studied the characteristics of the spheroids formed from the putative cancer stem cells (Stapelberg et al. 2005; Eguchi et al. 2015; Pasdar et al. 2015). One of the potential limitations of many of these studies is the difficulty of distinguishing spheres formed from a single cell, and therefore clonal, from those formed by aggregation of cells brought together by their migration or by external motion (Pastrana et al. 2011). Thus, spontaneously forming spheroids may not necessarily be clonal unless grown from a single cell per well and thus may be similar in makeup and behavior to spheroids generated in vitro. If so, the formation of the spheroid may represent the ability of single cells to move and aggregate and not the ability of stem cells to proliferate. Although spheroid formation studies have great potential interest for understanding mesothelioma, we will not consider this interesting field further here. Instead, the focus of this chapter will be on the behavior of 3D spheroids and thus will consider only studies in which the behavior (not the formation) of spheroids is studied.

In our laboratory, to generate 3D multicellular spheroids, we use the liquid overlay method, in which cells are added to nonadherent wells, lightly centrifuged to bring them into contact, and allowed to form into a spheroid. We consider a spheroid to be a stable multicellular structure that maintains its shape and can be pipetted into other wells. Mesothelioma cells appear to form spheroids readily in 24 h or sooner.

The numbers of cells in a spheroid can be adjusted for the purposes of the study. In our hands, to avoid cell death at baseline, we have studied baseline apoptosis over a range of spheroid sizes, from 1000 to 50,000 cells/spheroid (Barbone et al. 2008). In three different cell lines, 10,000 cells/spheroid was the largest size that did not show spontaneous cleavage of caspase-3 and was thus chosen as the standard spheroid size. However, when questions of drug penetrance arise, one can generate extremely small spheroids, called microspheroids, created from as few as 200–400 cells per spheroid. These are produced by allowing cells to settle from a suspension onto impressions in a mold (Napolitano et al. 2007; Barbone et al. 2008). If multicellular resistance persists in such small spheroids, drug penetrance is unlikely to explain the resistance.

MCS lend themselves to many variations. Cells can be grown with different matrix proteins or on matrix supports. Cells can be combined with other cells, such as macrophages or fibroblasts, to make heterospheroids or hybrid spheroids (Fig. 11.1). Spheroids of one cancer cell line can also be placed adjacent to other spheroids to test the invasiveness of the cancer cells into the other structure.

Fig. 11.1 Hybrid spheroid generated from a human mesothelioma cell line grown with human macrophages. This hybrid spheroid was formed by culturing 10,000 mesothelioma cells and 500 macrophages together in 96-well nonadherent wells. Confocal fluorescent microscopic image of the whole spheroid demonstrates mesothelioma cells (cytokeratin, *green*) and the macrophages (CD68, *red*). Staining of different cell types shows that the macrophages are well distributed throughout the structure. (Photograph by Nikita Kolhatkar, PhD)

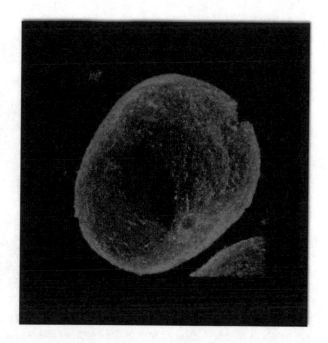

11.3.2   Tumor Fragment Spheroids

Tumor fragment spheroids (TFS) or explants are models by which tumor can be studied in a 3D setting ex vivo. We have chosen to study TFS in order to mimic the MCS in shape and size. In developing this model for mesothelioma, the tumor, obtained from the operating room after resection and either used fresh or after shipping overnight in transport media, is minced using scalpels under the cell culture hood. These TFS can be studied for months with viable mesothelioma cells (Kim et al. 2005). In addition, the TFS can be shown to include other cell types, such as macrophages (Fig. 11.2). Usually, we have studied mesothelioma TFS after culturing for 7–14 days, when they become rounded, indicating that they are viable (Kim et al. 2005). More recent studies of TFS grown from other tumors suggest that they may be studied in 2–3 days (Lao et al. 2015).

11.4   Spheroids for the Study of Cell Death

One characteristic that has been observed in many different tumors is that when cancer cells aggregate into spheroids, they acquire an increased resistance to cell death. The additional resistance has been termed "multicellular resistance" (Kobayashi et al. 1993). From early observations, particularly in the setting of radiation biology, it was proposed that the heterogeneity of the spheroid, in which portions were hypoxic, and cell-cell and cell-matrix connections might provide

Fig. 11.2 A two-week-old tumor fragment spheroid grown from human mesothelioma tumor showing macrophages (CD68, *brown*) interspersed with mesothelioma cells (cytokeratin, *pink*). In this ex vivo model of human mesothelioma, the macrophages are numerous and located adjacent to the mesothelioma cells. (Photograph by Ki Up Kim, MD)

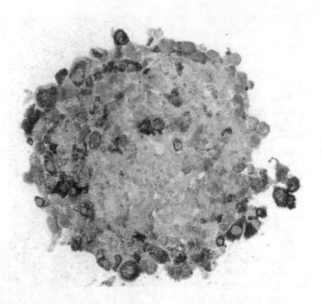

multicellular resistance (West and Sutherland 1987; Dubessy et al. 2000). Although penetration of drugs might account for some of the resistance to chemotherapeutic agents, a limitation of penetration could not explain resistance to radiation.

Cell survival within spheroids may underlie the metastatic potential of circulating tumor cell clusters, aggregates of cells in the bloodstream of cancer patients that appear to mediate metastasis. Circulating tumor cell clusters have been shown to have a much greater likelihood of producing a metastasis than single cells (Aceto et al. 2014). The clusters have been found to form at the site of the tumor and to contain polyclonal cells (Aceto et al. 2014; Cheung and Ewald 2016), reminiscent of the formation of multicellular spheroids. These structures are likely to provide a means of greater tumor cell survival in the bloodstream and in the distant tissue. Indeed, circulating tumor cells have been described in mesothelioma (Bobek et al. 2014; Yoneda et al. 2014; Raphael et al. 2015), but at this time no clusters have been reported.

11.5   Spheroids in Mesothelioma

Three-dimensional spheroid models may be particularly relevant to the study of mesothelioma. In fact, human mesothelioma is known to produce aggregates in the pleural fluid, a finding that was once used as a helpful clue in the discrimination of mesothelioma from adenocarcinoma (Whitaker 1977). In animal models of mesothelioma, tumor spheroids have also been observed. In a study of asbestos-induced peritoneal mesothelioma in rats, spheroids were described and noted to be similar to the spheroids described in human mesothelioma (Craighead et al. 1987). In a study of mouse peritoneal mesothelioma, tumor spheroids were found to contain tumor-associated macrophages, as did the tumor itself (Miselis et al. 2008). In a later study, it was noted that the spheroids appeared in the ascites before and after the tumor was established, suggesting that they may have played a role in the attachment and intraperitoneal spread of the tumor (Miselis et al. 2011). The spheroids contained tumor-associated macrophages, as did the tumor itself, and could induce tumors after transplantation. In another mouse mesothelioma study (Menges et al. 2014), tumor spheroids were found in the malignant ascites and thought to promote metastasis within the peritoneal cavity.

In fact, in a similar body cavity tumor, ovarian carcinoma, such spheroids have been described and found to exhibit resistance to chemotherapeutic drugs. They have been studied for a possible role in dissemination of tumor and implantation throughout the peritoneal space (Shield et al. 2009). It has been proposed that such spheroids form by aggregation of single cells in the peritoneal fluid, although spheroids have been shown to form spontaneously from monolayers and to acquire a resistance to cisplatin and paclitaxel that was reversed by dissociating the spheroids (Pease et al. 2012). Indeed, targeting ovarian cancer spheroids has become a focus of interest in the effort to control ovarian cancer (Shield et al. 2009).

It is also easy to produce spheroids from mesothelioma cell lines. In our experience, every mesothelioma cell line has readily formed spheroids within 24 h. Perhaps the ease of formation is a consequence of the cell-matrix adhesions and the ability of the mesothelioma to produce its own matrix. In our hands, normal mesothelial cells, which are known to produce matrix proteins (Kim et al. 2005), form spheroids in the same fashion. Indeed, we prefer to use spheroids without use of additional matrix, which appears to be unnecessary because the spheroids generate

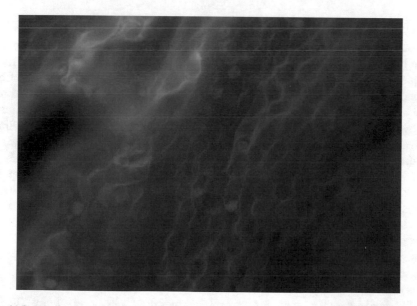

Fig. 11.3 Matrix of a multicellular spheroid. In this Hoechst 33342-stained section, the structure of a multicellular spheroid is seen supporting cells remaining after a short period of disaggregation with trypsin. The extensive matrix structure was generated by the cells themselves within 24 h in 3D. (Photograph by Dario Barbone, PhD)

their own (Fig. 11.3). When we attempted to produce spheroids from other cancers, including lung cancer cell lines, some of the cell lines failed to form intact spheroids within 24 h. Thus, we propose that mesothelioma, a tumor that produces spheroids in vivo and readily forms spheroids in vitro, may spread via spheroids in the pleural space and may be properly studied using 3D spheroid models.

Use of tumor fragment spheroids was possible in mesothelioma because tumor was available from surgical resection. Interestingly, efforts to generate TFS from lung cancer were largely unsuccessful because there was not enough tumor available after surgical resection (Fjellbirkeland et al. 1995). Early on, we attempted to grow cells from mesothelioma tumor, following disaggregation and growth on plastic or on matrix-coated plates. Although cells would attach and spread, the cancer cells would not continue to grow. Instead, we found that cells in the TFS remained alive for weeks and months and even demonstrated that they could proliferate (Kim et al. 2005). Thus, we concluded that tumor cells within the TFS were sustained by the matrix, the adjacent malignant cells, and perhaps the nonmalignant cells within the spheroid.

Certainly, the normal pleural mesothelium may best be modeled using a two-dimensional monolayer. However, when malignant pleural mesothelioma begins to form and becomes a solid tumor, we propose that the three-dimensional spheroid becomes a more relevant model.

11.6 Techniques for Studying Spheroids

Producing spheroids and studying them adds some challenges when compared to investigating monolayers. Even straightforward techniques may not directly translate from the monolayer to the spheroid. For example, annexin V staining, a technique we had found quite useful for studying apoptosis in cells disaggregated from monolayers, was not accurate in the cells disaggregated from spheroids (Barbone et al. 2008). The binding of annexin V was excessive and provided falsely high readings. Instead we have had to rely on nuclear morphology (a gold standard but time-consuming to quantitate), immunoblotting for caspase-3 or PARP cleavage, or fluorescent detection of cleaved caspase-3. In addition, measuring apoptosis in tumor fragment spheroids is complicated by the heterogeneity of the cell populations, necessitating a dual staining technique whereby the mesothelioma cells, stained for cytokeratin, can be distinguished from other cells (Kim et al. 2005). However, we found that other techniques worked well in spheroids, such as siRNA knockdown studies (Barbone et al. 2008; Barbone et al. 2011; Barbone et al. 2012; Barbone et al. 2015). RNA interference could be accomplished in the cells grown as monolayers, and the knockdown was maintained over the 24 h needed for the spheroids to form.

Spheroids may be used for screening studies of chemosensitivity (Kunz-Schughart et al. 2004; Friedrich et al. 2009). In mesothelioma, this has been reported on a microfluidic platform using single multicellular spheroids (Ruppen et al. 2014).

11.6.1 Mechanisms of Resistance to Cell Death

11.6.1.1 Survival Pathways

In our original study of mesothelioma spheroids, we investigated the role of the survival pathway PI3K/AKT/mTOR (Barbone et al. 2008). We had found that the AKT pathway contributed to the apoptotic resistance of mesothelioma in the tumor fragment spheroid model (Wilson et al. 2008), and we wished to test the role in the more tractable MCS model. The PI3K/AKT/mTOR pathway was restrained using several inhibitors, which all reduced resistance to TRAIL combination therapies. The common link was the inhibition of mTOR. Compared to the same cells cultured as monolayers, the mesothelioma cells grown in 3D consistently showed a decrease in phosphorylation of mTOR pathway proteins. Thus, it was something of a surprise to find that inhibition of the mTOR pathway decreased multicellular resistance in the spheroids but not in the monolayers. The answer may be that the level of activation of cells within spheroids was still significantly higher than that of normal non-malignant mesothelial cells. Another explanation might be that the activity of mTOR cannot be predicted from the phosphorylation status, at least in 3D.

In another study of spheroids (Daubriac et al. 2009), the focus was on the resistance to apoptosis at baseline, a resistance that counters the usual apoptosis upon detachment, or "anoikis." Similar to our study, the PI3K/AKT, ERK, and SAPK/JNK pathways were all noted to be hypophosphorylated in spheroids. Interestingly, the downregulation of the JNK pathway was found to be important for resisting anoikis. Activating this pathway with anisomycin led to apoptosis.

Finally, in a recent study (Manente et al. 2015), the estrogen receptor was shown to be upregulated in spheroids and in hypoxic mesothelioma cells. The estrogen receptor was upregulated in response to lactate in the hypoxic environment of the spheroid and could be targeted to suppress proliferation. Its role in the chemoresistance of the resting spheroid is not known, although it can be activated to sensitize to chemotherapy and, thus, targeting the estrogen receptor could presumably also target spheroid growth.

Again, the findings in these studies pointed to the differences between the activation and function of various survival pathways in spheroids compared to monolayers. Such differences may give insights into the actual tumor. The parallel use of tumor fragment spheroids can help determine which findings are relevant to the tumor (see section on Tumor Fragment Spheroids below).

11.6.1.2 Apoptotic Bcl-2 Family-Mediated Resistance

In earlier studies from our laboratory in 2D monolayers (Broaddus et al. 2005), a mitochondrial amplification role was found in the synergy between two apoptotic pathways, the death receptor pathway, induced by TRAIL, and the intrinsic pathway, induced by DNA damage or other injuries such as radiotherapy. However, when this combinatorial approach was tried in 3D spheroids, there was an intriguing lack of synergy. It was this evidence of acquired resistance in 3D that originally led us to pursue the mechanisms involved in cell death in 3D spheroids.

When investigated further (Barbone et al. 2011), the Bcl-2 family of proteins was found to have a different expression in spheroids than in monolayers. Interestingly, the striking and very surprising finding was the overexpression of BIM, a *pro*-apoptotic BH3 protein, in the spheroids from four different mesothelioma cell lines. However, it turned out that BIM was sequestered by anti-apoptotic proteins and its effect neutralized. The reason for the resistance was found to be an absence of the upregulation of NOXA, a BH3-only protein that acts to release BIM. Indeed, without NOXA, BIM could be released by a NOXA-like compound, ABT-737, which was developed to release BIM from its binding to the anti-apoptotic proteins, Bcl-2, Bcl-xL, and Bcl-w.

Thus, the spheroids, although *resistant* to chemotherapy and death, were also *primed* for death by a targeted approach to release BIM. The priming was confirmed by studying the cells disaggregated from monolayers and from spheroids; compared to cells from monolayers, the cells from spheroids showed sensitivity to agents (BAD, HRK, and ABT-737) that act by releasing BIM. This priming meant that, whereas spheroids were more resistant to single or combination apoptotic approaches than monolayers, the spheroids were *sensitive* to ABT-737 while the monolayers were not. Despite their protective armor of apoptotic resistance, the spheroids had developed a chink that could be capitalized upon. This finding suggests that understanding the 3D multicellular resistance may reveal vulnerabilities and lead to targeted approaches to therapy.

In parallel studies in tumor fragment spheroids (Barbone et al. 2011), we found that the ABT-737 was also effective at increasing the apoptotic response after chemotherapy but only in those tumors that expressed BIM. In mesotheliomas on a tissue microarray, BIM was found to be elevated in most (69%; 33/48) human mesothelioma tumors studied. We therefore proposed, based on our dual spheroid studies, that BIM could be a useful predictive marker for those mesotheliomas that would be expected to respond to ABT-737 or similar approaches designed to release BIM.

In the study of mesothelioma spheroids by Daubriac et al. (2009), spheroids were found to undergo apoptosis following activation of the JNK pathway, a process mediated by BIM. Presumably, BIM was activated or released from sequestration from its anti-apoptotic Bcl-2 family members.

Unfortunately, ABT-737 has the limiting side effect of thrombocytopenia, a consequence of inhibiting Bcl-xL, which turned out to be an important survival receptor for platelets. Efforts to develop related but safer agents that target only Bcl-2 and Bcl-w are under way, and recent studies in chronic lymphoid leukemia show promise (Cang et al. 2015).

11.6.1.3 Epigenetics

The cause of the lack of upregulation of NOXA was later found to be due to epigenetic regulation and could be restored by vorinostat (SAHA), a histone deacetylase inhibitor (Barbone et al. 2012). In fact, vorinostat has been the single most effective agent that we have found for eliminating spheroid multicellular resistance (Figs. 11.4 and 11.5). Interestingly, by itself, vorinostat had no obvious impact on spheroids. However, together with either bortezomib or cisplatin/pemetrexed, vorinostat was able to restore NOXA upregulation and reverse multicellular resistance of spheroids. Eliminating either NOXA or BIM blocked this effect.

In tumor fragment spheroids, vorinostat had a similar effect (Barbone et al. 2012). Following vorinostat, NOXA staining increased and, together with bortezomib or cisplatin/pemetrexed, vorinostat dramatically increased apoptosis of the tumor cells.

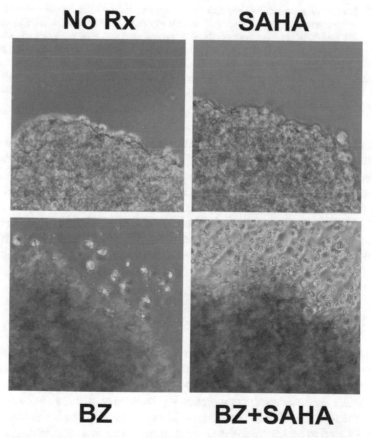

Fig. 11.4 Spheroids seen with phase contrast microscopy following treatment with vorinostat (SAHA). Mesothelioma spheroids are shown following 24 h of exposure to vehicle, vorinostat alone, bortezomib alone, and bortezomib together with vorinostat. The effect of vorinostat by itself is not evident but, when given with bortezomib, the effect is substantial. Cells are seen shedding from the spheroid as it disintegrates. (Photograph by Dario Barbone, PhD)

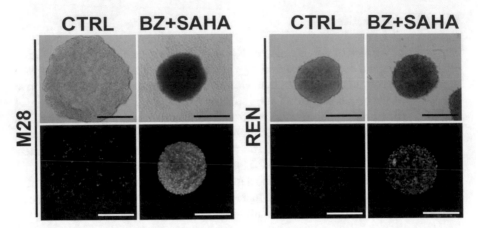

Fig. 11.5 Multicellular spheroids shown in phase contrast (*above*) and in fluorescence micros-copy (*below*) for cleaved caspase-3 after vehicle or the combination of bortezomib and vorinostat (SAHA). M28 and REN mesothelioma cells were grown as MCS. Where indicated, MCS were exposed to 25 nM bortezomib (BZ) in combination with 5 μM of vorinostat (SAHA) for 24 h. The whole MCS were then collected and stained for cleaved caspase-3 (*green*). Microscopic images of representative MCS show the appearance of increased death induced by BZ + SAHA. Spheroids exposed to BZ or to SAHA alone (not shown) were similar to control. Scale bar: 250 μm. (Photograph by Carlo Follo, PhD)

Although other studies in mesothelioma are few, there have been similar studies in spheroids of other tumor types. For example, vorinostat has been shown to enhance apoptosis in clear cell sarcoma spheroids (Liu et al. 2008), and activity of vorinostat was particularly noted in HCT116 colon carcinoma cells in the spheroid setting (Lobjois et al. 2009).

In related work, earlier studies of spheroids identified a role of DNA condensa-tion and chromatin structure in the resistance of spheroids to radiation (Gordon et al. 1990). These studies identified a difference in nuclear morphology, cell shape, and chromatin structure in spheroid cells compared to monolayer cells.

11.6.1.4   Calcium-Dependent Adhesion

Apoptosis can also be seen when cells are removed from their matrix, suffering a loss of contact that leads to an apoptotic death called anoikis. Resistance to anoikis is thought to be an important characteristic that allows for metastasis. In one study that examined this characteristic in mesothelioma (Daubriac et al. 2009), cell-cell contact and, in particular, the calcium-dependent adhesion that allows the formation of spher-oids were found to contribute to the survival of mesothelioma cells. When cells were plated on a nonadherent surface, they spontaneously aggregated into spheroids and demonstrated resistance to spontaneous apoptosis. When cells were incubated with the calcium chelator, EDTA, over 7 days, smaller spheroids formed and the level of apoptosis increased. Thus, the spontaneous aggregation of cells grown in a nonadher-ent setting allowed increased survival. The calcium-dependent binding of cells appears to be critical to the development and maintenance of resistance. It is not known whether the calcium-dependent binding is itself the source of survival or is a necessary step in forming a spheroid that then uses other pathways to become resistant.

Indeed, another study confirmed the resistance to anoikis in mesothelioma spheroids (Eguchi et al. 2015). These investigators attributed the resistance to anoikis and to chemotherapy to the activation of Src family kinases in the spheroids. Inhibition of Src family kinases with dasatinib abrogated the resistance to anoikis and also enhanced the apoptotic response to cisplatin.

11.6.1.5   Drug Penetrance

In another study of mesothelioma spheroids (Xiang et al. 2011), a significant multi-cellular resistance to an antibody conjugated to a toxin was described. After 24 h of exposure to a mesothelin-targeted antibody, all the cells in the monolayer had been killed, whereas only 50% of the cells grown in a spheroid had been killed. The difference in killing was not due to the expression of mesothelin, which was found to be expressed at the same level in both settings. The difference was found to be due to an incomplete penetration into the spheroid of the antibody, which remained limited to the outer surface without further penetration after 4 h of incubation. Investigation of the cell-cell interactions showed an increase in tight junctions and in the tight junction protein, E-cadherin, in spheroids. When expression was reduced, either by siRNA or by an antibody against E-cadherin given before the spheroid formed, the effectiveness of the anti-mesothelin antibody was increased.

In another related study of mesothelioma TFS (Bidlingmaier et al. 2009), a monoclonal single chain variable fragment antibody was able to penetrate the tumor fragments generated from three different human tumors. Thus, drug penetrance may depend on the type of antibody.

Spheroids may also demonstrate *increased* uptake of therapeutic agents. In one study of paclitaxel-loaded expansile nanoparticles (Lei et al. 2015), mesothelioma spheroids of one cell line readily took up the nanoparticles by endocytosis. Although spheroids were not directly compared to monolayers, the authors concluded that the spheroids were better models of the actual tumor, in which these nanoparticles are also avidly internalized.

The issue of penetration is one that must be considered as a cause or a contribution to the increased resistance of cells in spheroids. One can take steps to show that the agent entered the spheroid, as we have also shown for the TRAIL death receptor ligand into mesothelioma spheroids (Barbone et al. 2008); one can also test for the functional effect of the agent (Barbone et al. 2008). For example, in one study of lung cancer spheroids (Yang et al. 2009), it was possible to show that addition of bortezomib inhibited proteasome activity to the same extent in both spheroids and monolayers and that TRAIL cleaved BIM to the same extent, showing that penetration and activity of these agents were not impaired. Thus, resistance to the effect of bortezomib and TRAIL could be attributed to the effects of the spheroid rather than limitations to diffusion. In two studies (Barbone et al. 2008; Yang et al. 2009), we used microspheroids, created using as few as 250 cells, to show that multicellular resistance was similar to that of much larger spheroids and that diffusion was unlikely to explain the observed effect.

11.6.1.6 Gene Expression

The gene expression of spheroids has been compared to that of monolayers in an attempt to find clues to the mechanisms of multicellular resistance. Interestingly, although differences were found in several pathways, no clear smoking gun has been discovered.

In one study (Kim et al. 2012), pathways were found to be altered in a mesothelioma line studied as a spheroid compared to as a monolayer. The most upregulated and downregulated genes (112 upregulated; 30 downregulated) were analyzed for hierarchical clustering and gene ontology. Some of the downregulated genes were involved in apoptosis; otherwise, most genes were involved in membrane-related functions as well as immune function and leukocyte costimulation.

In a study from our laboratory (Barbone et al. 2016), the gene expression of three cell lines was compared when grown as spheroids versus monolayers. For the three lines, a total of 209 genes were differentially expressed (138 upregulated; 71 downregulated). Pathway analysis did not show a clear resistance pathway. When the differentially expressed genes were compared to two publicly available databases of mesothelioma (versus normal tissues), three genes were found to be upregulated in common between the three cell lines grown as spheroids and the 56 mesotheliomas. The three genes were argininosuccinate synthase 1 (ASS1), annexin A4 (ANXA4), and major vault protein (MVP, also known as lung resistance protein). The ASS1 protein was studied further and was found to be expressed by approximately one-half of the mesotheliomas on the tissue microarray. ASS1 expression was also found to contribute to cell survival, because *ASS1* knockdown by siRNA sensitized the spheroids that expressed ASS1 to chemotherapy. The finding of a role for ASS1 is interesting because mesothelioma has been reported to be an ASS1-deficient tumor (Delage et al. 2010; Wangpaichitr et al. 2014).

In other tumors, similar studies comparing gene expression in 3D and 2D are of interest. It has been recognized that gene expression in 3D may be more similar to that of the original tumor (Birgersdotter et al. 2005); yet, it has not been clear whether the gene expression differences underlie the multicellular resistance of the 3D spheroid. In a study of Hodgkin lymphoma, the gene expression of a 3D-cultured cell line was more similar to that of the tumor than the gene expression of the 2D suspension cells (Birgersdotter et al. 2007). In a similar study of glioblastoma, gene expression of the original tumor was compared to that of the cells from that tumor grown as spheroids and as monolayers (Ernst et al. 2009). The gene expression changes in the spheroids resembled those of the primary tumors, whereas the gene expression of the monolayers of cells derived from the same patients did not match well. A contrary view was reported in another study of solid tumors in which the gene expression of spheroids and of confluent monolayers was similar but different from that of the tumor. The authors concluded that the mechanisms of resistance of the spheroids are not likely to be the same as of the intractable (as opposed to more tractable) tumors (Steadman et al. 2008).

It appears that evidence is persuasive that the gene expression of cancer cells in 3D is more similar to that of the original tissue or tumor. Whether confluent monolayers are also similar is still to be determined. However, it may also be true that the gene expression does not determine the chemoresistance of the tumor. As described above, there appears to be more evidence supporting an epigenetic role than a genetic role in the acquired resistance seen in 3D.

11.6.1.7 Autophagy

Autophagy, a program of lysosomal degradation of cellular constituents, is triggered by nutrient insufficiency or stress and may be a means of survival of tumor cells. Much interest exists currently for determining whether inhibition of basal or stimulated autophagy will offer a therapeutic strategy for recalcitrant tumors such as mesothelioma.

Spheroids are logical models for studying autophagy, because they mimic the nutrient deficiency seen in the "avascular component" of a tumor. As of this writing, three studies have addressed this question using spheroids.

In the first study, Echeverry and colleagues (Echeverry et al. 2015) used spheroids to confirm their findings that blocking PI3K/mTOR, which led to an increase in autophagy in the monolayers, could be countered by blocking autophagy with chloroquine. The finding was of particular interest because spheroids are known to down-regulate the phosphorylation/activity of components of the PI3K/AKT pathway.

In the second study (Barbone et al. 2015), multicellular spheroids and tumor fragment spheroids were both studied. A PI3K/mTOR inhibitor was found to be effective in a subset of multicellular spheroids. Interestingly, this subset was not identified by its activation of the PI3K/mTOR pathway but by expression of a key autophagic protein, ATG13, and by a higher level of autophagy. In fact, the same finding was extended to human mesothelioma TFS by finding that the ex vivo tumor fragment spheroids that were responsive to the inhibitor were also the ones that expressed the ATG13 protein. This study suggested that ATG13 might be a better biomarker of sensitivity to PI3K/mTOR inhibition than phosphorylation of PI3K/mTOR pathway members.

In the third study (Follo et al. 2016), monolayers and multicellular spheroids from 6 mesothelioma cell lines, 25 tumor fragment spheroids and their matching formalin-fixed mesothelioma tissue, and, finally, human mesothelioma from 109 patients on a tissue microarray were all studied to learn how autophagy changed from one setting to another. Because autophagy can only be measured in living tissue by the inhibition of the autophagic process, another major goal was to find a marker that could be used in the formalin-fixed tumors and thus discover whether autophagy correlated with patient outcome. In the six mesothelioma cell lines, the autophagy of monolayers and spheroids differed markedly. In three of the cell lines, autophagy was higher in the monolayers than in the spheroids; in the other three lines, autophagy was higher in the spheroids than in the monolayers. For determining whether the monolayer or the spheroid was more representative of tumor biology, various markers were tested, and ATG13 was found to correlate with the autophagy in spheroids; interestingly, ATG13 could not be detected in the monolayers, even in the monolayers with high autophagy. Next, autophagy was measured in the tumor fragment spheroids, living tumor tissue in which the autophagic process could be inhibited and the level measured in the standard fashion, by the accumulation of LC3 (Fig. 11.6). Surprisingly, of the 25 TFS studied, approximately one-half had almost no autophagy, whereas the remainder had high autophagy (see Fig. 11.6). The putative marker of autophagy, ATG13, correlated well with the measured autophagy in the tumor fragment spheroids and also matched the ATG13 found in the original formalin-fixed tumor from which the tumor fragment spheroids were generated. At that point, the autophagic marker ATG13 was tested in the tissue microarray and found to be a robust marker of better outcome, both of survival and of progression-free survival, in patients with mesothelioma.

Presently, an explanation for the relationship between high autophagy and better clinical outcome is not known. However, the conclusions from this study are clear that, at least for the measurement of autophagy and its markers, the spheroid model reflects tumor behavior better than the monolayer. The multicellular spheroids enabled the discovery of the marker, ATG13. The tumor fragment spheroids allowed, for the first time, the measurement of autophagy in living mesothelioma tissue and the confirmation of the value of the marker.

11.7   Conclusions

Spheroids show resistance but also a vulnerability that can perhaps be targeted. They appear to be "addicted" to Bcl-2 anti-apoptotic proteins, because they die when BIM is released with ABT compounds. They respond to certain therapies that are not effective in cells grown in 2D. Phosphorylation of proteins, expression of Bcl-2 proteins, epigenetics, gene expression, and autophagy are each different in cells studied in 2D and in 3D.

However, one might ask, who is to say that the findings in a 3D setting are "better" than those seen in 2D? One way to address this question is to compare findings in the multicellular spheroids to those in the actual ex vivo tumor. Then, they can be compared to the findings in clinical samples. The best example of this is in the autophagy study (Follo et al. 2016), where a marker of autophagy was found in the multicellular spheroids, confirmed in the TFS, and then found to represent an independent marker of mesothelioma patient outcome.

It is best to be cautious about selecting a model. It may be that one model, the 2D monolayer, is better for some studies and that the other, the 3D spheroid, is better for others. The 2D monolayer offers the ultimate in speed, convenience, and scale, whereas 3D spheroid models are more cumbersome and slow, with many experimental techniques and protocols not yet applicable to 3D.

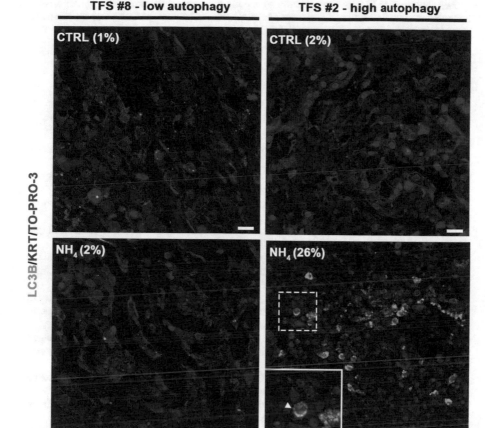

Fig. 11.6 Autophagic flux measured in actual mesothelioma ex vivo. In these tumor fragment spheroids grown from two different human mesotheliomas, autophagy was inhibited by ammonium chloride (NH_4^+) in order to measure the rate of autophagic flux by the accumulation of the autophagic protein LC3. In approximately half of the TFS in this study, few mesothelioma cells had LC3 accumulation after NH_4^+ and thus had low autophagic flux (*left*) and, in approximately half of the TFS, many mesothelioma cells had LC3 accumulation after NH_4^+ and thus had high autophagic flux (*right*). Using ex vivo tumor enabled measurement of autophagic flux for the first time in mesothelioma. Inset in lower right panel represents higher magnification of area circumscribed by dotted box in the same image. Scale bars: 10 μm. (Photograph by Carlo Follo, PhD)

However, we believe that the spheroid model offers mesothelioma researchers the opportunity for novel insights. Particularly, the liquid overlay technique of producing spheroids is straightforward for mesothelioma cells, which appear to adhere to each other with relish and form consistent spheroids in 24 h or less. Thus, we would recommend that spheroids be included in research laboratories as at least a complementary model to monolayers.

Acknowledgments We wish to acknowledge the funding sources that made this work possible, including the Department of Defense, the Mesothelioma Foundation (MARF), and the Simmons Foundation (a private, nonprofit organization founded by the Simmons Law Firm).

References

Aceto N, Bardia A, Miyamoto DT et al (2014) Circulating tumor cell clusters are oligoclonal precursors of breast cancer metastasis. Cell 158:1110–1122

Barbone D, Cheung P, Battula S et al (2012) Vorinostat eliminates multicellular resistance of mesothelioma 3D spheroids via restoration of Noxa expression. PLoS One 7:e52753

Barbone D, Follo C, Echeverry N et al (2015) Autophagy correlates with the therapeutic responsiveness of malignant pleural mesothelioma in 3D models. PLoS One 10:e0134825

Barbone D, Ryan JA, Kolhatkar N et al (2011) The Bcl-2 repertoire of mesothelioma spheroids underlies acquired apoptotic multicellular resistance. Cell Death Dis 2:e174

Barbone D, Van Dam L, Follo C et al (2016) Analysis of gene expression in 3D spheroids highlights a survival role for ASS1 in mesothelioma. PLoS One 11:e0150044

Barbone D, Yang TM, Morgan JR et al (2008) Mammalian target of rapamycin contributes to the acquired apoptotic resistance of human mesothelioma multicellular spheroids. J Biol Chem 283:13021–13030

Bidlingmaier S, He J, Wang Y et al (2009) Identification of MCAM/CD146 as the target antigen of a human monoclonal antibody that recognizes both epithelioid and sarcomatoid types of mesothelioma. Cancer Res 69:1570–1577

Birgersdotter A, Baumforth KR, Porwit A et al (2007) Three-dimensional culturing of the Hodgkin lymphoma cell-line L1236 induces a HL tissue-like gene expression pattern. Leuk Lymphoma 48:2042–2053

Birgersdotter A, Sandberg R, Ernberg I (2005) Gene expression perturbation in vitro--a growing case for three-dimensional (3D) culture systems. Semin Cancer Biol 15:405–412

Bobek V, Kacprzak G, Rzechonek A et al (2014) Detection and cultivation of circulating tumor cells in malignant pleural mesothelioma. Anticancer Res 34:2565–2569

Broaddus VC, Dansen TB, Abayasiriwardana KS et al (2005) Bid mediates apoptotic synergy between TRAIL and DNA damage. J Biol Chem 280:12486–12493

Cang S, Iragavarapu C, Savooji J et al (2015) ABT-199 (venetoclax) and BCL-2 inhibitors in clinical development. J Hematol Oncol 8:129

Cheung KJ, Ewald AJ (2016) A collective route to metastasis: seeding by tumor cell clusters. Science 352:167–169

Cortes-Dericks L, Froment L, Boesch R et al (2014) Cisplatin-resistant cells in malignant pleural mesothelioma cell lines show ALDH(high)CD44(+) phenotype and sphere-forming capacity. BMC Cancer 14:304

Cortes-Dericks L, Froment L, Kocher G et al (2016) Human lung-derived mesenchymal stem cell-conditioned medium exerts in vitro antitumor effects in malignant pleural mesothelioma cell lines. Stem Cell Res Ther 7:25

Craighead JE, Akley NJ, Gould LB et al (1987) Characteristics of tumors and tumor cells cultured from experimental asbestos-induced mesotheliomas in rats. Am J Pathol 129:448–462

Daubriac J, Fleury-Feith J, Kheuang L et al (2009) Malignant pleural mesothelioma cells resist anoikis as quiescent pluricellular aggregates. Cell Death Differ 16:1146–1155

Delage B, Fennell DA, Nicholson L et al (2010) Arginine deprivation and argininosuccinate synthetase expression in the treatment of cancer. Int J Cancer 126:2762–2772

Deng XB, Xiao L, Wu Y et al (2015) Inhibition of mesothelioma cancer stem-like cells with adenovirus-mediated NK4 gene therapy. Int J Cancer 137:481–490

Desoize B, Jardillier J (2000) Multicellular resistance: a paradigm for clinical resistance? Crit Rev Oncol Hematol 36:193–207

Dubessy C, Merlin JM, Marchal C et al (2000) Spheroids in radiobiology and photodynamic therapy. Crit Rev Oncol Hematol 36:179–192

Echeverry N, Ziltener G, Barbone D et al (2015) Inhibition of autophagy sensitizes malignant pleural mesothelioma cells to dual PI3K/mTOR inhibitors. Cell Death Dis 6:e1757

Eguchi R, Fujita Y, Tabata C et al (2015) Inhibition of Src family kinases overcomes anoikis resistance induced by spheroid formation and facilitates cisplatin-induced apoptosis in human mesothelioma cells. Oncol Rep 34:2305–2310

Ernst A, Hofmann S, Ahmadi R et al (2009) Genomic and expression profiling of glioblastoma stem cell-like spheroid cultures identifies novel tumor-relevant genes associated with survival. Clin Cancer Res 15:6541–6550

Fjellbirkeland L, Bjerkvig R, Laerum OD (1995) Tumour fragment spheroids from human non-small-cell lung cancer maintained in organ culture. Virchows Arch 426:169–178

Follo C, Barbone D, Richards WG et al (2016) Autophagy initiation correlates with the autophagic flux in 3D models of mesothelioma and with patient outcome. Autophagy 12:1180–1194

Friedrich J, Seidel C, Ebner R et al (2009) Spheroid-based drug screen: considerations and practical approach. Nat Protoc 4:309–324

Ghani FI, Yamazaki H, Iwata S et al (2011) Identification of cancer stem cell markers in human malignant mesothelioma cells. Biochem Biophys Res Commun 404:735–742

Gordon DJ, Milner AE, Beaney RP et al (1990) The increase in radioresistance of Chinese hamster cells cultured as spheroids is correlated to changes in nuclear morphology. Radiat Res 121:175–179

Hoda MA, Mohamed A, Ghanim B et al (2011) Temsirolimus inhibits malignant pleural mesothelioma growth in vitro and in vivo: synergism with chemotherapy. J Thorac Oncol 6:852–863

Jagirdar RM, Apostolidou E, Molyvdas PA et al (2016) Influence of AQP1 on cell adhesion, migration, and tumor sphere formation in malignant pleural mesothelioma is substratum- and histological-type dependent. Am J Phys Lung Cell Mol Phys 310:L489–L495

Katt ME, Placone AL, Wong AD et al (2016) In vitro tumor models: advantages, disadvantages, variables, and selecting the right platform. Front Bioeng Biotechnol 4:12

Kim H, Phung Y, Ho M (2012) Changes in global gene expression associated with 3D structure of tumors: an ex vivo matrix-free mesothelioma spheroid model. PLoS One 7:e39556

Kim KU, Wilson AD, Abayasiriwardana KS et al (2005) A novel in vitro model of human mesothelioma for studying tumor biology and apoptotic resistance. Am J Respir Cell Mol Biol 33:541–548

Kindler HL (2008) Systemic treatments for mesothelioma: standard and novel. Curr Treat Options in Oncol 9:171–179

Kobayashi H, Man S, Graham CH et al (1993) Acquired multicellular-mediated resistance to alkylating agents in cancer. Proc Natl Acad Sci U S A 90:3294–3298

Kunz-Schughart LA, Freyer JP, Hofstaedter F et al (2004) The use of 3-D cultures for high-throughput screening: the multicellular spheroid model. J Biomol Screen 9:273–285

Lao Z, Kelly CJ, Yang XY et al (2015) Improved methods to generate spheroid cultures from tumor cells, tumor cells & fibroblasts or tumor-fragments: microenvironment, microvesicles and miRNA. PLoS One 10:e0133895

Leek R, Grimes DR, Harris AL et al (2016) Methods: using three-dimensional culture (spheroids) as an in vitro model of tumour hypoxia. Adv Exp Med Biol 899:167–196

Lei H, Hofferberth SC, Liu R et al (2015) Paclitaxel-loaded expansile nanoparticles enhance chemotherapeutic drug delivery in mesothelioma 3-dimensional multicellular spheroids. J Thorac Cardiovasc Surg 149:1417–1424. discussion 1424-1425

Liu S, Cheng H, Kwan W et al (2008) Histone deacetylase inhibitors induce growth arrest, apoptosis, and differentiation in clear cell sarcoma models. Mol Cancer Ther 7:11751–11761

Lobjois V, Frongia C, Jozan S et al (2009) Cell cycle and apoptotic effects of SAHA are regulated by the cellular microenvironment in HCT116 multicellular tumour spheroids. Eur J Cancer 45:2402–2411

Manente AG, Pinton G, Zonca S et al (2015) Intracellular lactate-mediated induction of estrogen receptor beta (ERbeta) in biphasic malignant pleural mesothelioma cells. Oncotarget 6:25121–25134

Melaiu O, Stebbing J, Lombardo Y et al (2014) MSLN gene silencing has an anti-malignant effect on cell lines overexpressing mesothelin deriving from malignant pleural mesothelioma. PLoS One 9:e85935

Menges CW, Kadariya Y, Altomare D et al (2014) Tumor suppressor alterations cooperate to drive aggressive mesotheliomas with enriched cancer stem cells via a p53-miR-34a-c-Met axis. Cancer Res 74:1261–1271

Minchinton AI, Tannock IF (2006) Drug penetration in solid tumours. Nat Rev Cancer 6:583–592

Miselis NR, Wu ZJ, Van Rooijen N et al (2008) Targeting tumor-associated macrophages in an orthotopic murine model of diffuse malignant mesothelioma. Mol Cancer Ther 7:788–799

Miselis NR, Lau BW, Wu Z et al (2011) Kinetics of host cell recruitment during dissemination of diffuse malignant peritoneal mesothelioma. Cancer Microenviron 4:39–50

Napolitano AP, Chai P, Dean DM et al (2007) Dynamics of the self-assembly of complex cellular aggregates on micromolded nonadhesive hydrogels. Tissue Eng 13:2087–2094

Nath S, Devi GR (2016) Three-dimensional culture systems in cancer research: Focus on tumor spheroid model. Pharmacol Ther 163:94–108

Nishikawa S, Tanaka A, Matsuda A et al (2014) A molecular targeting against nuclear factor-kappaB, as a chemotherapeutic approach for human malignant mesothelioma. Cancer Med 3:416–425

Pasdar EA, Smits M, Stapelberg M et al (2015) Characterisation of mesothelioma-initiating cells and their susceptibility to anti-cancer agents. PLoS One 10:e0119549

Pastrana E, Silva-Vargas V, Doetsch F (2011) Eyes wide open: a critical review of sphere-formation as an assay for stem cells. Cell Stem Cell 8:486–498

Pease JC, Brewer M, Tirnauer JS (2012) Spontaneous spheroid budding from monolayers: a potential contribution to ovarian cancer dissemination. Biol Open 1:622–628

Raphael J, Massard C, Gong IY et al (2015) Detection of circulating tumour cells in peripheral blood of patients with malignant pleural mesothelioma. Cancer Biomark 15:151–156

Ruppen J, Cortes-Dericks L, Marconi E et al (2014) A microfluidic platform for chemoresistive testing of multicellular pleural cancer spheroids. Lab Chip 14:1198–1205

Schelch K, Hoda MA, Klikovits T et al (2014) Fibroblast growth factor receptor inhibition is active against mesothelioma and synergizes with radio- and chemotherapy. Am J Respir Crit Care Med 190:763–772

Shield K, Ackland ML, Ahmed N et al (2009) Multicellular spheroids in ovarian cancer metastases: biology and pathology. Gynecol Oncol 113:143–148

Stapelberg M, Gellert N, Swettenham E et al (2005) Alpha-tocopheryl succinate inhibits malignant mesothelioma by disrupting the fibroblast growth factor autocrine loop: mechanism and the role of oxidative stress. J Biol Chem 280:25369–25376

Steadman K, Stein WD, Litman T et al (2008) PolyHEMA spheroids are an inadequate model for the drug resistance of the intractable solid tumors. Cell Cycle 7:818–829

Sutherland RM, McCredie JA, Inch WR (1971) Growth of multicell spheroids in tissue culture as a model of nodular carcinomas. J Natl Cancer Inst 46:113–120

Varghese S, Whipple R, Martin SS et al (2012) Multipotent cancer stem cells derived from human malignant peritoneal mesothelioma promote tumorigenesis. PLoS One 7:e52825

Vogelzang NJ, Rusthoven JJ, Symanowski J et al (2003) Phase III study of pemetrexed in combination with cisplatin versus cisplatin alone in patients with malignant pleural mesothelioma. J Clin Oncol 21:2636–2644

Wangpaichitr M, Wu C, Bigford G et al (2014) Combination of arginine deprivation with TRAIL treatment as a targeted-therapy for mesothelioma. Anticancer Res 34:6991–6999

Weiswald LB, Bellet D, Dangles-Marie V (2015) Spherical cancer models in tumor biology. Neoplasia 17:1–15

West CM, Sutherland RM (1987) The radiation response of a human colon adenocarcinoma grown in monolayer, as spheroids, and in nude mice. Radiat Res 112:105–115

Whitaker D (1977) Cell aggregates in malignant mesothelioma. Acta Cytol 21:236–239

Wilson SM, Barbone D, Yang TM et al (2008) mTOR mediates survival signals in malignant mesothelioma grown as tumor fragment spheroids. Am J Respir Cell Mol Biol 39:576–583

Xiang X, Phung Y, Feng M et al (2011) The development and characterization of a human mesothelioma in vitro 3D model to investigate immunotoxin therapy. PLoS One 6:e14640

Yang TM, Barbone D, Fennell DA et al (2009) Bcl-2 family proteins contribute to apoptotic resistance in lung cancer multicellular spheroids. Am J Respir Cell Mol Biol 41:14–23

Yoneda K, Tanaka F, Kondo N et al (2014) Circulating tumor cells (CTCs) in malignant pleural mesothelioma (MPM). Ann Surg Oncol 21(Suppl 4):S472–S480

Chapter 12
Biomarkers of Response to Asbestos Exposure

Clementina Mesaros, Liwei Weng, and Ian A. Blair

Abstract Asbestos-related diseases (ARDs) resulting from exposure to asbestos include lung cancer and malignant mesothelioma (MM). This has significant health and economic implications that have been well documented. The 20–40-year latency periods of ARDs and their low incidence rates in the general population make preventative strategies and early treatment extremely challenging. The availability of well-validated diagnostic biomarkers of asbestos exposure would greatly facilitate both prevention and early treatment strategies. In this chapter, we have summarized the state of knowledge on biomarkers of response to asbestos exposure and highlighted recent advances, including the discovery of new specific biomarker based on the posttranslational modifications of the high mobility group box 1 (HMGB1) protein. Asbestos is inhaled and trapped primarily in lung tissue and so can only be detected in bronchoalveolar lavage fluid. This makes direct exposure assessments very difficult. In contrast, biomarkers of response, which reflect a change in biologic function in response to asbestos exposure, have proved to be more useful. MM is the major biological response to asbestos that can be readily monitored, and numerous studies have used this disease as confirmation of a prior asbestos exposure. There is some new evidence that an increase in serum nonacetylated HMGB1 can serve as a biological response biomarker of asbestos exposure; whereas acetylated serum HMGB1 is associated with progression to MM. Finally, we discuss the potential merit of combined use of a multiplexed serum lipid biomarker panel with serum protein biomarkers.

Keywords Malignant mesothelioma • Diagnostic • Mesothelin • Osteopontin • Fibulin-3 • High mobility group box 1 • Acetylation • Slow off-rate modified aptamers • Mass spectrometry

C. Mesaros • L. Weng • I.A. Blair (✉)
Penn SRP Center, Center of Excellence in Environmental Toxicology, Department of Systems Pharmacology and Translational Therapeutics, Perelman School of Medicine, University of Pennsylvania, 854 BRB II/III, 421 Curie Boulevard, Philadelphia, PA 19104-6160, USA
e-mail: ianblair@mail.med.upenn.edu

J.R. Testa (ed.), *Asbestos and Mesothelioma*, Current Cancer Research,
DOI 10.1007/978-3-319-53560-9_12

12.1 Biomarkers of Malignant Mesothelioma (MM) and Other Asbestos-Related Diseases (ARDs)

Studies with animal models (Guo et al. 2014; Xu et al. 2014; Kalra et al. 2015) together with genetic (Testa et al. 2011; Carbone et al. 2013; Cheung et al. 2013; Carbone et al. 2015; Ohar et al. 2016) and epidemiological research (Becklake 1976; Lemen et al. 1980; Britton 2002; Stayner et al. 2013; Prazakova et al. 2014) have shown unequivocally that asbestos exposure can lead to ARDs such as MM and lung cancer as well as pulmonary fibrosis. MM is a heterogeneous, aggressive cancer that is mainly observed on the serosal surfaces of the pleura and to a lesser extent in the peritoneum as well as much less commonly in the lining of the testes and pericardium (Montjoy et al. 2009). Surgery can result in long-term benefit for early stage MMs, where there is a better chance that most or all of the cancer can be removed (Lang-Lazdunski 2014). Unfortunately, treatment of later stages of MM is not curative, and so the focus is more on palliative care (Sterman and Albelda 2005). The National Institute for Occupational Safety and Health analysis of the annual cause of death records for 1999–2005 (the most recent years available) revealed that there were 18,068 deaths from MM in the USA, with the number of reported MM deaths increasing from 2482 in 1999 to 2704 in 2005 (Bang et al. 2009). However, the annual death rate was stable at 14.1/million in 1999 and 14.0/million in 2005. Asbestos is still mined in Brazil, Canada, China, Kazakhstan, Russia, and Zimbabwe even though its use is restricted in many Western countries (Frank and Joshi 2014). Therefore, prolonged latency periods from exposure to diagnosis coupled with the ongoing mining and use of asbestos have led to the increasing prevalence of this deadly disease worldwide (Linton et al. 2012; Stayner et al. 2013). Although the occupational exposure to asbestos has declined in the USA through restrictions on its use, there are risks for nonoccupational environmental exposures at old mining sites such as Libby, Montana (Peipins et al. 2003), and old asbestos industrial manufacturing sites such as the BoRit superfund site in Ambler, PA (http://www.boritcag.org).

Early detection of ARDs, when surgical removal of tumors is more successful, provides an attractive therapeutic approach. However, most clinical cases result from exposures that occurred decades earlier (Selikoff et al. 1980; Reid et al. 2014). This means that the discovery and validation of biomarkers of response to asbestos exposure would greatly facilitate the detection of asbestos-exposed individuals prior to the onset of ARDs (Mesaros et al. 2015). This would allow the exposed individuals to be more closely monitored for any sign of disease and allow treatment before progression to inoperable cancer occurs. In addition, biological response biomarker assays conducted in populations living proximal to a site contaminated with asbestos (such as the BoRit site in Ambler) would allow the efficacy of site remediation to be assessed.

12.2 Asbestos Exposure and Biomarkers of Oxidative Stress

There is significant experimental evidence to suggest that oxidative stress is involved in the cellular response to asbestos exposure (Fung et al. 1997; Swain et al. 2004; Schurkes et al. 2004) and in the etiology of asbestos-induced pulmonary fibrosis (Cheresh et al. 2015; Marczynski et al. 2000b). Isoprostanes (Milne et al. 2005) and 8-oxo-2′-deoxyguanosine (dGuo) (Mesaros et al. 2012) are widely used as biomarkers of oxidative stress, although isoprostanes are the only rigorously validated biomarkers of oxidative stress (Kadiiska et al. 2005). Several studies have explored the use of isoprostanes (Pelclova et al. 2008) or 8-oxo-dGuo (Marczynski et al. 2000a; Valavanidis et al. 2009; Hanaoka et al. 1993; Yoshida et al. 2001; Pilger and Rudiger 2006; Chew and Toyokuni 2015) as biomarkers of asbestos exposure. Regrettably, neither of these biomarkers can distinguish asbestos exposure from other causes of oxidative stress such as cigarette smoking (Navarro-Compan et al. 2013; Mesaros et al. 2012; Ellegaard and Poulsen 2016) and atherosclerosis (Victor et al. 2009; Serban and Dragan 2014; Schulze and Lee, 2005; Armstrong et al. 2011; Peluso et al. 2012).

Inhaled asbestos fibers, which are typically longer (typically >5 μm) than they are wide (typically <2 μm diameter) (Boulanger et al. 2014), infiltrate the lung, reach the pleural surface, and are engulfed by phagocytic cells – primarily macrophages (Pooley 1972). It has been suggested that macrophages exposed to asbestos undergo frustrated phagocytosis of the elongated fibers. This process then causes chronic production of reactive oxygen species (ROS), activation of the nuclear factor kappa-light-chain-enhancer of activated B cells (NF-κB) pathway, and cytokine release (Ramos-Nino et al. 2006). DNA damage caused by this ROS production (and subsequent mutagenesis) is one mechanism that could be involved in MM carcinogenesis (Mossman et al. 2013). This could occur through the direct action of ROS on DNA or through ROS-derived lipid peroxide-mediated DNA damage (Blair 2008).

Asbestos is also known to activate the nucleotide-binding oligomerization domain (NOD)-like receptor family, pyrin domain containing 3 (NLRP3) inflammasome, which promotes the release of interleukin (IL)-1β and IL-18 (Hillegass et al. 2013). Only a small proportion of patients who have been exposed to asbestos develop MM. Consequently, the disease is thought to result from an interaction of genetic and environmental factors. For example, cyclin-dependent kinase inhibitor 4a (p16INK4a) and ARF tumor suppressor (p14ARF) genes are frequently inactivated somatically in MMs, and approximately 50% of MM tumors exhibit inactivation of the neurofibromin type 2 gene (*NF2*) due to a combination of somatic nonsense or missense mutations and loss of the remaining wild-type allele (Cheng et al. 1994; Bianchi et al. 1995; Altomare et al. 2011; Sekido 2013; de Assis et al. 2014). In addition, mice with germline heterozygous inactivating mutations of these genes develop MM at an accelerated rate compared to genetically normal littermates when exposed to asbestos through intraperitoneal injections. Moreover, germline and sporadic mutations of the tumor suppressor, breast cancer susceptibility (BRCA)-1 associated protein-1 (BAP1) gene, results in a predisposition for MM (Testa et al. 2011; Carbone et al. 2013; Cheung et al. 2013).

12.3 Biomarkers of Response to Asbestos Exposure

Asbestos fibers are not normally present in urine or plasma but they can appear in bronchoalveolar lavage (BAL) fluid. Quantification of asbestos fibers in BAL provides a qualitative/categorical approach to exposure assessment but has not been useful as a predictive biomarker (Sartorelli et al. 2007). This means that it is necessary to analyze biomarkers of response to asbestos fibers rather than directly quantifying the numbers of fibers. Before being implemented as a diagnostics test in clinical settings, biological response biomarkers must first be fully characterized and validated in large sample sets. Candidate biomarkers of exposure to asbestos often lack diagnostic utility because of poor sensitivity and/or inadequate specificity through confounding exposures or individual variability. Additional problems can arise from bioanalytical issues such as pre-analytic stability, inconsistent sample preparation, inconsistent sample processing, or inadequate technology. This means that robust and reproducible bioanalytical assay methodology is required for accurate and reproducible biomarker analysis. Rigorously validated assays for response biomarkers of exposure to asbestos could serve a critical role in early detection of ARDs and in monitoring novel approaches to treatment.

The major route of exposure to asbestos is thought to be through inhalation although there is now some evidence that asbestos can be transported in water (Wu et al. 2015), so it could potentially also be absorbed orally. Inhaled fibers are transported throughout the respiratory system, penetrate pleural cells in the lining of the lung, and induce oxidative stress as noted above. Proteins involved in the immune response, cell proliferation, and the generation of fibrotic tissue are showing promise as potential biomarkers of asbestos exposure. Other factors likely to impact risk of ARDs include common environmental variables, germline genetic factors (Testa et al. 2011), and differential expression of genes that interact with such variables (Hillegass et al. 2010).

We have reviewed the current status of biomarkers of response of human populations exposed to asbestos. The review is focused primarily on MM biomarkers as this is a disease that arises primarily from asbestos exposure. Validation of the more promising MM biomarkers in larger population studies will facilitate early detection of the disease, improve preventative measures, and help assess the efficacy of novel therapies.

12.4 Mesothelin as a Biomarker of MM

Mesothelin is a 40-kDa glycoprotein, which results from proteolytic cleavage of a 69-kDa mesothelin precursor, and is overexpressed in several types of cancer including MM. The soluble form, soluble mesothelin-related protein (SMRP), sometimes known as soluble mesothelin-related peptide, has emerged as a potential biomarker in serum or urine for the early detection of MM (Creaney et al. 2010a; Creaney et al. 2010b). A number of enzyme-linked immunosorbent assay (ELISA) kits have been developed to analyze SMRP including the MESOMARK serum assay, which is a US Food and Drug Administration (FDA)-approved biomarker for use as an aid in the monitoring of patients with epithelioid and biphasic MM (Table 12.1) (Beyer et al. 2007). A meta-analysis of 30 studies revealed a mean sensitivity of 66% and specificity 97% for SMRP as a serum biomarker of MM when compared with healthy controls (Fig. 12.1) (Cui et al. 2014).

A study conducted in Australia with a sandwich ELISA using two monoclonal antibodies showed increased levels of SMRP in MM patients when compared with healthy controls (Robinson et al. 2003). However, the small sample size did not permit adequate statistical power. A study on the occupational exposure to asbestos in the Czech Republic showed that subjects who had been exposed to asbestos with benign lung disease had higher serum levels of SMRP than normal subjects. Individuals with benign disease had lower serum SMRP levels than subjects with MM (Jakubec et al. 2015). A Turkish biomarker study analyzed serum SMRP in 24 patients with MM from naturally occurring asbestos, 279 subjects with pleural plaques, 123 healthy exposed, and 120 control subjects. This study revealed that serum SMRP had a sensitivity of 63% and specificity of only 74% for detecting the MM patients in this population (Bayram et al. 2014).

Several other studies have found higher levels of serum SMRP in asbestos-exposed individuals than unexposed controls (Pass et al. 2008; Rodriguez Portal et al.

Table 12.1 Response biomarkers of asbestos exposure

Asbestos biomarker	Abbrev	Description	Refrences
Soluble mesothelin-related peptide or soluble mesothelin-related protein	SMRP	Mesothelin and SMRP are 40-kDa glycoproteins from proteolytic cleavage of the 69-kDa mesothelin precursor protein	Robinson et al. (2003)
Osteopontin	None	A 32-kDa integrin-binding protein involved in tumorigenesis, progression, and metastasis	Pass et al. (2005)
Fibulin-3	None	Fibulin-3 is a 57-kDa protein that belongs to a family of extracellular proteins expressed in the basement membranes of blood vessels	Pass et al. (2012)
Nonacetylated high mobility group box 1	HMGB1	HMGB1 is a 30-kDa chromatin protein. The unmodified protein has a nuclear location	Tabata et al. (2013a)
Acetylated high mobility group box 1	Acetylated HMGB1	Lysine hyperacetylation within two nuclear localization signals (Fig. 12.4) causes translocation of HMGB1 into the cytosol	Napolitano et al. (2016)
Proteomic biomarkers	None	A panel of 13 high abundance serum proteins identified by Slow Off-rate Modified Aptamer (SOMAmer) technology	Ostroff et al. (2012)

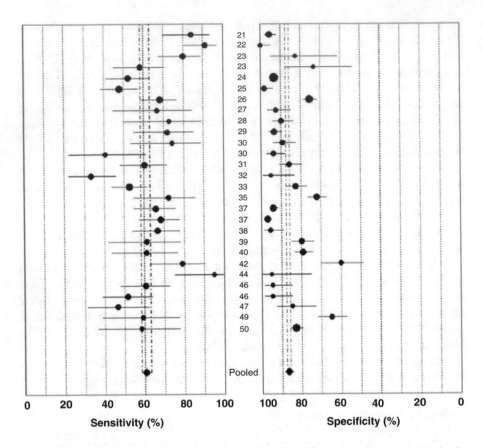

Fig. 12.1 Forest plots of estimates of sensitivity and specificity for soluble mesothelin family proteins in serum for diagnosing malignant pleural mesothelioma. The point estimates of sensitivity and specificity from each study are shown as solid circles. Error bars are 95% CIs. Numbers indicate the reference numbers of studies cited in the original reference list. Modified with permission from Cui et al. (2014)

2009; Marini et al. 2011). One of these studies (Marini et al. 2011) also examined the correlation between mesothelin (SMRP) levels and frequency of micronuclei in blood. A statistically significant positive correlation of the SMRP levels with the frequency of mononuclei in the mononucleated lymphocytes was observed.

Another Australian study measured serum SMRP in a cohort of 514 asbestos-exposed subjects in which the severity of ARDs was assessed separately (Park et al. 2012). The serum SMRP level in the population with compensable ARDs was positively associated with disability assessment. Conversely, the mean SMRP level in healthy asbestos-exposed subjects was significantly lower than those with pleural plaques and in subjects with ARDs who received compensation. The authors concluded that serum SMRP levels correlated with the severity of compensable ARDs and that serum SMRP could potentially be applied to monitor the progress of ARDs.

One known potential problem apart from the variable sensitivity and specificity of serum SMRP assays (de Assis et al. 2014) is the increased expression of SMRP in ovarian cancer (Wu et al. 2014). Additional confounding issues include the effects of sample storage, body mass index, glomerular filtration rate, age, and smoking status (Park et al. 2010).

12.5 Osteopontin as a Biomarker of MM

Osteopontin is a 32-kDa protein that is encoded by the *SPP1* gene (secreted phosphoprotein 1) in humans (Table 12.1). It is an integrin-binding glycoprotein involved in tumorigenesis, progression, and metastasis that is overexpressed in lung cancer, MM, and several other types of cancer (Denhardt and Chambers 1994). High levels of osteopontin are correlated with tumor progression and metastasis. In a rat model, osteopontin was upregulated in asbestos-induced tumors (Sandhu et al. 2000). There is a report that osteopontin levels in plasma or serum were able to differentiate between healthy subjects exposed to asbestos and MM patients (Grigoriu et al. 2007). A number of other human population studies have reported the serum levels of osteopontin in asbestos-exposed subjects. In one study, osteopontin levels were reported for 69 asbestos-exposed subjects, 45 healthy controls, and 76 patients with surgically staged MM (Pass et al. 2005). Serum osteopontin levels were significantly higher in the group with pleural MM than in the group with exposure to asbestos but without MM. An analysis of serum osteopontin levels comparing the receiver operating characteristic (ROC) curve in the group exposed to asbestos with that of the group with MM had a sensitivity of 77.6% and a specificity of 85.5% (Pass et al. 2005). Another study, which was conducted in Turkey, had 120 healthy controls and 123 subjects exposed to naturally occurring asbestos (Bayram et al. 2014). The difference in the levels of osteopontin was significant ($p < 0.05$) in controls versus asbestos-exposed individuals but was not useful for predicting malignant transformation.

A large study analyzed SMRP and osteopontin levels in asbestos-exposed workers ($n = 1894$) together with a smaller number of unexposed controls ($n = 102$) (Felten et al. 2014). The levels of osteopontin were not significantly different between the two groups. This study also found no correlation between osteopontin levels with the length of the asbestos exposure. A systematic review and meta-analysis of six studies was conducted in order to evaluate the diagnostic accuracy of circulating osteopontin for MM (Hu et al. 2014). The overall mean diagnostic sensitivity and specificity were 65% and 81%, respectively (Fig. 12.2). The area under the ROC curve (AUC) was 0.83, and the diagnostic accuracy of both serum and plasma osteopontin was comparable. The authors concluded that osteopontin was an effective marker for MM diagnosis but that more studies with larger sample sizes and better designs were needed in order to rigorously assess its diagnostic power.

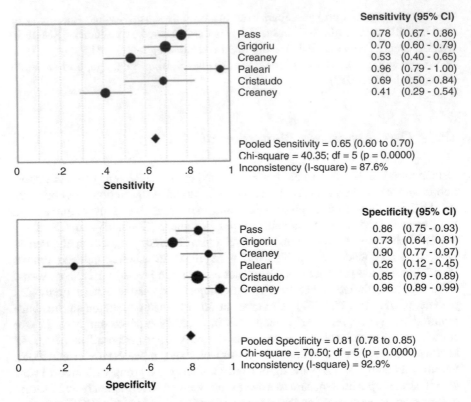

Fig. 12.2 Forest plots to estimate sensitivity and specificity of osteopontin from six studies. Each solid circle represents an eligible study. The size of the solid circle reflects the sample size of each eligible study. Error bars represent 95% CI. *Solid diamond* symbols represent mean pooled sensitivity and specificity. Reprinted with permission from Hu et al. (2014)

12.6   Fibulin-3 as a Biomarker of MM

Fibulin-3 is a 57-kDa protein, which belongs to a family of extracellular proteins expressed on the basement membranes of blood vessels. It has emerged as a potential plasma protein from the studies of Pass et al. as a biomarker of asbestos exposure with the capability of distinguishing between exposed and disease states within multiple cohorts (Table 12.1) (Pass et al. 2012). Unusually, in matched samples, fibulin-3 levels were lower in serum than in plasma probably due to the presence of thrombin cleavage sites within fibulin-3. It was also found that fibulin-3 was not able to distinguish between patients with MM and asbestosis because serum levels were elevated in both groups (Corradi et al. 2013). Plasma fibulin-3 was significantly elevated in MM patients from a Sydney patient cohort, but not a Vienna patient cohort (Fig. 12.3) (Kirschner et al. 2015).

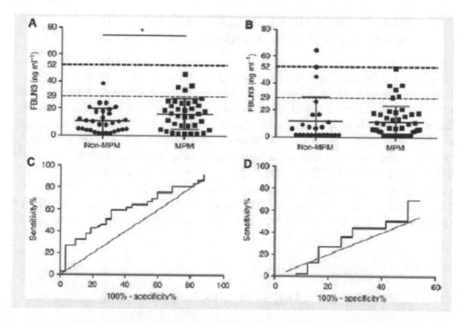

Fig. 12.3 Fibulin-3 in patient plasma. Plasma fibulin-3 protein levels in the Sydney (**a**) and Vienna cohorts (**b**). Mean levels in both cohorts were below those previously reported. Mean ± s.d. are represented by the lines in the scatter plots, and the cutoffs applied in the original study (Pass et al. 2012) are indicated by dotted lines. The diagnostic accuracy of plasma fibulin-3 was low in both investigated cohorts: (**c**) Sydney cohort AUC = 0.63 (95% CI, 0.50–0.76) and (**d**) Vienna cohort AUC = 0.56 (95% CI, 0.41–0.71). Reprinted with permission from Kirschner et al. (2015)

In addition, the diagnostic accuracy was low, which raised questions as to whether fibulin-3 actually has diagnostic value (Kirschner et al. 2015). However, in another recent study, patients with fibulin-3 levels >34.25 ng/mL before treatment had more than four times higher probability for developing progressive disease within 18 months than patients with levels ≤34.25 ng/mL (Kovac et al. 2015). In addition, patients with fibulin-3 levels >34.25 ng/mL after treatment had increased odds for progressive disease within 18 months even if they had a complete response or stable disease. The authors concluded that a combination of serum SMRP and plasma fibulin-3 levels might be helpful in detecting the progression of MM. Clearly, additional validation studies will be required to fully elucidate the utility of fibulin-3 as a dependable biomarker of asbestos exposure in human populations. It would be interesting to assess multiplexed assays with other protein biomarkers for MM (Kovac et al. 2015; Creaney et al. 2015). In fact, a recent study has demonstrated that compared to an asbestos exposure group of 48 subjects, a group of 42 MM patients had significantly higher mean epidermal growth factor (EGFR), thioredoxin-1 (TRX), SMRP, and fibulin-3 levels (Demir et al. 2016).

12.7   High Mobility Group Box (HMGB) 1 Protein as a Biomarker of MM and Asbestos Exposure

HMGB1 is a 30-kDa DNA-binding nonhistone protein that is present in nucleus (Lotze and Tracey 2005). It consists of 215 amino acid residues that are organized into three domains, which include two tandem HMG box domains (A box and B box) that are arranged in an L-shaped configuration, and a C-terminal tail of 30 amino acid residues (Fig. 12.4). The nuclear localization of HMGB1 is due to the presence of two lysine-rich nuclear localization sequences (NLSs), spanning amino acids 28–44 (NLS1) and 179–185 (NLS2) (Fig. 12.4) (Lotze and Tracey 2005). HMGB1 is released from macrophages and monocytes by endogenous pro-inflammatory cyto-kines such as tumor necrosis factor (TNF), interleukin [IL]-1β, and interferon [IFN]-γ (Wang et al. 2004). Because its N-terminus lacks a signal sequence, HMGB1 cannot

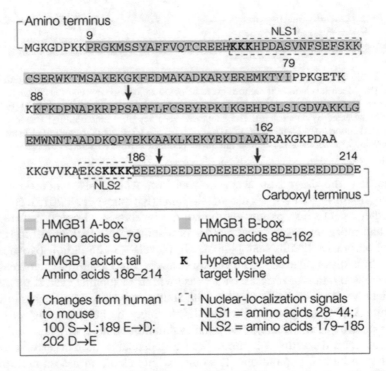

Fig. 12.4   HMGB1 structure. A linear diagram of high-mobility group box 1 protein (HMGB1) is shown, including the residues that constitute the A-box (*pink*), B-box (*purple*), and acidic tail (*green*). The proximal A-box and B-box of HMGB1 both contain putative nuclear-emigration sig-nals, as identified by binding to the nuclear exportin chromosome-region maintenance 1. HMGB1 also contains 43 lysine residues, some of which are frequently acetylated in lipopolysaccharide-activated macrophages (shown in *bold*). These lysine residues are found within two nuclear-local-ization signals (indicated by *dashed boxes*): NLS1, which spans amino acids 28–44; and NLS2, which spans amino acids 179–185. Reprinted with permission from Lotze and Tracey (2005)

be released via the classical endoplasmic reticulum-Golgi secretory pathway. Instead, activated macrophages/monocytes acetylate the HMGB1 at three lysine residues in the NLS1 region and five lysine residues in the NLS2 region (Fig. 12.4) (Lotze and Tracey 2005), which leads to translocation into the cytoplasm and release into the extracellular milieu (Bonaldi et al. 2003; Chen et al. 2005).

The HMGB1 protein, which has a regulatory role in inflammatory immune responses, has received substantial attention as a potential biomarker of MM (Qi et al. 2013) (Table 12.1). Gene expression profiling of mesothelial cells exposed to asbestos has shown upregulation of many genes targeted by HMGB1 (Qi et al. 2013). Furthermore, exposing mice to asbestos resulted in increased serum levels of HMGB1 for 10 or more weeks after crocidolite exposure, but returned to background levels within 8 weeks after chrysotile exposure. Continuous administration of chrysotile was required for sustained high serum levels of HMGB1 (Qi et al. 2013). One study found elevated serum levels of HMGB1, in asbestos-exposed individuals when compared with both smoking and nonsmoking controls (Yang et al. 2010), indicating that serum HMGB1 could be exploited for assessing asbestos exposure in human populations. In agreement with this finding, elevated serum levels of HMGB1 have been found in MM patients (Jube et al. 2012; Tabata et al. 2013b; Yamada et al. 2011).

More recently, it was found that serum HMGB1 is extensively acetylated in the serum of MM patients (Napolitano et al. 2016). The quantification of HMGB1 has generally been conducted using immunoassay-based methodology such as ELISAs, which cannot readily distinguish the nonacetylated and acetylated forms (Zhou et al. 2016; Yamada et al. 2003; Zangar et al. 2006; Barnay-Verdier et al. 2011; Bergmann et al. 2016). Development of high-specificity liquid chromatography-mass spectrometry (LC-MS)-based methods by Antoine and his colleagues (Antoine et al. 2012; Ge et al. 2014; Napolitano et al. 2016) made it possible to distinguish the HMGB1 hyperacetylated forms from the unmodified form normally found in the nucleus (Lotze and Tracey 2005). The MS-based methods are based upon the use of electrospray ionization (ESI) analysis of intact HMGB1 protein followed by spectral deconvolution (Fig. 12.5) (Napolitano et al. 2016) or by the use of Glu-C protease digestion of the HMGB1 followed by LC-ESI/tandem mass spectrometry (MS/MS) analysis of the hyperacetylated NLS2-derived decapeptide $K^{180}SKKKKEEEE^{189}$, which contains five acetylated lysine residues (Fig. 12.6) (Ge et al. 2014). LC-MS analysis of synthetic acetylated peptide from the NLS2 region of HMGB1–K(Ac)SK(Ac)K(Ac)K(Ac)K(Ac)EEEE – revealed that it could be rapidly adsorbed on plastic surfaces (Antoine et al. 2012). As a result, glass vials were required throughout the assay procedure. To minimize losses during LC-MS analysis, a desalted tryptic digest of human serum albumin was used as a proteinaceous carrier for the Glu-C-derived peptides.

Hyperacetylated and nonacetylated HMGB1 (together referred to as total HMGB1) were analyzed blindly in blood collected from MM patients ($n = 22$), individuals with verified chronic asbestos exposure ($n = 20$), patients with benign pleural effusions ($n = 13$), malignant pleural effusions not due to MM ($n = 25$), and healthy control subjects ($n = 20$) (Napolitano et al. 2016). Blood levels of previously

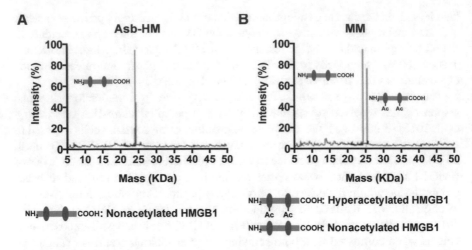

Fig. 12.5 Asbestos-exposed human mesothelial (HM) and malignant mesothelioma (MM) cells release different HMGB1 isoforms. (**a**) Representative spectrum of whole protein ESI/MS analysis of HMGB1 in crocidolite asbestos-exposed HM, where only nonacetylated HMGB1 was detected. (**b**) Representative spectrum of whole protein ESI/MS spectrum of HMGB1 in MM cells where both hyperacetylated and nonacetylated HMGB1 were detected. Reprinted with permission from Napolitano et al. (2016)

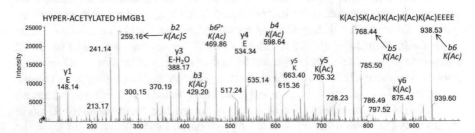

Fig. 12.6 Diagnostic LC–MS/MS spectrum of Glu-C-derived peptide confirming the identification of hyper-acetylated HMGB1 derived from inflammatory cells present in patient sera during acetaminophen hepatotoxicity. Amino acids, b and y ions and peptide sequences are indicated on each spectrum. Acetylated lysine residues within HMGB1 are represented by K(Ac). Reprinted with permission from Antoine et al. (2012)

proposed biomarkers (fibulin-3, SMRP, and osteopontin) were also analyzed in the non-healthy individuals. HMGB1 serum levels reliably distinguished MM patients, asbestos-exposed individuals, and unexposed controls (Napolitano et al. 2016). Total HMGB1 was significantly higher in MM patients and asbestos-exposed individuals compared with healthy controls. Hyperacetylated HMGB1 was significantly higher in MM patients compared with asbestos-exposed individuals and healthy controls and did not vary with tumor stage. At the cutoff value of 2.00 ng/mL, the sensitivity and specificity of serum hyperacetylated HMGB1 in differentiating MM patients from asbestos-exposed individuals and healthy controls was 100%, outperforming other previously proposed biomarkers. Furthermore, by combining HMGB1 and fibulin-3, increased sensitivity and specificity was obtained for differentiating MM patients from patients with cytologically benign or malignant non-mesothelioma pleural effusion. If confirmed by other groups, these results are clearly highly significant and clinically relevant because they provide the first biomarker of asbestos exposure and indicate that hyperacetylated HMGB1 is an accurate biomarker to differentiate MM patients from individuals occupationally exposed to asbestos and unexposed controls. More extensive studies will reveal whether these exciting new findings offer an approach to distinguish subjects exposed to asbestos from those who have progressed to MM.

12.8 Proteomic Biomarkers of MM

A targeted proteomics approach using Slow Off-rate Modified Aptamer (SOMAmer) technology (Ostroff et al. 2012) was employed for the discovery, verification, and validation of MM biomarkers. SOMAmers have slow specific off-rates for dissociation of targeted analytes, which results in highly selective protein detection. This makes it possible to simultaneously quantify over 1000 proteins in unfractionated biologic samples (Vaught et al. 2010). The biomarker study by Ostroff and colleagues used serum from 117 MM cases and 142 asbestos-exposed control individuals. An initial set of 64 candidate high abundance protein biomarkers was discovered. A training set identified a panel of 13-protein biomarkers for the validation studies (Table 12.1). In a paired sample analysis, the sensitivity (91%) and specificity (94%) of the 13-protein panel and the AUC of the ROC curve of 0.99 were far superior to those observed for serum SMRP (Fig. 12.7). The 13-protein panel consists of both inflammatory and proliferative proteins, which are involved in biological processes that are strongly associated with asbestos-induced malignancy. Further validation studies will be required to determine whether this panel will be useful for screening and diagnosis of high-risk individuals.

12.9 Conclusions and Future Perspectives

There is a compelling need to rigorously validate the serum and plasma proteins that are upregulated in MM as a panel of useful biological response biomarkers of asbestos exposure (Table 12.1). In spite of the ban on mining it in the USA, asbestos is still being mined in other parts of the world where there are poor controls on potential exposure of workers to asbestos (Linton et al. 2012). Furthermore, the 20–40-year latency period before ARDs are detected means that they will continue to be a public health problem in the USA for many years (Carbone et al. 2012). A reliable biomarker panel capable of assessing whether a particular individual is at risk for ARDs would be a useful clinical tool in screening, diagnosis, and prevention. Perhaps more importantly, such a diagnostic biomarker panel could help alleviate

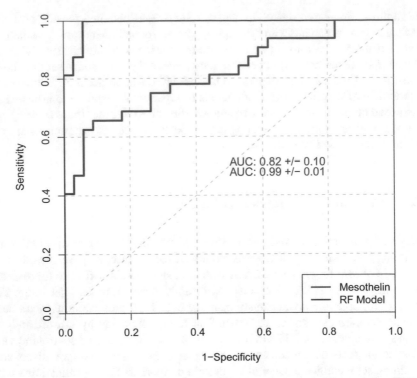

Fig. 12.7 ROC curves comparing 13-protein MM biomarker panel to mesothelin (SMRP). Performance of the 13-protein random forest (RF) classifier panel (*red*) compared to a commercial mesothelin (SMRP) assay (*blue*) on the same cohort of 32 MM cases and 34 asbestos-exposed controls. ROC curves are plotted with corresponding AUC values and 95% confidence intervals. Reprinted with permission from Ostroff et al. (2012)

concerns about possible environmental exposure as well as help to ensure that effective removal of asbestos from the environment has been implemented. In the past, response biomarker studies have focused on small molecule biomarkers of oxidative stress, signaling factors for cell-mediated and humoral immune responses, and growth factors generated in response to inhalation of asbestos fibers. These studies were able to elucidate many of the important factors involved with the pathogenesis of ARDs as well as guide efforts for developing effective asbestos exposure biomarkers. This has led to the potentially exciting observation that acetylated HMGB1 may be a highly specific biomarker of MM and that elevated nonacetylated HMGB1 might be a useful response biomarker of asbestos exposure.

The discovery of acetylated HMGB1 in MM patients has highlighted the potential utility of LC-MS-based methodology, which is more specific than ELISA-based procedures as also evidenced in our recent studies of apolipoprotein A-I (Wang et al. 2015). Furthermore, LC-MS methodology can be readily adapted to multiplexing, so that multiple candidate proteins can be quantified with high sensitivity and specificity in a single analysis (Mesaros and Blair 2016). Another approach that could be applied to the discovery of biomarkers of response resulting from asbestos exposure involves the implementation of untargeted serum lipidomics using ultrahigh-performance LC coupled with high-resolution MS (Snyder et al. 2015). This could lead to the discovery of a panel of serum lipid biomarkers of response to asbestos exposure that could be validated in more extensive biomarker studies. A serum lipid biomarker panel when combined with serum protein biomarkers would provide an extremely rigorous approach to monitoring populations at risk for environmental asbestos exposure such as near the BoRit site in Pennsylvania and the disused mine in Libby, Montana. Finally, highly specific and sensitive LC-MS assays of rigorously validated MM biomarkers would be extremely effective in assessing the impact of novel approaches to the treatment of MM such as the immune checkpoint inhibitors (Lievense et al. 2014; Ceresoli et al. 2016).

Acknowledgments This work was supported by NIH grants P42ES023720, P30ES013508, and T32ES019851. The authors have no competing financial interests to disclose.

References

Altomare DA, Menges CW, Xu J et al (2011) Losses of both products of the Cdkn2a/Arf locus contribute to asbestos-induced mesothelioma development and cooperate to accelerate tumorigenesis. PLoS One 6:e18828

Antoine DJ, Jenkins RE, Dear JW et al (2012) Molecular forms of HMGB1 and keratin-18 as mechanistic biomarkers for mode of cell death and prognosis during clinical acetaminophen hepatotoxicity. J Hepatol 56:1070–1079

Armstrong AW, Voyles SV, Armstrong EJ et al (2011) Angiogenesis and oxidative stress: common mechanisms linking psoriasis with atherosclerosis. J Dermatol Sci 63:1–9

Bang KM, Mazurek JM, Storey E et al (2009) Malignant mesothelioma mortality-United States, 1999–2005. MMWR Morb Mortal Wkly Rep 58:393–396

Barnay-Verdier S, Gaillard C, Messmer M et al (2011) PCA-ELISA: a sensitive method to quantify free and masked forms of HMGB1. Cytokine 55:4–7

Bayram M, Dongel I, Akbas A et al (2014) Serum biomarkers in patients with mesothelioma and pleural plaques and healthy subjects exposed to naturally occurring asbestos. Lung 192:197–203

Becklake MR (1976) Asbestos-related diseases of the lung and other organs: their epidemiology and implications for clinical practice. Am Rev Respir Dis 114:187–227

Bergmann C, Strohbuecker L, Lotfi R et al (2016) High mobility group box 1 is increased in the sera of psoriatic patients with disease progression. J Eur Acad Dermatol Venereol 30:435–441

Beyer HL, Geschwindt RD, Glover CL et al (2007) MESOMARK: a potential test for malignant pleural mesothelioma. Clin Chem 53:666–672

Bianchi AB, Mitsunaga SI, Cheng JQ et al (1995) High frequency of inactivating mutations in the neurofibromatosis type 2 gene (NF2) in primary malignant mesotheliomas. Proc Natl Acad Sci U S A 92:10854–10858

Blair IA (2008) DNA adducts with lipid peroxidation products. J Biol Chem 283:15545–15549

Bonaldi T, Talamo F, Scaffidi P et al (2003) Monocytic cells hyperacetylate chromatin protein HMGB1 to redirect it towards secretion. EMBO J 22:5551–5560

Boulanger G, Andujar P, Pairon JC et al (2014) Quantification of short and long asbestos fibers to assess asbestos exposure: a review of fiber size toxicity. Environ Health 13:59

Britton M (2002) The epidemiology of mesothelioma. Semin Oncol 29:18–25

Carbone M, Flores EG, Emi M et al (2015) Combined genetic and genealogic studies uncover a large BAP1 cancer syndrome kindred tracing back nine generations to a common ancestor from the 1700s. PLoS Genet 11:e1005633

Carbone M, Ly BH, Dodson RF et al (2012) Malignant mesothelioma: facts, myths, and hypotheses. J Cell Physiol 227:44–58

Carbone M, Yang H, Pass HI et al (2013) BAP1 and cancer. Nat Rev Cancer 13:153–159

Ceresoli GL, Bonomi M, Sauta MG (2016) Immune checkpoint inhibitors in malignant pleural mesothelioma: promises and challenges. Expert Rev Anticancer Ther 16:673–675

Chen G, Li J, Qiang X et al (2005) Suppression of HMGB1 release by stearoyl lysophosphatidyl-choline: an additional mechanism for its therapeutic effects in experimental sepsis. J Lipid Res 46:623–627

Cheng JQ, Jhanwar SC, Klein WM et al (1994) p16 alterations and deletion mapping of 9p21-p22 in malignant mesothelioma. Cancer Res 54:5547–5551

Cheresh P, Morales-Nebreda L, Kim SJ et al (2015) Asbestos-induced pulmonary fibrosis is augmented in 8-oxoguanine DNA glycosylase knockout mice. Am J Respir Cell Mol Biol 52:25–36

Cheung M, Talarchek J, Schindeler K et al (2013) Further evidence for germline BAP1 mutations predisposing to melanoma and malignant mesothelioma. Cancer Genet 206:206–210

Chew SH, Toyokuni S (2015) Malignant mesothelioma as an oxidative stress-induced cancer: an update. Free Radic Biol Med 86:166–178

Corradi M, Goldoni M, Alinovi R et al (2013) YKL-40 and mesothelin in the blood of patients with malignant mesothelioma, lung cancer and asbestosis. Anticancer Res 33:5517–5524

Creaney J, Dick IM, Robinson BW (2015) Comparison of mesothelin and fibulin-3 in pleural fluid and serum as markers in malignant mesothelioma. Curr Opin Pulm Med 21:352–356

Creaney J, Musk AW, Robinson BW (2010a) Sensitivity of urinary mesothelin in patients with malignant mesothelioma. J Thorac Oncol 5:1461–1466

Creaney J, Olsen NJ, Brims F et al (2010b) Serum mesothelin for early detection of asbestos-induced cancer malignant mesothelioma. Cancer Epidemiol Biomark Prev 19:2238–2246

Cui A, Jin XG, Zhai K et al (2014) Diagnostic values of soluble mesothelin-related peptides for malignant pleural mesothelioma: updated meta-analysis. BMJ Open 4:e004145

de Assis LV, Locatelli J, Isoldi MC (2014) The role of key genes and pathways involved in the tumorigenesis of malignant mesothelioma. Biochim Biophys Acta 1845:232–247

Demir M, Kaya H, Taylan M et al (2016) Evaluation of new biomarkers in the prediction of malignant mesothelioma in subjects with environmental asbestos exposure. Lung 194:409–417

Denhardt DT, Chambers AF (1994) Overcoming obstacles to metastasis--defenses against host defenses: osteopontin (OPN) as a shield against attack by cytotoxic host cells. J Cell Biochem 56:48–51

Ellegaard PK, Poulsen HE (2016) Tobacco smoking and oxidative stress to DNA: a meta-analysis of studies using chromatographic and immunological methods. Scand J Clin Lab Invest 76:151–158

Felten MK, Khatab K, Knoll L et al (2014) Changes of mesothelin and osteopontin levels over time in formerly asbestos-exposed power industry workers. Int Arch Occup Environ Health 87:195–204

Frank AL, Joshi TK (2014) The global spread of asbestos. Ann Glob Health 80:257–262

Fung H, Kow YW, Van HB et al (1997) Patterns of 8-hydroxydeoxyguanosine formation in DNA and indications of oxidative stress in rat and human pleural mesothelial cells after exposure to crocidolite asbestos. Carcinogenesis 18:825–832

Ge X, Antoine DJ, Lu Y et al (2014) High Mobility Group Box-1 (HMGB1) participates in the pathogenesis of alcoholic liver disease (ALD). J Biol Chem 289:22672–22691

Grigoriu BD, Scherpereel A, Devos P et al (2007) Utility of osteopontin and serum mesothelin in malignant pleural mesothelioma diagnosis and prognosis assessment. Clin Cancer Res 13:2928–2935

Guo Y, Chirieac LR, Bueno R et al (2014) Tsc1-Tp53 loss induces mesothelioma in mice, and evidence for this mechanism in human mesothelioma. Oncogene 33:3151–3160

Hanaoka T, Tsugane S, Yamano Y et al (1993) Quantitative analysis of 8-hydroxyguanine in peripheral blood cells: an application for asbestosis patients. Int Arch Occup Environ Health 65:S215–S217

Hillegass JM, Miller JM, Macpherson MB et al (2013) Asbestos and erionite prime and activate the NLRP3 inflammasome that stimulates autocrine cytokine release in human mesothelial cells. Part Fibre Toxicol 10:39

Hillegass JM, Shukla A, Lathrop SA et al (2010) Inflammation precedes the development of human malignant mesotheliomas in a SCID mouse xenograft model. Ann N Y Acad Sci 1203:7–14

Hu ZD, Liu XF, Liu XC et al (2014) Diagnostic accuracy of osteopontin for malignant pleural mesothelioma: a systematic review and meta-analysis. Clin Chim Acta 433:44–48

Jakubec P, Pelclova D, Smolkova P et al (2015) Significance of serum mesothelin in an asbestos-exposed population in the Czech Republic. Biomed Pap Med Fac Univ Palacky Olomouc Czech Repub 159:472–479

Jube S, Rivera ZS, Bianchi ME et al (2012) Cancer cell secretion of the DAMP protein HMGB1 supports progression in malignant mesothelioma. Cancer Res 72:3290–3301

Kadiiska MB, Gladen BC, Baird DD et al (2005) Biomarkers of oxidative stress study II: are oxidation products of lipids, proteins, and DNA markers of CCl4 poisoning? Free Radic Biol Med 38:698–710

Kalra N, Zhang J, Thomas A et al (2015) Mesothelioma patient derived tumor xenografts with defined BAP1 mutations that mimic the molecular characteristics of human malignant mesothelioma. BMC Cancer 15:376

Kirschner MB, Pulford E, Hoda MA et al (2015) Fibulin-3 levels in malignant pleural mesothelioma are associated with prognosis but not diagnosis. Br J Cancer 113:963–969

Kovac V, Dodic-Fikfak M, Arneric N et al (2015) Fibulin-3 as a biomarker of response to treatment in malignant mesothelioma. Radiol Oncol 49:279–285

Lang-Lazdunski L (2014) Surgery for malignant pleural mesothelioma: why, when and what? Lung Cancer 84:103–109

Lemen RA, Dement JM, Wagoner JK (1980) Epidemiology of asbestos-related diseases. Environ Health Perspect 34:1–11

Lievense LA, Hegmans JP, Aerts JG (2014) Biomarkers for immune checkpoint inhibitors. Lancet Oncol 15:e1

Linton A, Vardy J, Clarke S et al (2012) The ticking time-bomb of asbestos: its insidious role in the development of malignant mesothelioma. Crit Rev Oncol Hematol 84:200–212

Lotze MT, Tracey KJ (2005) High-mobility group box 1 protein (HMGB1): nuclear weapon in the immune arsenal. Nat Rev Immunol 5:331–342

Marczynski B, Kraus T, Rozynek P et al (2000a) Association between 8-hydroxy-2′-deoxyguanosine levels in DNA of workers highly exposed to asbestos and their clinical data, occupational and non-occupational confounding factors, and cancer. Mutat Res 468:203–212

Marczynski B, Rozynek P, Kraus T et al (2000b) Levels of 8-hydroxy-2′-deoxyguanosine in DNA of white blood cells from workers highly exposed to asbestos in Germany. Mutat Res 468:195–202

Marini V, Michelazzi L, Cioe A et al (2011) Exposure to asbestos: correlation between blood levels of mesothelin and frequency of micronuclei in peripheral blood lymphocytes. Mutat Res 721:114–117

Mesaros C, Arora JS, Wholer A et al (2012) 8-Oxo-2′-deoxyguanosine as a biomarker of tobacco-smoking-induced oxidative stress. Free Radic Biol Med 53:610–617

Mesaros C, Blair IA (2016) Mass spectrometry-based approaches to targeted quantitative proteomics in cardiovascular disease. Clin Proteomics 13:20

Mesaros C, Worth AJ, Snyder NW et al (2015) Bioanalytical techniques for detecting biomarkers of response to human asbestos exposure. Bioanalysis 7:1157–1173

Milne GL, Musiek ES, Morrow JD (2005) F2-Isoprostanes as markers of oxidative stress in vivo: an overview. Biomarkers 10(Suppl 1):S10–S23

Montjoy C, Parker J, Petsonk L et al (2009) Mesothelioma review. W V Med J 105:13–16

Mossman BT, Shukla A, Heintz NH et al (2013) New insights into understanding the mechanisms, pathogenesis, and management of malignant mesotheliomas. Am J Pathol 182:1065–1077

Napolitano A, Antoine DJ, Pellegrini L et al (2016) HMGB1 and its hyperacetylated isoform are sensitive and specific serum biomarkers to detect asbestos exposure and to identify mesothelioma patients. Clin Cancer Res 22(12):3087–3096

Navarro-Compan V, Melguizo-Madrid E, Hernandez-Cruz B et al (2013) Interaction between oxidative stress and smoking is associated with an increased risk of rheumatoid arthritis: a case-control study. Rheumatology (Oxford) 52:487–493

Ohar JA, Cheung M, Talarchek J et al (2016) Germline BAP1 mutational landscape of asbestos-exposed malignant mesothelioma patients with family history of cancer. Cancer Res 76:206–215

Ostroff RM, Mehan MR, Stewart A et al (2012) Early detection of malignant pleural mesothelioma in asbestos-exposed individuals with a noninvasive proteomics-based surveillance tool. PLoS One 7:e46091

Park EK, Thomas PS, Creaney J et al (2010) Factors affecting soluble mesothelin related protein levels in an asbestos-exposed population. Clin Chem Lab Med 48:869–874

Park EK, Yates DH, Creaney J et al (2012) Association of biomarker levels with severity of asbestos-related diseases. Saf Health Work 3:17–21

Pass HI, Levin SM, Harbut MR et al (2012) Fibulin-3 as a blood and effusion biomarker for pleural mesothelioma. N Engl J Med 367:1417–1427

Pass HI, Lott D, Lonardo F et al (2005) Asbestos exposure, pleural mesothelioma, and serum osteopontin levels. N Engl J Med 353:1564–1573

Pass HI, Wali A, Tang N et al (2008) Soluble mesothelin-related peptide level elevation in mesothelioma serum and pleural effusions. Ann Thorac Surg 85:265–272

Peipins LA, Lewin M, Campolucci S et al (2003) Radiographic abnormalities and exposure to asbestos-contaminated vermiculite in the community of Libby, Montana, USA. Environ Health Perspect 111:1753–1759

Pelclova D, Fenclova Z, Kacer P et al (2008) Increased 8-isoprostane, a marker of oxidative stress in exhaled breath condensate in subjects with asbestos exposure. Ind Health 46:484–489

Peluso I, Morabito G, Urban L et al (2012) Oxidative stress in atherosclerosis development: the central role of LDL and oxidative burst. Endocr Metab Immune Disord Drug Targets 12:351–360

Pilger A, Rudiger HW (2006) 8-Hydroxy-2′-deoxyguanosine as a marker of oxidative DNA damage related to occupational and environmental exposures. Int Arch Occup Environ Health 80:1–15

Pooley FD (1972) Electron microscope characteristics of inhaled chrysotile asbestos fibre. Br J Ind Med 29:146–153

Prazakova S, Thomas PS, Sandrini A et al (2014) Asbestos and the lung in the 21st Century: an update. Clin Respir J 8:1–10

Qi F, Okimoto G, Jube S et al (2013) Continuous exposure to chrysotile asbestos can cause transformation of human mesothelial cells via HMGB1 and TNF-alpha signaling. Am J Pathol 183:1654–1666

Ramos-Nino ME, Testa JR, Altomare DA et al (2006) Cellular and molecular parameters of mesothelioma. J Cell Biochem 98:723–734

Reid A, de Klerk NH, Magnani C et al (2014) Mesothelioma risk after 40 years since first exposure to asbestos: a pooled analysis. Thorax 69:843–850

Robinson BW, Creaney J, Lake R et al (2003) Mesothelin-family proteins and diagnosis of mesothelioma. Lancet 362:1612–1616

Rodriguez Portal JA, Rodriguez BE, Rodriguez RD et al (2009) Serum levels of soluble mesothelin-related peptides in malignant and nonmalignant asbestos-related pleural disease: relation with past asbestos exposure. Cancer Epidemiol Biomark Prev 18:646–650

Sandhu H, Dehnen W, Roller M et al (2000) MRNA Expression patterns in different stages of asbestos-induced carcinogenesis in rats. Carcinogenesis 21:1023–1029

Sartorelli P, Romeo R, Scancarello G et al (2007) Measurement of asbestos fibre concentrations in fluid of repeated bronchoalveolar lavages of exposed workers. Ann Occup Hyg 51:495–500

Schulze PC, Lee RT (2005) Oxidative stress and atherosclerosis. Curr Atheroscler Rep 7:242–248

Schurkes C, Brock W, Abel J et al (2004) Induction of 8-hydroxydeoxyguanosine by man made vitreous fibres and crocidolite asbestos administered intraperitoneally in rats. Mutat Res 553:59–65

Sekido Y (2013) Molecular pathogenesis of malignant mesothelioma. Carcinogenesis 34:1413–1419

Selikoff IJ, Hammond EC, Seidman H (1980) Latency of asbestos disease among insulation workers in the United States and Canada. Cancer 46:2736–2740

Serban C, Dragan S (2014) The relationship between inflammatory and oxidative stress biomarkers, atherosclerosis and rheumatic diseases. Curr Pharm Des 20:585–600

Snyder NW, Mesaros C, Blair IA (2015) Translational metabolomics in cancer research. Biomark Med 9:821–834

Stayner L, Welch LS, Lemen R (2013) The worldwide pandemic of asbestos-related diseases. Annu Rev Public Health 34:205–216

Sterman DH, Albelda SM (2005) Advances in the diagnosis, evaluation, and management of malignant pleural mesothelioma. Respirology 10:266–283

Swain WA, O'Byrne KJ, Faux SP (2004) Activation of p38 MAP kinase by asbestos in rat mesothelial cells is mediated by oxidative stress. Am J Phys Lung Cell Mol Phys 286:L859–L865

Tabata C, Kanemura S, Tabata R et al (2013a) Serum HMGB1 as a diagnostic marker for malignant peritoneal mesothelioma. J Clin Gastroenterol 47:684–688

Tabata C, Shibata E, Tabata R et al (2013b) Serum HMGB1 as a prognostic marker for malignant pleural mesothelioma. BMC Cancer 13:205–211

Testa JR, Cheung M, Pei J et al (2011) Germline BAP1 mutations predispose to malignant mesothelioma. Nat Genet 43:1022–1025

Valavanidis A, Vlachogianni T, Fiotakis C (2009) 8-Hydroxy-2'-deoxyguanosine (8-OHdG): a critical biomarker of oxidative stress and carcinogenesis. J Environ Sci Health C Environ Carcinog Ecotoxicol Rev 27:120–139

Vaught JD, Bock C, Carter J et al (2010) Expanding the chemistry of DNA for in vitro selection. J Am Chem Soc 132:4141–4151

Victor VM, Rocha M, Sola E et al (2009) Oxidative stress, endothelial dysfunction and atherosclerosis. Curr Pharm Des 15:2988–3002

Wang H, Yang H, Tracey KJ (2004) Extracellular role of HMGB1 in inflammation and sepsis. J Intern Med 255:320–331

Wang Q, Zhang S, Guo L et al (2015) Serum apolipoprotein A-1 quantification by LC-MS with a SILAC internal standard reveals reduced levels in smokers. Bioanalysis 7:2895–2911

Wu L, Ortiz C, Xu Y et al (2015) In situ liquid cell observations of asbestos fiber diffusion in water. Environ Sci Technol 49:13340–13349

Wu X, Li D, Liu L et al (2014) Serum soluble mesothelin-related peptide (SMRP): a potential diagnostic and monitoring marker for epithelial ovarian cancer. Arch Gynecol Obstet 289:1309–1314

Xu J, Kadariya Y, Cheung M et al (2014) Germline mutation of Bap1 accelerates development of asbestos-induced malignant mesothelioma. Cancer Res 74:4388–4397

Yamada S, Inoue K, Yakabe K et al (2003) High mobility group protein 1 (HMGB1) quantified by ELISA with a monoclonal antibody that does not cross-react with HMGB2. Clin Chem 49:1535–1537

Yamada S, Tabata C, Tabata R et al (2011) Clinical significance of pleural effusion mesothelin in malignant pleural mesothelioma. Clin Chem Lab Med 49:1721–1726

Yang H, Rivera Z, Jube S et al (2010) Programmed necrosis induced by asbestos in human mesothelial cells causes high-mobility group box 1 protein release and resultant inflammation. Proc Natl Acad Sci U S A 107:12611–12616

Yoshida R, Ogawa Y, Shioji I et al (2001) Urinary 8-oxo-7,8-dihydro-2'-deoxyguanosine and biopyrrins levels among construction workers with asbestos exposure history. Ind Health 39:186–188

Zangar RC, Daly DS, White AM (2006) ELISA microarray technology as a high-throughput system for cancer biomarker validation. Expert Rev Proteomics 3:37–44

Zhou Q, Zhu Z, Hu X et al (2016) HMGB1: A critical mediator for oxidized-low density lipoproteins induced atherosclerosis. Int J Cardiol 202:956–957

Chapter 13
Surgery Approaches in Mesothelioma

Andrea Wolf and Raja Flores

Abstract The role of surgical resection in malignant pleural mesothelioma (MPM) is controversial, but cancer-directed surgery has yielded long-term survivors and demonstrated 15% 5-year survival. The two operations developed for surgical resection, extrapleural pneumonectomy (EPP), and radical or extended pleurectomy/decortication (P/D) are described. In addition, this chapter summarizes the preoperative, perioperative, and postoperative management of these patients and the results of studies evaluating both procedures. Data and clinical experience suggest that P/D is better tolerated by patients, and evidence suggests survival is not worse. Although EPP is still performed in selected cases, the authors advocate radical P/D for most patients with MPM.

Keywords Malignant pleural mesothelioma • Surgical resection • Extrapleural pneumonectomy • Pleurectomy/decortication

13.1 Introduction

Surgery has several roles in the diagnosis and treatment of malignant pleural mesothelioma (MPM). Early in the course of identification of a patient with MPM, surgical biopsy via pleuroscopy or video-assisted thoracoscopic surgery (VATS) is critical to distinguishing MPM from pleural dissemination of metastatic disease and identifying the histologic cell type of tumor (epithelial, sarcomatoid, biphasic, or other). The role of surgical resection in MPM is controversial, but cancer-directed surgery for MPM is associated with a 15% 5-year survival (Yan et al. 2009; Taioli et al. 2015a).

Two operations have been developed for surgical resection of MPM: (1) extrapleural pneumonectomy (EPP), an en bloc resection of the lung, parietal and visceral pleurae, diaphragm, and pericardium (Fig. 13.1); and (2) radical or extended

A. Wolf • R. Flores (✉)
Mount Sinai Health System, Thoracic Surgery Department, Icahn School of Medicine,
New York, NY 10029-5674, USA
e-mail: raja.flores@mountsinai.org

© Springer International Publishing AG 2017
J.R. Testa (ed.), *Asbestos and Mesothelioma*, Current Cancer Research,
DOI 10.1007/978-3-319-53560-9_13

pleurectomy/decortication (P/D), the removal of the parietal and visceral pleurae, with resection of the diaphragm and/or pericardium if involved with tumor, but always preservation of the underlying lung. Various patient-, surgeon-, and center-related factors influence which operation is preferred. Most studies evaluating the surgical treatment of MPM have focused exclusively on either EPP or P/D in the context of multimodality therapy. Adjuvant treatments include preoperative or post-operative chemotherapy, intracavitary chemotherapy or photodynamic therapy, pre-operative or postoperative external beam radiation, and now immunologic therapy (Pass et al. 1997; Weder et al. 2004; Flores et al. 2006; Richards et al. 2006; Kindler et al. 2012; de Perrot et al. 2016).

Left untreated, the median overall survival of patients with MPM is 7 months (Sugarbaker and Wolf 2010). Numerous studies have supported curative intent surgery as part of multimodality therapy (Sugarbaker and Wolf 2010; Wolf et al. 2010b; Sugarbaker et al. 2011; Taioli et al. 2014). While more than 40% of MPM patients seen at large tertiary referral centers are offered surgical resec-tion, fewer patients are offered cancer-directed surgery in the general popula-tion (Flores et al. 2010). Flores and colleagues reported that cancer-directed surgery was performed in only 22% of 5937 patients with MPM in the Surveillance, Epidemiology, and End Results (SEER) dataset between 1990 and 2004 (Flores et al. 2010). Patients who underwent surgery experienced a median overall survival of 11 months (compared to 7 months without surgery, $p < 0.0001$), and cancer-directed surgery was an independent predictor of improved survival (HR 0.68, 95% CI 0.63–0.74). In more comprehensive recent

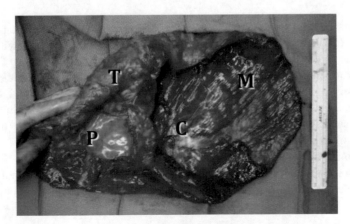

Fig. 13.1 Surgical resection of MPM by extrapleural pneumonectomy (EPP). Depicted is an en bloc resection of the lung, parietal and visceral pleurae, diaphragm, and pericardium. Abbreviations: *T* lung with tumor involving the fused visceral and parietal pleura, *P* pericardium, *C* central tendon of the diaphragm, and *M* muscle of the diaphragm

SEER analyses of MPM patients diagnosed between 1973 and 2009, cancer-directed surgery was predictive of longer survival (Taioli et al. 2015a, c).

Many clinicians advocate surgical resection for MPM patients who have favorable disease characteristics. Favorable prognostic factors are epithelial histology, female gender, and earlier stage. In a retrospective study in 945 patients, epithelial histology, female gender, earlier stage, lack of smoking or asbestos exposure, and left-sided disease were associated with longer survival (Flores et al. 2007). Women experience longer survival compared to men, but this finding may be unique to younger women and those with epithelial tumors. Women under the age of 50 with early-stage MPM demonstrated a median survival longer than 30 months with EPP (Wolf et al. 2010b). In a SEER analysis of 14,229 MPM patients diagnosed in the USA between 1973 and 2009, female gender was a significant predictor of longer survival, independent of age, stage, race, and treatment (adjusted HR 0.78, 95% CI 0.75–0.82) (Taioli et al. 2014). For men and women, higher stage disease and non-epithelial histology are associated with lower survival (Wolf et al. 2010b; Flores et al. 2007).

13.2 Surgical Resection in MPM

13.2.1 EPP

The technique of EPP was first described by Irving Sarot in 1949 with a series of tuberculosis patients treated at the Mount Sinai Hospital in New York City (Sarot 1949). The British surgeon, Butchart, first described the use of EPP for MPM in 1976, in a series in which the perioperative mortality rate was 31% (Butchart et al. 1976). Improvements have been made in the years since Butchart's series in preoperative patient risk stratification, operative technique, anesthesia, monitoring, and early identification of complications. These have dramatically reduced the mortality of EPP, with rates of 2.2–7% reported in modern series (Sugarbaker et al. 1999; Flores et al. 2008a; Wolf et al. 2009; Flores 2009; Sugarbaker and Wolf 2010; Cao et al. 2014).

13.2.2 P/D

As EPP was criticized for a period of time after Butchart's series reported prohibitive mortality, there was a renewed interest in lung-sparing resection with P/D (McCormack et al. 1982). Many surgeons feel strongly that macroscopic complete resection can be accomplished with less morbidity and mortality through this operation (Flores 2016).

13.3   Preoperative Evaluation

13.3.1   EPP

MPM patients being evaluated for EPP are staged with positron emission tomography-computed tomography (PET-CT) to evaluate for nodal or distant metastases. Higher PET avidity of the pleural tumor has been associated with lower survival (Flores 2005). Enlarged or PET-avid mediastinal lymph nodes are evaluated with endobronchial ultrasound (EBUS) or cervical mediastinoscopy. Some clinicians routinely stage the mediastinum in all patients, while others have abandoned this practice because of the variable nodal drainage of the pleura with unpredictable pattern of nodal metastases and lack of sensitivity of cervical mediastinoscopy for detecting extrapleural nodal spread of MPM (Flores et al. 2008b; Sugarbaker et al. 2014). Chest magnetic resonance imaging (MRI) is often performed to evaluate for diffuse chest wall and subdiaphragmatic or mediastinal invasion of tumor (Patz et al. 1992). The presence of subdiaphragmatic extension of tumor and/or ascites warrants further evaluation with staging laparoscopy as intra-abdominal tumor would preclude surgical resection.

The remaining preoperative evaluation is to determine the patient's ability to tolerate EPP (Sugarbaker and Wolf 2010). Pulmonary function tests, including spirometry and diffusion lung capacity, should be performed. Quantitative ventilation/perfusion scan ("split function" test) is done to assess perfusion to the affected lung. The product of the fraction of perfusion to the contralateral lung (which will remain following pneumonectomy) and the forced expiratory volume in 1 s (FEV1) is the predicted postoperative FEV1. While many clinicians recommend a value of at least 800 cc for pneumonectomy, the added morbidity of extrapleural, diaphragmatic, and pericardial resection has led most surgeons to consider a higher level, such as 1.2 L, for average-sized patients (Wolf et al. 2009). A cardiac stress test to rule out inducible myocardial ischemia from coronary artery disease and an echocardiogram with Doppler estimation of pulmonary artery pressure based on tricuspid regurgitation should be performed. A patient with pre-existing pulmonary hypertension may not survive the added right ventricular strain of pneumonectomy. Finally, duplex ultrasound of the lower extremity veins to rule out deep vein thrombosis (DVT) is also recommended. MPM patients have a high incidence of occult DVT, and preoperative treatment with anticoagulation (and possibly inferior vena cava filter) may reduce the risk of fatal pulmonary embolus following pneumonectomy.

13.3.2   P/D

The preoperative evaluation for radical or extended pleurectomy/decortication is identical to that for EPP. Staging, in particular, follows the procedure outlined above. Comorbidities such as poor pulmonary function, high pulmonary arterial pressures, coronary disease, and reduced ventricular function may not preclude P/D to the same extent as would be for EPP. Nevertheless, it is sometimes difficult to predict whether P/D or EPP will be required for resection in certain patients and having a thorough understanding of the patient's physiology allows for better intra-operative decision-making.

13.4 Perioperative Management

13.4.1 EPP

In preparation for EPP, the anesthesia team places routine monitors, lines, and an epidural catheter for regional pain control postoperatively (Ng and Hartigan 2008). An arterial line is needed due to rapid hemodynamic changes; large bore IV access, including a central line, is recommended. If there is any concern regarding pulmonary hypertension, a Swan-Ganz catheter is floated with caution to pull this back prior to pulmonary artery division. Central lines should be placed on the operative side to avoid pneumothorax on the side of the ventilated (and postoperatively, only) lung. Lung isolation with double-lumen endotracheal tube (preferred) or bronchial blocker is obtained, with the latter pulled back prior to division of the bronchus. Finally, a nasogastric tube is inserted to facilitate intraoperative identification of the esophagus and to decompress the stomach postoperatively. Disruption of vagal fibers to the bronchus often causes mild postoperative esophageal dysmotility, and nasogastric decompression may prevent life-threatening aspiration after pneumonectomy in the early postoperative period.

13.4.2 P/D

The same anesthetic preparation is made for P/D, particularly given the possibility that the operative plan may change from P/D to EPP. Routine lines and monitors are required, but with less need for a Swan-Ganz catheter. The gastric tube for P/D is usually placed orally and removed before extubation at the end of the case. Bleeding may be more profuse in P/D because of the visceral pleurectomy (see below); thus, transfusion may be needed. Air leak lost through the chest tubes following visceral pleurectomy may make it difficult to inflate the lung. If the lung is expanded, even high volumes "lost" (as reflected by lower return volumes in the ventilator bellows) do not prohibit gas exchange. As long as oxygenation is adequate, ventilation typically occurs through the circuit as well as the lung surface (out the tube), and the result is normal plasma oxygen with slight hypocapnea.

13.5 Technique of Surgery

13.5.1 EPP

The basic technique of EPP is fairly standard, although surgeons may vary specific steps. An extended posterolateral thoracotomy, incorporating prior pleuroscopy or VATS incisions if possible, is performed with many surgeons resecting the sixth rib. The tumor is separated from the endothoracic fascia by dissecting the extrapleural plane. The dissection is continued posteriorly, anteriorly, superiorly, and inferiorly. The posterior borders of dissection are the azygous vein on the right and the aorta on the left. Caution not to dissect beyond these borders is necessary to avoid avulsion of the azygous vein/tributaries or intercostal aortic branches.

Apically, the subclavian vessels must be identified. As the dissection is continued down the superior mediastinum, caution should be taken near the superior vena cava on the right and the aortic arch on the left. Anteriorly, the thymic fat and pericardium form the border for dissection. A large pericardial effusion is suggestive of transpericardial invasion. The anterior pericardium is incised, and the inner surface is palpated for evidence of intrapericardial tumor.

If no invasion of critical mediastinal structures is identified, the anterior pericardial incision is continued inferiorly to the medial border of the diaphragm. The diaphragmatic attachments to the chest wall are bluntly dissected with the fingers or with the aid of the Cobb. On the right, caution is exercised in the area of the inferior vena cava deep in the costophrenic recess posteriorly as the inferior pulmonary ligament is divided. On the left, a rim of diaphragmatic crus is preserved to decrease the risk of postoperative gastric herniation. Phrenic vessels are clipped and/or coagulated as the diaphragm is resected. The pericardial incision is continued posteriorly and continued superiorly to divide the remaining posterior pericardium.

The hilum is approached last. The superior and inferior pulmonary veins are divided within the pericardium. The right pulmonary artery is divided within the pericardium, but, on the left, the intrapericardial segment of pulmonary artery is quite short, and the artery is generally divided extrapericardially. Peribronchial lymph nodes are swept up with the main stem bronchus, and the latter is closed with a heavy wire stapler and divided sharply. A lymph node dissection is performed for lymph nodes in the aortopulmonary, paratracheal, subcarinal, inferior pulmonary ligament, periesophageal, and any palpable locations (such as internal mammary or diaphragmatic). The bronchus can be buttressed with thymic tissue or omentum mobilized on a vascularized flap. It is preferable to avoid intercostal muscle pedicle, particularly if the rib is removed.

The diaphragm is reconstructed with a 2 mm Gore-Tex patch secured to the chest wall. If an omental flap is mobilized for bronchial stump coverage, it must be advanced through a fenestration in the diaphragmatic patch (Wolf et al. 2009). A 0.1 mm lo Gore-Tex or Dacron patch is fenestrated and secured to the pericardial edges in a loose, floppy fashion (Fig. 13.2). The fenestrations must be large enough to prohibit tamponade but small enough not to allow herniation of any part of the

Fig. 13.2 Reconstruction of diaphragm with Gore-Tex patch during EPP procedure. Patch is fenestrated and secured to the pericardial edges in a loose, floppy fashion

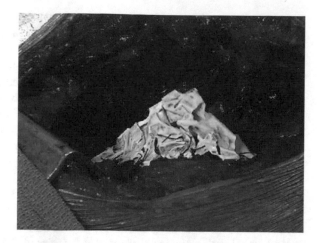

heart, such as the atrial appendage. The inferior portion of the pericardial patch is secured to the diaphragmatic patch as well as to the pericardial rim to prevent post-operative herniation of intra-abdominal contents.

The extrapleural dissection is associated with larger fluid shifts than seen with standard pneumonectomy in addition to higher risk of bleeding or chylothorax. The pneumonectomy space may fill more rapidly after EPP than with standard pneumo-nectomy and, combined with pericardial and diaphragmatic resection/reconstruc-tion, may lead to a more mobile mediastinum. This mandates strict management of the pneumonectomy space with the many options available, including chest tube without suction, balanced drainage, intrapleural pressure monitoring, and/or inter-mittent aspiration of fluid/air (Wolf et al. 2010a).

13.5.2 P/D

The initial approach, thoracotomy, and extrapleural dissection for P/D are similar to that of EPP. The extrapleural dissection comprises the parietal pleurectomy portion of the P/D. As the mediastinum is approached, the tumor is resected off the pericar-dium to the hilar cuff, if possible. If resection of the pericardium is required, it is preferable to delay opening the pericardium until a greater surface area of tumor is mobilized as pericardial entry may precipitate arrhythmias and hemodynamic insta-bility. Likewise, the dissection of the diaphragm off the chest wall is delayed until the extent of tumor can be assessed. If the tumor can be peeled or excised off the diaphragm, every attempt to preserve the diaphragm should be made.

The next step, the visceral pleurectomy, is equivalent to a decortication. A blade on a long handle is used to incise the tumor overlying the lung with caution not to injure the underlying lung parenchyma (a step that is easier with bulkier tumor and with prior talcpleurodesis). A plane is developed bluntly under the tumor using the

Pearson scissors, and Kochers are placed on the tumor to facilitate blunt dissection (e.g., using a sponge on a stick or laparotomy pad) of the underlying lung parenchyma away from the tumor. The dissection is carried out, often tediously, throughout the lung surfaces, with caution in the fissures not to injure the underlying pulmonary vessels. If the diaphragm is densely involved with tumor, the lower lobe pleura/tumor is bluntly dissected off to be resected en bloc with the diaphragm. The dissection is continued inferiorly toward the inferior ligament, superiorly, anteriorly, and posteriorly to encircle the hilum.

As noted above, blood loss may be substantial during P/D. Packing with laparotomy pads in areas that are not being dissected can tamponade bleeding, as can having the anesthesiologist inflate the lung (positive pressure can impede brisk bleeding). Argon beam coagulation or water-based bipolar sealants, such as Aquamantys, can be used as well. Finally, the hilum can be encircled with a red rubber catheter as a tourniquet if there is uncontrolled bleeding to allow time for coagulation, ligation, or repair of a vessel (Wolf et al. 2009). As pneumonectomy is the "bail-out" solution to catastrophic bleeding and/or major vessel injury, the possibility of EPP must be considered in patients undergoing P/D.

As the dissection continues to the hilar cuff, the pleura thins out and it is gently peeled off the hilar structures. The specimen is frequently removed in pieces. The lung can often be retracted out of the bulky tumor, and the inferior shell can be swept down toward the diaphragm. If the diaphragm can be preserved, even in the event of minimal residual disease, postoperative lung function and performance status are better. If there is extensive diaphragmatic invasion, resection and reconstruction are completed as described for EPP above. Likewise, if the pericardium is removed due to invasion, it is reconstructed as above. Three chest tubes are usually left to manage the pleural space, straight tubes anteriorly and posteriorly with a right-angle tube over the diaphragm.

13.6 Postoperative Management

13.6.1 EPP

Surgery should be performed at medical centers experienced with the postoperative management of patients undergoing EPP. This involves members of the surgery, nursing, anesthesia, and critical care teams. Patients should be extubated to avoid positive pressure on the bronchial stump but monitored in the intensive care unit during the early postoperative period. Prompt recognition of subtle clinical changes, such as a shifting mediastinum, can prevent life-threatening complications (Wolf et al. 2010a). Immediate identification of complications with appropriate intervention can prevent postoperative mortality (Sugarbaker et al. 2004). Finally, careful management of fluid status and pulmonary toilet is mandated in caring for these patients. Figure 13.3 depicts the preoperative (a) and baseline 6-month postoperative (b) imaging for a patient who successfully underwent EPP for MPM.

Fig. 13.3 Imaging of patient who underwent successful EPP for MPM. Preoperative (**a**) and baseline 6-month postoperative (**b**) images are depicted

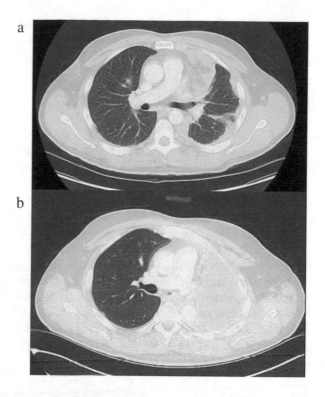

Most of the complications described after EPP result from injury to structures during resection. Vocal cord paralysis due to resection and/or cautery of the recurrent laryngeal nerve can lead to poor cough and subsequent aspiration. If vocal cord paresis occurs, all efforts to medialize the affected vocal cord must be made to maximize effectiveness of pulmonary toilet. The extrapleural dissection for EPP frequently disturbs the sympathetic nerves, with mild but refractory vasoplegia resulting in the early postoperative period. This is frequently compounded by use of thoracic epidural anesthesia but not responsive to stopping infusion of anesthetic. Treatment with oral vasoconstrictors, such as phenylephrine, is effective, and these can typically be weaned in the days to weeks after surgery. Unnecessary and/or excessive fluid resuscitation in response to this benign source of hypotension should be avoided as this may precipitate right heart failure, atrial fibrillation, and/or pulmonary edema in these single-lung patients.

The most common complication after EPP is supraventricular arrhythmia, such as atrial fibrillation. Major morbidities, such as tamponade, cardiac or gastric herniation, patch dehiscence, myocardial infarction, chylothorax, and pulmonary embolus, occur more rarely (Sugarbaker et al. 2011). DVT is more common in MPM patients, and routine screening or higher suspicion of early signs of venous thromboembolism is needed to minimize potentially fatal emboli in a patient with one lung. Bronchopleural fistula can occur weeks to months (and sometimes longer) after EPP and usually manifests with fever, wet cough, malaise, and unexplained drop in fluid level in the pneumonectomy space.

13.6.2   P/D

The postoperative management of P/D patients is similar to that of EPP although with less risk of pulmonary edema, right heart failure, and mediastinal shift. The remaining cardiac, pulmonary, infectious, renal, and hematologic complications that occur with EPP can also occur with P/D. The major complications unique to P/D are prolonged air leak and mucous plugging with atelectasis. Air leak is controlled with tubes, which can be placed to a Heimlich valve for more portable use. Doxycycline pleurodesis at the bedside (with tubes hung on a pole instead of clamped) has been used with limited success. Mucous plugging is frequent, and prevention or treatment requires aggressive pulmonary toilet, with bronchoscopic suction if needed. One should be wary of a large air leak that disappears suddenly, as this is often the result of total atelectasis of that lung and can be diagnosed by chest x-ray. In contrast, if the air leak resolves and the lung is expanded, the tube is ready for removal. Figure 13.4 depicts the preoperative (a) and 2-year postoperative (b) imaging of a patient who underwent successful P/D for MPM.

Fig. 13.4 Imaging of MPM patient who underwent successful pleurectomy/decortication (P/D). Preoperative (**a**) and 2-year postoperative (**b**) images are shown

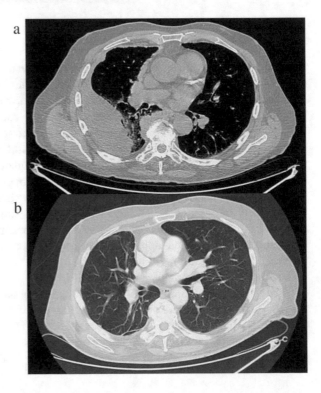

13.7 Outcomes of Surgery in MPM

13.7.1 EPP

As EPP has generally been performed in the context of multimodality therapy, results reported for this operation reflect outcomes for EPP and adjuvant treatment, such as chemotherapy, radiation therapy, or immunologic therapy. In one series of 183 patients who underwent EPP with adjuvant chemotherapy and radiation, perioperative mortality was 3.8% and morbidity was 50% (combined major and minor complications) (Sugarbaker et al. 1999). Median survival for those who did not die perioperatively was 19 months. Epithelial cell type, negative resection margins, and lack of extrapleural nodal disease were associated with a median long-term survival of 51 months.

In a phase I study of EPP with heated intraoperative chemotherapy (HIOC), the median survival for patients who received cisplatin doses of 175–200 mg/m^2 was 26 months (Sugarbaker et al. 2013). For patients with epithelial stage I or II disease, median survival was 39 months, compared to 15 months for those with stage III epithelial disease. In a larger phase II series of 121 patients who underwent EPP with HIOC, overall median survival was 12.8 months, with a median survival of 21 months for patients with early-stage disease (Tilleman et al. 2009).

In a Scottish study of 302 MPM patients, those with stage I–II disease treated with EPP and adjuvant chemotherapy had a median survival of 35 months (Aziz et al. 2002). Those treated with EPP alone experienced a survival of 13 months. In a Turkish study of 20 patients undergoing EPP followed by adjuvant radiation and platinum-based chemotherapy, median survival was 17 months (Batirel et al. 2008). Yan and colleagues published a retrospective review of 70 patients undergoing EPP followed by chemotherapy and/or radiation, in which patients experienced a median survival of 20 months (Yan et al. 2009). Adjuvant radiation and adjuvant pemetrexed-based chemotherapy were independently associated with longer survival.

A Swiss study of 19 patients who underwent EPP after induction chemotherapy and followed by adjuvant radiation reported a median survival of 23 months, with 13 patients completing the full regimen (Weder et al. 2004). In a large, multicenter prospective Swiss trial, the same investigators enrolled 61 patients, of whom 58 (95%) completed induction chemotherapy, 45 (74%) underwent EPP, and 36 (59%) received at least a portion of adjuvant radiotherapy (Weder et al. 2007). Median survival was 19.8 months for all patients and 23 months for the subgroup who underwent EPP after induction chemotherapy.

We reported a phase II trial of induction chemotherapy followed by EPP followed by adjuvant hemithoracic radiation (Flores et al. 2006). While median overall survival for all patients was 19 months, the eight patients who completed chemotherapy and EPP experienced a median survival of 35 months. A similar phase II trial involving multiple centers, and with cisplatin-pemetrexed instead of cisplatin-gemcitabine, enrolled 77 patients, with 40 (52%) patients completing the full regimen (Krug et al. 2009). Perioperative mortality was 3.7% and local recurrence occurred in 14% of patients. The median overall survival for all patients was 16.8 months and was 29 months for those who completed the full regimen. De Perrot published similar results in a retrospective analysis of 60 patients who underwent cisplatin-based chemotherapy followed by EPP with adjuvant hemithoracic radiation (de Perrot et al. 2009). Median survival for all patients was 14 months. Of the 30 patients (50%) who completed the full treatment regimen, those with node-negative final pathology demonstrated a median survival of 59 months. The same investigators conducted a phase I/II trial enrolling 25 patients to undergo EPP within 1 week of administering 25 Gy external beam intensity-modulated radiation therapy (IMRT) with patients found to have mediastinal nodal disease undergoing postoperative adjuvant chemotherapy (Cho et al. 2014). There was one (4%) postoperative death. With a median follow-up of 23 months, 3-year survival was 84% for patients with epithelial disease and 13% for those with non-epithelial (all biphasic) disease.

Despite advances in adjuvant therapy, local control remains the major barrier to long-term survival in MPM after EPP. Recurrence occurs in most patients, generally locoregional with rare hematogenous metastases. In the largest series to describe recurrence patterns after EPP-based multimodality therapy, Baldini and colleagues reported recurrence in 75% of 158 evaluable patients (nine died perioperatively, and location of recurrence was not available for another two patients) (Baldini et al. 2015). Fifty-four patients, or 72% of all episodes of recurrence, occurred in the ipsilateral hemithorax or mediastinum as the first site. The remaining distribution of recurrence was in the abdomen (53%), contralateral chest (38%), and distant sites (7%), with many patients presenting with multiple sites of simultaneous recurrence. The authors concluded that the ipsilateral chest is the most common site of treatment failure after EPP-based multimodality therapy. Flores reported a slightly different pattern of treatment failure in a retrospective review of 663 patients undergoing surgery-based multimodality therapy on various protocols (Flores et al. 2008a). Fifty-seven percent of 385 patients undergoing EPP recurred, with 33% of treatment failures occurring in the ipsilateral chest or pericardium as the first site of recurrence. The distribution site of first treatment failure was the abdomen (31%), contralateral chest (22%), abdomen and chest (8%), and bone (3%).

13.7.2   P/D

Treatment failure after P/D is most commonly found in ipsilateral chest, with 95% of sites of first recurrence occurring in the ipsilateral hemithorax and/or mediastinum in a series evaluating this question in 59 MPM patients undergoing P/D (Wolf et al. 2012). Similarly, in our series comparing EPP to P/D, 65% of first recurrences were local (Flores et al. 2008a). In an effort to decrease risk of local recurrence, various methods have been employed for adjuvant therapy, just as in EPP. In one prospective phase I/II trial, 44 patients underwent P/D with

HIOC, resulting in a median survival of 13 months for all resected patients and 18 months in the 35 patients who received higher doses of cisplatin HIOC (175–450 mg/m^2) (Richards et al. 2006).

Some have considered the remaining lung after P/D to be a limitation of adjuvant therapy in the form of external beam radiation. Several studies have demonstrated, however, that traditional hemithoracic radiation can be given safely following P/D. In the largest retrospective series of 123 patients, using a median of 42.5 Gy hemithoracic radiation after P/D, local control was seen in 42% of patients, and median survival was 13.5 months (Gupta et al. 2005). The same group reported 1- and 2-year survival of 75% and 53%, respectively, using 46.8 Gy IMRT following P/D (Rosenzweig et al. 2012). Grade 3 or 4 pneumonitis occurred in 20% of patients.

13.7.3 Data Comparing EPP to P/D

P/D is associated with better short-term outcomes than EPP in the form of perioperative morbidity and mortality. One study evaluating these results in the Society of Thoracic Surgeons Database found higher rates of acute respiratory distress syndrome, reintubation, unexpected reoperation, sepsis, and mortality after EPP compared to P/D (Burt et al. 2014).

The high risk of EPP without clear demonstration of survival benefit has led many clinicians to advocate against EPP (Treasure et al. 2011). The Mesothelioma and Radical Surgery (MARS) trial was designed to compare EPP to no surgery for MPM, but randomization was not successful in this effort. Subsequent exploratory analyses evaluating long-term outcomes lacked adequate power to draw meaningful conclusions. In the largest retrospective study comparing EPP to P/D, cumulative survival for patients with early-stage disease was found to be higher with curative-intent P/D compared to EPP (Flores et al. 2008a). For later-stage disease, EPP conferred higher cumulative survival.

Several studies have sought to compare EPP to P/D. One recent meta-analysis found significantly lower mortality and a trend toward higher cumulative survival with P/D but only included a small portion of the published literature comparing the two operations (Cao et al. 2014). A more recent meta-analysis including all English-language observational studies from 1990 to 2014 that compared the two surgical procedures analyzed 24 datasets, including 1391 patients undergoing EPP and 1512 undergoing P/D (Taioli et al. 2015b). The percentage of non-epithelial cases and the use and types of adjuvant treatment varied from study to study. There was significantly higher 30-day mortality associated with EPP (4.5% vs. 1.7%, $p < 0.05$) with little heterogeneity between studies. Among the 17 studies that reported median survival, 53% reported higher median survival with EPP (and 47% with P/D). Of the seven studies reporting at least 2-year survival, survival was similar for the cohorts, but there was significant heterogeneity among studies (Taioli et al. 2015b).

13.8 Conclusions

MPM is universally fatal without treatment. Surgery-based therapy has been associated with long-term survivors and has demonstrated 15% 5-year survival in series involving all patients (all stages and all risk factor status). While there is no standard-of-care treatment that is universally accepted, more evidence is accumulating that surgical resection has a prominent role in the context of multimodality therapy. P/D is better tolerated by patients, and evidence suggests that survival is no worse. As recurrence patterns are generally local regardless of operation, leaving the patient with two lungs after first surgery may well improve his ability to tolerate further therapy upon recurrent disease. Without a substantial benefit in terms of long-term outcomes, the added risk of EPP may not be worthwhile for most MPM patients.

Conflicts of Interest The authors declare no conflicts of interest to disclose.

References

Aziz T, Jilaihawi A, Prakash D (2002) The management of malignant pleural mesothelioma; single centre experience in 10 years. Eur J Cardiothorac Surg 22:298–305

Baldini EH, Richards WG, Gill RR et al (2015) Updated patterns of failure after multimodality therapy for malignant pleural mesothelioma. J Thorac Cardiovasc Surg 149:1374–1381

Batirel HF, Metintas M, Caglar HB et al (2008) Trimodality treatment of malignant pleural mesothelioma. J Thorac Oncol 3:499–504

Burt BM, Cameron RB, Mollberg NM et al (2014) Malignant pleural mesothelioma and the Society of Thoracic Surgeons Database: an analysis of surgical morbidity and mortality. J Thorac Cardiovasc Surg 148:30–35

Butchart EG, Ashcroft T, Barnsley WC et al (1976) Pleuropneumonectomy in the management of diffuse malignant mesothelioma of the pleura. Experience with 29 patients. Thorax 31:15–24

Cao C, Tian D, Park J et al (2014) A systematic review and meta-analysis of surgical treatments for malignant pleural mesothelioma. Lung Cancer 83:240–245

Cho BC, Feld R, Leighl N et al (2014) A feasibility study evaluating Surgery for Mesothelioma After Radiation Therapy: the "SMART" approach for resectable malignant pleural mesothelioma. J Thorac Oncol 9:397–402

de Perrot M, Feld R, Cho BC et al (2009) Trimodality therapy with induction chemotherapy followed by extrapleural pneumonectomy and adjuvant high-dose hemithoracic radiation for malignant pleural mesothelioma. J Clin Oncol 27:1413–1418

de Perrot M, Feld R, Leighl NB et al (2016) Accelerated hemithoracic radiation followed by extrapleural pneumonectomy for malignant pleural mesothelioma. J Thorac Cardiovasc Surg 151:468–473

Flores RM (2005) The role of PET in the surgical management of malignant pleural mesothelioma. Lung Cancer 49(Suppl 1):S27–S32

Flores RM, Krug LM, Rosenzweig KE et al (2006) Induction chemotherapy, extrapleural pneumonectomy, and postoperative high-dose radiotherapy for locally advanced malignant pleural mesothelioma: a phase II trial. J Thorac Oncol 1:289–295

Flores RM, Zakowski M, Venkatraman E et al (2007) Prognostic factors in the treatment of malignant pleural mesothelioma at a large tertiary referral center. J Thorac Oncol 2:957–965

Flores RM, Pass HI, Seshan VE et al (2008a) Extrapleural pneumonectomy versus pleurectomy/decortication in the surgical management of malignant pleural mesothelioma: results in 663 patients. J Thorac Cardiovasc Surg 135:620–626. 6 e1–3

Flores RM, Routledge T, Seshan VE et al (2008b) The impact of lymph node station on survival in 348 patients with surgically resected malignant pleural mesothelioma: implications for revision of the American Joint Committee on Cancer staging system. J Thorac Cardiovasc Surg 136:605–610

Flores RM (2009) Surgical options in malignant pleural mesothelioma: extrapleural pneumonectomy or pleurectomy/decortication. Semin Thorac Cardiovasc Surg 21:149–153

Flores RM, Riedel E, Donington JS et al (2010) Frequency of use and predictors of cancer-directed surgery in the management of malignant pleural mesothelioma in a community-based (Surveillance, Epidemiology, and End Results [SEER]) population. J Thorac Oncol 5:1649–1654

Flores RM (2016) Pleurectomy decortication for mesothelioma: the procedure of choice when possible. J Thorac Cardiovasc Surg 151:310–312

Gupta V, Mychalczak B, Krug L et al (2005) Hemithoracic radiation therapy after pleurectomy/decortication for malignant pleural mesothelioma. Int J Radiat Oncol Biol Phys 63:1045–1052

Kindler HL, Karrison TG, Gandara DR et al (2012) Multicenter, double-blind, placebo-controlled, randomized phase II trial of gemcitabine/cisplatin plus bevacizumab or placebo in patients with malignant mesothelioma. J Clin Oncol 30:2509–2515

Krug LM, Pass HI, Rusch VW et al (2009) Multicenter phase II trial of neoadjuvant pemetrexed plus cisplatin followed by extrapleural pneumonectomy and radiation for malignant pleural mesothelioma. J Clin Oncol 27:3007–3013

McCormack PM, Nagasaki F, Hilaris BS et al (1982) Surgical treatment of pleural mesothelioma. J Thorac Cardiovasc Surg 84:834–842

Ng JM, Hartigan PM (2008) Anesthetic management of patients undergoing extrapleural pneumonectomy for mesothelioma. Curr Opin Anaesthesiol 21:21–27

Pass HI, Temeck BK, Kranda K et al (1997) Phase III randomized trial of surgery with or without intraoperative photodynamic therapy and postoperative immunochemotherapy for malignant pleural mesothelioma. Ann Surg Oncol 4:628–633

Patz EF Jr, Shaffer K, Piwnica-Worms DR et al (1992) Malignant pleural mesothelioma: value of CT and MR imaging in predicting resectability. AJR Am J Roentgenol 159:961–966

Richards WG, Zellos L, Bueno R et al (2006) Phase I to II study of pleurectomy/decortication and intraoperative intracavitary hyperthermic cisplatin lavage for mesothelioma. J Clin Oncol 24:1561–1567

Rosenzweig KE, Zauderer MG, Laser B et al (2012) Pleural intensity-modulated radiotherapy for malignant pleural mesothelioma. Int J Radiat Oncol Biol Phys 83:1278–1283

Sarot IA (1949) Extrapleural pneumonectomy and pleurectomy in pulmonary tuberculosis. Thorax 4:173–223

Sugarbaker DJ, Flores RM, Jaklitsch MT et al (1999) Resection margins, extrapleural nodal status, and cell type determine postoperative long-term survival in trimodality therapy of malignant pleural mesothelioma: results in 183 patients. J Thorac Cardiovasc Surg 117:54–63. discussion p 65

Sugarbaker DJ, Jaklitsch MT, Bueno R et al (2004) Prevention, early detection, and management of complications after 328 consecutive extrapleural pneumonectomies. J Thorac Cardiovasc Surg 128:138–146

Sugarbaker DJ, Wolf AS (2010) Surgery for malignant pleural mesothelioma. Expert Rev Respir Med 4:363–372

Sugarbaker DJ, Wolf AS, Chirieac LR et al (2011) Clinical and pathological features of three-year survivors of malignant pleural mesothelioma following extrapleural pneumonectomy. Eur J Cardiothorac Surg 40:298–303

Sugarbaker DJ, Gill RR, Yeap BY et al (2013) Hyperthermic intraoperative pleural cisplatin chemotherapy extends interval to recurrence and survival among low-risk patients with malignant pleural mesothelioma undergoing surgical macroscopic complete resection. J Thorac Cardiovasc Surg 45:955–963

Sugarbaker DJ, Richards WG, Bueno R (2014) Extrapleural pneumonectomy in the treatment of epithelioid malignant pleural mesothelioma: novel prognostic implications of combined N1 and N2 nodal involvement based on experience in 529 patients. Ann Surg 260:577–580. discussion pp 80–82

Taioli E, Wolf AS, Camacho-Rivera M et al (2014) Women with malignant pleural mesothelioma have a threefold better survival rate than men. Ann Thorac Surg 98:1020–1024

Taioli E, Wolf AS, Camacho-Rivera M et al (2015a) Determinants of survival in malignant pleural mesothelioma: a Surveillance, Epidemiology, and End Results (SEER) study of 14,228 Patients. PLoS One 10:e0145039

Taioli E, Wolf AS, Flores RM (2015b) Meta-analysis of survival after pleurectomy decortication versus extrapleural pneumonectomy in mesothelioma. Ann Thorac Surg 99:472–480

Taioli E, Wolf AS, Moline JM et al (2015c) Frequency of surgery in black patients with malignant pleural mesothelioma. Dis Markers 2015:282145

Tilleman TR, Richards WG, Zellos L et al (2009) Extrapleural pneumonectomy followed by intracavitary intraoperative hyperthermic cisplatin with pharmacologic cytoprotection for treatment of malignant pleural mesothelioma: a phase II prospective study. J Thorac Cardiovasc Surg 138:405–411

Treasure T, Lang-Lazdunski L, Waller D et al (2011) Extra-pleural pneumonectomy versus no extra-pleural pneumonectomy for patients with malignant pleural mesothelioma: clinical outcomes of the Mesothelioma and Radical Surgery (MARS) randomised feasibility study. Lancet Oncol 12:763–772

Weder W, Kestenholz P, Taverna C et al (2004) Neoadjuvant chemotherapy followed by extrapleural pneumonectomy in malignant pleural mesothelioma. J Clin Oncol 22:3451–3457

Weder W, Stahel RA, Bernhard J et al (2007) Multicenter trial of neo-adjuvant chemotherapy followed by extrapleural pneumonectomy in malignant pleural mesothelioma. Ann Oncol 18:1196–1202

Wolf AS, Daniel J, Sugarbaker DJ (2009) Surgical techniques for multimodality treatment of malignant pleural mesothelioma: extrapleural pneumonectomy and pleurectomy/decortication. Semin Thorac Cardiovasc Surg 21:132–148

Wolf AS, Jacobson FL, Tilleman TR et al (2010a) Managing the pneumonectomy space after extrapleural pneumonectomy: postoperative intrathoracic pressure monitoring. Eur J Cardiothorac Surg 37:770–775

Wolf AS, Richards WG, Tilleman TR et al (2010b) Characteristics of malignant pleural mesothelioma in women. Ann Thorac Surg 90:949–956. discussion p 956

Wolf AS, Gill RR, Baldini EH et al (2012) Patterns of recurrence following pleurectomy/decortication for malignant pleural mesothelioma. In: Abstracts of 11th International Conference of the International Mesothelioma Interest Group

Yan TD, Boyer M, Tin MM et al (2009) Extrapleural pneumonectomy for malignant pleural mesothelioma: outcomes of treatment and prognostic factors. J Thorac Cardiovasc Surg 138:619–624

Chapter 14
Radiotherapy and Photodynamic Therapy for Malignant Pleural Mesothelioma

Charles B. Simone II, Theresa M. Busch, and Keith A. Cengel

Abstract Ionizing radiotherapy (RT) and non-ionizing radiotherapy (photodynamic therapy, PDT) play important roles in both the palliative and definitive treatment settings for patients with malignant pleural mesothelioma (MPM). As the technological sophistication of RT planning and delivery devices increases, the ability of RT to provide durable local control has become increasingly important. Similarly, PDT, which combines a photosensitizer, light, and molecular oxygen, is increasingly being used to treat thoracic malignancies, including MPM. This chapter discusses the mechanistic and logistical basics of RT and PDT and the use of these therapies in the increasingly multidisciplinary care of patients with MPM. In addition, the major clinical trials that support the use of RT and PDT in the care of patients with MPM are reviewed and discussed. Finally, the potential for future improvements and new directions for RT and PDT is described.

Keywords Mesothelioma • Ionizing radiotherapy • Non-ionizing radiotherapy • Photodynamic therapy • Surgical cytoreduction • Palliative radiotherapy • Normal tissue radiotolerance • Photosensitizers • Adjuvant and neoadjuvant hemithoracic radiotherapies • Florescence-guided resection

C.B. Simone II
Department of Radiation Oncology, Hospital of the University of Pennsylvania, Perelman School of Medicine, Philadelphia, PA 19104, USA

Department of Radiation Oncology, University of Maryland Medical Center, Baltimore, MD 21201, USA

T.M. Busch • K.A. Cengel (✉)
Department of Radiation Oncology, Hospital of the University of Pennsylvania, Perelman School of Medicine, Philadelphia, PA 19104, USA
e-mail: keith.cengel@uphs.upenn.edu

© Springer International Publishing AG 2017
J.R. Testa (ed.), *Asbestos and Mesothelioma*, Current Cancer Research,
DOI 10.1007/978-3-319-53560-9_14

14.1 Introduction and General Considerations

The treatment of patients with malignant pleural mesothelioma (MPM) is often palliative in nature, although therapy with definitive intent can be appropriate in selected patients. MPM can present with significant dyspnea due to an effusion and/or mass effect from pleural tumor. Other common symptoms include pain and anorexia. Because no single therapy is sufficient to manage most MPM patients, their care is of necessity multidisciplinary in nature. Aside from ionizing radiotherapy (RT), palliative therapies include physiologically directed therapies such as drainage of pleural effusion, medically directed therapies such as chemotherapy, and symptom-directed therapies such as narcotic analgesics. Median survivals with palliative therapies vary considerably with the stage of disease at presentation, but generally range from 6 to 14 months. Anatomically, the pleural and MPM tumor envelops the relatively radiosensitive lung parenchyma. Patients with MPM frequently experience pain and mass effects that can be difficult to palliate with surgery or chemotherapy alone. In this setting, it is important to note that the local response rates for RT meet or far exceed those of chemotherapy, and the RT can be significantly less detrimental to patient quality of life than a large and potentially morbid surgical procedure. Multidisciplinary MPM management with definitive intent typically involves surgical cytoreduction. Both RT and photodynamic therapy (PDT) have been used in attempts to increase local control and allow lung-sparing procedures to be performed.

14.2 Ionizing Versus Non-ionizing Radiotherapy

14.2.1 Fundamental Principles of RT

In RT, high-energy photons (X-rays, gamma rays) or particles (electrons, protons, heavy ions) are used to create specific distributions of ionization (absorbed dose) in patients. The therapeutic index of RT derives from a combination of spatial and radiobiological cancer cell selectivity. Spatial selectivity for cancer tissues is achieved using highly specialized equipment that modulates the fluence/energy profile of ionizing radiation delivered to create dose distributions in which the tumor tissues receive more dose than the surrounding normal tissues. Radiobiologic cancer selectivity is achieved by fractionating the radiation dose over days to weeks, typically delivering one radiation dose per weekday. In general, increases in the volume of irradiated normal tissue and/or the intrinsic normal tissue radiosensitivity require the total dose to be delivered in a larger number of fractions to mitigate the risk of radiation-induced normal tissue toxicity. Thus, for highly conformal treatment of relatively small tumors with acceptable normal tissue doses, RT to a total dose of 50–60 Gy can be completed in 3–5 fractions with a low (5–10%) risk of grade 1–3 complications and a very low (~1%) risk of grade 4–5 complications. In thoracic radiation oncology, this is exemplified by stereotactic body radiotherapy (SBRT) of peripheral, early stage lung cancers (Chang et al. 2015). Conversely, 28

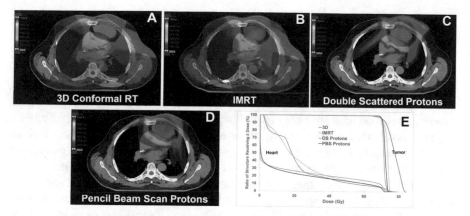

Fig. 14.1 Dose distributions produced by different RT techniques. (**a–d**) Dose color wash images for a patient with an anterior mediastinal MPM recurrence treated to 70 Gy in 35 fractions planned using 3D conformal, IMRT, double scattered (DS) protons or pencil-beam scanned (PBS) protons as indicated. (**e**) Dose volume histogram demonstrating the increasing conformality of dose to tumor provided by IMRT and protons as compared to 3D conformal RT and the increased sparing of normal tissues (e.g., the heart) with proton techniques

fractions are required to deliver a 50.4-Gy dose to a large proportion of the pleura and the risk of grade 1–3 complications increases to 15–20% (Rimner et al. 2016).

For patients with MPM, RT can be delivered using a wide variety of radiation forms (e.g., photons, electrons, protons, etc.) and an even wider array of techniques. Photon (X-ray) radiotherapy is typically delivered using a linear accelerator (LINAC), and the most basic forms of RT (2D or 3D) typically consist of geometric field shapes (portals) defined by multileaf collimator (MLC) blocks delivered from 1 to 4 beam angles (Fig. 14.1a). More complex dose distributions can be achieved using an intensity modulated radiotherapy (IMRT) technique, in which the fluence across each portal is modulated by using multiple different MLC configurations per portal. While this can create highly conformal dose distributions with convex or concave geometry, the dose gradients are achieved at the cost of increased volume of normal tissues receiving a lower RT dose (Fig. 14.1b). Additional conformality, and increased volume of normal tissue receiving a lower RT dose, is achieved by moving the gantry in a rotational arc, whereas the MLC is adjusted continuously while the beam is delivered in a technique called volumetric modulated arc radiotherapy (VMAT). Other mechanical solutions for modulating photon RT doses include CyberKnife and TomoTherapy, but these also suffer from the fundamental problem of increased low dose to normal tissues. Thus, the physical characteristics of photons fundamentally limit the dose distributions that can be achieved, even as the technology to plan and deliver RT increases in sophistication. Charged particle radiotherapy using protons has the potential to provide a greater degree of spatial control over radiation dose distribution and permit the delivery of increasing doses of ionizing radiation to malignant tumors while sparing dose to critical normal tissues (Fig. 14.1c, d, e). Early experience using proton RT for patients with MPM has been quite promising (Li et al. 2015; Pan et al. 2015). Nevertheless, there remain significant technological hurdles to overcome before the true potential of proton RT can be realized.

14.2.2   Fundamental Principles of PDT

In contrast to ionizing RT, PDT combines non-ionizing radiation (visible or near-infrared light), a photosensitizing agent (PS), and molecular oxygen to produce cellular cytotoxicity. The essential mechanism for PDT cytotoxicity involves the capture of light energy by the photosensitizer and transfer of this energy to oxygen, thus creating excited singlet-state oxygen and other reactive oxygen species. The excited oxygen species then mediate tumor cytotoxicity through direct mechanisms such as tumor cell apoptosis or necrosis, as well as indirect mechanisms, such as damage to the tumor's blood supply. In addition to the tumor cell (direct) and tumor microenvironment (indirect) effects that act to produce local tumor control, PDT can act to stimulate an antitumor immune response that affects both local and systemic disease controls. Thus, the response to PDT is complex and depends upon many factors, including the specific photosensitizer used, the dose and subcellular localization of the photosensitizer, the light dose and fluence rate, the timing between photosensitizer and light delivery, the presence of oxygen, and the underlying molecular abnormalities in the neoplastic cell and the underlying host antitumor immune balance.

As noted above, the three main components of PDT are light, PS, and oxygen. Monochromatic light with a wavelength designed to match peak absorption for a specific PS is typically produced by a laser and delivered using a variety of applicators. Treating limited areas of the pleura can be achieved using either a microlens or cylindrically diffusing optical fiber. Treating the entire pleura is achieved using a custom-designed, spherically diffusing light probe, in conjunction with isotropic light detectors that measure the dose of light in real time (Fig. 14.2). The PS is typically delivered intravenously and has the potential to selectively accumulate in tumors as compared to normal tissues. Indeed, initial preclinical evidence suggested that PS can be more selectively retained in tumors than in some normal tissues. However, in patients with either serosal (peritoneal or pleural)-based spread of malignancy, the uptake ratio of tumor as compared to clinically relevant normal tissues such as the lung or bowel may not be as dramatic as predicted by preclinical models (Cengel et al. 2007). Emerging technologies have the potential to increase the tumor cell selectivity of PDT by combining PS into molecularly targeted, multifunctional nanoparticles or by conjugating PS to antitumor antibodies. In addition to light and PS, oxygen is required for effective PDT-mediated cytotoxicity. Preclinical studies of cancer cells and tissues under a variety of oxygen concentrations demonstrate that pretreatment tumor/cellular hypoxia significantly decreases PDT efficacy. Studies of PDT and tumor hypoxia in clinical samples confirm the relationship between hypoxia and decreased PDT efficacy, but they also suggest that the intra- and inter-patient heterogeneity in tumor hypoxia may hinder a universal or one-fit solution to this problem. Moreover, it is important to consider that PDT itself consumes oxygen and that the rate of molecular oxygen consumption by PDT depends on the fluence rate of the light (amount of light energy delivered to an area as a function of time). At high fluence rates, the consumption of oxygen can lead to increased tumor hypoxia during treatment and decrease the PDT efficacy that can be compounded by PDT-induced vascular damage/shutdown. However, the vascular

Fig. 14.2 PDT techniques and apparatus for MPM. PDT is performed using a spherical light diffuser (*top panel*) and delivered to the resection bed for all pleural surfaces with the assistance of diluted intralipid as a light scattering medium (*middle panel*). Light dose is measured in real time using isotropic detectors and displayed on a monitor (*bottom panel*)

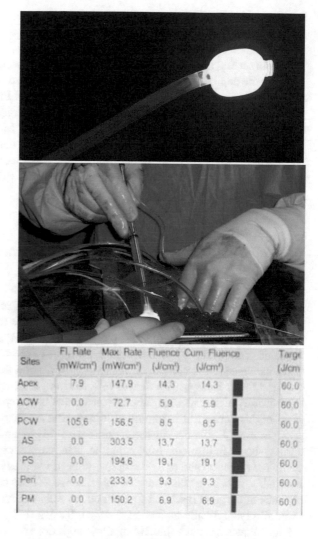

Sites	Fl. Rate (mW/cm²)	Max. Rate (mW/cm²)	Fluence (J/cm²)	Cum. Fluence (J/cm²)		Target (J/cm
Apex	7.9	147.9	14.3	14.3	▮	60.0
ACW	0.0	72.7	5.9	5.9	▮	60.0
PCW	105.6	156.5	8.5	8.5	▮	60.0
AS	0.0	303.5	13.7	13.7	▮	60.0
PS	0.0	194.6	19.1	19.1	▮	60.0
Peri	0.0	233.3	9.3	9.3	▮	60.0
PM	0.0	150.2	6.9	6.9	▮	60.0

anatomy and other tumor and/or patient-specific factors are likely to affect the absolute value for this fluence rate limit. Adding real-time monitoring of tumor blood flow and tissue oxygenation might allow modulation of light doses to ameliorate these effects. Such technology to improve PDT dosimetry is under development, along with methods to more accurately measure light, PS, and even $^1O_2$ in real time.

PDT has several potential advantages when compared with conventional therapies. Unlike ionizing RT and many chemotherapy agents, PDT with typical photosensitizers targets neither tumor deoxyribonucleic acid specifically nor rapidly dividing cells more generally. Thus, PDT-induced secondary cancers are highly unlikely to occur, and PDT-mediated cytotoxicity is not intrinsically linked to RT or cytotoxic chemotherapy sensitivity. PDT can also be repeated to the same site without compromising efficacy or increasing toxicity, and PDT does not compromise the ability to administer other treatment modalities in patients with recurrent or residual disease. By combining (partially) tumor selective destruction with the ability to treat and conform to relatively large surface areas, PDT is especially attractive for use in serosal malignancies such as MPM. Moreover, the intrinsic, physical limitation in the depth of effective visible light penetration through tissue (2–10 mm for red light) limits PDT damage to deeper structures and thereby provides additional potential for tumor cell selectivity while reducing toxicity to the underlying organs such as the lung. This property allows for treatment of relatively large surface areas with acceptable toxicity while simultaneously limiting the usefulness to cancers that are relatively superficial (<1 cm in tumor thickness). Consequently, surgical exposure and debulking is typically required for optimal PDT efficacy when treating deeper-seeded, bulkier cancers.

14.2.3   RT, PDT, and Surgical Cytoreduction

Definitive approaches to managing patients with MPM typically involve combinations of multiple standard treatment modalities and must address both widespread local disease and the high risk of systemic disease. This is made more challenging because the potential morbidity of highly aggressive local treatment strategies can limit the implementation of aggressive systemic treatment strategies and vice versa. Nevertheless, in patients with a good performance status and few comorbidities, therapy with definitive intention (and higher RT doses) can lead to significantly higher median survivals than have been reported with palliative therapies. In this context, it is important to note that no single modality, including surgery, is highly effective in the treatment of MPM and that the strategy in any surgery-based multimodal treatment plan is to use surgery to achieve a macroscopic complete resection and to then employ other modalities in an attempt to control the inevitably present residual microscopic disease. RT has been used definitively in the absence of surgical resection in selected patients to treat bulky areas of disease or even all glycolytically active (FDG-avid) disease (Feigen et al. 2011), but current RT techniques are not sufficient to allow high dose RT to all pleural surfaces without unacceptable toxicity. Accordingly, definitive radiotherapy is frequently associated with surgical therapy, and this section will discuss the role of PDT and RT in the surgically based multimodality therapy of patients with MPM.

In the overwhelming majority of MPM patients, even the most aggressive surgical resection results in high rates of local relapse. For this reason, both RT and PDT have been used to treat microscopic residual disease following surgery that was performed with the goal of achieving a macroscopically complete resection (MCR). One strategy for MCR involves an extrapleural pneumonectomy (EPP), in which the parietal pleura, diaphragm, pericardium, and lung are resected en bloc. The other commonly used strategy is the lung-sparing pleurectomy/decortication (P/D), which when performed with the intent of achieving an MCR is often referred to as an extended P/D (eP/D) or radical pleurectomy. As there is no surgical procedure

accepted as the standard of care for pleural malignancies, there is certainly no procedure acknowledged as the standard cytoreductive operation, and both EPP and
eP/D are performed at high-volume MPM surgical centers (see chapter Surgery
Approaches in Mesothelioma of this volume by Wolf and Flores).

14.3   Palliative RT for Patients with MPM

Patients with MPM often experience severe pain and/or dyspnea. The etiology of
pain is likely to be multifactorial but can include pain due to invasion of structures
such as the chest wall or diaphragm by tumor, as well as pain due to a malignant
pleural effusion. The dyspnea is also multifactorial, but can arise from compressive
atelectasis of the lung by a combination of mass and pleural effusion, decreased
lung compliance/ventilation due to circumferential involvement of the lung by
tumor, and alteration in ventilation perfusion matching. In general, palliative RT
aims to identify and alleviate the most proximal or significant cause of distress. This
section will discuss techniques and results for palliative RT in patients with MPM.

14.3.1   The Problem of Normal Tissue Radiotolerance

As noted above, the essence of the problem with MPM is that the radiotolerance of
the normal thoracic tissues is insufficient to allow for effective tumoricidal RT doses
to all pleural surfaces using conventional radiation therapy (photons and electrons)
while preserving normal/sufficient cardiopulmonary function. Proton radiotherapy
may allow for an unprecedented degree of RT conformality due to increased spatial
control of dose deposition. Early reports of proton RT as a part of a multimodality
management schema (including sequential chemotherapy) demonstrate the potential to achieve dramatic and long-lasting clinical benefits for patients with MPM (Li
et al. 2015). Nevertheless, several technological challenges remain that must be
overcome before proton RT can be used to treat the entirety of the pleura while sparing the underlying lung. Until these are surmounted, proton or photon RT is typically limited to treatment of the peripheral pleural in the definitive/surgical setting
or to treating specific, symptomatic regions in the palliative setting.

14.3.2   RT for Palliation of Pain in Patients with MPM

While RT is frequently used for palliation of symptoms in patients with MPM, there
are few robust studies in the literature that describe response rates or define the optimal dose/fractionation. In a retrospective review of RT in 54 patients with advanced
MPM, the infield radiologic response rate was 43% at 2 months, which compares

favorably with objective response rates for multi-agent chemotherapy (Jenkins et al. 2011). It should be noted that MPM tumors can take several months to reach minimal size following RT, so that this 2-month time point may underestimate the true RT objective response rate. In addition, pain response frequently occurs prior to or in the absence of objective tumor shrinkage. Indeed, a systematic literature review noted that the reported RT response rates for pain range from 50 to 69%, although the supporting studies are largely retrospective or descriptive in nature (Macleod et al. 2014). Therefore, Macleod and colleagues undertook a phase II trial (SYSTEMS) of RT for pain palliation in 40 patients recruited at three oncology centers in the UK of whom 35 received RT (MacLeod et al. 2015). Of the 30 patients who were assessable at week 5 after receiving 20 Gy in 5 daily fractions, 47% experienced an improvement in pain scores. Of note, 14/19 patients achieved either a partial response or stable disease by modified RECIST 1.1 criteria for an overall response rate of 74% at 12 weeks. These encouraging results have led the investigators to initiate the SYSTEMS-2 trial, a randomized trial of 20 Gy/5 fractions vs. 36 Gy in 6 fractions to determine whether dose escalation might improve pain palliation.

14.4   Definitive PDT for Patients with MPM

14.4.1   Porfimer Sodium-Mediated PDT

Unlike lung cancer, in which PDT can be delivered as monotherapy or as part of multi-modality therapy, PDT for MPM only has a role in definitive therapy as part of a multimodality treatment regimen. When combined with surgery, PDT is generally well tolerated, but it does result in localized inflammation and fluid accumulation in the immediate postoperative setting and may modestly extend hospital stay beyond what is seen with the surgical procedure alone. Trials using porfimer sodium comprise the majority of the clinical experience with pleural PDT. In the early 1990s, several phase 1 and 2 studies were performed at the US National Cancer Institute and the Roswell Park Cancer Institute. Pass and colleagues performed a phase 1 trial of pleural PDT in patients with pleural malignancies (40 MPM, 8 NSCLC, 6 sarcoma/fibrous tumor of the pleura) using 2 mg/kg porfimer sodium and a drug light interval of 24–48 h (Pass et al. 1994). The surgery was an EPP in the majority of patients, and the protocol required the tumor to be surgically resectable such that any residual disease had a thickness of ≤5 mm. Fifty-four patients were enrolled, of which 42 went on to have intraoperative PDT, while the remaining 12 patients were unable to complete PDT due to inability to resect to within 5 mm (9 patients) or intraoperative complications (3 patients). The time between PS dosing and light delivery (drug-light interval) was 48 hours for the first 33 patients and 24 h for the remaining 9 patients. Light (630 nm) was delivered using combined intralipid plus spherical light diffuser, as described above (Fig. 14.2), and light dose was measured using a real-time, four-position, non-isotropic dosimetry system. Two out of three patients treated with a 24-h drug light interval and 32.5 J/cm^2 experienced esophageal perforations that were considered dose-limiting toxicities (DLT), and the maximally tolerated dose was 30 J/cm^2 with a 24-h drug light interval. While not designed to measure overall survival, the median survival for the overall cohort was 13 months, which was considered promising and worthy of further study. Similarly, Takita and colleagues treated 40 patients with MPM using surgical resection (33 P/D, 7 EPP) and intraoperative porfimer sodium-mediated PDT and a drug light interval of 48 hour, with 20–30 J/cm^2 of 630 nm light (Moskal et al. 1998). The median survival was 36 months for stage I–II patients ($n = 13$) and 10 months for patients with more advanced disease ($n = 24$) ($p < 0.0001$). On multivariate analysis, PDT dose was determined to be an independent prognostic indicator for overall survival ($p < 0.009$).

Based on the promising phase 1 results, Pass and colleagues performed a randomized phase 3 study in which patients with surgically resectable MPM confined to one hemithorax were randomly assigned to receive intraoperative PDT using porfimer sodium and drug light interval of 24 h versus no intraoperative adjuvant therapy (Pass et al. 1997). Patients on both arms received postoperative, adjuvant chemoimmunotherapy using tamoxifen, cisplatin, and subcutaneous interferon alpha. Of the 48 patients who completed therapy (25 PDT, 23 non-PDT), 26 patients had tumor resected via EPP (14 PDT, 11 non-PDT) and 23 patients had tumor resected via P/D (11 PDT, 12 non-PDT). With a median potential follow-up among all patients (regardless of survival) of 23 months from surgery, there was no difference in the median overall survival in the PDT group versus the non-PDT group (14.1 vs. 14.4 months, respectively). Similarly, no difference was detected in the median recurrence-free survival (8.5 vs. 7.7 months, respectively).

Continued evolution of the pleural PDT technique at the University of Pennsylvania led to the initiation of a pilot trial of porfimer sodium-mediated PDT for patients with malignant pleural disease using a seven-detector, isotropic light dosimetry system. All patients received PDT using porfimer sodium, a 24-h drug light interval, and 60-J/cm^2 light which was determined to be the equivalent of 30 J/cm^2 using the older, non-isotropic detector system. When survival was compared between 14 patients receiving EPP with intraoperative PDT and 14 receiving radical pleurectomy (current terminology = eP/D) with intraoperative PDT, the median overall survival for the EPP patients was 8.4 months, while the median overall survival for the eP/D-PDT patients had not been reached with a 2.1-year median follow-up. A follow-up study that included 38 patients with MPM (37/38 stage III/IV), treated using eP/D-PDT as described above, demonstrated a median overall survival of 31.7 months in all patients and a 41.2-month median overall survival in the subgroup of patients with epithelial histology (Friedberg et al. 2012). Finally, a recent extension of this work detailing the results of eP/D-PDT in 73 patients with epithelial MPM demonstrated a 3-year overall survival among all patients, with a 7.3-year overall survival in the 19 N0 patients (Friedberg et al. 2016). Interestingly, there was a clear separation between the progression-free survival and overall survival curves for patients with epithelial MPM, which is unusual when compared to other surgical series. The reasons for the differences between this experience and prior porfimer sodium-mediated PDT trials remain an area of active investigation, but may be related to improvements in both PDT and surgical techniques. Of note, in the phase 3 randomized trial, the median survival of patients receiving EPP was 11 months, while the survival of patients receiving eP/D was 22 months ($p = 0.07$), but the effect of PDT on survival within each surgical-type cohort was not analyzed. Moreover, a pilot study comparing PDT with hyperbaric oxygen (HBO) to surgery alone demonstrated a superior overall survival for PDT/HBO (Matzi et al. 2004), and a randomized trial of eP/D with or without porfimer sodium-mediated PDT in patients with epithelial MPM is currently ongoing (NCT02153229).

14.4.2   PPDT Using Other Photosensitizers

The second-generation photosensitizer mTHPC has been evaluated in patients with MPM in several clinical studies. In a pilot study of eight patients who received EPP-PDT using 0.3 mg/kg of mTHPC with a 48-h drug light interval and 10 J/cm² of 652-nm light (Ris et al. 1996), seven patients had local control of their disease by CT scan, but developed distant metastases or contralateral disease 4 to 18 months after the procedure. Pass and colleagues reported on a phase 1 study of EPP-PDT in which patients with MPM received 0.075 mg/kg to 0.15 mg/kg mTHPC with a drug light interval of 4 or 6 days (Schouwink et al. 2001). The dose-limiting toxicity including PDT-related death was reached at a dose level including 0.15 mg/kg mTHPC, a drug light interval of 4 days, and light fluence of 10 J/cm². In a parallel trial conducted with a similar design at the University of Pennsylvania, 26 patients were treated with surgical resection (7 EPP, 19 eP/D) and intraoperative mTHPC-mediated PDT (Friedberg et al. 2003). In this study, two out of three patients treated at the 0.1 mg/kg mTHPC/10 J/cm² dose level with a 4-day drug light interval experienced a cyto-kine-related capillary leak syndrome that was felt to be definitely related to protocol therapy and eventually lead to patient demise, suggesting that PDT with an intact lung might have a slightly different therapeutic index. Despite the use of the second-generation photosensitizer, the median overall survival in both of these trials was 10–12.4 months. Thus, while second-generation sensitizers may have pharmaco-logically and biophysically superior properties, initial attempts have shown no demonstrable clinical advantage as compared to initial trials with porfimer sodium.

14.5   Definitive RT for Patients with MPM

As noted above, definitive RT approaches to patients with MPM almost exclusively involve multimodality approaches including surgical cytoreduction. Following sur-gical cytoreduction by either EPP or eP/D, hemithoracic RT has been used in an attempt to diminish the risk of local recurrence.

14.5.1 Adjuvant Hemithoracic RT Following EPP

Several techniques for irradiation of the chest wall after EPP have been described. Using 3D conformal photon (X-ray) RT techniques, it is possible to treat the entire hemithorax to a total dose of 30–40 Gy with boost doses in high-risk regions of up to 60 Gy. These techniques generally lead to significant toxicity to achieve what are typically subtherapeutic doses with multiple long-term complications, including radiation pneumonitis, pulmonary fibrosis, pulmonary vascular damage, esophagitis, pericarditis, and pneumothorax. More modern techniques include mixed photon-electron (Yajnik et al. 2003) and hemithoracic IMRT techniques (Forster et al. 2003). Although the mixed photon-electron technique results in a decrease in the volume of contralateral lung exposed to lower RT doses (Hill-Kayser et al. 2009), the majority of current studies use IMRT or VMAT approaches due to the increased conformality and consistency in delivery. It should be noted that there is a significant learning curve for treatment planning in these cases, with experienced centers demonstrating clearly superior plans in terms of dose to target vs. normal tissues (Patel et al. 2012).

Outcomes following delivery of therapeutic doses of radiation to the involved hemithorax have demonstrated promising local control and serious but potentially tolerable toxicities. Multiple centers have reported on results of similar protocols comprised of neoadjuvant chemotherapy, EPP, and postoperative hemithoracic RT (Weder et al. 2007; Krug et al. 2009; de Perrot et al. 2009; Van Schil et al. 2010; Federico et al. 2013; Gomez et al. 2013; Thieke et al. 2015; Hasegawa et al. 2016) (Table 14.1). These studies have typically included about 2/3 earlier stage (AJCC 7th edition stage I/II) MPM patients treated with total doses of 50–60 Gy in 1.8–2-

Table 14.1 Selected large studies of EPP followed by hemithoracic RT

Citation	Total no. patients (%)			Stage I/II vs. III/IV	RT dose (Gy)	Overall survival (mos.)	
	Initial	EPP	RT			ITT	RT
Weder et al. (2007)	61 (100)	45 (74)	36 (59)	64% vs. 26%	50–60	19.8	NR
Krug et al. (2009)	77 (100)	57 (74)	40 (59)	52% vs. 48%	54	16.8	29.1
de Perrot et al. (2009)	60 (100)	45 (75)	30 (50)	58% vs. 42%	50-60	14	59 (N0), 14 (N+)
Van Schil et al. (2010)	58 (100)	42 (72)	37 (64)	88% vs. 12%	54	18.4	32.9
Gomez et al. (2013)	NR	136 (100)	86 (64)	50% N0, 50% N+	45–60	NR	14.7
Federico et al. (2013)	54 (100)	45 (83)	25 (46)	60% vs. 40%	50.4–54	15.5	NR
Thieke et al. (2015)	NR	NR	62	NR	50–54	NR	20.4
Hasegawa et al. (2016)	42 (100)	30 (71)	17 (40)	64% vs. 36%	54	19.9	39

Gy fractions. Median overall survival for all patients under an intention to treat analysis that includes all patients who started chemotherapy ranged from 14 to 20 months. When patients who did not complete the full course of trimodality treatment are excluded, median overall survivals are significantly improved to 15–40 months. However, 70–75% of patients did not undergo surgery primarily due to disease progression on chemotherapy (EPP column in Table 14.1), and only 40–60% of patients completed the full trimodality course (RT column in Table 14.1). As mentioned above, there is a relatively steep learning curve required to produce RT plans that minimize the dose to normal tissue, and even at experienced centers there remains a significant rate of radiation pneumonitis that is fatal in 3–10% of treated patients. Indeed, in one trial, 46% of patients developed radiation pneumonitis, and analysis of these data suggests that low-dose spread to the contralateral lung can result in potentially fatal pulmonary toxicity (Allen et al. 2006).

In non-randomized comparisons of institutional data, patients who complete RT have superior progression-free and overall survival when compared to patients who only complete EPP. However, there is an obvious potential for bias in these results, since patients who undergo EPP without RT are often too moribund to receive RT or have rapidly progressive disease. In an attempt to quantify the potential magnitude of benefit of post-EPP RT, the Swiss Group for Clinical Cancer Research (SAKK) conducted a randomized clinical trial of preoperative chemotherapy followed by EPP with or without RT at 14 centers in Switzerland, Belgium, and Germany (Stahel et al. 2015). In this trial, 151 patients with stage I–III MPM received preoperative chemotherapy consisting of cisplatin/pemetrexed every 21 days for three cycles. Following chemotherapy, 113 (75%) underwent EPP, and 96 of these patients achieved an MCR. Of these 96 patients, 54 underwent randomization to postoperative IMRT (27 in each group). Final analysis of these data failed to demonstrate a statistically significant improvement in overall survival. Critiques of this study noted that the radiotherapy cohort consisted of only 27 patients out of the original 151 who were treated at 14 centers with three different dose/fractionation schemes without central radiotherapy quality assurance and also noted the aforementioned impact of center RT experienced on quality of plans. In addition, the OS for all 151 patients was 15 months, which is on the lower end of the intention to treat (ITT) overall survivals noted in Table 14.1. Nevertheless, these findings, along with the generally superior results of protocols using lung-sparing surgery, raise a cautionary note for the future of EPP/RT in the management of patients with MPM.

14.5.2 Adjuvant Hemithoracic RT Following eP/D

As lung-sparing MCR procedures have become more common, the need to develop additional technologies to reduce the rate of local recurrence following surgical cytoreduction is increasingly urgent. PDT (discussed above), hyperthermic chemotherapy, and hyperthermia povidone iodine can be used intraoperatively. Postoperative RT cannot be delivered to all pleural surfaces, including the major/

minor fissures, even with the most advanced RT techniques/technology. However, the group at Memorial Sloan Kettering Cancer Center in New York has pioneered a technique using IMRT to treat the peripheral pleural space that carries the highest risk of local recurrence. In the recently published IMPRINT study, 45 patients with MPM were treated with neoadjuvant chemotherapy, 21 of which underwent lung-sparing surgery (Rimner et al. 2016). Of these, 16 underwent postoperative RT. Among 27 patients treated with RT (median dose: 46.8 Gy), the median overall survival was 23.7 months. Similar results have been reported by other groups, with 20 patients experiencing a 33-month median overall survival in one trial and 20 patients experiencing a median overall survival of 28.4 months in another trial (Chance et al. 2015; Minatel et al. 2014). Taken together, these results suggest that IMRT can be used following lung-sparing surgery with potentially promising results on a par or perhaps even superior to those achieved with EPP and RT with lower rates of toxicities than were previously reported with older RT delivery techniques.

14.5.3 Neoadjuvant Hemithoracic RT Followed by EPP

Preoperative radiotherapy has been used in other thoracic malignancies, including lung and esophageal cancer, with significant success. To test the feasibility and outcomes of this approach in patients with clinically node negative MPM, de Perrot and colleagues initiated a trial in which patients received 25 Gy in 5 daily fractions to the entire hemithorax with a simultaneous infield boost of 5 Gy to areas of high-risk disease (de Perrot et al. 2016). This was followed 6 days later by EPP and resulted in a median overall survival of 36 months in the entire patient cohort (ITT). In patients with epithelial MPM, the median overall survival was 51 months. Although this number should be interpreted with some caution, since the majority of patients are censored prior to 3 years, these results suggest that the fully mature data will continue to demonstrate the potential clinical promise of this approach.

14.5.4 Adjuvant Prophylactic Radiotherapy to Interventional Sites

MPM has a propensity to seed interventional sites. To reduce this risk, superficial (orthovoltage X-rays or electrons) RT is often employed in prophylactic tract irradiation (PIT). The reported rates of intervention site metastases in the absence of RT vary considerably, with the control (no prophylactic radiation) arm of the three published, randomized clinical trials of prophylactic intervention site RT showing 10–40% of patients developing intervention site metastases (Boutin et al. 1995; Bydder et al. 2004; O'Rourke et al. 2007) (Table 14.2). Overall, while many radiotherapists recommend prophylactic intervention site RT, more study is needed to identify which patients might benefit most from this therapy. A multicenter

Table 14.2 Randomized trials of prophylactic irradiation of surgical tracts (PIT) in patients with MPM

Citation	No. patients	RT details	Tract relapse rate (%)		p-value
			No PIT	PIT	
Boutin et al. (1995)	20	21 Gy/3 Fx <15 days post procedure	40	0	<0.001
Bydder et al. (2004)	43	10 Gy/1 Fx < 15 days post procedure	10	7	n.s.
O'Rourke et al. (2007)	61	21 Gy/3 Fx < 21 days post procedure	13	10	n.s.
Bayman et al. (2016)	374	21 Gy/3 Fx	Pending study completion		

randomized phase 3 trial of PIT vs. observation was initiated with full accrual anticipated in 2016 (Bayman et al. 2016). Given its size, this trial should significantly improve our understanding of the potential benefits of PIT in patients with MPM.

14.6   New Horizons for Patients with MPM

14.6.1   RT Technology Meets Tumor Biology

Increases in the technological sophistication of RT planning and delivery will continue to outline new uses of RT in the management of patients with MPM. Currently, the ability to place high doses of RT with precision using technologies such as SBRT allows treatment to sites of oligometastases and oligoprogression in an attempt to provide local control at multiple disease sites. Going forward, technologies such as image-guided, stereotactic proton RT will only increase the ability to create such "pockets" of local control. The major challenge in this respect is to better identify which patients or circumstances this local control might translate to changing the natural history of the disease and therefore affect patient survival. In addition, the potential effects of localized RT on systemic host-antitumor immunity are only beginning to be explored. Ongoing studies such as those with definitive RT to oligometastases or RT with immunotherapeutic drugs such as checkpoint inhibitors will help to clarify some of these questions, but clearly more studies are needed.

14.6.2   Molecularly Targeted PDT and Fluorescence-Guided Resection

As the signaling mechanisms of PDT-mediated cytotoxicity are further elucidated, new molecular targets will continue to develop that may improve the therapeutic index of PDT. Currently, agents directed against EGFR and angiogenesis have shown promise in preclinical testing. Another potential mechanism for enhancing the efficacy of PDT is through improving the PS targeting to tumor vs. normal tissue, using strategies such as nanoparticle-based PS delivery vehicles combined with molecular targeting. In addition, as fluorescence-guided resection agents are tested and perfected in thoracic oncology (Okusanya et al. 2015), the development of theranostic PDT strategies will follow in which the surgeon can "see it, resect it, and treat the residual." Moreover, current preclinical development of multifunctional nanoparticles that provide for cancer cell targeting with inhibition of critical signaling pathways with PS that can be used for theranostic PDT has the potential to revolutionize surgical and adjuvant therapy approaches in MPM patients.

Declaration of Interests The authors declare no potential conflict of interest.

References

Allen AM, Czerminska M, Janne PA et al (2006) Fatal pneumonitis associated with intensity-modulated radiation therapy for mesothelioma. Int J Radiat Oncol Biol Phys 65:640–645

Bayman N, Ardron D, Ashcroft L et al (2016) Protocol for PIT: a phase III trial of prophylactic irradiation of tracts in patients with malignant pleural mesothelioma following invasive chest wall intervention. BMJ Open 6:e010589

Boutin C, Rey F, Viallat JR (1995) Prevention of malignant seeding after invasive diagnostic procedures in patients with pleural mesothelioma. A randomized trial of local radiotherapy. Chest 108:754–758

Bydder S, Phillips M, Joseph DJ et al (2004) A randomised trial of single-dose radiotherapy to prevent procedure tract metastasis by malignant mesothelioma. Br J Cancer 91:9–10

Cengel KA, Glatstein E, Hahn SM (2007) Intraperitoneal photodynamic therapy. Cancer Treat Res 134:493–514

Chance WW, Rice DC, Allen PK et al (2015) Hemithoracic intensity modulated radiation therapy after pleurectomy/decortication for malignant pleural mesothelioma: toxicity, patterns of failure, and a matched survival analysis. Int J Radiat Oncol Biol Phys 91:149–156

Chang JY, Senan S, Paul MA et al (2015) Stereotactic ablative radiotherapy versus lobectomy for operable stage I non-small-cell lung cancer: a pooled analysis of two randomised trials. Lancet Oncol 16:630–637

de Perrot M, Feld R, Cho BC et al (2009) Trimodality therapy with induction chemotherapy followed by extrapleural pneumonectomy and adjuvant high-dose hemithoracic radiation for malignant pleural mesothelioma. J Clin Oncol 27:1413–1418

de Perrot M, Feld R, Leighl NB et al (2016) Accelerated hemithoracic radiation followed by extrapleural pneumonectomy for malignant pleural mesothelioma. J Thorac Cardiovasc Surg 151:468–473

Federico R, Adolfo F, Giuseppe M et al (2013) Phase II trial of neoadjuvant pemetrexed plus cisplatin followed by surgery and radiation in the treatment of pleural mesothelioma. BMC Cancer 13:22

Feigen M, Lee ST, Lawford C et al (2011) Establishing locoregional control of malignant pleural mesothelioma using high-dose radiotherapy and (18) F-FDG PET/CT scan correlation. J Med Imaging Radiat Oncol 55:320–332

Forster KM, Smythe WR, Starkschall G et al (2003) Intensity-modulated radiotherapy following extrapleural pneumonectomy for the treatment of malignant mesothelioma: clinical implementation. Int J Radiat Oncol Biol Phys 55:606–616

Friedberg JS, Culligan MJ, Mick R et al (2012) Radical pleurectomy and intraoperative photodynamic therapy for malignant pleural mesothelioma. Ann Thorac Surg 93:1658–1665. discussion 1665–1657

Friedberg JS, Mick R, Stevenson J et al (2003) A phase I study of Foscan-mediated photodynamic therapy and surgery in patients with mesothelioma. Ann Thorac Surg 75:952–959

Friedberg JS, Simone CB 2nd, Culligan MJ et al (2016) Extended pleurectomy-decortication-based treatment for advanced stage epithelial mesothelioma yielding a median survival of nearly three years. Ann Thorac Surg. [Epub ahead of print]

Gomez DR, Hong DS, Allen PK et al (2013) Patterns of failure, toxicity, and survival after extrapleural pneumonectomy and hemithoracic intensity-modulated radiation therapy for malignant pleural mesothelioma. J Thorac Oncol 8:238–245

Hasegawa S, Okada M, Tanaka F et al (2016) Trimodality strategy for treating malignant pleural mesothelioma: results of a feasibility study of induction pemetrexed plus cisplatin followed by extrapleural pneumonectomy and postoperative hemithoracic radiation (Japan Mesothelioma Interest Group 0601 Trial). Int J Clin Oncol 21:523–530

Hill-Kayser CE, Avery S, Mesina CF et al (2009) Hemithoracic radiotherapy after extrapleural pneumonectomy for malignant pleural mesothelioma: a dosimetric comparison of two well-described techniques. J Thorac Oncol 4:1431–1437

Jenkins P, Milliner R, Salmon C (2011) Re-evaluating the role of palliative radiotherapy in malignant pleural mesothelioma. Eur J Cancer 47:2143–2149

Krug LM, Pass HI, Rusch VW et al (2009) Multicenter phase II trial of neoadjuvant pemetrexed plus cisplatin followed by extrapleural pneumonectomy and radiation for malignant pleural mesothelioma. J Clin Oncol 27:3007–3013

Li Y, Alley E, Friedberg J et al (2015) Prospective assessment of proton therapy for malignant pleural mesothelioma. International Association for the Study of Lung Cancer Annual Meeting, Denver, CO

MacLeod N, Chalmers A, O'Rourke N et al (2015) Is radiotherapy useful for treating pain in mesothelioma?: a phase II trial. J Thorac Oncol 10:944–950

Macleod N, Price A, O'Rourke N et al (2014) Radiotherapy for the treatment of pain in malignant pleural mesothelioma: a systematic review. Lung Cancer 83:133–138

Matzi V, Maier A, Woltsche M et al (2004) Polyhematoporphyrin-mediated photodynamic therapy and decortication in palliation of malignant pleural mesothelioma: a clinical pilot study. Interact Cardiovasc Thorac Surg 3:52–56

Minatel E, Trovo M, Polesel J et al (2014) Radical pleurectomy/decortication followed by high dose of radiation therapy for malignant pleural mesothelioma. Final results with long-term follow-up. Lung Cancer 83:78–82

Moskal TL, Dougherty TJ, Urschel JD et al (1998) Operation and photodynamic therapy for pleural mesothelioma: 6-year follow-up. Ann Thorac Surg 66:1128–1133

O'Rourke N, Garcia JC, Paul J et al (2007) A randomised controlled trial of intervention site radiotherapy in malignant pleural mesothelioma. Radiother Oncol 84:18–22

Okusanya OT, DeJesus EM, Jiang JX et al (2015) Intraoperative molecular imaging can identify lung adenocarcinomas during pulmonary resection. J Thorac Cardiovasc Surg 150:28–35.e1

Pan HY, Jiang S, Sutton J et al (2015) Early experience with intensity modulated proton therapy for lung-intact mesothelioma: a case series. Pract Radiat Oncol 5:e345–e353

Pass HI, DeLaney TF, Tochner Z et al (1994) Intrapleural photodynamic therapy: results of a phase I trial. Ann Surg Oncol 1:28–37

Pass HI, Temeck BK, Kranda K et al (1997) Phase III randomized trial of surgery with or without intraoperative photodynamic therapy and postoperative immunochemotherapy for malignant pleural mesothelioma. Ann Surg Oncol 4:628–633

Patel PR, Yoo S, Broadwater G et al (2012) Effect of increasing experience on dosimetric and clinical outcomes in the management of malignant pleural mesothelioma with intensity-modulated radiation therapy. Int J Radiat Oncol Biol Phys 83:362–368

Rimner A, Zauderer MG, Gomez DR et al (2016) Phase II study of hemithoracic intensity-modulated pleural radiation therapy (IMPRINT) as part of lung-sparing multimodality therapy in patients with malignant pleural mesothelioma. J Clin Oncol 34:2761–2768

Ris H, Altermatt H, Nachbur B et al (1996) Intraoperative photodynamic therapy with m-tetrahydroxyphenylchlorin for chest malignancies. Lasers Surg Med 18:39–45

Schouwink H, Rutgers ET, van der Sijp J et al (2001) Intraoperative photodynamic therapy after pleuropneumonectomy in patients with malignant pleural mesothelioma: dose finding and toxicity results. Chest 120:1167–1174

Stahel RA, Riesterer O, Xyrafas A et al (2015) Neoadjuvant chemotherapy and extrapleural pneumonectomy of malignant pleural mesothelioma with or without hemithoracic radiotherapy (SAKK 17/04): a randomised, international, multicentre phase 2 trial. Lancet Oncol 16:1651–1658

Thieke C, Nicolay NH, Sterzing F et al (2015) Long-term results in malignant pleural mesothelioma treated with neoadjuvant chemotherapy, extrapleural pneumonectomy and intensity-modulated radiotherapy. Radiat Oncol 10:267

Van Schil PE, Baas P, Gaafar R et al (2010) Trimodality therapy for malignant pleural mesothelioma: results from an EORTC phase II multicentre trial. Eur Respir J 36(6):1362–1369

Weder W, Stahel RA, Bernhard J et al (2007) Multicenter trial of neo-adjuvant chemotherapy followed by extrapleural pneumonectomy in malignant pleural mesothelioma. Ann Oncol 18:1196–1202

Yajnik S, Rosenzweig KE, Mychalczak B et al (2003) Hemithoracic radiation after extrapleural pneumonectomy for malignant pleural mesothelioma. Int J Radiat Oncol Biol Phys 56:1319–1326

Chapter 15
Standard Chemotherapy Options and Clinical Trials of Novel Agents for Mesothelioma

Marjorie G. Zauderer

Abstract Despite recent dramatic advances in many solid tumors, malignant meso-thelioma remains challenging to treat. Historically, because of the modest number of cases globally and the substantial geographic distribution of patients, large randomized clinical trials were difficult and lengthy to complete, and thus, interest from pharmaceutical companies was limited. Additionally, financial support from various funding agencies is limited for this orphan disease. Consequently, most studies of systemic therapy for mesothelioma were small phase II trials. Despite these limitations, several standards of care were established. This chapter reviews standard cytotoxic chemotherapy treatment for malignant mesothelioma and discusses many novel agents recently and currently under investigation in clinical trials. The roles of surgery, radiation treatment, and combined modality therapy are covered in accompanying chapters. Furthermore, the ongoing development of immunotherapeutic agents is discussed in an accompanying chapter by Hassan and colleagues.

Keywords Chemotherapy • Cytotoxic agents • Novel agents • Angiogenesis • PI3K/mTOR • NF2 • BAP1 • Clinical trials

15.1 Standard Frontline Therapy

While numerous agents were studied for the treatment of mesothelioma (Table 15.1), the results were generally disappointing, with minimal improvement in response rates and unclear implications for survival (Alberts et al. 1988; Baas et al. 2003, 2000; Bajorin et al. 1987; Belani et al. 2004; Boutin et al. 1987; Cowan et al. 1988; Falkson et al. 1992; Kindler et al. 1999, 2005, 2001; Kosty et al. 2001; Lerner et al. 1983; Maksymiuk et al. 1998; Martensson and

M.G. Zauderer (✉)
Department of Medicine, Memorial Sloan Kettering Cancer Center and Weill Cornell Medical College, New York, NY 10065, USA
e-mail: zauderem@mskcc.org

© Springer International Publishing AG 2017
J.R. Testa (ed.), *Asbestos and Mesothelioma*, Current Cancer Research,
DOI 10.1007/978-3-319-53560-9_15

Table 15.1 Previously investigated agents with minimal efficacy

Agent	Year	N	Response rate (%)	Median survival months
Capecitabine (1)	2004	27	4	4.9
Carboplatin (2)	1986	17	12	Not reported
Carboplatin (3)	1990	31	16	8
Carboplatin (4)	1990	40	5	7.1
Cisplatin (5)	1985	24	13	5
Cisplatin (6)	1988	35	14	7.5
Cyclophosphamide (7)	1985	21	0	Not reported
Docetaxel (8)	2002	30	10	12
Docetaxel (9)	2004	19	5	4
Doxorubicin (10)	1983	51	14	7.5
Doxorubicin (7)	1985	21	0	Not reported
Doxorubicin (11)	2001	10	0	4.8
Edatrexate (12)	1999	20	25	9.6
Edatrexate (12)	1999	38	16	6.6
Etoposide (13)	1997	49	4	7.3
Etoposide (13)	1997	45	7	9.5
Gemcitabine (14)	2001	17	0	4.7
Gemcitabine (15)	1999	27	7	8
Ifosfamide (16)	1992	26	8	6.5
Ifosfamide (17)	1988	17	24	9
Ifosfamide (18)	1992	40	3	6.9
Irinotecan (19)	2005	28	0	7.9
Liposomal daunorubicin (20)	2001	14	0	6
Liposomal doxorubicin (21)	2000	24	0	9
Liposomal doxorubicin (22)	2000	33	6	13
Liposomal doxorubicin (23)	2002	15	7	Not reported
Methotrexate (24)	1992	63	37	11
Mitomycin C (25)	1987	19	21	Not reported
Paclitaxel (26)	1996	25	0	9
Paclitaxel (27)	1999	35	9	5
Pemetrexed (28)	2003	21	10	8
Pemetrexed (28)	2003	43	16	13
Raltitrexed (29)	2003	25	21	7
Temozolomide (30)	2002	27	4	8.2
Topotecan (31)	1998	22	0	8
Vinblastine (32)	1988	20	0	3
Vincristine (33)	1989	23	0	7
Vindesine (34)	1987	17	6	Not reported
Vinorelbine (35)	2000	29	24	10.6

Table 15.2 Results from trials with cisplatin ± antifolate

Agent(s)/arm	N	RR (%)	Median TTP months	Median OS months	One-year survival (%)
Pemetrexed + cisplatin	226	41	5.7	12.1	50
vs.		$p < 0.001$	$p = 0.001$	$p = 0.02$	$p = 0.012$
Cisplatin (intention to treat) (36)	222	17	3.9	9.3	38
Pemetrexed + cisplatin	168	46	6.1	13.3	57
vs.		$p < 0.001$	$p = 0.001$	$p = 0.05$	$p = 0.01$
Cisplatin (vitamin supplementation) (36)	163	20	3.9	10	42
Raltitrexed + cisplatin	126	24	Not reported	11.2	46
vs.		$p = 0.06$		$p = 0.056$	$p = 0.056$
Cisplatin (37)	124	14		8.8	39

OS overall survival, *RR* response rate, *TTP* time to progression

Sorenson 1989; Mbidde et al. 1986; Mintzer et al. 1985; Oh et al. 2000; Otterson et al. 2004; Raghavan et al. 1990; Sahmoud et al. 1997; Scagliotti et al. 2003; Skubitz 2002; Solheim et al. 1992; Sorensen et al. 1985; Steele et al. 2001, 2000; van Meerbeeck et al. 1996, 1999, 2002; Vogelzang et al. 1990, 1999; Vorobiof et al. 2002; Zidar et al. 1988, 1992). It was not until 2003 that a standard first-line treatment regimen was established. In a 456-patient phase III randomized clinical trial, chemotherapy-naïve patients with unresectable malignant pleural mesothelioma were randomized to receive either cisplatin and pemetrexed or cisplatin alone (Vogelzang et al. 2003). Median overall survival with cisplatin and pemetrexed was 12.1 months versus 9.3 months with cisplatin alone ($p = 0.02$ two-sided log-rank test). The hazard ratio for death of patients in the cisplatin and pemetrexed arm versus the cisplatin control arm was 0.77. The chemotherapy combination arm had a response rate of 41.3% versus 16.7% with cisplatin alone ($p < 0.0001$). While the demonstrated improvement in survival is modest, this clinical trial established cisplatin and pemetrexed as the standard systemic therapy for mesothelioma and achieved FDA approval for this indication in 2004. Subsequently, other studies have confirmed these results and a similar survival benefit of about 3 months with cisplatin and pemetrexed or raltitrexed, another antimetabolite agent (Table 15.2) (Porta 2006; van Meerbeeck et al. 2005).

Unfortunately, over the next 10 years, the field of systemic therapy for mesothelioma largely plateaued. Several subsequent studies evaluated and established the use of carboplatin with pemetrexed for patients who could not receive cisplatin (Castagneto et al. 2008; Ceresoli et al. 2006; Katirtzoglou et al. 2010; Santoro ct al. 2008). In the pemetrexed expanded access program, 861 chemotherapy-naïve patients received carboplatin and pemetrexed with a response rate of 21.7% (95% CI 18.8–24.8%) and a disease control rate of 75.8% (95% CI 72.6–78.8%) (Santoro et al.

Table 15.3 Efficacy of carboplatin with pemetrexed

Author/year	N	RR (%)	DCR (%)	Median TTP months	Median OS months
Ceresoli 2006 (40)	102	18.6	65.7	6.5	12.7
Castagneto 2008 (41)	76	25	64	8	14
Katirtzoglou 2010 (42)	62	29	83.9	7	14

DCR disease control rate (stable disease + partial response + complete response), *OS* overall survival, *RR* response rate, *TTP* time to progression

Table 15.4 Efficacy of cisplatin and gemcitabine

Author/year	N	RR (%)	DCR (%)	Median PFS months	Median OS months
van Haarst et al. 2002 (44)	32	16	88	Not reported	9.4
Nowak et al. 2002 (45)	52	33	93	Not reported	11.2
Castagneto et al. 2005 (46)	35	26	66	8	13
Kalmadi et al. 2008(47)	50	12	62	6	10

DCR disease control rate (stable disease + partial response + complete response), *OS* overall survival, *PFS* progression-free survival, *RR* response rate

2008). One-year survival was 64% (95% CI 53.3–74.6%). Three single-arm phase II studies also supported the use of carboplatin with pemetrexed (Castagneto et al. 2008; Ceresoli et al. 2006; Katirtzoglou et al. 2010). The size of these studies varied from 62 to 102 patients and median overall survival spanned 12.7 months to 14 months, which is consistent with the phase III trial of cisplatin and pemetrexed. Response rates with this combination were modest, but a significant fraction of patients achieved prolonged stable disease (Table 15.3). Additionally, a pooled analysis of two of the three trials demonstrated similar outcomes and toxicity among patients 70 years of age and older versus those younger than 70 years (Ceresoli et al. 2008).

Cisplatin in combination with gemcitabine remains a viable alternative for any patients who cannot receive pemetrexed as established by several single-arm phase II clinical trials (Table 15.4) (Castagneto et al. 2005; Kalmadi et al. 2008; Nowak et al. 2002; van Haarst et al. 2002). One multicenter phase II study conducted in the Netherlands and Germany enrolled 32 chemotherapy-naïve patients with malignant pleural mesothelioma to receive cisplatin and gemcitabine (van Haarst et al. 2002). The partial response rate was 16% (95% CI 1–31%) with 72% achieving stable disease. Overall median survival was 9.4 months (95% CI 7.3–11.4 months). Similarly, in an Australian multicenter phase II study, 53 chemotherapy-naïve malignant mesothelioma patients were treated with cisplatin and gemcitabine (Nowak et al. 2002). No complete responses were achieved, but 33% (95% CI 20–46%) had a partial response and median overall survival was 11.2 months. The response rate was comparable in an Italian study of this combination, with 26% (95% CI 12.5–43.2%) achieving partial response and a median overall survival of 13 months (Castagneto et al. 2005). Additionally, in a Southwest Oncology Group (SWOG) phase II study, there was a response rate of 12% (95% CI 5–24%) among

50 chemotherapy-naïve malignant mesothelioma patients, including one confirmed complete response (Kalmadi et al. 2008). As with the combination of cisplatin and pemetrexed, carboplatin can be substituted for cisplatin in combination with gemcitabine based on a multicenter phase II study in which 50 patients received carboplatin and gemcitabine (Favaretto et al. 2003). In this study, the observed response rate was 26% (95% CI 15–40%) and median overall survival was 66 weeks.

Finally, in 2015, the benefits of targeting angiogenesis in mesothelioma were realized with the results of the French Mesothelioma Avastin Cisplatin Pemetrexed Study (MAPS NCT00651456) trial (Zalcman et al. 2016). In MAPS, 448 chemotherapy-naïve patients were randomly assigned to receive cisplatin, pemetrexed, and bevacizumab with bevacizumab maintenance versus cisplatin and pemetrexed. Randomization was stratified by histology, performance status, study center, and smoking status, and the two arms were well balanced. Median overall survival with the three-drug combination was 18.8 months (95% CI 15.9–22.6) versus 16.1 months (95% CI 14.0–17.9). The relative hazard ratio was 0.77 (95% CI 0.62–0.95, $p = 0.0167$). Toxicity, not surprisingly, was greater among those who received triplet therapy and led to more toxicity-related discontinuation. However, despite early discontinuation and post-study treatment actually favoring the doublet arm, the triplet arm was still superior with respect to survival.

Of note, a previous multicenter double-blind randomized phase II trial of gemcitabine and cisplatin with bevacizumab or placebo failed to demonstrate benefit with the addition of bevacizumab (Kindler et al. 2012). In the gemcitabine trial, the response rates were 24.5% and 21.8% ($p = 0.74$) for the bevacizumab and placebo arms, respectively. There were no statistically significant differences in median progression-free or overall survival. In addition, a multicenter phase II study of cisplatin, pemetrexed, and bevacizumab did not meet its primary endpoint of 33% improvement in progression-free survival at 6 months using historical controls with cisplatin and pemetrexed (Dowell et al. 2012). While these data are somewhat conflicting, the survival benefit demonstrated in MAPS justifies the addition of bevacizumab to cisplatin and pemetrexed (Zauderer 2016). Regulatory approval in the United States is currently pending, but the triplet combination has already been added to the National Comprehensive Cancer Network's Mesothelioma Guidelines.

15.2   Standard Second-Line Therapy Options

With the routine use of platinum and pemetrexed, many patients remain fit for second-line therapy, but the limited efficacy data for agents in this setting leave oncologists with several options but no universally accepted standard (Table 15.5). If patients had a good initial response to treatment and more than 6 months have elapsed since initial treatment, data support rechallenging patients with pemetrexed-based therapy (Bearz et al. 2012; Ceresoli et al. 2011; Janne et al. 2006; Razak et al. 2008; Taylor et al. 2008). In an analysis of the phase IIIB expanded access program for pemetrexed, there was a response rate of 5.5% (95% CI 1.5–13.4%) and disease control rate of

Table 15.5 Efficacy of agents often used as salvage therapy

Agent	Setting	N	RR (%)	DCR (%)	Median OS months
Pemetrexed (53)	Re-treatment case series	4	75	100	Not reported
Pemetrexed-based (54)	Re-treatment retrospective	30	17	66	13.6
Pemetrexed-based (55)	Re-treatment observational	31	19	48	10.5
Pemetrexed (56)	Re-treatment retrospective	73	5.5	46.6	4.1
Pemetrexed-based (56)	Re-treatment retrospective	80	32.5	68.8	7.6
Pemetrexed (57)	Initial treatment observational	247	10.5	59.1	14.1
Pemetrexed (57)	Salvage treatment observational	396	12.1	58.1	Not estimable
Vinorelbine (59)	Salvage treatment phase II	63	16	84	9.6
Vinorelbine (61)	Salvage retrospective	59	15.2	49.1	6.2
Vinorelbine (63)	Salvage retrospective	45	0	42	5.4
Gemcitabine (63)	Salvage retrospective	27	4	26	4.9
Gemcitabine (15)	Initial treatment phase II	27	7	63	8
Gemcitabine (14)	Initial treatment phase II	17	0	Not reported	4.7

DCR disease control rate (stable disease + partial response + complete response), *OS* overall survival, *RR* response rate, *TTP* time to progression

46.6% with single-agent pemetrexed in previously treated patients (Janne et al. 2006). Similarly, in the International Expanded Access Program, the response rate was 10.5% (95% CI 7–15%) in chemotherapy-naïve patients and 12.1% (95% CI 9.1–15.7) in the pretreated patients (Taylor et al. 2008). In a small observational study, 31 patients who had previously received pemetrexed-based chemotherapy and achieved a complete response, partial response, or stable disease were re-treated with pemetrexed-based chemotherapy (Ceresoli et al. 2011). Fifteen patients received pemetrexed alone and 16 received pemetrexed with a platinum agent. One patient achieved a complete response, and partial response was achieved in five patients for an objective response rate of 19%. Twenty-nine percent achieved stable disease giving a disease control rate of 48%. In a retrospective analysis, 30 patients were re-treated with pemetrexed-based chemotherapy and achieved a disease control rate of 66% (Bearz et al. 2012). Similar to the observational study, only patients who had initially responded to pemetrexed-based therapy with a partial response or stable disease were included. Thus, in a very select patient population, re-treatment with pemetrexed-based chemotherapy is a reasonable second-line therapy option.

Other agents have also been extensively studied and used, although there is no proven survival benefit. From the retrospective analysis of post-study treatment of patients from the phase III trial of cisplatin and pemetrexed, receipt of additional chemotherapy was common and vinorelbine and gemcitabine were the most frequently used agents in those who had received pemetrexed (Manegold et al. 2005). When controlling for performance status and histology, those who received post-study chemotherapy had significantly longer survival than those who did not receive further chemotherapy.

One prospective clinical trial assessed the efficacy of weekly vinorelbine in 63 previously treated patients with malignant pleural mesothelioma (Stebbing et al. 2009). There were no complete responses, and the partial response rate was 10%. Sixty-eight percent of patients had stable disease without progression for 6 months. Median overall survival was 9.6 months (95% CI 7.3–11.8 months). While these data are intriguing, there are several limitations of this study. First, all of the included patients were classified as low risk according to the EORTC prognostic score (Fennell et al. 2005), and the survival of such patients in the absence of cytotoxic therapy is not known. Second, these patients had relatively indolent disease as evidenced by the median interval of 6 months between first-line therapy and treatment on this study. Finally, it is unclear what fraction of these patients received pemetrexed or raltitrexed as their initial therapy. Another small single-arm study evaluated weekly vinorelbine in 59 previously treated patients with malignant pleural mesothelioma who had progression after at least one pemetrexed-based chemotherapy regimen (Zucali et al. 2014). In this cohort, the response rate was 15.2%, and 33.9% of patients achieved stable disease. Median overall survival was 6.2 months (range 0.8–27.8 months). Certainly, the modest efficacy supports the use of vinorelbine as second-line treatment for mesothelioma. Additionally, ongoing efforts to establish a biomarker for vinorelbine efficacy may help optimize patient selection for this particular treatment (Busacca et al. 2012).

Gemcitabine has also been studied in two single-arm phase II clinical trials. In one trial, 27 chemotherapy-naïve malignant pleural mesothelioma patients received weekly gemcitabine (van Meerbeeck et al. 1999). There were two partial responses, giving a response rate of 7% (95% CI 1–24%). Median overall survival was 8 months (95% CI 5–12 months), with 33% of patients alive at 1 year. The CALGB conducted a multicenter phase II trial of gemcitabine in chemotherapy-naïve patients with similar modest results (Kindler et al. 2001). There were no responses among the 17 enrolled patients and median overall survival was 4.7 months (95% CI 3.1–12.9 months), with 24% alive at 1 year. Thus, the activity of single-agent gemcitabine is low, even in previously untreated patients. These findings were confirmed in a retrospective analysis of a single-institution experience with vinorelbine and gemcitabine as second- or third-line therapy for malignant pleural mesothelioma (Zauderer et al. 2014). Among 56 evaluable patients, there was a very low response rate of 2% (95% CI 0–10%), with a single patient achieving a partial response with gemcitabine. A large fraction of patients had stable disease but only for a short duration. Additionally, toxicity was significant, with 46% of patients experiencing at least one episode of grade 3–4 toxicity and 38% experiencing at least one episode of grade 3–4 nonhematologic toxicity.

Another small single-arm trial evaluated the combination of gemcitabine and vinorelbine in pemetrexed-pretreated patients with malignant pleural mesothelioma (Zucali et al. 2008). Thirty patients were enrolled and 29 were evaluable for response. Three patients (10%, 95% CI 2.1–26.5%) achieved partial response, and ten patients (33.3%, 95% CI 17/3–52.8%) achieved stable disease. The median overall survival was 10.9 months (range 0.8–25.3 months). Nonhematologic toxicity was mild, and grade 3–4 neutropenia was 10%.

Certainly the activity of these agents in the second-line setting is intriguing and justifies use. Hopefully biomarkers, such as BRCA1 expression for vinorelbine, can be used to better select patients. However, there remains a tremendous unmet need for novel therapeutics. Given the limitations on drug development resources for this orphan disease, future mesothelioma clinical trials must carefully plan evaluation of agents with strong biologic rationale, in the appropriate clinical context, and use an optimized trial design. Only through such efforts will clinically meaningful advances be made. Meanwhile, for those who are ineligible for clinical trials or unable to access them, re-treatment with pemetrexed, gemcitabine, and vinorelbine all remain viable therapeutic options.

15.3 Novel Agent Development: Agents Explored in Recently Completed and Ongoing Clinical Trials

In addition to incorporating bevacizumab into routine use in the first-line setting, efforts to further advance the development and study of new drugs with strong biologic rationale must continue. While oncogene addiction drives some cancers, most molecular alterations in mesothelioma occur in tumor suppressors, and it is challenging to identify a clear corresponding drug target. Thankfully, as several large randomized trials have been successfully executed and next-generation sequencing has facilitated a more robust understanding of common molecular alterations and dependencies in mesothelioma (Bott et al. 2011; Bueno et al. 2016; Illei et al. 2003; Lu et al. 1994; Thurneysen et al. 2009), many more trials are underway. Some notable examples of prior and ongoing investigations (Table 15.6) with agents to exploit

Table 15.6 Ongoing clinical trials of novel agents for mesothelioma

Agent	NCT #	Phase	Setting
ADI-PEG20	02029690	Phase II/III	First line
Cediranib	01064648	Phase I/II	First line
GSK3052230	01868022	Phase I	First line
LY3023414	01655225	Phase I	First line and salvage
TRC102	02535312	Phase I/II	First line
NGR-hTNF	01358084	Phase II	Maintenance
Nintedanib	02863055	Phase II	Maintenance
Alisertib	02293055	Phase II	Salvage
Nintedanib	02568449	Phase II	Salvage
Tazemetostat	02860286	Phase II	Salvage

the biologic underpinnings of mesothelioma development and propagation are detailed below, excluding immunotherapeutics, which are discussed in the accompanying chapter Immunotherapeutic Approaches to Mesothelioma.

15.3.1 Angiogenesis

Vascular epithelial growth factor (VEGF) and its cognate receptors are highly expressed in mesothelioma (Ohta et al. 1999), and the addition of VEGF to mesothelioma cell lines leads to dose-dependent cell proliferation, whereas the addition of VEGF inhibitors attenuates mesothelioma cell growth (Loganathan et al. 2011; Masood et al. 2003; Strizzi et al. 2001). Furthermore, in patients, high levels of VEGF correlate with poor survival, while decreasing VEGF during treatment correlates with improved survival (Edwards et al. 2001; Kao et al. 2012). Thus, many inhibitors of angiogenesis have been studied in mesothelioma. While the single-agent efficacy of these compounds in the second-line setting has been modest, the recently demonstrated survival benefit in MAPS has reinvigorated these avenues of investigation.

15.3.1.1 Sorafenib

Sorafenib, a potent inhibitor of VEGF receptors, cKIT, and the ras/raf/MEK pathway, was evaluated in a CALBG single-arm phase II trial (CALGB 30307) (Dubey et al. 2010). Fifty evaluable patients with malignant mesothelioma received sorafenib and 6% achieved a partial response rate (95% CI 1.3–16.6%), with 54% achieving stable disease (95% CI 39.3–68.2%). Median overall survival was 9.7 months. While this cohort included patients who were both chemotherapy naïve and previously treated, there was not a statistically significant difference in survival among these two subgroups. In the UK, 53 patients who had previously received pemetrexed-based chemotherapy were treated with sorafenib in a multicenter phase II study (Papa et al. 2013). The partial response rate was identical at 6%, with 62% having disease control at 8 weeks. Median overall survival was similar at 9.0 months (95% CI 6.7–11.3 months).

15.3.1.2 Vatalanib

Vatalanib, an inhibitor of several VEGF receptors and PDGF receptors, was studied in a single-arm phase II CALGB study (CALGB 30107) (Jahan et al. 2012). Among 47 chemotherapy-naïve patients with unresectable malignant mesothelioma, 6.4% (95% CI 2.2–5.3%) achieved a partial response and 72.3% achieved stable disease. Median overall survival was 10 months (95% CI 6.3–14.4). These results were comparable to those from the sorafenib studies (Dubey et al. 2010; Papa et al. 2013).

15.3.1.3   Sunitinib

Sunitinib, a multitargeted tyrosine kinase inhibitor of VEGF and PDGF receptor, was evaluated in 53 patients with malignant pleural mesothelioma who had progression of disease after prior chemotherapy (Nowak et al. 2012). Partial response and stable disease were achieved in 12% (95% CI 6–23%) and 65%, respectively. Median overall survival was 6.1 months (95% CI 3.8–8.5). Thirty-five patients were enrolled on a National Cancer Institute of Canada Clinical Trials Group phase II study of sunitinib (Laurie et al. 2011). Cohort 1, with 17 patients, included previously treated patients who had received at least one platinum-based regimen and no more than three prior regimens. Cohort 2, with 18 patients, enrolled only those who were chemotherapy naïve. Unfortunately, no responses were observed in previously treated patients. Among the previously untreated patients, there was one partial response and ten patients had stable disease for a median of 4.5 months (range 2.5–12.7). The median overall survival was 8.3 months and 6.7 months in cohorts 1 and 2, respectively.

15.3.1.4   Thalidomide

Thalidomide was also revisited as an anticancer agent for its putative effects on angiogenesis (Bartlett et al. 2004; Fine et al. 2000; Folkman 1971), which is known to be important in mesothelioma (Kumar-Singh et al. 1997b, 1999; Linder et al. 1998; Ohta et al. 1999; Van et al. 2012). In a small phase I/II trial of patients with progressive malignant pleural mesothelioma, 27.5% of patients (11/40) achieved stable disease for 6 months or more (Baas et al. 2005). Based on these results, a large randomized phase III study of thalidomide versus active supportive care for maintenance in malignant mesothelioma after first-line therapy was conducted (Buikhuisen et al. 2013). Two hundred and twenty-two patients who had completed a minimum of four cycles of pemetrexed-based chemotherapy without progression of disease were randomized to thalidomide or active supportive care. The median time to progression in the thalidomide group was 3.6 months (95% CI 3.2–4.1) vs. 3.5 months (95% CI 2.3–4.8) in the active supportive care group with a hazard ratio of 0.95 (95% CI 0.73–1.20, $p = 0.72$). While the investigators looked for factors other than lack of efficacy to explain these findings, they were unable to identify an alternative explanation.

Two parallel single-arm phase II studies of thalidomide were conducted in Australia (Kao et al. 2012). Chemotherapy-naïve patients were enrolled to arm A in which they received thalidomide, cisplatin, and gemcitabine. Previously treated patients or those ineligible to receive cisplatin were enrolled to arm B and treated with thalidomide alone. While treatment was well tolerated with few grade 3 or 4 adverse events, efficacy was disappointing. There was a response rate of 13% (95% CI 4–33%) in arm A and 0% (95% CI 0–16%) in arm B. One-year survival was 39% and 31%, respectively, for arms A and B.

15.3.1.5   Axitinib

Axitinib is an oral inhibitor of the tyrosine kinase receptor for VEGF and has shown activity against solid tumors with a manageable toxicity profile. An open-label, single-center phase II study randomized patients to receive cisplatin and pemetrexed with or without axitinib (Buikhuisen et al. 2016). Thirty-two patients were enrolled, but only 25 were randomized and there was no statistically significant difference between response rate (36% vs. 18%, p = 0.85), progression-free survival (5.8 months vs. 8.3 months, $p = 0.73$), or overall survival in the two arms (18.9 months vs. 18.5 months, $p = 0.77$), respectively, for axitinib and chemotherapy only. There was a statistically significant increase in microvessel density in the before and after treatment tumor biopsy samples in those treated with cisplatin and pemetrexed (p < 0.0001), and there was an increase in the number of immature blood vessels ($p = 0.0003$). In the axitinib group, however, microvessel density and the number of mature blood vessels were the same after treatment.

15.3.1.6   NGR-hTNF

Tumor necrosis factor-alpha (TNF-alpha) has powerful antitumor activity by causing clustering of death domain-containing receptors, which leads to caspase activation and ultimately apoptosis (Carswell et al. 1975; Lejeune et al. 2006). Developing TNF-alpha for clinical use has been hampered by severe toxicities with systemic administration (Creaven et al. 1989; Gamm et al. 1991; Kimura et al. 1987; Mittelman et al. 1992; Schwartz et al. 1989; Wiedenmann et al. 1989). To overcome this limitation, NGR-hTNF was created by fusing the N-terminal of TNF-alpha with the C-terminal of NGR, a cyclic tumor-homing peptide, which is a selective ligand of an aminopeptide overexpressed in tumor blood vessel cells (Colombo et al. 2002; Corti and Ponzoni 2004; Curnis et al. 2002, 2000). NGR-hTNF thus selectively disrupts the aberrant development of new blood vessels from preexisting blood vessels (Rangel et al. 2007) and is a promising anti-angiogenic agent.

Two phase I trials established a safe and possibly efficacious dose of NGR-hTNF (Gregorc et al. 2010a; van Laarhoven et al. 2010). A phase II study evaluated NGR-hTNF in previously treated patients with malignant pleural mesothelioma (Gregorc et al. 2010b). The primary endpoint was the 12-week progression-free rate. Forty-three patients were enrolled in the triweekly dosing cohort and 14 in the weekly dosing cohort. The triweekly cohort had 44% disease control rate and the weekly cohort had 50% disease control rate. Median overall survival was 11.6 months (95% CI 5.6–17.6) and had not been reached (95% CI 2.3–17.0) in the triweekly and weekly cohorts, respectively. NGR-hTNF was well tolerated and adverse reactions were usually infusion related and generally short lived. Based on these results, the authors recommended further investigation with the weekly dosing for patients with advanced malignant pleural mesothelioma. There is an ongoing randomized phase

II clinical trial of NGR-hTNF versus placebo as maintenance therapy after nonprogression on six cycles of pemetrexed-based chemotherapy (NCT01358084). The primary endpoint of this study is progression-free survival with overall survival, response rate, safety, and quality of life metrics as secondary endpoints. The planned enrollment is 100 patients and recruitment is ongoing.

15.3.1.7 Cediranib

There were also two phase II trials evaluating cediranib, an oral tyrosine kinase inhibitor of VEGFR1–3, which demonstrated minimal to modest efficacy (Campbell et al. 2012; Garland et al. 2011). In SWOG study S0509, among 47 evaluable patients with previously treated malignant pleural mesothelioma, 9% achieved partial response, including marked shrinkage for two patients with bulky tumors, and 34% achieved stable disease for a disease control rate of 43% and median overall survival of 9.5 months (95% CI 5.6–19.7 months) (Garland et al. 2011). In the University of Chicago Consortium study, a response rate of 10% was observed among 50 evaluable patients with malignant mesothelioma, with a median duration of 6.5 months (range 4.0–9.8 months) (Campbell et al. 2012). The median overall survival in this cohort was 4.4 months (95% CI 0.9–41.7 months). Unlike the SWOG study, the University of Chicago Consortium trial included both previously treated and chemotherapy-naïve patients, but virtually identical response rates were observed. Despite the similarities, the authors articulated different conclusions. While the University of Chicago Consortium concluded that the modest activity and high toxicity observed did not justify further study of cediranib, the SWOG authors noted that further study of lower dose cediranib in combination with cytotoxic chemotherapy was warranted given the uncommon but dramatic responses observed. Thus, there is an ongoing phase I/II trial evaluating cediranib in combination with pemetrexed and cisplatin (NCT01064648).

15.3.1.8 Nintedanib

Nintedanib is an oral, twice-daily triple kinase inhibitor of VEGF receptors 1–3, platelet-derived growth factor receptors alpha/beta, and fibroblast growth factor receptors 1–3 (Epstein Shochet et al. 2016; Hilberg et al. 2008; Kudo et al. 2011; Roth et al. 2009). This drug is already approved for the treatment of idiopathic pulmonary fibrosis (Epstein Shochet et al. 2016). Additionally, in the European Union, nintedanib in combination with docetaxel is an approved treatment for locally advanced, metastatic, or locally recurrent non-small cell lung cancer, particularly adenocarcinoma, after first-line chemotherapy (Popat et al. 2015; Reck et al. 2014; Syrios et al. 2015). There are currently three accruing clinical trials that will evaluate the role of nintedanib for the treatment of mesothelioma.

First, there is an ongoing phase II/III trial of nintedanib vs. placebo in combination with cisplatin and pemetrexed (NCT01907100) as initial therapy in patients with unresectable malignant pleural mesothelioma (Scagliotti et al. 2016). Accrual for the planned 537 patients is ongoing. The primary endpoint is progression-free survival, with overall survival as the secondary endpoint. The study design is adaptive so that based on interim analysis after the first 87 patients, the final accrual goal can be modified to ensure sufficient power for the planned progression-free and overall survival analyses. The European Organisation for Research and Treatment of Cancer (EORTC) is conducting a study of nintedanib as maintenance therapy in a randomized double-blind phase II trial (NCT02863055). In this trial, 116 patients who do not progress after four to six cycles of platinum-pemetrexed chemotherapy will be randomized to nintedanib or placebo. The primary endpoint is progression-free survival, with overall survival and overall response as secondary outcomes. The Karmanos Cancer Institute is also conducting a multicenter, single-arm phase II study of nintedanib in patients with malignant pleural mesothelioma who have previously received platinum-based chemotherapy (NCT02568449). Plans for this study are to enroll 55 patients, with a primary objective of assessing progression-free survival at 4 months. Secondary objectives include response rate, overall survival, and toxicity.

15.4   Cell Signaling Inhibitors

Despite the activity of many small molecule inhibitors in other solid tumors, these agents have not yet demonstrated activity in mesothelioma. For example, clinical trials with erlotinib, gefitinib, and imatinib did not demonstrate clinically meaningful activity (Garland et al. 2007; Govindan et al. 2005; Mathy et al. 2005; Tsao et al. 2014). However, as knowledge rapidly expands regarding the key molecular disruptions that drive mesothelioma development and persistence, therapies that target functions of relevance are being investigated. In particular, as next-generation sequencing and tumor microenvironment profiling have revealed consistently altered pathways in mesothelioma (Bott et al. 2011; Bueno et al. 2016), exploiting those dependencies has become a great focus of mesothelioma research.

15.4.1   Everolimus

Several tumor suppressor genes are commonly lost in mesothelioma (Bott et al. 2011; Bueno et al. 2016; Kaufman and Pass 2008). The neurofibromatosis type 2 (NF2) gene is frequently absent in mesothelioma. Merlin, encoded by NF2, mediates contact-dependent inhibition of cellular proliferation through inhibition of mTOR (Moriya et al. 2014; Okada et al. 2005). Knockout experiments in mesothelioma models show that loss of Merlin leads to unchecked mTOR activity, which can be abrogated by mTOR inhibition (Lopez-Lago et al. 2009; Ranzato et al. 2009). Furthermore, two mTOR inhibitors, sirolimus and temsirolimus, demonstrated activity in preclinical models (Hartman et al. 2010; Hoda et al. 2011). These discoveries were the preclinical rationale for two clinical trials of everolimus, an oral mTOR inhibitor, in mesothelioma (NCT01024946 and NCT00770120). Everolimus is an oral inhibitor of mTOR already approved for use in renal cell carcinoma (Motzer et al. 2008), giant cell astrocytomas associated with tuberous sclerosis (Franz et al. 2013), angiomyolipoma associated with tuberous sclerosis (Bissler et al. 2013), pancreatic neuroendocrine tumors (Pavel et al. 2011; Yao et al. 2010, 2011), and in combination with exemestane in breast cancer (Baselga et al. 2012; Dancey 2010; Lebwohl et al. 2013).

Unfortunately, the Memorial Sloan Kettering Cancer Center study (NCT01024946) of everolimus in malignant pleural mesotheliomas with Merlin loss closed early and no results have been reported. A SWOG study (NCT00770120) successfully enrolled 59 malignant pleural mesothelioma patients previously treated with platinum (Ou et al. 2015). The primary endpoint of this single-arm phase II trial was 4-month progression-free survival. The response rate was 2% (95% CI 0–12%), the median overall survival was 6.3 months (95% CI 4–8 months), and the 4-month progression-free survival rate was 29% (95% CI 16–39%), which fell short of the prespecified threshold of 50% for being worthy of further study. As this population was treated irrespective of Merlin/NF2 status, the lack of biomarker selection of patients may have contributed to the lack of activity. Additionally, combination strategies inhibiting both PI3K and mTOR may be necessary to elicit clinically meaningful responses (Cedres et al. 2012; Fruman and Rommel 2014; Ladanyi et al. 2012; Syrios et al. 2015; Zhou et al. 2014).

15.4.2 Apitolisib

Given the lack of efficacy of mTOR inhibition and an increased understanding of the feedback mechanism through PI3K, dual inhibitors of PI3K and mTOR have been explored (Ladanyi et al. 2012; Zhou et al. 2014). Apitolisib is an oral dual catalytic site inhibitor of PI3K and mTOR (Sutherlin et al. 2011). A recent phase I trial of apitolisib in advanced solid tumors included an expansion cohort in malignant pleural mesothelioma (Dolly et al. 2013, 2016). After establishing the maximum tolerated dose, 27 mesothelioma patients were treated. Of the 26 evaluable patients, two achieved confirmed partial responses and 20 patients achieved stable disease. Median time on the trial was 4 months (range 0.5–38.9 months) with a significant fraction of patients (29.6%) on study for more than 6 months. Interestingly, if all mesothelioma patients on this trial are included in the response analysis, the response rate is 12%. While the response rate is modest, it compares favorably to other second-line agents. Further investigations of pulse dosing and combinations with cytotoxic therapy are being planned.

15.4.3   LY3023414

LY3023414 is an oral dual kinase inhibitor of PI3K and mTOR and binds to the ATP active site of PI3K to competitively inhibit phosphorylation of PIP2. Preclinical studies demonstrated antitumor efficacy, so a phase I clinical trial was undertaken (NCT01655225). After an initial dose escalation and safety run-in, two cohorts were opened for malignant mesothelioma: (1) chemotherapy-naïve patients who receive LY3023414 in combination with cisplatin and pemetrexed in a dose escalation fashion and (2) previously treated patients who receive LY3023414 alone. Accrual to this study is ongoing, and results are anticipated some time in 2017.

15.4.4   GSK3052230

Fibroblast growth factor (FGF) signaling is important for the initiation and growth of several tumor types with roles in the regulation of cell growth and differentiation, regulation of angiogenesis, and participation in tumor-stromal interactions (Grose and Dickson 2005; Turner and Grose 2010). There are 22 distinct FGF proteins whose downstream effects are mediated by four different FGF receptors (FGFR) (Beenken and Mohammadi 2009; Itoh 2007), and deregulation of this signaling occurs in several tumors through a variety of mechanisms including activating mutations (di Martino et al. 2009; Dutt et al. 2008; Liao et al. 2013), chromosomal translocations (Avet-Loiseau et al. 1998; Wu et al. 2013), and amplification (Dutt et al. 2011; Goke et al. 2013; Turner et al. 2010; Weiss et al. 2010). Mesothelioma, in particular, has high levels of FGF2 (Davidson et al. 2004; Kumar-Singh et al. 1999; Li et al. 2011), and FGFR1 drives mesothelioma growth (Marek et al. 2014). Additionally, high levels of FGF ligands correlate with poor clinical outcomes, thereby making inhibition of FGF signaling an attractive therapeutic target.

GSK3052230 includes the extracellular domains of FGFR1 linked to a modified hinge and native Fc regions of IgG1. Thus, GSK3052230 acts as a fusion trap protein sequestering FGFs and inhibiting FGFR signaling. In a panel of mesothelioma cell lines and tumor xenografts, GSK3052230 demonstrated antiproliferative effects (Blackwell et al. 2016). A phase I study of GSK3052230 as single-agent therapy in patients with metastatic or locally advanced solid tumors was conducted (Tolcher et al. 2016). These observations and the previously established single-agent safety of GSK3052230 led to the inclusion of a mesothelioma arm in the ongoing phase IB trial of GSK3052230 in combination with chemotherapy (NCT01868022). Chemotherapy-naïve patients with malignant pleural mesothelioma receive cisplatin and pemetrexed along with GSK3052230. The primary endpoints are safety and the overall response rate. Preliminary results have been presented in abstract form with an identified maximum tolerated dose of 15 mg/kg of GSK3052230, but response data are still immature (Garrido et al. 2015; Garrido et al. 2014; Lopez et al. 2014).

15.5   Epigenetic Modification

In addition to the burgeoning knowledge regarding specific genetic alterations, there is a growing appreciation of the role of epigenetic changes in carcinogenesis and cancer progression (Dawson et al. 2012; Yoo and Jones 2006). Much ongoing work focuses on distinct epigenetic pathways that affect DNA methylation and chromatin remodeling. Some epigenetic agents are already approved for the treatment of cancer (Duvic et al. 2007; Duvic and Vu 2007), while others are currently under investigation. Two compounds with epigenetic targets are of particular interest in mesothelioma.

15.5.1   Vorinostat

The histone family of proteins controls the structural elements of chromatin, and DNA transcription can occur only when chromatin is decondensed. Thus, compounds that control the condensation and decondensation of chromatin can have a profound impact on gene transcription. Specifically, histone deacetylases (HDACs) remove lysine residues from histone tails and associated proteins and thus prevent gene transcription (Minucci and Pelicci 2006; Paik and Krug 2010). Substantial preclinical data show that blocking histone deacetylation can lead to more apoptosis, cell cycle arrest, inhibition of angiogenesis, and immune modulation in mesothelioma and other malignancies (Bolden et al. 2006; Cao et al. 2001; Ellis et al. 2009; Kumar-Singh et al. 1997a; Neuzil et al. 2004; Shao et al. 2007; Symanowski et al. 2009; Vandermeers et al. 2009). Vorinostat is an oral HDAC inhibitor that is approved for the treatment of cutaneous T-cell lymphoma (Duvic et al. 2007; Duvic and Vu 2007). In a phase I dose escalation study of vorinostat in patients with both solid tumor and hematologic malignancies, 13 patients had malignant pleural mesothelioma (Kelly et al. 2005). Among these 13 patients, six continued on study for more than 4 months and two patients had radiographic partial responses, including one heavily pretreated patient.

Based on these data (Kelly et al. 2005), a large randomized phase III trial was undertaken in patients with progressive or relapsed mesothelioma who had previously received pemetrexed-based chemotherapy (NCT00128102) (Krug et al. 2015). Six hundred and sixty patients were randomized to vorinostat or placebo. Median overall survival with vorinostat was 30.7 weeks (95% CI 26.7–36.1) compared to 27.1 weeks (95% CI 23.1–31.9) with placebo (hazard ratio 0.98, 95% CI 0.83–1.17, $p = 0.86$). While vorinostat did not improve survival, as the largest randomized trial to date in mesothelioma, this study demonstrated the feasibility of conducting such studies in this patient population and has contributed to the subsequent willingness of pharmaceutical companies to pursue drugs in this space.

15.5.2   Tazemetostat

While the high frequency of BAP1 alterations in mesothelioma was discovered more than 5 years ago, the therapeutic strategy to exploit this common alteration remains elusive (Bott et al. 2011; Bueno et al. 2016; Guo et al. 2015; Ladanyi et al. 2012). ASXL1 is a known interaction partner of BAP1 in the formation of a polycomb deubiquitinase complex (Margueron and Reinberg 2011; Sahtoe et al. 2016), and using a knockout model system, loss of *Bap1* and *Asxl1* was found to have inverse effects on gene expression, opposite effects on *HoxA* gene expression (Abdel-Wahab et al. 2012), and opposite impact on levels of trimethylated histone H3 lysine 27 (H3K27me3) (Abdel-Wahab et al. 2013; LaFave et al. 2015). Silencing of BAP1 led to increased H3K27me3 and dysregulation of genes implicated in EZH2-dependent regulation. In mouse models, knockout of *Ezh2* abrogated the myelodysplastic syndrome induced by *Bap1* loss (Dey et al. 2012; LaFave et al. 2015). To validate the genetic data, *Bap1* knockout mice were treated with tazemetostat, a small molecular EZH2 inhibitor (Campbell et al. 2015), and the myelodysplastic syndrome improved. These observations were validated in several mesothelioma cell lines, with tazemetostat impairing cell growth in *BAP1*-deficient cells while having little impact on *BAP1* wild-type cells. Additionally, EZH2 inhibition was already under investigation (Takawa et al. 2011) and showing preliminary efficacy signals in lymphoma (Knutson et al. 2012; McCabe et al. 2012) and malignant rhabdoid tumors (Knutson et al. 2013).

These discoveries were the preclinical rationale for an ongoing phase II multicenter single-arm clinical trial of tazemetostat in malignant mesothelioma with loss of BAP1 (NCT02860286). There is an initial 12-patient pharmacokinetic cohort in this study to ensure that a new formulation of this oral medication has similar bioavailability and half-life. Subsequently, 55 additional patients with mesothelioma that has molecular evidence of *BAP1* loss of function mutation, either by lack of nuclear BAP1 staining by immunohistochemistry or evidence of loss of function by gene sequencing, are eligible to receive oral tazemetostat. The primary endpoint of this study is to assess the disease control rate at 12 weeks. Target accrual should be reached in November 2018.

15.6   Cell Cycle Disruption Agents

Disruption of the cell cycle by interfering with the formation and function of key structures and steps in cell cycle progression and cell division has long been an active area for the development of cancer therapeutics (Evan and Vousden 2001; Hartwell and Kastan 1994; Kastan and Bartek 2004; Vermeulen et al. 2003). In fact, several traditional cytotoxic chemotherapy agents target such structures critical for cell division.

15.6.1 Bortezomib

Bortezomib is a proteasome 20S inhibitor and is already an established treatment for multiple myeloma in multiple clinical settings (Garderet et al. 2012; Jacobus et al. 2016; Kumar et al. 2012; Orlowski et al. 2016, 2007; Palumbo et al. 2010; Rosinol et al. 2012; Sonneveld et al. 2013, 2012). By transcriptionally upregulating the proapoptotic protein family Noxa, bcl-2-interacting mediator of cell death, and p53 upregulated modulator of apoptosis, bortezomib activates the intrinsic apoptotic pathway (Busacca et al. 2013; Fennell et al. 2008). In several preclinical mesothelioma models, bortezomib has demonstrated promising activity (Gordon et al. 2008; Sartore-Bianchi et al. 2007). These findings led to a single-arm phase II trial by the Ireland Cooperative Oncology Research Group (Fennell et al. 2012). Ten mesothelioma patients were accrued in the first-line setting and 23 in the second-line setting. In the first-line setting, there were no partial or complete responses and only one patient with stable disease. In the second-line setting, one patient had a partial response. There was also a single-arm phase II study of bortezomib in combination with cisplatin and pemetrexed conducted by the EORTC (O'Brien et al. 2013). The response rate among the 82 chemotherapy-naïve patients was 27.4%, including two complete responses and 21 partial responses. Median overall survival was 13.5 months (95% CI 10.5–15). The primary endpoint was the progression-free survival rate at 18 weeks, which was 53% and did not meet the prespecified threshold of 67.5%.

15.6.2 CBP501

Unlike normal cells, which repair most DNA damage at the G1 checkpoint, cancer cells typically disrupt the G1 checkpoint. Thus, they are more dependent on the G2 checkpoint (Kawabe 2004), and disruption of the G2 checkpoint becomes an attractive drug target. CBP501 inhibits several kinases involved in cell cycle arrest at G2 (Peng et al. 1997). By phosphorylating a serine on CDC25C, the transition from G2 to M by CDC/cyclin B is blocked. In combination with chemotherapy in cell lines, CBP501 increases the fraction of cells in G1 and thereby increases the cytotoxicity of cisplatin (Peng et al. 1997).

These observations were the preclinical rationale for a large randomized phase II trial of cisplatin and pemetrexed with or without CBP501 (NCT00700336). Blinding was not used, as the major toxicity of CBP501 is an infusion-related urticarial rash (Shapiro et al. 2011). In this study, 65 chemotherapy-naïve patients with unresectable malignant pleural mesothelioma were randomized to CBP501 versus placebo in a 2 to 1 ratio. The primary endpoint was the number of patients with progression-free survival equal to or greater than 4 months. For those treated with CBP501, 63% had progression-free survival equal or greater than 4 months, 31% (95% CI 17–47.6%) achieved a partial response, and median overall survival was 13.3 months

(95% CI 9.2–16.3). In the chemotherapy alone arm, 39% had progression-free survival equal or greater than 4 months, 10% (95% CI 1.2–31.7%) achieved a partial response, and median overall survival was 12.8 months (95% CI 6.5–16.1). While this trial met its prespecified endpoint of 60% achieving progression-free survival of 4 months or greater, because of the response rate and overall survival, the authors concluded that CBP501 did not improve the efficacy of cisplatin and pemetrexed for malignant pleural mesothelioma.

15.6.3   TRC102

Base excision repair (BER) is used by malignant cells to avoid the destruction that can be caused by antimetabolite and alkylating chemotherapies. When bases are damaged or abnormal bases incorporated, BER repairs them. Thus, blocking BER could improve the efficacy of chemotherapies that cause this type of DNA damage (Liu and Gerson 2004). TRC102, methoxyamine hydrochloride, is a small molecule inhibitor of BER that rapidly interrupts the BER pathway leading to the accumulation of DNA strand breaks which in turn cause apoptosis (Liuzzi and Talpaert-Borle 1985; Liuzzi et al. 1987). Because BER response is triggered by the pemetrexed-induced incorporation of uracil into DNA (Bulgar et al. 2012), TRC102 is an attractive drug to evaluate in combination with pemetrexed. A multicenter, open-label phase I study with 28 advanced solid tumor patients identified the maximum tolerated dose (MTD) of TRC102 as 60 mg/m²/day × 4 days when given in combination with pemetrexed (Gordon et al. 2013). There was a modest efficacy signal in the phase I trial, so a subsequent phase I/II trial is ongoing to evaluate TRC102 in combination with cisplatin and pemetrexed (NCT02535312). The primary objectives of this study are to establish the maximum tolerated dose of TRC102 in combination with both cisplatin and pemetrexed and then evaluate the efficacy of the combination. While most clinical trials that add a new drug to the standard cisplatin-pemetrexed combination exclude patients who previously received these agents, in an interesting twist, this clinical trial has a specific arm for prior pemetrexed recipients.

15.6.4   Alisertib

The Aurora kinase family of proteins are serine/threonine kinases that play a key role in the appropriate functioning of mitosis (Bolanos-Garcia 2005) with effects on centrosome function, spindle assembly, chromosome segregation, and mitotic entry (Barr and Gergely 2007; Carvajal et al. 2006; Marumoto et al. 2003). Specifically, preclinical experiments to disrupt the function of Aurora kinase A lead to cell death (Gorgun et al. 2010; Huck et al. 2010; Marumoto et al. 2003), and antitumor activity of Aurora kinase A inhibitors has been observed in several tumor types including mesothelioma (Crispi et al. 2010; Dar et al. 2008; Hook et al. 2012; Hoque et al. 2003; Mazumdar et al. 2009; Zhang et al. 2008). Alisertib is an oral selective inhibitor of Aurora kinase A (Manfredi et al. 2011) that has demonstrated activity against a variety of tumor types (Carol et al. 2011; Manfredi et al. 2011; Maris et al. 2010; Sells et al. 2015; Tomita and Mori 2010; Wang et al. 2015). Based on this preclinical rationale and using the already established MTD from phase I trials (Falchook et al. 2014), there is an ongoing phase II study of alisertib as salvage therapy in malignant mesothelioma (NCT02293005). Patients with unresectable mesothelioma who have previously received at least one prior pemetrexed-based chemotherapy regimen receive alisertib for a week every 21 days. The primary endpoint is disease control at 4 months using Simon's minimax two-stage design, and the secondary objective is response rate at 6 weeks. Enrollment is planned for 58 patients and is ongoing.

15.6.5   ADI-PEG20

Argininosuccinate synthase 1 (ASS1) is the rate-limiting enzyme for the synthesis of arginine, which is a key amino acid in several pathways related to tumorigenesis, such as the synthesis of polyamines, nitric oxide, and creatine (Jobgen et al. 2006; Leuzzi et al. 2008). In a variety of cancers, including mesothelioma (Szlosarek et al. 2006), ASS1 expression is frequently lost (Delage et al. 2010). Thus, depriving ASS1-deficient cells of arginine can induce lethality (Locke et al. 2016), as there is no mechanism for arginine biosynthesis. Using the arginine depleter mycoplasma-derived pegylated arginine deiminase (ADI-PEG20), this approach has shown both tolerability and efficacy in a few cancers (Ascierto et al. 2005; Glazer et al. 2010; Izzo et al. 2004; Synakiewicz et al. 2014; Yang et al. 2010).

Because of the frequent loss of ASS1 in mesothelioma, especially in sarcomatoid and biphasic histologies (Szlosarek et al. 2006), a biomarker-driven randomized phase II trial of ADI-PEG20 in patients with mesothelioma was conducted (NCT01279967) (Szlosarek et al. 2016). Sixty-eight patients with ASS1-deficient malignant pleural mesothelioma were eligible for randomization to weekly ADI-PEG20 or placebo. No complete or partial responses were observed. Among patients evaluable at 4 months, 52% had stable disease with ADI-PEG20, while 22% had stable disease with placebo. Median progression-free and overall survivals were 3.2 and 11.5 versus 2.0 and 11.1 months for ADI-PEG20 and placebo, respectively. The progression-free survival hazard ratio, adjusted for randomization stratification factors, was 0.47 (95% CI 0.25–0.86). Of note, one patient did have a dramatic 40% reduction in the maximum standardized uptake of his mesothelioma on this trial (Szlosarek et al. 2013). Based on this modest but statistically significant difference in progression-free survival, the authors concluded that ADI-PEG20 was worthy of further study.

In particular, given the potentiation of antifolate cytotoxicity with ADI-PEG20 in ASS1-negative cell lines (Allen et al. 2014), there has been interest in studying ADI-PEG20 in combination with pemetrexed-based chemotherapy. A phase I clinical trial of ADI-PEG20 in combination with cisplatin and pemetrexed is ongoing and includes patients with ASS1-deficient mesothelioma, non-squamous non-small cell lung cancer, metastatic uveal melanoma, hepatocellular carcinoma, glioma, and sarcomatoid cancers (NCT02029690). Based on the safety and preliminary efficacy signal seen in this phase I trial, a phase II/III randomized placebo-controlled study of ADI-PEG20 in combination with cisplatin and peme-trexed for chemotherapy-naïve patients with ASS1-deficient malignant pleural mesothelioma was launched (NCT02709512). The primary endpoint of this trial is response rate, with progression-free survival as a secondary endpoint. The planned accrual is 386 patients and is estimated to finish in October 2019.

15.7 Immunotherapy

Many novel immunotherapy agents are currently under development and investigation in mesothelioma, including checkpoint inhibitors, the WT1 vaccine SLS-001, anti-mesothelin directed antibodies, antibody-drug conjugates, and mesothelin-directed T-cell CARs. The field of immunotherapy continues to expand and evolve rapidly, and a separate chapter has been devoted to a thorough discussion of these agents and approaches.

15.8 Conclusions and Future Directions

The use of pemetrexed and platinum is a widely accepted standard for the initial treatment of mesothelioma, and the addition of bevacizumab is increasingly perva-sive. Not for lack of attempts, no agent has yet shown a survival benefit in the second-line setting. Several options are available including vinorelbine, gem-citabine, and re-treatment with pemetrexed-based therapy. Given the near universal lethality, clinical trial enrollment should be strongly encouraged at every stage of treatment for this disease. Additionally, research must focus on agents with strong biologic rationale, and clinical trials must be optimally designed to successfully enroll patients and answer clinically meaningful questions so that care can be rap-idly advanced to raise, rather than shift, survival curves.

While the many ongoing endeavors in mesothelioma are intriguing and most have solid foundations in preclinical research, some are pursuing questions with limited applicability to rapidly evolving patient care. For example, in an era when most patients will likely receive frontline bevacizumab based on MAPS (Zalcman et al. 2016), the applicability of the results of the ongoing nintedanib second-line trial (NCT02568449), which excludes patients who have received prior VEGF-directed therapy, is unclear. It is possible that nintedanib may improve survival as part of initial therapy or maintenance, but none of the ongoing trials will clarify how to use both bevacizumab and nintedanib and a head-to-head comparison is unlikely since the ultimate impact of such inquiry would be limited to an incremental advance. Similar vulnerabilities exist with ongoing clinical trials of other agents. Researchers for other uncommon diseases have successfully banded together to form consortiums through which clinically meaningful trials are rapidly executed. Such cooperation and organization is long overdue for mesothelioma and is likely the only way to break through the current therapeutic plateau in this disease.

Declaration of Interests The author declares no potential conflict of interest.

References

Abdel-Wahab O, Adli M, LaFave LM et al (2012) ASXL1 mutations promote myeloid transformation through loss of PRC2-mediated gene repression. Cancer Cell 22:180–193

Abdel-Wahab O, Gao J, Adli M et al (2013) Deletion of Asxl1 results in myelodysplasia and severe developmental defects in vivo. J Exp Med 210:2641–2659

Alberts AS, Falkson G, Van Zyl L (1988) Malignant pleural mesothelioma: phase II pilot study of ifosfamide and mesna. J Natl Cancer Inst 80:698–700

Allen MD, Luong P, Hudson C et al (2014) Prognostic and therapeutic impact of argininosuccinate synthetase 1 control in bladder cancer as monitored longitudinally by PET imaging. Cancer Res 74:896–907

Ascierto PA, Scala S, Castello G et al (2005) Pegylated arginine deiminase treatment of patients with metastatic melanoma: results from phase I and II studies. J Clin Oncol 23:7660–7668

Avet-Loiseau H, Li JY, Facon T et al (1998) High incidence of translocations t(11;14)(q13;q32) and t(4;14)(p16;q32) in patients with plasma cell malignancies. Cancer Res 58:5640–5645

Baas P, Ardizzoni A, Grossi F et al (2003) The activity of raltitrexed (Tomudex) in malignant pleural mesothelioma: an EORTC phase II study (08992). Eur J Cancer 39:353–357

Baas P, Boogerd W, Dalesio O et al (2005) Thalidomide in patients with malignant pleural mesothelioma. Lung Cancer 48:291–296

Baas P, van Meerbeeck J, Groen H et al (2000) Caelyx in malignant mesothelioma: a phase II EORTC study. Ann Oncol 11:697–700

Bajorin D, Kelsen D, Mintzer DM (1987) Phase II trial of mitomycin in malignant mesothelioma. Cancer Treat Rep 71:857–858

Barr AR, Gergely F (2007) Aurora-A: the maker and breaker of spindle poles. J Cell Sci 120:2987–2996

Bartlett JB, Dredge K, Dalgleish AG (2004) The evolution of thalidomide and its IMiD derivatives as anticancer agents. Nat Rev Cancer 4:314–322

Baselga J, Campone M, Piccart M et al (2012) Everolimus in postmenopausal hormone-receptor-positive advanced breast cancer. N Engl J Med 366:520–529

Bearz A, Talamini R, Rossoni G et al (2012) Re-challenge with pemetrexed in advanced mesothelioma: a multi-institutional experience. BMC Res Notes 5:482

Beenken A, Mohammadi M (2009) The FGF family: biology, pathophysiology and therapy. Nat Rev Drug Discov 8:235–253

Belani CP, Adak S, Aisner S et al (2004) Docetaxel for malignant mesothelioma: phase II study of the Eastern Cooperative Oncology Group. Clin Lung Cancer 6:43–47

Bissler JJ, Kingswood JC, Radzikowska E et al (2013) Everolimus for angiomyolipoma associated with tuberous sclerosis complex or sporadic lymphangioleiomyomatosis (EXIST-2): a multicentre, randomised, double-blind, placebo-controlled trial. Lancet 381:817–824

Blackwell C, Sherk C, Fricko M et al (2016) Inhibition of FGF/FGFR autocrine signaling in mesothelioma with the FGF ligand trap, FP-1039/GSK3052230. Oncotarget 7:39861–39871

Bolanos-Garcia VM (2005) Aurora kinases. Int J Biochem Cell Biol 37:1572–1577

Bolden JE, Peart MJ, Johnstone RW (2006) Anticancer activities of histone deacetylase inhibitors. Nat Rev Drug Discov 5:769–784

Bott M, Brevet M, Taylor BS et al (2011) The nuclear deubiquitinase BAP1 is commonly inactivated by somatic mutations and 3p21.1 losses in malignant pleural mesothelioma. Nat Genet 43:668–672

Boutin C, Irisson M, Guerin JC et al (1987) Phase II trial of vindesine in malignant pleural mesothelioma. Cancer Treat Rep 71:205–206

Bueno R, Stawiski EW, Goldstein LD et al (2016) Comprehensive genomic analysis of malignant pleural mesothelioma identifies recurrent mutations, gene fusions and splicing alterations. Nat Genet 48:407–416

Buikhuisen WA, Burgers JA, Vincent AD et al (2013) Thalidomide versus active supportive care for maintenance in patients with malignant mesothelioma after first-line chemotherapy (NVALT 5): an open-label, multicentre, randomised phase 3 study. Lancet Oncol 14:543–551

Buikhuisen WA, Scharpfenecker M, Griffioen AW et al (2016) A randomized phase II study adding axitinib to pemetrexed-cisplatin in patients with malignant pleural mesothelioma: a single-center trial combining clinical and translational outcomes. J Thorac Oncol 11:758–768

Bulgar AD, Weeks LD, Miao Y et al (2012) Removal of uracil by uracil DNA glycosylase limits pemetrexed cytotoxicity: overriding the limit with methoxyamine to inhibit base excision repair. Cell Death Dis 3:e252

Busacca S, Chacko AD, Klabatsa A et al (2013) BAK and NOXA are critical determinants of mitochondrial apoptosis induced by bortezomib in mesothelioma. PLoS One 8:e65489

Busacca S, Sheaff M, Arthur K et al (2012) BRCA1 is an essential mediator of vinorelbine-induced apoptosis in mesothelioma. J Pathol 227:200–208

Campbell JE, Kuntz KW, Knutson SK et al (2015) EPZ011989, A Potent, Orally-Available EZH2 Inhibitor with Robust in Vivo Activity. ACS Med Chem Lett 6:491–495

Campbell NP, Kunnavakkam R, Leighl N et al (2012) Cediranib in patients with malignant mesothelioma: a phase II trial of the University of Chicago Phase II Consortium. Lung Cancer 78:76–80

Cao XX, Mohuiddin I, Ece F et al (2001) Histone deacetylase inhibitor downregulation of bcl-xl gene expression leads to apoptotic cell death in mesothelioma. Am J Respir Cell Mol Biol 25:562–568

Carol H, Boehm I, Reynolds CP et al (2011) Efficacy and pharmacokinetic/pharmacodynamic evaluation of the Aurora kinase A inhibitor MLN8237 against preclinical models of pediatric cancer. Cancer Chemother Pharmacol 68:1291–1304

Carswell EA, Old LJ, Kassel RL et al (1975) An endotoxin-induced serum factor that causes necrosis of tumors. Proc Natl Acad Sci U S A 72:3666–3670

Carvajal RD, Tse A, Schwartz GK (2006) Aurora kinases: new targets for cancer therapy. Clin Cancer Res 12:6869–6875

Castagneto B, Botta M, Aitini E et al (2008) Phase II study of pemetrexed in combination with carboplatin in patients with malignant pleural mesothelioma (MPM). Ann Oncol 19:370–373

Castagneto B, Zai S, Dongiovanni D et al (2005) Cisplatin and gemcitabine in malignant pleural mesothelioma: a phase II study. Am J Clin Oncol 28:223–226

Cedres S, Montero MA, Martinez P et al (2012) Exploratory analysis of activation of PTEN-PI3K pathway and downstream proteins in malignant pleural mesothelioma (MPM). Lung Cancer 77:192–198

Ceresoli GL, Castagneto B, Zucali PA et al (2008) Pemetrexed plus carboplatin in elderly patients with malignant pleural mesothelioma: combined analysis of two phase II trials. Br J Cancer 99:51–56

Ceresoli GL, Zucali PA, De Vincenzo F et al (2011) Retreatment with pemetrexed-based chemotherapy in patients with malignant pleural mesothelioma. Lung Cancer 72:73–77

Ceresoli GL, Zucali PA, Favaretto AG et al (2006) Phase II study of pemetrexed plus carboplatin in malignant pleural mesothelioma. J Clin Oncol 24:1443–1448

Colombo G, Curnis F, De Mori GM et al (2002) Structure-activity relationships of linear and cyclic peptides containing the NGR tumor-homing motif. J Biol Chem 277:47891–47897

Corti A, Ponzoni M (2004) Tumor vascular targeting with tumor necrosis factor alpha and chemotherapeutic drugs. Ann N Y Acad Sci 1028:104–112

Cowan JD, Green S, Lucas J et al (1988) Phase II trial of five day intravenous infusion vinblastine sulfate in patients with diffuse malignant mesothelioma: a Southwest Oncology Group study. Investig New Drugs 6:247–248

Creaven PJ, Brenner DE, Cowens JW et al (1989) A phase I clinical trial of recombinant human tumor necrosis factor given daily for five days. Cancer Chemother Pharmacol 23:186–191

Crispi S, Fagliarone C, Biroccio A et al (2010) Antiproliferative effect of Aurora kinase targeting in mesothelioma. Lung Cancer 70:271–279

Curnis F, Arrigoni G, Sacchi A et al (2002) Differential binding of drugs containing the NGR motif to CD13 isoforms in tumor vessels, epithelia, and myeloid cells. Cancer Res 62:867–874

Curnis F, Sacchi A, Borgna L et al (2000) Enhancement of tumor necrosis factor alpha antitumor immunotherapeutic properties by targeted delivery to aminopeptidase N (CD13). Nat Biotechnol 18:1185–1190

Dancey J (2010) mTOR signaling and drug development in cancer. Nat Rev Clin Oncol 7:209–219

Dar AA, Zaika A, Piazuelo MB et al (2008) Frequent overexpression of Aurora Kinase A in upper gastrointestinal adenocarcinomas correlates with potent antiapoptotic functions. Cancer 112:1688–1698

Davidson B, Vintman L, Zcharia E et al (2004) Heparanase and basic fibroblast growth factor are co-expressed in malignant mesothelioma. Clin Exp Metastasis 21:469–476

Dawson MA, Kouzarides T, Huntly BJ (2012) Targeting epigenetic readers in cancer. N Engl J Med 367:647–657

Delage B, Fennell DA, Nicholson L et al (2010) Arginine deprivation and argininosuccinate synthetase expression in the treatment of cancer. Int J Cancer 126:2762–2772

Dey A, Seshasayee D, Noubade R et al (2012) Loss of the tumor suppressor BAP1 causes myeloid transformation. Science 337:1541–1546

di Martino E, L'Hote CG, Kennedy W et al (2009) Mutant fibroblast growth factor receptor 3 induces intracellular signaling and cellular transformation in a cell type- and mutation-specific manner. Oncogene 28:4306–4316

Dolly SO, Krug LM, Wagner AJ et al (2013) Evaluation of tolerability and anti-tumor activity of Gdc-0980, an oral Pi3k/mtor inhibitor, administered to patients with advanced malignant pleural mesothelioma (MPM). J Thorac Oncol 8:S307–S308

Dolly SO, Wagner AJ, Bendell JC et al (2016) Phase I study of apitolisib (GDC-0980), dual phosphatidylinositol-3-kinase and mammalian target of rapamycin kinase inhibitor, in patients with advanced solid tumors. Clin Cancer Res 22:2874–2884

Dowell JE, Dunphy FR, Taub RN et al (2012) A multicenter phase II study of cisplatin, pemetrexed, and bevacizumab in patients with advanced malignant mesothelioma. Lung Cancer 77:567–571

Dubey S, Janne PA, Krug L et al (2010) A phase II study of sorafenib in malignant mesothelioma: results of Cancer and Leukemia Group B 30307. J Thorac Oncol 5:1655–1661

Dutt A, Ramos AH, Hammerman PS et al (2011) Inhibitor-sensitive FGFR1 amplification in human non-small cell lung cancer. PLoS One 6:e20351

Dutt A, Salvesen HB, Chen TH et al (2008) Drug-sensitive FGFR2 mutations in endometrial carcinoma. Proc Natl Acad Sci U S A 105:8713–8717

Duvic M, Talpur R, Ni X et al (2007) Phase 2 trial of oral vorinostat (suberoylanilide hydroxamic acid, SAHA) for refractory cutaneous T-cell lymphoma (CTCL). Blood 109:31–39

Duvic M, Vu J (2007) Vorinostat: a new oral histone deacetylase inhibitor approved for cutaneous T-cell lymphoma. Expert Opin Investig Drugs 16:1111–1120

Edwards JG, Cox G, Andi A et al (2001) Angiogenesis is an independent prognostic factor in malignant mesothelioma. Br J Cancer 85:863–868

Ellis L, Atadja PW, Johnstone RW (2009) Epigenetics in cancer: targeting chromatin modifications. Mol Cancer Ther 8:1409–1420

Epstein Shochet G, Israeli-Shani L, Koslow M et al (2016) Nintedanib (BIBF 1120) blocks the tumor promoting signals of lung fibroblast soluble microenvironment. Lung Cancer 96:7–14

Evan GI, Vousden KH (2001) Proliferation, cell cycle and apoptosis in cancer. Nature 411:342–348

Falchook G, Kurzrock R, Gouw L et al (2014) Investigational aurora A kinase inhibitor alisertib (MLN8237) as an enteric-coated tablet formulation in non-hematologic malignancies: phase 1 dose-escalation study. Investig New Drugs 32:1181–1187

Falkson G, Hunt M, Borden EC et al (1992) An extended phase II trial of ifosfamide plus mesna in malignant mesothelioma. Investig New Drugs 10:337–343

Favaretto AG, Aversa SM, Paccagnella A et al (2003) Gemcitabine combined with carboplatin in patients with malignant pleural mesothelioma: a multicentric phase II study. Cancer 97:2791–2797

Fennell DA, Gaudino G, O'Byrne KJ et al (2008) Advances in the systemic therapy of malignant pleural mesothelioma. Nat Clin Pract Oncol 5:136–147

Fennell DA, McDowell C, Busacca S et al (2012) Phase II clinical trial of first or second-line treatment with bortezomib in patients with malignant pleural mesothelioma. J Thorac Oncol 7:1466–1470

Fennell DA, Parmar A, Shamash J et al (2005) Statistical validation of the EORTC prognostic model for malignant pleural mesothelioma based on three consecutive phase II trials. J Clin Oncol 23:184–189

Fine HA, Figg WD, Jaeckle K et al (2000) Phase II trial of the antiangiogenic agent thalidomide in patients with recurrent high-grade gliomas. J Clin Oncol 18:708–715

Folkman J (1971) Tumor angiogenesis: therapeutic implications. N Engl J Med 285:1182–1186

Franz DN, Belousova E, Sparagana S et al (2013) Efficacy and safety of everolimus for subependymal giant cell astrocytomas associated with tuberous sclerosis complex (EXIST-1): a multicentre, randomised, placebo-controlled phase 3 trial. Lancet 381:125–132

Fruman DA, Rommel C (2014) PI3K and cancer: lessons, challenges and opportunities. Nat Rev Drug Discov 13:140–156

Gamm H, Lindemann A, Mertelsmann R et al (1991) Phase I trial of recombinant human tumour necrosis factor alpha in patients with advanced malignancy. Eur J Cancer 27:856–863

Gardcret L, Iacobelli S, Moreau P et al (2012) Superiority of the triple combination of bortezomib-thalidomide-dexamethasone over the dual combination of thalidomide-dexamethasone in patients with multiple myeloma progressing or relapsing after autologous transplantation: the MMVAR/IFM 2005-04 Randomized Phase III Trial from the Chronic Leukemia Working Party of the European Group for Blood and Marrow Transplantation. J Clin Oncol 30:2475–2482

Garland LL, Chansky K, Wozniak AJ et al (2011) Phase II study of cediranib in patients with malignant pleural mesothelioma: SWOG S0509. J Thorac Oncol 6:1938–1945

Garland LL, Rankin C, Gandara DR et al (2007) Phase II study of erlotinib in patients with malignant pleural mesothelioma: a Southwest Oncology Group Study. J Clin Oncol 25:2406–2413

Garrido P, Delgado I, Felip E et al (2015) FP1039/GSK3052230 with chemotherapy in patients with fibroblast growth factor (FGF) pathway deregulated squamous NSCLC or MPM. J Thorac Oncol 10:S403–S403

Garrido P, Felip E, Delord JP et al (2014) Multi-arm, nonrandomized, open-label phase Ib study to evaluate FP1039/GSK3052230 with chemotherapy in NSCLC and MPM with deregulated FGF pathway signaling. Ann Oncol 25. (abstract)

Glazer ES, Piccirillo M, Albino V et al (2010) Phase II study of pegylated arginine deiminase for nonresectable and metastatic hepatocellular carcinoma. J Clin Oncol 28:2220–2226

Goke F, Bode M, Franzen A et al (2013) Fibroblast growth factor receptor 1 amplification is a common event in squamous cell carcinoma of the head and neck. Mod Pathol 26:1298–1306

Gordon GJ, Mani M, Maulik G et al (2008) Preclinical studies of the proteasome inhibitor bortezomib in malignant pleural mesothelioma. Cancer Chemother Pharmacol 61:549–558

Gordon MS, Rosen LS, Mendelson D et al (2013) A phase 1 study of TRC102, an inhibitor of base excision repair, and pemetrexed in patients with advanced solid tumors. Investig New Drugs 31:714–723

Gorgun G, Calabrese E, Hideshima T et al (2010) A novel Aurora-A kinase inhibitor MLN8237 induces cytotoxicity and cell-cycle arrest in multiple myeloma. Blood 115:5202–5213

Govindan R, Kratzke RA, Herndon JE 2nd et al (2005) Gefitinib in patients with malignant mesothelioma: a phase II study by the Cancer and Leukemia Group B. Clin Cancer Res 11:2300–2304

Gregorc V, Citterio G, Vitali G et al (2010a) Defining the optimal biological dose of NGR-hTNF, a selective vascular targeting agent, in advanced solid tumours. Eur J Cancer 46:198–206

Gregorc V, Zucali PA, Santoro A et al (2010b) Phase II study of asparagine-glycine-arginine-human tumor necrosis factor alpha, a selective vascular targeting agent, in previously treated patients with malignant pleural mesothelioma. J Clin Oncol 28:2604–2611

Grose R, Dickson C (2005) Fibroblast growth factor signaling in tumorigenesis. Cytokine Growth Factor Rev 16:179–186

Guo G, Chmielecki J, Goparaju C et al (2015) Whole-exome sequencing reveals frequent genetic alterations in *BAP1*, *NF2*, *CDKN2A*, and *CUL1* in malignant pleural mesothelioma. Cancer Res 75:264–269

Hartman ML, Esposito JM, Yeap BY et al (2010) Combined treatment with cisplatin and sirolimus to enhance cell death in human mesothelioma. J Thorac Cardiovasc Surg 139:1233–1240

Hartwell LH, Kastan MB (1994) Cell cycle control and cancer. Science 266:1821–1828

Hilberg F, Roth GJ, Krssak M et al (2008) BIBF 1120: triple angiokinase inhibitor with sustained receptor blockade and good antitumor efficacy. Cancer Res 68:4774–4782

Hoda MA, Mohamed A, Ghanim B et al (2011) Temsirolimus inhibits malignant pleural mesothelioma growth in vitro and in vivo: synergism with chemotherapy. J Thorac Oncol 6:852–863

Hook KE, Garza SJ, Lira ME et al (2012) An integrated genomic approach to identify predictive biomarkers of response to the aurora kinase inhibitor PF-03814735. Mol Cancer Ther 11:710–719

Hoque A, Carter J, Xia W et al (2003) Loss of aurora A/STK15/BTAK overexpression correlates with transition of in situ to invasive ductal carcinoma of the breast. Cancer Epidemiol Biomark Prev 12:1518–1522

Huck JJ, Zhang M, McDonald A et al (2010) MLN8054, an inhibitor of aurora A kinase, induces senescence in human tumor cells both in vitro and in vivo. Mol Cancer Res 8:373–384

Illei PB, Ladanyi M, Rusch VW et al (2003) The use of CDKN2A deletion as a diagnostic marker for malignant mesothelioma in body cavity effusions. Cancer 99:51–56

Itoh N (2007) The Fgf families in humans, mice, and zebrafish: their evolutional processes and roles in development, metabolism, and disease. Biol Pharm Bull 30:1819–1825

Izzo F, Marra P, Beneduce G et al (2004) Pegylated arginine deiminase treatment of patients with unresectable hepatocellular carcinoma: results from phase I/II studies. J Clin Oncol 22:1815–1822

Jacobus SJ, Rajkumar SV, Weiss M et al (2016) Randomized phase III trial of consolidation therapy with bortezomib-lenalidomide-Dexamethasone (VRd) vs bortezomib-dexamethasone (Vd) for patients with multiple myeloma who have completed a dexamethasone based induction regimen. Blood Cancer J 6:e448

Jahan T, Gu L, Kratzke R et al (2012) Vatalanib in malignant mesothelioma: a phase II trial by the Cancer and Leukemia Group B (CALGB 30107). Lung Cancer 76:393–396

Janne PA, Wozniak AJ, Belani CP et al (2006) Pemetrexed alone or in combination with cisplatin in previously treated malignant pleural mesothelioma: outcomes from a phase IIIB expanded access program. J Thorac Oncol 1:506–512

Jobgen WS, Fried SK, Fu WJ et al (2006) Regulatory role for the arginine-nitric oxide pathway in metabolism of energy substrates. J Nutr Biochem 17:571–588

Kalmadi SR, Rankin C, Kraut MJ et al (2008) Gemcitabine and cisplatin in unresectable malignant mesothelioma of the pleura: a phase II study of the Southwest Oncology Group (SWOG 9810). Lung Cancer 60:259–263

Kao SC, Harvie R, Paturi F et al (2012) The predictive role of serum VEGF in an advanced malignant mesothelioma patient cohort treated with thalidomide alone or combined with cisplatin/gemcitabine. Lung Cancer 75:248–254

Kastan MB, Bartek J (2004) Cell-cycle checkpoints and cancer. Nature 432:316–323

Katirtzoglou N, Gkiozos I, Makrilia N et al (2010) Carboplatin plus pemetrexed as first-line treatment of patients with malignant pleural mesothelioma: a phase II study. Clin Lung Cancer 11:30–35

Kaufman AJ, Pass HI (2008) Current concepts in malignant pleural mesothelioma. Expert Rev Anticancer Ther 8:293–303

Kawabe T (2004) G2 checkpoint abrogators as anticancer drugs. Mol Cancer Ther 3:513–519

Kelly WK, O'Connor OA, Krug LM et al (2005) Phase I study of an oral histone deacetylase inhibitor, suberoylanilide hydroxamic acid, in patients with advanced cancer. J Clin Oncol 23:3923–3931

Kimura K, Taguchi T, Urushizaki I et al (1987) Phase I study of recombinant human tumor necrosis factor. Cancer Chemother Pharmacol 20:223–229

Kindler HL, Belani CP, Herndon JE 2nd et al (1999) Edatrexate (10-ethyl-deaza-aminopterin) (NSC #626715) with or without leucovorin rescue for malignant mesothelioma. Sequential phase II trials by the cancer and leukemia group B. Cancer 86:1985–1991

Kindler HL, Herndon JE, Zhang C et al (2005) Irinotecan for malignant mesothelioma A phase II trial by the Cancer and Leukemia Group B. Lung Cancer 48:423–428

Kindler HL, Karrison TG, Gandara DR et al (2012) Multicenter, double-blind, placebo-controlled, randomized phase II trial of gemcitabine/cisplatin plus bevacizumab or placebo in patients with malignant mesothelioma. J Clin Oncol 30:2509–2515

Kindler HL, Millard F, Herndon JE 2nd et al (2001) Gemcitabine for malignant mesothelioma: A phase II trial by the Cancer and Leukemia Group B. Lung Cancer 31:311–317

Knutson SK, Warholic NM, Wigle TJ et al (2013) Durable tumor regression in genetically altered malignant rhabdoid tumors by inhibition of methyltransferase EZH2. Proc Natl Acad Sci U S A 110:7922–7927

Knutson SK, Wigle TJ, Warholic NM et al (2012) A selective inhibitor of EZH2 blocks H3K27 methylation and kills mutant lymphoma cells. Nat Chem Biol 8:890–896

Kosty MP, Herndon JE 2nd, Vogelzang NJ et al (2001) High-dose doxorubicin, dexrazoxane, and GM-CSF in malignant mesothelioma: a phase II study-Cancer and Leukemia Group B 9631. Lung Cancer 34:289–295

Krug LM, Kindler HL, Calvert H et al (2015) Vorinostat in patients with advanced malignant pleural mesothelioma who have progressed on previous chemotherapy (VANTAGE-014): a phase 3, double-blind, randomised, placebo-controlled trial. Lancet Oncol 16:447–456

Kudo K, Arao T, Tanaka K et al (2011) Antitumor activity of BIBF 1120, a triple angiokinase inhibitor, and use of VEGFR2 + pTyr + peripheral blood leukocytes as a pharmacodynamic biomarker in vivo. Clin Cancer Res 17:1373–1381

Kumar S, Flinn I, Richardson PG et al (2012) Randomized, multicenter, phase 2 study (EVOLUTION) of combinations of bortezomib, dexamethasone, cyclophosphamide, and lenalidomide in previously untreated multiple myeloma. Blood 119:4375–4382

Kumar-Singh S, Segers K, Rodeck U et al (1997a) WT1 mutation in malignant mesothelioma and WT1 immunoreactivity in relation to p53 and growth factor receptor expression, cell-type transition, and prognosis. J Pathol 181:67–74

Kumar-Singh S, Vermeulen PB, Weyler J et al (1997b) Evaluation of tumour angiogenesis as a prognostic marker in malignant mesothelioma. J Pathol 182:211–216

Kumar-Singh S, Weyler J, Martin MJ et al (1999) Angiogenic cytokines in mesothelioma: a study of VEGF, FGF-1 and -2, and TGF beta expression. J Pathol 189:72–78

Ladanyi M, Zauderer MG, Krug LM et al (2012) New strategies in pleural mesothelioma: BAP1 and NF2 as novel targets for therapeutic development and risk assessment. Clin Cancer Res 18:4485–4490

LaFave LM, Beguelin W, Koche R et al (2015) Loss of BAP1 function leads to EZH2-dependent transformation. Nat Med 21:1344–1349

Laurie SA, Gupta A, Chu Q et al (2011) Brief report: a phase II study of sunitinib in malignant pleural mesothelioma. the NCIC Clinical Trials Group. J Thorac Oncol 6:1950–1954

Lebwohl D, Anak O, Sahmoud T et al (2013) Development of everolimus, a novel oral mTOR inhibitor, across a spectrum of diseases. Ann N Y Acad Sci 1291:14–32

Lejeune FJ, Lienard D, Matter M et al (2006) Efficiency of recombinant human TNF in human cancer therapy. Cancer Immun 6:6

Lerner HJ, Schoenfeld DA, Martin A et al (1983) Malignant mesothelioma. The Eastern Cooperative Oncology Group (ECOG) experience. Cancer 52:1981–1985

Leuzzi V, Alessandri MG, Casarano M et al (2008) Arginine and glycine stimulate creatine synthesis in creatine transporter 1-deficient lymphoblasts. Anal Biochem 375:153–155

Li Q, Wang W, Yamada T et al (2011) Pleural mesothelioma instigates tumor-associated fibroblasts to promote progression via a malignant cytokine network. Am J Pathol 179:1483–1493

Liao RG, Jung J, Tchaicha J et al (2013) Inhibitor-sensitive FGFR2 and FGFR3 mutations in lung squamous cell carcinoma. Cancer Res 73:5195–5205

Linder C, Linder S, Munck-Wikland E et al (1998) Independent expression of serum vascular endothelial growth factor (VEGF) and basic fibroblast growth factor (bFGF) in patients with carcinoma and sarcoma. Anticancer Res 18:2063–2068

Liu L, Gerson SL (2004) Therapeutic impact of methoxyamine: blocking repair of abasic sites in the base excision repair pathway. Curr Opin Investig Drugs 5:623–627

Liuzzi M, Talpaert-Borle M (1985) A new approach to the study of the base-excision repair pathway using methoxyamine. J Biol Chem 260:5252–5258

Liuzzi M, Weinfeld M, Paterson MC (1987) Selective inhibition by methoxyamine of the apurinic/apyrimidinic endonuclease activity associated with pyrimidine dimer-DNA glycosylases from Micrococcus luteus and bacteriophage T4. Biochemistry 26:3315–3321

Locke M, Ghazaly E, Freitas MO et al (2016) Inhibition of the polyamine synthesis pathway is synthetically lethal with loss of argininosuccinate synthase 1. Cell Rep 16:1604–1613

Loganathan S, Kanteti R, Siddiqui SS et al (2011) Role of protein kinase C beta and vascular endothelial growth factor receptor in malignant pleural mesothelioma: therapeutic implications and the usefulness of *Caenorhabditis elegans* model organism. J Carcinog 10:4

Lopez PG, Felip E, Delord JP et al (2014) Multiarm, nonrandomized, open-label phase IB study to evaluate FP1039/GSK3052230 with chemotherapy in NSCLC and MPM with deregulated FCT pathway signaling. J Clin Oncol 32. (abstract)

Lopez-Lago MA, Okada T, Murillo MM et al (2009) Loss of the tumor suppressor gene NF2, encoding merlin, constitutively activates integrin-dependent mTORC1 signaling. Mol Cell Biol 29:4235–4249

Lu YY, Jhanwar SC, Cheng JQ et al (1994) Deletion mapping of the short arm of chromosome 3 in human malignant mesothelioma. Genes Chromosom Cancer 9:76–80

Maksymiuk AW, Marschke RF Jr, Tazelaar HD et al (1998) Phase II trial of topotecan for the treatment of mesothelioma. Am J Clin Oncol 21:610–613

Manegold C, Symanowski J, Gatzemeier U et al (2005) Second-line (post-study) chemotherapy received by patients treated in the phase III trial of pemetrexed plus cisplatin versus cisplatin alone in malignant pleural mesothelioma. Ann Oncol 16:923–927

Manfredi MG, Ecsedy JA, Chakravarty A et al (2011) Characterization of Alisertib (MLN8237), an investigational small-molecule inhibitor of aurora A kinase using novel in vivo pharmacodynamic assays. Clin Cancer Res 17:7614–7624

Marek LA, Hinz TK, von Massenhausen A et al (2014) Nonamplified FGFR1 is a growth driver in malignant pleural mesothelioma. Mol Cancer Res 12:1460–1469

Margueron R, Reinberg D (2011) The Polycomb complex PRC2 and its mark in life. Nature 469:343–349

Maris JM, Morton CL, Gorlick R et al (2010) Initial testing of the aurora kinase A inhibitor MLN8237 by the Pediatric Preclinical Testing Program (PPTP). Pediatr Blood Cancer 55:26–34

Martensson G, Sorenson S (1989) A phase II study of vincristine in malignant mesothelioma--a negative report. Cancer Chemother Pharmacol 24:133–134

Marumoto T, Honda S, Hara T et al (2003) Aurora-A kinase maintains the fidelity of early and late mitotic events in HeLa cells. J Biol Chem 278:51786–51795

Masood R, Kundra A, Zhu S et al (2003) Malignant mesothelioma growth inhibition by agents that target the VEGF and VEGF-C autocrine loops. Int J Cancer 104:603–610

Mathy A, Baas P, Dalesio O et al (2005) Limited efficacy of imatinib mesylate in malignant mesothelioma: a phase II trial. Lung Cancer 50:83–86

Mazumdar A, Henderson YC, El-Naggar AK et al (2009) Aurora kinase A inhibition and paclitaxel as targeted combination therapy for head and neck squamous cell carcinoma. Head Neck 31:625–634

Mbidde EK, Harland SJ, Calvert AH et al (1986) Phase II trial of carboplatin (JM8) in treatment of patients with malignant mesothelioma. Cancer Chemother Pharmacol 18:284–285

McCabe MT, Ott HM, Ganji G et al (2012) EZH2 inhibition as a therapeutic strategy for lymphoma with EZH2-activating mutations. Nature 492:108–112

Mintzer DM, Kelsen D, Frimmer D et al (1985) Phase II trial of high-dose cisplatin in patients with malignant mesothelioma. Cancer Treat Rep 69:711–712

Minucci S, Pelicci PG (2006) Histone deacetylase inhibitors and the promise of epigenetic (and more) treatments for cancer. Nat Rev Cancer 6:38–51

Mittelman A, Puccio C, Gafney E et al (1992) A phase I pharmacokinetic study of recombinant human tumor necrosis factor administered by a 5-day continuous infusion. Investig New Drugs 10:183–190

Moriya M, Yamada T, Tamura M et al (2014) Antitumor effect and antiangiogenic potential of the mTOR inhibitor temsirolimus against malignant pleural mesothelioma. Oncol Rep 31:1109–1115

Motzer RJ, Escudier B, Oudard S et al (2008) Efficacy of everolimus in advanced renal cell carcinoma: a double-blind, randomised, placebo-controlled phase III trial. Lancet 372:449–456

Neuzil J, Swettenham E, Gellert N (2004) Sensitization of mesothelioma to TRAIL apoptosis by inhibition of histone deacetylase: role of Bcl-xL down-regulation. Biochem Biophys Res Commun 314:186–191

Nowak AK, Byrne MJ, Williamson R et al (2002) A multicentre phase II study of cisplatin and gemcitabine for malignant mesothelioma. Br J Cancer 87:491–496

Nowak AK, Millward MJ, Creaney J et al (2012) A phase II study of intermittent sunitinib malate as second-line therapy in progressive malignant pleural mesothelioma. J Thorac Oncol 7:1449–1456

O'Brien ME, Gaafar RM, Popat S et al (2013) Phase II study of first-line bortezomib and cisplatin in malignant pleural mesothelioma and prospective validation of progression free survival rate as a primary end-point for mesothelioma clinical trials (European Organisation for Research and Treatment of Cancer 08052). Eur J Cancer 49:2815–2822

Oh Y, Perez-Soler R, Fossella FV et al (2000) Phase II study of intravenous Doxil in malignant pleural mesothelioma. Investig New Drugs 18:243–245

Ohta Y, Shridhar V, Bright RK et al (1999) VEGF and VEGF type C play an important role in angiogenesis and lymphangiogenesis in human malignant mesothelioma tumours. Br J Cancer 81:54–61

Okada T, Lopez-Lago M, Giancotti FG (2005) Merlin/NF-2 mediates contact inhibition of growth by suppressing recruitment of Rac to the plasma membrane. J Cell Biol 171:361–371

Orlowski RZ, Nagler A, Sonneveld P et al (2016) Final overall survival results of a randomized trial comparing bortezomib plus pegylated liposomal doxorubicin with bortezomib alone in patients with relapsed or refractory multiple myeloma. Cancer 122:2050–2056

Orlowski RZ, Nagler A, Sonneveld P et al (2007) Randomized phase III study of pegylated liposomal doxorubicin plus bortezomib compared with bortezomib alone in relapsed or refractory multiple myeloma: combination therapy improves time to progression. J Clin Oncol 25:3892–3901

Otterson GA, Herndon JE 2nd, Watson D et al (2004) Capecitabine in malignant mesothelioma: a phase II trial by the Cancer and Leukemia Group B (39807). Lung Cancer 44:251–259

Ou SH, Moon J, Garland LL et al (2015) SWOG S0722: phase II study of mTOR inhibitor everolimus (RAD001) in advanced malignant pleural mesothelioma (MPM). J Thorac Oncol 10:387–391

Paik PK, Krug LM (2010) Histone deacetylase inhibitors in malignant pleural mesothelioma: preclinical rationale and clinical trials. J Thorac Oncol 5:275–279

Palumbo A, Bringhen S, Rossi D et al (2010) Bortezomib-melphalan-prednisone-thalidomide followed by maintenance with bortezomib-thalidomide compared with bortezomib-melphalan-prednisone for initial treatment of multiple myeloma: a randomized controlled trial. J Clin Oncol 28:5101–5109

Papa S, Popat S, Shah R et al (2013) Phase 2 study of sorafenib in malignant mesothelioma previously treated with platinum-containing chemotherapy. J Thorac Oncol 8:783–787

Pavel ME, Hainsworth JD, Baudin E et al (2011) Everolimus plus octreotide long-acting repeatable for the treatment of advanced neuroendocrine tumours associated with carcinoid syndrome (RADIANT-2): a randomised, placebo-controlled, phase 3 study. Lancet 378:2005–2012

Peng CY, Graves PR, Thoma RS et al (1997) Mitotic and G2 checkpoint control: regulation of 14-3-3 protein binding by phosphorylation of Cdc25C on serine-216. Science 277:1501–1505

Popat S, Mellemgaard A, Fahrbach K et al (2015) Nintedanib plus docetaxel as second-line therapy in patients with non-small-cell lung cancer: a network meta-analysis. Future Oncol 11:409–420

Porta C (2006) Adding raltitrexed to cisplatin improves overall survival in people with malignant pleural mesothelioma. Cancer Treat Rev 32:229–233

Raghavan D, Gianoutsos P, Bishop J et al (1990) Phase II trial of carboplatin in the management of malignant mesothelioma. J Clin Oncol 8:151–154

Rangel R, Sun Y, Guzman-Rojas L et al (2007) Impaired angiogenesis in aminopeptidase N-null mice. Proc Natl Acad Sci U S A 104:4588–4593

Ranzato E, Grosso S, Patrone M et al (2009) Spreading of mesothelioma cells is rapamycin-sensitive and requires continuing translation. J Cell Biochem 108:867–876

Razak AR, Chatten KJ, Hughes AN (2008) Retreatment with pemetrexed-based chemotherapy in malignant pleural mesothelioma (MPM): a second line treatment option. Lung Cancer 60:294–297

Reck M, Kaiser R, Mellemgaard A et al (2014) Docetaxel plus nintedanib versus docetaxel plus placebo in patients with previously treated non-small-cell lung cancer (LUME-Lung 1): a phase 3, double-blind, randomised controlled trial. Lancet Oncol 15:143–155

Rosinol L, Oriol A, Teruel AI et al (2012) Superiority of bortezomib, thalidomide, and dexamethasone (VTD) as induction pretransplantation therapy in multiple myeloma: a randomized phase 3 PETHEMA/GEM study. Blood 120:1589–1596

Roth GJ, Heckel A, Colbatzky F et al (2009) Design, synthesis, and evaluation of indolinones as triple angiokinase inhibitors and the discovery of a highly specific 6-methoxycarbonyl-substituted indolinone (BIBF 1120). J Med Chem 52:4466–4480

Sahmoud T, Postmus PE, van Pottelsberghe C et al (1997) Etoposide in malignant pleural mesothelioma: two phase II trials of the EORTC Lung Cancer Cooperative Group. Eur J Cancer 33:2211–2215

Sahtoe DD, van Dijk WJ, Ekkebus R et al (2016) BAP1/ASXL1 recruitment and activation for H2A deubiquitination. Nat Commun 7:10292

Santoro A, O'Brien ME, Stahel RA et al (2008) Pemetrexed plus cisplatin or pemetrexed plus carboplatin for chemonaive patients with malignant pleural mesothelioma: results of the International Expanded Access Program. J Thorac Oncol 3:756–763

Sartore-Bianchi A, Gasparri F, Galvani A et al (2007) Bortezomib inhibits nuclear factor-kappaB dependent survival and has potent in vivo activity in mesothelioma. Clin Cancer Res 13:5942–5951

Scagliotti GV, Gaafar R, Nowak A et al (2016) P2.01: LUME-MeSO: phase II/III study of Nintedanib + Pemetrexed/Cisplatin in patients with malignant pleural mesothelioma: track: SCLC, mesothelioma, thymoma. J Thorac Oncol 11:S216

Scagliotti GV, Shin DM, Kindler HL et al (2003) Phase II study of pemetrexed with and without folic acid and vitamin B12 as front-line therapy in malignant pleural mesothelioma. J Clin Oncol 21:1556–1561

Schwartz JE, Scuderi P, Wiggins C et al (1989) A phase I trial of recombinant tumor necrosis factor (rTNF) administered by continuous intravenous infusion in patients with disseminated malignancy. Biotherapy 1:207–214

Sells TB, Chau R, Ecsedy JA et al (2015) MLN8054 and Alisertib (MLN8237): discovery of selective oral aurora A inhibitors. ACS Med Chem Lett 6:630–634

Shao Y, Lu J, Cheng C et al (2007) Reversible histone acetylation involved in transcriptional regulation of WT1 gene. Acta Biochim Biophys Sin Shanghai 39:931–938

Shapiro GI, Tibes R, Gordon MS et al (2011) Phase I studies of CBP501, a G2 checkpoint abrogator, as monotherapy and in combination with cisplatin in patients with advanced solid tumors. Clin Cancer Res 17:3431–3442

Skubitz KM (2002) Phase II trial of pegylated-liposomal doxorubicin (Doxil) in mesothelioma. Cancer Investig 20:693–699

Solheim OP, Saeter G, Finnanger AM et al (1992) High-dose methotrexate in the treatment of malignant mesothelioma of the pleura. A phase II study. Br J Cancer 65:956–960

Sonneveld P, Goldschmidt H, Rosinol L et al (2013) Bortezomib-based versus nonbortezomib-based induction treatment before autologous stem-cell transplantation in patients with previously untreated multiple myeloma: a meta-analysis of phase III randomized, controlled trials. J Clin Oncol 31:3279–3287

Sonneveld P, Schmidt-Wolf IG, van der Holt B et al (2012) Bortezomib induction and maintenance treatment in patients with newly diagnosed multiple myeloma: results of the randomized phase III HOVON-65/GMMG-HD4 trial. J Clin Oncol 30:2946–2955

Sorensen PG, Bach F, Bork E et al (1985) Randomized trial of doxorubicin versus cyclophosphamide in diffuse malignant pleural mesothelioma. Cancer Treat Rep 69:1431–1432

Stebbing J, Powles T, McPherson K et al (2009) The efficacy and safety of weekly vinorelbine in relapsed malignant pleural mesothelioma. Lung Cancer 63:94–97

Steele JP, O'Doherty CA, Shamash J et al (2001) Phase II trial of liposomal daunorubicin in malignant pleural mesothelioma. Ann Oncol 12:497–499

Steele JP, Shamash J, Evans MT et al (2000) Phase II study of vinorelbine in patients with malignant pleural mesothelioma. J Clin Oncol 18:3912–3917

Strizzi L, Catalano A, Vianale G et al (2001) Vascular endothelial growth factor is an autocrine growth factor in human malignant mesothelioma. J Pathol 193:468–475

Sutherlin DP, Bao L, Berry M et al (2011) Discovery of a potent, selective, and orally available class I phosphatidylinositol 3-kinase (PI3K)/mammalian target of rapamycin (mTOR) kinase inhibitor (GDC-0980) for the treatment of cancer. J Med Chem 54:7579–7587

Symanowski J, Vogelzang N, Zawel L et al (2009) A histone deacetylase inhibitor LBH589 downregulates XIAP in mesothelioma cell lines which is likely responsible for increased apoptosis with TRAIL. J Thorac Oncol 4:149–160

Synakiewicz A, Stachowicz-Stencel T, Adamkiewicz-Drozynska E (2014) The role of arginine and the modified arginine deiminase enzyme ADI-PEG 20 in cancer therapy with special emphasis on Phase I/II clinical trials. Expert Opin Investig Drugs 23:1517–1529

Syrios J, Nintos G, Georgoulias V (2015) Nintedanib in combination with docetaxel for second-line treatment of advanced non-small-cell lung cancer. Expert Rev Anticancer Ther 15:875–884

Szlosarek PW, Klabatsa A, Pallaska A et al (2006) In vivo loss of expression of argininosuccinate synthetase in malignant pleural mesothelioma is a biomarker for susceptibility to arginine depletion. Clin Cancer Res 12:7126–7131

Szlosarek PW, Luong P, Phillips MM et al (2013) Metabolic response to pegylated arginine deiminase in mesothelioma with promoter methylation of argininosuccinate synthetase. J Clin Oncol 31:e111–e113

Szlosarek PW, Steele JP, Nolan L et al (2016) Arginine deprivation with pegylated arginine deiminase in patients with argininosuccinate synthetase 1-deficient malignant pleural mesothelioma: a randomized clinical trial. JAMA Oncol. [Epub ahead of print]

Takawa M, Masuda K, Kunizaki M et al (2011) Validation of the histone methyltransferase EZH2 as a therapeutic target for various types of human cancer and as a prognostic marker. Cancer Sci 102:1298–1305

Taylor P, Castagneto B, Dark G et al (2008) Single-agent pemetrexed for chemonaive and pre-treated patients with malignant pleural mesothelioma: results of an International Expanded Access Program. J Thorac Oncol 3:764–771

Thurneysen C, Opitz I, Kurtz S et al (2009) Functional inactivation of NF2/merlin in human meso-thelioma. Lung Cancer 64:140–147

Tolcher AW, Papadopoulos KP, Patnaik A et al (2016) A phase I, first in human study of FP-1039 (GSK3052230), a novel FGF ligand trap, in patients with advanced solid tumors. Ann Oncol 27:526–532

Tomita M, Mori N (2010) Aurora A selective inhibitor MLN8237 suppresses the growth and sur-vival of HTLV-1-infected T-cells in vitro. Cancer Sci 101:1204–1211

Tsao AS, Harun N, Lee JJ et al (2014) Phase I trial of cisplatin, pemetrexed, and imatinib mesylate in chemonaive patients with unresectable malignant pleural mesothelioma. Clin Lung Cancer 15:197–201

Turner N, Grose R (2010) Fibroblast growth factor signalling: from development to cancer. Nat Rev Cancer 10:116–129

Turner N, Pearson A, Sharpe R et al (2010) FGFR1 amplification drives endocrine therapy resis-tance and is a therapeutic target in breast cancer. Cancer Res 70:2085–2094

van Haarst JM, Baas P, Manegold C et al (2002) Multicentre phase II study of gemcitabine and cisplatin in malignant pleural mesothelioma. Br J Cancer 86:342–345

van Laarhoven HW, Fiedler W, Desar IM et al (2010) Phase I clinical and magnetic resonance imaging study of the vascular agent NGR-hTNF in patients with advanced cancers (European Organization for Research and Treatment of Cancer Study 16041). Clin Cancer Res 16:1315–1323

van Meerbeeck J, Debruyne C, van Zandwijk N et al (1996) Paclitaxel for malignant pleural meso-thelioma: a phase II study of the EORTC Lung Cancer Cooperative Group. Br J Cancer 74:961–963

van Meerbeeck JP, Baas P, Debruyne C et al (1999) A Phase II study of gemcitabine in patients with malignant pleural mesothelioma. European Organization for Research and Treatment of Cancer Lung Cancer Cooperative Group. Cancer 85:2577–2582

van Meerbeeck JP, Baas P, Debruyne C et al (2002) A phase II EORTC study of temozolomide in patients with malignant pleural mesothelioma. Eur J Cancer 38:779–783

van Meerbeeck JP, Gaafar R, Manegold C et al (2005) Randomized phase III study of cisplatin with or without raltitrexed in patients with malignant pleural mesothelioma: an intergroup study of the European Organisation for Research and Treatment of Cancer Lung Cancer Group and the National Cancer Institute of Canada. J Clin Oncol 23:6881–6889

Van TT, Hanibuchi M, Goto H et al (2012) SU6668, a multiple tyrosine kinase inhibitor, inhibits progression of human malignant pleural mesothelioma in an orthotopic model. Respirology 17:984–990

Vandermeers F, Hubert P, Delvenne P et al (2009) Valproate, in combination with pemetrexed and cisplatin, provides additional efficacy to the treatment of malignant mesothelioma. Clin Cancer Res 15:2818–2828

Vermeulen K, Van Bockstaele DR, Berneman ZN (2003) The cell cycle: a review of regulation, deregulation and therapeutic targets in cancer. Cell Prolif 36:131–149

Vogelzang NJ, Goutsou M, Corson JM et al (1990) Carboplatin in malignant mesothelioma: a phase II study of the Cancer and Leukemia Group B. Cancer Chemother Pharmacol 27:239–242

Vogelzang NJ, Herndon JE 2nd, Miller A et al (1999) High-dose paclitaxel plus G-CSF for malig-nant mesothelioma: CALGB phase II study 9234. Ann Oncol 10:597–600

Vogelzang NJ, Rusthoven JJ, Symanowski J et al (2003) Phase III study of pemetrexed in combina-tion with cisplatin versus cisplatin alone in patients with malignant pleural mesothelioma. J Clin Oncol 21:2636–2644

Vorobiof DA, Rapoport BL, Chasen MR et al (2002) Malignant pleural mesothelioma: a phase II trial with docetaxel. Ann Oncol 13:412–415

Wang F, Li H, Yan XG et al (2015) Alisertib induces cell cycle arrest and autophagy and suppresses epithelial-to-mesenchymal transition involving PI3K/Akt/mTOR and sirtuin 1-mediated signaling pathways in human pancreatic cancer cells. Drug Des Develop Ther 9:575–601

Weiss J, Sos ML, Seidel D et al (2010) Frequent and focal FGFR1 amplification associates with therapeutically tractable FGFR1 dependency in squamous cell lung cancer. Sci Transl Med 2:62ra93

Wiedenmann B, Reichardt P, Rath U et al (1989) Phase-I trial of intravenous continuous infusion of tumor necrosis factor in advanced metastatic carcinomas. J Cancer Res Clin Oncol 115:189–192

Wu YM, Su F, Kalyana-Sundaram S et al (2013) Identification of targetable FGFR gene fusions in diverse cancers. Cancer Discov 3:636–647

Yang TS, Lu SN, Chao Y et al (2010) A randomised phase II study of pegylated arginine deiminase (ADI-PEG 20) in Asian advanced hepatocellular carcinoma patients. Br J Cancer 103:954–960

Yao JC, Lombard-Bohas C, Baudin E et al (2010) Daily oral everolimus activity in patients with metastatic pancreatic neuroendocrine tumors after failure of cytotoxic chemotherapy: a phase II trial. J Clin Oncol 28:69–76

Yao JC, Shah MH, Ito T et al (2011) Everolimus for advanced pancreatic neuroendocrine tumors. N Engl J Med 364:514–523

Yoo CB, Jones PA (2006) Epigenetic therapy of cancer: past, present and future. Nat Rev Drug Discov 5:37–50

Zalcman G, Mazieres J, Margery J et al (2016) Bevacizumab for newly diagnosed pleural mesothelioma in the Mesothelioma Avastin Cisplatin Pemetrexed Study (MAPS): a randomised, controlled, open-label, phase 3 trial. Lancet 387:1405–1414

Zauderer MG (2016) A new standard for malignant pleural mesothelioma. Lancet 387:1352–1354

Zauderer MG, Kass SL, Woo K et al (2014) Vinorelbine and gemcitabine as second- or third-line therapy for malignant pleural mesothelioma. Lung Cancer 84:271–274

Zhang XH, Rao M, Loprieato JA et al (2008) Aurora A, Aurora B and survivin are novel targets of transcriptional regulation by histone deacetylase inhibitors in non-small cell lung cancer. Cancer Biol Ther 7:1388–1397

Zhou S, Liu L, Li H et al (2014) Multipoint targeting of the PI3K/mTOR pathway in mesothelioma. Br J Cancer 110:2479–2488

Zidar BL, Green S, Pierce HI et al (1988) A phase II evaluation of cisplatin in unresectable diffuse malignant mesothelioma: a Southwest Oncology Group Study. Investig New Drugs 6:223–226

Zidar BL, Metch B, Balcerzak SP et al (1992) A phase II evaluation of ifosfamide and mesna in unresectable diffuse malignant mesothelioma. A Southwest Oncology Group study. Cancer 70:2547–2551

Zucali PA, Ceresoli GL, Garassino I et al (2008) Gemcitabine and vinorelbine in pemetrexed-pretreated patients with malignant pleural mesothelioma. Cancer 112:1555–1561

Zucali PA, Perrino M, Lorenzi E et al (2014) Vinorelbine in pemetrexed-pretreated patients with malignant pleural mesothelioma. Lung Cancer 84:265–270

Chapter 16
Immunotherapeutic Approaches to Mesothelioma

Anish Thomas, Madhuri Badrinath, and Raffit Hassan

Abstract Several lines of evidence indicate the activation of a host humoral and cellular response in mesothelioma patients. Tumor cells employ a number of mechanisms to promote immune tolerance and to escape host immune surveillance. These include immune checkpoints—molecules expressed on the surface of immune cells and tumor cells—that curb effector T-cell responses. The emerging category of drugs that inhibit immune checkpoints and their ligands have shown preliminary clinical activity in patients with mesothelioma. Among antigen-specific approaches, therapies targeting a tumor differentiation antigen mesothelin, which is differentially expressed in mesothelioma, are farthest along in clinical development. Included among the mesothelin-targeted immunotherapies that are under clinical investigation are immunotoxins, tumor vaccine, chimeric antigen receptor T cell, and antibody-based therapies. Of these, the monoclonal antibody amatuximab and an antibody-drug conjugate anetumab ravtansine are undergoing registration trials. Ongoing research is focused on better understanding the antitumor responses to immune-based approaches and to prospectively identify patients who are more likely to respond to these interventions. Parallel efforts are also investigating ways to therapeutically improve mesothelioma immunogenicity.

Keywords Mesothelioma • Immunotherapy • Mesothelin-targeted immunotherapies • Programmed death 1/programmed death ligand 1 pathway • Immunotoxins • Vaccines • Chimeric antigen receptor T cells • Antibody-drug conjugates • Chimeric monoclonal antibody • Immune checkpoint blockades

A. Thomas • M. Badrinath • R. Hassan (✉)
Thoracic and GI Oncology Branch, Center for Cancer Research, National Cancer Institute, Bethesda, MD, USA
e-mail: hassanr@mail.nih.gov

© Springer International Publishing AG 2017
J.R. Testa (ed.), *Asbestos and Mesothelioma*, Current Cancer Research,
DOI 10.1007/978-3-319-53560-9_16

16.1 Introduction

Although generally not considered a particularly immunogenic tumor unlike melanoma or renal cell carcinoma, there is considerable evidence from clinical reports and animal models that an immune response—both cellular (T lymphocyte mediated) and humoral (antibody mediated)—can be elicited to mesothelioma. For example, cases of pleural mesothelioma have been reported with transient spontaneous regression associated with tumor tissue infiltration with mononuclear cells and serological evidence of antitumor reactivity (Robinson et al. 2001). Serological studies have defined antigens expressed by mesothelioma cells that elicit an effective immune response (Robinson et al. 1998). One of the target antigens identified, mesothelin, is a glycosyl-phosphatidylinositol-anchored glycoprotein present on the cell surface; mesothelin elicits a humoral immune response in over one third of patients with mesothelioma (Ho et al. 2005). Finally, the presence of an inflammatory response—as indicated by lymphoid infiltration—has been reported to be a good prognostic indicator in patients with mesothelioma (Leigh and Webster 1982). Recent studies have shown that the type of tumor-infiltrating immune cells is important in this context. Specifically, tumors with low CD163+ tumor-associated macrophages and high CD20+ lymphocyte infiltration had better prognosis (Ujiie et al. 2015).

Despite the immune responses, spontaneous tumor regressions rarely occur, indicating the ability of the mesothelioma tumor cells to promote immune tolerance and escape host immune surveillance. The immune system actively inhibits the formation and progression of transformed cells and ultimately "shapes" nascent tumors by forcing the selective evolution of tumor cells that can evade the immune response, a phenomenon called tumor immunoediting (Dunn et al. 2002). Tumors also utilize a number of pathways/mechanisms to inhibit immune responses, including local immune suppression, induction of tolerance, systemic dysfunction in T-cell signaling, and expression of immune checkpoints (Drake et al. 2006). The programmed death 1 (PD1)/programmed death ligand 1 (PDL1) pathway is an immune checkpoint and a critical mediator of peripheral immune tolerance (Dong et al. 1999). PDL1 is expressed by many components of the immune system including antigen-presenting cells and T cells (Dong et al. 1999). Many tumors, including mesothelioma, express PDL1, and its expression is a marker of poor prognosis mesothelioma (Mansfield et al. 2014; Khanna et al. 2016). T cells that express PD1, the receptor for PDL1, undergo apoptosis when PD1 and PDL1 bind, and tumors that express PDL1 blunt antitumor immunity through T-cell apoptosis (Dong et al. 2002). PDL1 can be adaptively expressed in response to interferon-γ or constitutively expressed due to signal pathway abnormalities that result from mutations (Pardoll 2012).

Preliminary clinical evidence suggests that immunotherapy—in particular mesothelin-targeted therapies and immune checkpoint blockade—can produce tumor control in some patients with mesothelioma. This chapter will focus on these two approaches, which are furthest along in terms of clinical evaluation. Among the approaches that are not covered in this chapter include dendritic cell-based immunotherapy (Cornelissen et al. 2016) and oncolytic virotherapy (Boisgerault et al. 2015).

16.2   Mesothelin-Targeted Immunotherapies

Mesothelin is overexpressed in malignant mesothelioma and is an attractive antigen target for immunotherapies considering its high expression in mesothelioma and limited expression on normal tissue (Hassan et al. 2004; Pastan and Hassan 2014). In normal tissues, mesothelin is expressed in a single layer of mesothelial cells lining the pleura, peritoneum, and pericardium (Ordonez 2003a). Mesothelin is expressed in almost all epithelial mesotheliomas as well as the epithelial component of biphasic tumors, but it is absent in sarcomatoid mesotheliomas (Ordonez 2003b). The role of mesothelin in cancer is still unclear and may be cancer-type specific. Mice in which the mesothelin gene had been inactivated had no detectable abnormalities (Bera and Pastan 2000). Mesothelin binds to CA125, and it is believed that this interaction mediates cell adhesion and metastatic spread of cancer (Rump et al. 2004). Mesothelin expression promotes invasion in malignant pleural mesothelioma and aggressiveness with poor outcomes in other thoracic cancers (Servais et al. 2012). Multiple phase I and ongoing phase II clinical trials using a number of approaches to target mesothelioma—including immunotoxins, tumor vaccine, chimeric T cells containing single-chain variable fragments (scFv) that recognize mesothelin, and antibody-based therapies—have demonstrated the safety and feasibility of targeting mesothelin-expressing cancer cells for the treatment of advanced mesothelioma.

16.3   Immunotoxins

Immunotoxins are highly targeted therapies such as antibody-drug conjugates that utilize a toxin payload rather than a chemotherapy payload to kill cancer cells. Anti-mesothelin immunotoxin consists of an anti-mesothelin variable fragment linked to PE38, a portion of *Pseudomonas* exotoxin A, and it is cytotoxic to mesothelin-expressing cell lines (Chowdhury et al. 1998). The first mesothelin-directed agent to enter the clinic was the immunotoxin SS1P. After binding to mesothelin on the cell surface, SS1P is internalized and undergoes processing in the endocytic compartment of the cell, leading to inhibition of protein synthesis and ultimately cell death.

Two different schedules of administration of SS1P monotherapy were evaluated in phase I clinical trials. In one trial, SS1P was administered as a bolus infusion over a 30-minute time frame, and in the other it was administered as a continuous infusion for 10 days (Hassan et al. 2007a; Kreitman et al. 2009). SS1P was well tolerated in these clinical trials, with similar dose-limiting toxicity of pleuritic at the highest dose level. The maximum tolerated dose with the bolus infusion was 45 mcg/kg. As a single agent, clinical activity was modest, and there was no significant advantage of continuous infusion over bolus dosing. The most commonly reported adverse events (AEs) in the phase I trials were hypoalbuminemia and fatigue.

Based on the hypothesis that limited tumor penetration might limit the activity of SS1P monotherapy, a subsequent phase I trial evaluated the combination of chemotherapy—which could disrupt the close packing of tumor, allowing better penetration of immunotoxin into the tumor—with SS1P (Zhang et al. 2007; Hassan et al. 2014b). Twenty-four patients received SS1P at four dose levels from 25 to 55 mcg/kg in combination with standard doses of cisplatin and pemetrexed (Hassan et al. 2014b). Fatigue was the dose-limiting toxicity at the highest dose level. The maximum tolerated dose was established as 45 mcg/kg. Among 20 evaluable patients, 12 (60%) had a partial response, 3 had stable disease, and 5 had progressive disease. Of 13 patients who received the MTD, 10 (77%) had a partial response, 1 had stable disease, and 2 had progressive disease. The study showed that the combination of SS1P with chemotherapy was feasible with no overlapping toxicities. In this small study in a well-selected patient population, response rates to treatment were superior to historical controls.

Another factor that limited the efficacy of immunotoxins was the development of human antibody response to immunotoxins. In these early clinical trials described above, approximately 90% of patients developed antibodies to SS1P after three doses. Development of neutralizing antibodies correlated with markedly lower SS1P levels and precluded administration of additional cycles of SS1P. In fact, the combination trial with chemotherapy showed that concurrent chemotherapy does not affect the rate of antibody formation (Hassan et al. 2014b). Among the strategies that are being explored to minimize immunogenicity and allow for repeated therapeutic administration of immunotoxin include modification of the immunotoxin protein structure to decrease its immunogenicity (Liu et al. 2012) and modulation of the host immune system (Mossoba et al. 2011). A pilot study in ten patients showed that host immune depletion can effectively delay anti-immunotoxin antibody formation (Hassan et al. 2013). This was based on preclinical studies in immunocompetent Balb/C mice immunized with SS1P, which showed that administration of pentostatin and cyclophosphamide depleted T and B cells and thereby completely abrogated the development of anti-SS1P antibodies. Among ten patients who received pentostatin and cyclophosphamide to deplete T cells and B cells before SS1P, only two patients (20%) developed anti-SS1P antibodies after cycle 1. Three patients with heavily pretreated advanced mesothelioma had durable partial responses (Hassan et al. 2013).

An alternative strategy that is being explored to minimize immunogenicity of immunotoxins involves identifying and mutilating the immunogenic epitopes of the immunotoxin to produce less immunogenic molecules. RG7787 is a mesothelin-targeted immunotoxin that consists of a humanized anti-MSLN Fab fragment with a newly designed PE (PE24). When compared to SS1P, RG7787 has decreased immunogenicity and reduced nonspecific toxicity (Alewine et al. 2014). In vivo and in vitro data indicated that RG7787 is synergistic in combination with nab-Paclitaxel against primary human mesothelioma cells (Zhang et al. 2016). An ongoing phase I clinical trial is evaluating the safety and efficacy of LMB-100 (previously RG7787) in patients with previously treated pleural and peritoneal mesothelioma.

16.4 Vaccines

Mesothelin is an immunogenic protein that can elicit an antitumor immune response. CRS-207 is a *Listeria monocytogenes* (Lm)-based vaccine that stimulates both innate and adaptive immunity. It is engineered to secrete mesothelin into the cytosol of infected antigen presentation cells (Brockstedt et al. 2004). The bacteria retain potency of the fully virulent pathogen, but have vastly reduced toxicity, as compared with wild-type *Listeria* due to selective deletion of two virulence factors, ActA (ΔactA) and Internalin B (ΔinlB). In preclinical studies, CRS-207 uptake by phagocytes in the liver resulted in local inflammatory responses and activation and recruitment of natural killer and T cells and was associated with increased survival of mice bearing hepatic metastases (Le et al. 2012). In a phase I clinical trial, CRS-207 was well tolerated up to the maximum planned dose, with minor adverse events that were consistent with transient cytokine release and resulted in induction of mesothelin-specific T-cell responses (Le et al. 2012). An ongoing phase I clinical trial is evaluating the safety and efficacy of a combination of CRS-207 and chemotherapy for frontline therapy of malignant pleural mesothelioma.

16.5 Chimeric Antigen Receptor T Cells

Chimeric antigen receptors (CARs) are synthetic receptors that target T cells to cell-surface antigens and augment T-cell function and persistence. CARs consist of an ectodomain (commonly derived from a scFv), a hinge, a transmembrane domain, and an endodomain (typically comprising signaling domains derived from CD3ζ and costimulatory receptors). Mesothelin CAR T cells are generated by modifying autologous patient T cells to express a mesothelin-binding T-cell receptor linked to appropriate co-signaling molecules, so that binding of these T cells to mesothelin on cancer cells activates the cells to attack the tumor (Morello et al. 2016). One approach to modifying T cells involves transfection of mRNA that encodes the mesothelin CAR, which results in transient CAR expression for a few days (Morello et al. 2016). This approach is, however, limited by transient expression of the CAR that may limit long-term efficacy.

Preliminary clinical evidence indicates that adoptive transfer of mRNA CAR T cells that target mesothelin is feasible and safe without overt evidence of off-tumor on-target toxicity against normal tissues (Beatty et al. 2014). In a report of two patients with mesothelin-expressing tumors (including one patient with mesothelioma), mesothelin CAR T cells persisted transiently within the peripheral blood after intravenous administration and migrated to primary and metastatic tumor sites. Mesothelin CAR T cells elicited an antitumor immune response and modest clinical activity was observed. The potential for immunogenicity of CARs derived from murine antibodies is exemplified by a report of a patient who developed anaphylaxis and cardiac arrest after repeated administration of mesothelin CAR T cells. The use of fully human mesothelin CAR might reduce the risk of developing such an anti-CAR antibody response (Lanitis et al. 2012; Morello et al. 2016). Several clinical trials of systemic administration of mesothelin CAR T cells are underway.

In orthotopic models, intrapleural administration of mesothelin CAR T cells has been shown to be superior to systemic administration in terms of antitumor efficacy and functional T-cell persistence (Adusumilli et al. 2014). Additionally, antitumor activity was also observed in extra-thoracic tumor sites. Based on this data, an ongoing phase I clinical trial is evaluating the safety of intrapleural administration of mesothelin-targeted CAR T cells in patients with primary or secondary pleural malignancies.

16.6 Antibody-Drug Conjugates

Antibody-drug conjugates consist of monoclonal antibodies that are specific to tumor cell-surface proteins conjugated to cytotoxic agents via a linker (Thomas et al. 2016). Anetumab ravtansine is an antibody-drug conjugate that consists of a human anti-mesothelin antibody conjugated to the maytansinoid analogue DM4 via a disulfide-containing linker. Anetumab ravtansine is bound and internalized by mesothelin-expressing cells, resulting in degradation of the disulfide-based linker and release of the DM4 metabolite. Maytansinoid analogues target tubulin and fragment microtubules. In preclinical studies, the antitumor efficacy of anetumab ravtansine generally correlated with mesothelin expression and was superior to that of standard chemotherapy (Golfier et al. 2014). A phase I clinical trial of anetumab ravtansine enrolled patients with multiple tumor types that are known to have high expression of mesothelin. Keratitis and neuropathy were the dose-limiting toxicities, and the maximum tolerated dose was 6.5 mg/kg, administered intravenously every 3 weeks. Five of 16 (31%) mesothelioma patients treated at the maximum tolerated drug dose had durable partial responses. An ongoing phase II registration trial is evaluating the efficacy of anetumab ravtansine versus navelbine in the second-line treatment of patients with malignant pleural mesothelioma.

16.7 Chimeric Monoclonal Antibody

Amatuximab is a chimeric high-affinity monoclonal IgG1/k antibody targeting mesothelin. Amatuximab mediates inhibition of mesothelin-dependent cell adhesion and antibody-dependent cellular cytotoxicity in preclinical studies (Hassan et al. 2007b). Treatment with amatuximab in combination with chemotherapy led to a marked reduction in tumor growth of mesothelin-expressing tumors in nude mice compared to chemotherapy or amatuximab treatment alone (Hassan et al. 2014a). In a phase I trial, patients with multiple primary tumors were treated with amatuximab intravenously on days 1, 8, 15, and 22. Dose-limiting toxicity observed at 400 mg/m^2 included transaminitis and serum sickness. The maximum tolerated dose was defined as 200 mg/m^2.

On the basis of its synergy with chemotherapy in preclinical studies, amatuximab was evaluated in combination with chemotherapy in patients with unresectable malignant pleural mesothelioma. Amatuximab (5 mg/kg) was administered on days 1 and 8, with standard doses of pemetrexed and cisplatin in 21-day cycles for up to 6 cycles. Combination therapy resulted in no overlapping toxicities, and 33 of 89 (40%) patients had partial responses. The median overall survival was 14.8 months, which compared favorably to historical controls. Exposure-response analyses showed that treatment with amatuximab had a positive effect on overall survival. Patients who had higher than median exposure to amatuximab had significantly longer overall survival than patients with lower than median exposure to amatuximab (Gupta et al. 2016). Based on these results, a randomized phase II registration trial of chemotherapy with or without amatuximab in newly diagnosed patients with malignant pleural mesothelioma is underway.

16.8 Immune Checkpoint Blockade

As described in the introduction, immune checkpoints are molecules expressed on the surface of immune cells including T lymphocytes that modulate the immune responses via inhibitory or stimulatory signaling to T cells. Extensively studied immune checkpoints include the cytotoxic T-lymphocyte antigen-4 (CTLA-4) and PD1. Activation of both receptors causes downregulation and inhibition of immune responses.

Several cancer types, including non-small cell lung cancer and melanoma, employ PDL1 expression to generate an immunosuppressive tumor microenvironment and avoid T-cell cytolysis. A few studies have used immunohistochemistry to evaluate expression of PDL1 in malignant mesothelioma. For example, Mansfeld and colleagues found expression of PDL1 in 42 of 106 (40%) mesotheliomas (Mansfield et al. 2014). Sarcomatoid mesotheliomas tended to express PDL1 more commonly than epithelioid mesotheliomas. Patients with PDL1-expressing tumors had significantly lower overall survival compared with patients whose tumors did not (median 5 months versus 14.5 months, respectively). Another group observed PDL1 positivity in 20% of 119 cases evaluated (Cedres et al. 2015). As with the previous study, there was a significant association between PDL1 expression and histology, with non-epithelioid tumors having a higher frequency of PDL1 expression. Median overall survival in patients with PDL1-positive tumors was 4.8 months versus 16 months for patients with PDL1-negative tumors. While these two studies consisted largely of patients with pleural mesothelioma, a third investigation evaluated 65 patients, of which 44 had peritoneal mesothelioma (Khanna et al. 2016). Sixty-three percent of tumors were PDL1 positive, with similar frequency of expression in pleural and peritoneal mesothelioma. PDL1 expression was associated with slightly inferior overall survival (median 23 months versus 33 months, respectfully, although this difference was not statistically significant). Due to technical and evaluative challenges, among others, immunohistochemistry-based PDL1 assessment in general has not been a robust determinant of tumor response to anti-PD1/PDL1-based immunotherapy.

In addition to tumor tissues, malignant effusions of mesothelioma patients have also been shown to contain PDL1-positive tumor cells as well as PD1- and PDL1-positive immune cells. Lymphocytes present in malignant mesothelioma effusions induce PDL1 expression on tumor cells, which in turn could be targeted using the patient's own NK cells in the presence of anti-PDL1 antibody (Khanna et al. 2016).

Preliminary reports indicate clinical activity of PD1 and PDL1 inhibition in a subset of patients with mesothelioma. Safety and efficacy of a PD1 inhibitor, pembrolizumab, was evaluated in the KEYNOTE-028 study (Alley et al. 2015). Malignant pleural mesothelioma patients who had failed standard therapy and whose tumors expressed PDL1 in ≥1% of cells in tumor nests or PDL1-positive bands in stroma as determined by an immunohistochemistry at a central laboratory were eligible. Forty-five percent of patients who were screened (38 of 84) had PDL1-positive tumors. Pembrolizumab was administered at 10 mg/kg intravenously every 2 weeks for up to 2 years or until disease progression or unacceptable toxicity. Preliminary overall response rate (this included both confirmed and unconfirmed responses) was 24% (6 of 25 patients); 13 of 25 patients (52%) had stable disease, providing a disease control rate of 76%. The most common treatment-related adverse events were nausea, fatigue, and decreased appetite. Immune-related adverse events included transaminitis and uveitis. In the NivoMes trial, the PD1 inhibitor nivolumab yielded an overall response rate of 28% (5 of 18) patients (Quispel-Janssen et al. 2016). In the JAVELIN study, the PDL1 antibody avelumab was evaluated in patients with unresectable pleural or peritoneal mesothelioma (Hassan et al. 2016). Avelumab was administered at 10 mg/kg intravenously every 2 weeks until disease progression or unacceptable toxicity. The most common treatment-related adverse events were infusion-related reaction, fatigue, chills, and pyrexia. Unconfirmed responses were observed in 5 of 53 (9.4%) patients. Stable disease was observed in 25 patients (47%), and median progression free survival was 17.1 weeks. In contrast to PD1/PDL1 axis inhibitors, the CTLA-4 inhibitor tremelimumab showed no benefit compared to best supportive care in patients with malignant pleural mesothelioma and was poorly tolerated (Kindler et al. 2016).

16.9   Conclusions

Mesothelioma, unlike melanoma, was thought to be a non-immunogenic tumor until recently. However, several lines of evidence suggest that mesothelioma tumors are under immunosurveillance. Preliminary clinical evidence suggests that immunotherapy can produce tumor control in some patients with mesothelioma. Various therapies targeting mesothelin and immune checkpoint inhibition are immune-based approaches that are farthest along in clinical testing in patients with mesothelioma. Based on preliminary clinical and translational data, both of these approaches appear to be promising therapeutic strategy in patients with mesothelioma.

Acknowledgment This work was supported in part by the intramural research program of the National Cancer Institute.

References

Adusumilli PS, Cherkassky L, Villena-Vargas J et al (2014) Regional delivery of mesothelin-targeted CAR T cell therapy generates potent and long-lasting CD4-dependent tumor immunity. Sci Transl Med 6:261ra151

Alewine C, Xiang L, Yamori T et al (2014) Efficacy of RG7787, a next-generation mesothelin-targeted immunotoxin, against triple-negative breast and gastric cancers. Mol Cancer Thera 13:2653–2661

Alley EW, Molife LR, Santoro A, et al. (2015) Clinical safety and efficacy of pembrolizumab (MK-3475) in patients with malignant pleural mesothelioma: preliminary results from KEYNOTE-028 AACR Annual Meeting 2015 Abstract CT103

Beatty GL, Haas AR, Maus MV et al (2014) Mesothelin-specific chimeric antigen receptor mRNA-engineered T cells induce antitumor activity in solid malignancies. Cancer Immunol Res 2:112–120

Bera TK, Pastan I (2000) Mesothelin is not required for normal mouse development or reproduction. Mol Cell Biol 20:2902–2906

Boisgerault N, Achard C, Delaunay T et al (2015) Oncolytic virotherapy for human malignant mesothelioma: recent advances. Oncolytic Virother 4:133–140

Brockstedt DG, Giedlin MA, Leong ML, Bahjat KS, Gao Y, Luckett W, Liu WQ, Cook DN, Portnoy DA, Dubensky TW (2004) Listeria-based cancer vaccines that segregate immunogenicity from toxicity. Proc Natl Acad Sci U S A 101(38):13832–13837. doi:10.1073/pnas.040635101

Cedres S, Ponce-Aix S, Zugazagoitia J et al (2015) Analysis of expression of programmed cell death 1 ligand 1 (PD-L1) in malignant pleural mesothelioma (MPM). PLoS One 10:e0121071

Chowdhury PS, Viner JL, Beers R et al (1998) Isolation of a high-affinity stable single-chain Fv specific for mesothelin from DNA-immunized mice by phage display and construction of a recombinant immunotoxin with anti-tumor activity. Proc Natl Acad Sci U S A 95:669–674

Cornelissen R, Hegmans JPJJ, Maat APWM et al (2016) Extended tumor control after dendritic cell vaccination with low-dose cyclophosphamide as adjuvant treatment in patients with malignant pleural mesothelioma. Am J Resp Crit Care 193:1023–1031

Dong H, Strome SE, Salomao DR et al (2002) Tumor-associated B7-H1 promotes T-cell apoptosis: a potential mechanism of immune evasion. Nat Med 8:793–800

Dong H, Zhu G, Tamada K et al (1999) B7-H1, a third member of the B7 family, co-stimulates T-cell proliferation and interleukin-10 secretion. Nat Med 5:1365–1369

Drake CG, Jaffee E, Pardoll DM (2006) Mechanisms of immune evasion by tumors. Adv Immunol 90:51–81

Dunn GP, Bruce AT, Ikeda H et al (2002) Cancer immunoediting: from immunosurveillance to tumor escape. Nat Immunol 3(11):991–998

Golfier S, Kopitz C, Kahnert A et al (2014) Anetumab ravtansine: a novel mesothelin-targeting antibody-drug conjugate cures tumors with heterogeneous target expression favored by bystander effect. Mol Cancer Ther 13:1537–1548

Gupta A, Hussein Z, Hassan R et al (2016) Population pharmacokinetics and exposure-response relationship of amatuximab, an anti-mesothelin monoclonal antibody, in patients with malignant pleural mesothelioma and its application in dose selection. Cancer Chemother Pharmacol 77:733–743

Hassan R, Bera T, Pastan I (2004) Mesothelin: a new target for immunotherapy. Clin Cancer Res 10:3937–3942

Hassan R, Bullock S, Premkumar A et al (2007a) Phase I study of SS1P a recombinant anti-mesothelin immunotoxin given as a bolus IV infusion to patients with mesothelin-expressing mesothelioma, ovarian, and pancreatic cancers. Clin Cancer Res 13:5144–5149

Hassan R, Ebel W, Routhier EL et al (2007b) Preclinical evaluation of MORAb-009, a chimeric antibody targeting tumor-associated mesothelin. Cancer Immun 7:20

Hassan R, Kindler HL, Jahan T et al (2014a) Phase II clinical trial of amatuximab, a chimeric antimesothelin antibody with pemetrexed and cisplatin in advanced unresectable pleural mesothelioma. Clin Cancer Res 20:5927–5936

Hassan R, Miller AC, Sharon E et al (2013) Major cancer regressions in mesothelioma after treatment with an anti-mesothelin immunotoxin and immune suppression. Sci Transl Med 5:208ra147

Hassan R, Sharon E, Thomas A et al (2014b) Phase 1 study of the antimesothelin immunotoxin SS1P in combination with pemetrexed and cisplatin for front-line therapy of pleural mesothelioma and correlation of tumor response with serum mesothelin, megakaryocyte potentiating factor, and cancer antigen 125. Cancer 120:3311–3319

Hassan R, Thomas A, Patel M et al (2016) Avelumab (MSB0010718C; anti-PD-L1) in patients with advanced unresectable mesothelioma from the JAVELIN solid tumor phase Ib trial: safety, clinical activity, and PD-L1 expression. J Clin Oncol 34(suppl.; abstr 8503)

Ho M, Hassan R, Zhang JL et al (2005) Humoral immune response to mesothelin in mesothelioma and ovarian cancer patients. Clin Cancer Res 11:3814–3820

Khanna S, Thomas A, Abate-Daga D et al (2016) Malignant mesothelioma effusions are infiltrated by CD3+ T cells highly expressing PD-L1 and the PD-L1+ tumor cells within these effusions are susceptible to ADCC by the anti-PD-L1 antibody avelumab. J Thorac Oncol 11:1993–2005

Kindler H, Scherpereel A, Calabro L et al (2016) Tremelimumab as second- or third-line treatment of unresectable malignant mesothelioma (MM): results from the global, double-blind, placebo-controlled DETERMINE study. J Clin Oncol 34(suppl; abstr 8502)

Kreitman RJ, Hassan R, FitzGerald DJ et al (2009) Phase I trial of continuous infusion anti-mesothelin recombinant immunotoxin SS1P. Clin Cancer Res 15:5274–5279

Lanitis E, Poussin M, Hagemann IS et al (2012) Redirected antitumor activity of primary human lymphocytes transduced with a fully human anti-mesothelin chimeric receptor. Mol Ther 20:633–643

Le DT, Brockstedt DG, Nir-Paz R et al (2012) A live-attenuated Listeria vaccine (ANZ-100) and a live-attenuated Listeria vaccine expressing mesothelin (CRS-207) for advanced cancers: phase I studies of safety and immune induction. Clin Cancer Res 18:858–868

Leigh RA, Webster I (1982) Lymphocytic infiltration of pleural mesothelioma and its significance for survival. S Afr Med J 61:1007–1009

Liu W, Onda M, Lee B, Kreitman RJ, Hassan R, Xiang L, Pastan I (2012) Recombinant immunotoxin engineered for low immunogenicity and antigenicity by identifying and silencing human B-cell epitopes. Proc Natl Acad Sci U S A 109(29):11782–11787. doi:10.1073/pnas.1209292109

Mansfield AS, Roden AC, Peikert T et al (2014) B7-H1 expression in malignant pleural mesothelioma is associated with sarcomatoid histology and poor prognosis. J Thorac Oncol 9:1036–1040

Morello A, Sadelain M, Adusumilli PS (2016) Mesothelin-targeted CARs: driving T cells to solid tumors. Cancer Discovery 6:133–146

Mossoba ME, Onda M, Taylor J et al (2011) Pentostatin plus cyclophosphamide safely and effectively prevents immunotoxin immunogenicity in murine hosts. Clin Cancer Res 17:3697–3705

Ordonez NG (2003a) Application of mesothelin immunostaining in tumor diagnosis. Am J Surg Pathol 27:1418–1428

Ordonez NG (2003b) Value of mesothelin immunostaining in the diagnosis of mesothelioma. Mod Pathol 16:192–197

Pardoll DM (2012) The blockade of immune checkpoints in cancer immunotherapy. Nat Rev Cancer 12(4):252–264. doi:10.1038/nrc3239

Pastan I, Hassan R (2014) Discovery of mesothelin and exploiting it as a target for immunotherapy. Cancer Res 74:2907–2912

Quispel-Janssen J, Zimmerman M, Buikhuisen W, et al. (2016) MS04.07: Nivolumab in malignant pleural mesothelioma (NIVOMES): an interim analysis. In: 13th international conference of the International Mesothelioma Interest Group.

Robinson BW, Robinson C, Lake RA (2001) Localised spontaneous regression in mesothelioma -- possible immunological mechanism. Lung Cancer 32:197–201

Robinson C, Robinson BWS, Lake RA (1998) Sera from patients with malignant mesothelioma can contain autoantibodies. Lung Cancer 20:175–184

Rump A, Morikawa Y, Tanaka M et al (2004) Binding of ovarian cancer antigen CA125/MUC16 to mesothelin mediates cell adhesion. J Biol Chem 279:9190–9198

Servais EL, Colovos C, Rodriguez L et al (2012) Mesothelin overexpression promotes mesothelioma cell invasion and MMP-9 secretion in an orthotopic mouse model and in epithelioid pleural mesothelioma patients. Clin Cancer Res 18:2478–2489

Thomas A, Teicher BA, Hassan R (2016) Antibody-drug conjugates for cancer therapy. Lancet Oncol 17:e254–e262

Ujiie H, Kadota K, Nitadori JI et al (2015) The tumoral and stromal immune microenvironment in malignant pleural mesothelioma: a comprehensive analysis reveals prognostic immune markers. Oncoimmunology 4:e1009285

Zhang J, Khanna S, Jiang Q et al (2016) Efficacy of anti-mesothelin immunotoxin RG7787 plus nab-paclitaxel against mesothelioma patient derived xenografts and mesothelin as a biomarker of tumor response. Clin Cancer Res. doi:10.1158/1078-0432.CCR-16-1667 [Epub ahead of print]

Zhang Y, Xiang L, Hassan R et al (2007) Immunotoxin and Taxol synergy results from a decrease in shed mesothelin levels in the extracellular space of tumors. Proc Natl Acad Sci U S A 104:17099–17104

Chapter 17
Challenges Facing Mesothelioma Patients and Their Families: Medical/Legal Intersections

Kirk Hartley and Mary Hesdorffer

Abstract To enhance foresight for patients and their physicians, and to encourage mutual understanding of likely medical/legal events, this chapter addresses medical/legal aspects of lawsuits to obtain compensation for a mesothelioma possibly caused—in whole or in part—by intake of asbestos fibers. The chapter includes overview information on (1) the approximately 2000 US mesothelioma lawsuits filed in each of 2014 and 2015, (2) factors to consider when thinking about a mesothelioma lawsuit and considering lawyers for such a lawsuit, (3) the economics of mesothelioma claims, and (4) "asbestos trusts" and mesothelioma compensation. Also addressed are trial and pretrial "discovery" processes, including emotional and stress factors that may arise from actual or potential conflicting thoughts and priorities generated by simultaneously going through litigation and therapy. Medical data and medical record disclosure issues will arise when lawsuits and claims to trusts are asserted, including demands by lawyers and/or trusts for experts to have access to portions of biopsy samples or other biologic materials used to diagnose mesothelioma. Genetic testing for the person and/or family also may be requested, as was done during pretrial processes for an early 2016 mesothelioma trial which included expert testimony regarding the possible significance of germ line (inherited) genetic characteristics of the person afflicted by mesothelioma. Other pretrial discovery processes arise from the issues that will be resolved in trial. In mesothelioma cases, the overall issue typically is the "cause" of the tumor, as that term is defined and utilized in legal systems. Because of scientific issues about when and how asbestos intake can lead to mesothelioma, persons with mesothelioma and family members should expect to become involved in legal system processes aimed at collecting testimony and documents about the possible amounts

K. Hartley (✉)
LSP Group LLC, 445 West Erie Street—Suite 102, Chicago, IL 60654, USA
e-mail: khartley@lspgrp.com

M. Hesdorffer
Mesothelioma Applied Research Foundation, 1317 King Street, Alexandria, VA 22314, USA
e-mail: info@curemeso.org

© Springer International Publishing AG 2017
J.R. Testa (ed.), *Asbestos and Mesothelioma*, Current Cancer Research,
DOI 10.1007/978-3-319-53560-9_17

and sources of asbestos intake for a particular person. Treating doctors and scientists may be called upon to provide expert testimony regarding which "exposures" to which asbestos products might or might not be deemed "enough" to be a legal cause of the mesothelioma. In addition, some lawyers and other professionals (e.g., actuaries) are starting to pay attention to "molecular science," including developments at the intersections between science and law regarding biomarkers, possible signatures in somatic mutation patterns, and individual variability, including the impact of individual variability for workplace regulations and "toxic tort" lawsuits. Most lawsuits settle without a trial, but each year, perhaps 40–100 mesothelioma cases will at least start a trial against some of the entities named as defendants, and these cases will generate the most pretrial discovery activity. In addition, trial dates are catalysts for settlements, so there also are extensive pretrial discovery processes for hundreds of cases set for trial each year.

Keywords Asbestos exposure and litigation • Medical/legal aspects of mesothelioma • Lawsuits and compensation • Mesothelioma causation • Genetic testing

17.1 Background to and Relevance of this Chapter

Mesothelioma and litigation are so often related that this and other treatises include chapters with medical/legal information. This chapter is believed to be a first-of-its-kind compilation of objective medical/legal information that is relevant as treatment of mesothelioma moves into the age of genomics and precision medicine, with some data and comments on other asbestos-related lawsuits and trust claims. The chapter presents a multidisciplinary and nonpartisan view of medical/legal topics that may well be encountered by many of the persons diagnosed with mesothelioma and their treating physicians and/or other members of hospital staffs. The topics also are relevant to family members and to patient advocates, including plaintiff lawyers.

This chapter is timely for patients who may very naturally wonder about the economics of a lawsuit and the related burdens of a lawsuit. Unfortunately, mesotheliomas continue to occur in larger than expected numbers, and therefore the economics of mesothelioma claiming is significant for financial stakeholders on all sides. As a result, mesothelioma claims have been and remain subject to extensive social media and general media articles, some of which are disguised forms of advertising to persons considering whether to file a lawsuit. In addition, patients and physicians may work together more smoothly if both understand that social media and regular media often repeat inaccurate assertions issued by partisan advocates on various sides of issues.

The chapter also is timely for physicians and patients because the increasing arrival of "precision medicine" means new medical/legal issues are arising for persons with mesothelioma and their treating and consulting physicians. In general, the new issues arise around access to genetic information. The issues occur because treatment of mesothelioma increasingly involves the use of tests that assess genetic information. Such testing increasingly is conducted as part of clinical trials of stand-alone "precision medicine" therapies, trials involving "immunotherapy," and/or trials of new combinations of drugs and therapies. Some tests are focused on genetic findings of the tumor itself (i.e., somatic cells). Such tests require access to tumor tissue taken during biopsies. Other tests assess heritable (germ line) genetic information obtained from non-cancerous cells. Laboratories perform germ line tests by examining healthy cells found in blood, saliva, and bodily fluids or by using non-cancerous tissue in addition to tumor tissue. The tests may be performed by laboratories found at major medical centers or may be performed by private laboratories that provide fee-for-service tests.

The results of genetic tests are starting to become part of pretrial discovery processes and trial issues. For example, January 2016 brought the first mesothelioma product liability trial with expert trial testimony regarding the possible role(s) of germ line *BAP1* mutations in the development of a mesothelioma in a particular person. The trial involved a woman with a pleural mesothelioma who was a member of a family with a reported four instances of mesothelioma among her first-degree siblings and their children. In addition, some lawyers are monitoring efforts to find "signature" patterns of somatic mutations. We anticipate that physicians caring for patients with a diagnosis of mesothelioma, having read through this chapter, will be able to clarify for patients the impact of genetic testing on mesothelioma lawsuits in the context of what is known today.

17.2   Overview Information Regarding Mesothelioma Lawsuits and Trust Claims

17.2.1   Statistics Regarding Mesothelioma and Other Asbestos Lawsuits

Asbestos litigation is a notable component of the overall litigation industry. Each year, there are multiple litigation conferences at which lawyers, judges, and a few medical experts meet, talk, and debate about the asbestos litigation industry, including talks about changes and development in tactics, and presentation of litigation statistics. Court systems generate few if any statistics for specific subtypes of litigation, and so most asbestos litigation statistics are generated from private datasets generated by law firms or others involved in asbestos litigation. Typically the datasets are limited to a specific state or court system. However, as of 2016, aggregate national asbestos statistics for the past 2 years were presented by a consulting firm (kcic.com) that assists corporate defendants with tracking

Table 17.1 Asbestos complaints by disease in the USA in 2014 and 2015

Disease from complaint[a]	2014	2015	Percent change
Mesothelioma	2012	2102	4.5%
Lung cancer	1092	1062	−2.7%
Nonmalignant	998	758	−24.0%
Unknown	408	339	−16.9%
Other cancer	132	145	9.8%
Pneumoconiosis	88	44	−50.0%
Silicosis	90	15	−83.3%
Total	4820	4465	

[a]When more than one disease is alleged, the highest level of malignancy is used for purposes of reporting

asbestos-related lawsuits. The database itself is not public, but on February 18, 2016, the firm published on its blog numerous charts drawn from the database as of November, 2015 (Terrell 2015), and later added an update with December 2015 data (Potter 2016). Within the community of asbestos lawyers, the data are valued and viewed as reasonably consistent with other state-specific and court-specific data. A broad view chart presenting the aggregate numbers is shown in Table 17.1.

As shown in Table 17.1, mesothelioma claims are not decreasing. As to non-mesothelioma "lung cancer" claims, they appear constant for this 2-year time period, after some fluctuation in 2012–2014 that was driven primarily by a group of about 650 lung cancer case filings in 2013 and 2014 by one law firm (Heather Isringhausen Gvillo, Legal Newsline 2014a), which also represented many persons in claiming against the Zadroga Trust created to compensate some persons injured by the events of September 11, 2001 (Napoli and Crosby 2011). Some plaintiff lawyers express serious interest in pressing lung cancer against "asbestos trusts" and/or in lawsuits for persons with "good facts," meaning factors such as indisputable evidence of asbestos exposure in "meaningful" amounts, and little or no tobacco use and/or 15 or more years without tobacco use. Claims involving "other cancers" (e.g., laryngeal or colon) also may be increasing, and more might be expected due to a recent federal court ruling that allowed a kidney cancer lawsuit to proceed ahead to trial. The authors are not aware of any lawsuits or trust claims involving heart diseases and asbestos (e.g., Harding et al. 2012).

17.2.2   Average Mesothelioma Recoveries and Other Economics of Mesothelioma Claiming

The adverse economic impacts of mesothelioma can be severe for the afflicted person and their family, and so patients and family members tend to seek answers to questions about average recoveries if litigation is undertaken. Due to limitations on publicly available data about lawsuits, and a lack of public data about settlements, it is simply not possible to provide an objective "average number" calculated from comprehensive, verifiable data. Indeed, there are multiple reasons to question the veracity of the few public suggestions about "average" numbers for mesothelioma recoveries, and all projections and estimates should be considered with caution. Selected views and data are, however, provided.

Despite the lack of comprehensive, verifiable data, some will still ask for a view on an "average" recovery by a person with mesothelioma allegedly caused by asbestos. For current claimants (as opposed to past or future claimants), the subjective view of one author (K.H.) is that persons with well-documented asbestos exposures through occupational work with or around asbestos will on average obtain a total gross recovery (before expenses) in the range of $1.5–2.2 million, if represented by well-prepared plaintiff lawyers who can credibly take a case to trial against one or more defendants. Under that view, a net recovery for the person or family may run from $500,000 to $1.5 million, depending on the expenses of the case and the terms of a contingency fee agreement with a plaintiff's law firm. The amounts recovered for other persons with other fact patterns typically may be expected to be lower, because settlement monies or trial verdicts typically are mainly paid by defendants for which there is evidence that its products (1) were used at work by the person with mesothelioma, resulting in excess exposure to asbestos or (2) were used in significant amount by a family member who then "brought home" some amount of asbestos fibers, thereby producing some degree of excess intake of fibers.

17.2.3 General Guidelines About Hiring Lawyers and Mesothelioma Litigation

Marketing of lawsuits to asbestos-exposed persons has become its own industry. Unfortunately, a result is that too many persons with cancer are lured to websites purporting to provide advocacy, expert advice, "support," and access to "top medical specialists." In our opinion, these assertions often are only barely true, and instead many of the websites are primarily about seeking out persons to become clients for some plaintiff law firms. This is not a complaint about the filing of lawsuits; they are often well-founded and much needed to provide economic resources to persons with cancer and/or their spouses or children. The complaint instead is that the client recruiting process too often diverts patients away from better sources of medical information and results in less than optimal medical care choices. For example, a patient may be diverted away from expert care fairly close to home and toward a doctor or medical center with which financial relationships have been developed. In some instances, this type of situation may needlessly delay care, and in some instances, it may decrease overall survival for a person with an aggressive mesothelioma. In other instances, persons may be discouraged from participating in clinical trials that need patient participation in order to advance research against this rare disease.

The confusion may also grow as to hiring lawyers. In April 2014, Kantar Media reported on the general growth of television advertising by "meso lawyers" and that some plaintiff lawyers who actually handle lawsuits are attacking other lawyers who do not really want to handle lawsuits and instead just seek to recruit clients and then refer them to other lawyers. Kantar explained, "From the Great Recession in 2008 onwards, the upward trend of trial lawyer TV advertising continued unabated even while the rest of the advertising industry took a hit. This ad category has grown by 68% over the past eight years from $531 million in 2008 to nearly $900 million for 2015. Legal services has grown six times faster than all other advertising sectors, according to a recent Kantar Media CMAG study for the U.S. Chamber of Commerce, while doubling its share of local spot advertising."

Kantar also reported on the newer trend of ads that encourage hiring local lawyers instead of "national recruiting firms" that do not want to actually handle lawsuits. Kantar explained: Geoffrey Fieger, a plaintiffs' attorney based in Detroit, MI, has published ads that state the following attack on lawyers who advertise for cases but do not actually handle lawsuits: "Every day, people are forced to settle for less than they need or deserve. Why? Because their lawyer doesn't really try cases; they only advertise on TV and never go to court." (Geoffrey Perieira, Trial lawyer on trial lawyer (April 14, 2016), available at: http://us.kantar.com/tech/tv/2016/lawyer-tv-ads-about-lawyers/).

In our opinion, some patients, doctors, and researchers have been duped into providing quotes and interviews for websites not fully understanding the nature of the relationship between these marketing sites and the financial rewards for each patient recruited into situations that may be suboptimal for the patient. For example, well-intentioned statements may be taken out of context and/or used simply to draw patients to a law firm. These quotes and interviews add an air of credibility to a site that may look like a nonprofit advocacy organization, but in fact may be part of a for-profit business model that is only barely disclosed upon careful investigation. Accordingly, it is important to check to see if a website provider is a 501(c)(3) charity and, if so, how it is rated by an independent body such as Charity Navigator.

17.2.4 Precision Medical/Legal Interactions for Persons with Mesothelioma

Principles of precision medicine seem appropriate for doctor/patient/lawyer interactions about medical/legal situations. We think this concern especially applies to treating physicians with patients who look to and/or completely depend on physicians for medical advice. From our combined 50+ years of hands-on experience with asbestos litigation and care of persons with mesothelioma, it appears to us that patients assume/think doctors are knowledgeable about asbestos litigation, but our observation is that in fact most physicians and researchers understand very little about asbestos litigation and asbestos-containing products. Therefore, we urge patients, family members, physicians, researchers, and lawyers to diligently seek to use precision when discussing possible claims and when recording information about "asbestos exposure" and imparting information about the patient's disease status. Simply put, as advocates, trial lawyers for both defendants and plaintiffs are expert at taking a statement out of context and putting a headline spin around an imprecise statement. With those principles in mind, we set out below some explanations of relevant facts about asbestos-containing products and issues in asbestos litigation.

Just as medical groups create databases of information for use in treating future patients, the better plaintiff law firms create databases of information that can be used to better serve future clients. Their databases may contain, for example, information about the types, sources, and amounts of asbestos products in use at particular facilities. This information can then be used in lawsuits filed by particular persons. Consider, for example, a pipe fitter with mesothelioma. He may have been a union worker sent to work on renovation products at numerous large industrial facilities in a region, with many persons present as employees or contractors. For such facilities, a plaintiff firm in that geographic area likely will have invested in years of building a database of documents of sales records and invoices obtained from the facility through the litigation discovery process. The plaintiff firm also will have built a database of past testimony about asbestos use at the facilities. For example, the firm may have testimony from the persons who installed asbestos-containing pipe insulation at a refinery in 1965 and who saw labels on boxes that identified the company that supplied the product. Or the firm may have similar testimony from persons who installed products during the construction of high-rise buildings, power plants, or school buildings. The firm may also know the whereabouts of retired employees able and willing to provide testimony about products installed decades in the past or the practice of a company to purchase all of its products from supplier "X." Similar processes and data sources also exist for navy ships and shipyards (see http://bldg92.org/media/uploads/Archives%20Finding%20Aids/MC24_Trezza%20Finding%20Aid.pdf).

Consider also a very different fact pattern, such as a woman with mesothelioma, apparently "caused" in whole or in part by asbestos fibers "brought home" or into a family car from products her husband worked with in the course of his work. That husband/worker may have been a union worker of the sort described above, and so the law firm's knowledge may be critical to the recovery of the wife, especially if the husband died before the woman developed mesothelioma. Or consider a different fact pattern, such as the husband having worked at only two or three facilities, and also assume the facilities have never before been at issue in a lawsuit. Cases of that sort will require extensive de novo investigation as to the past or current presence of asbestos at the facilities where the husband worked and that investigation may or may not reveal evidence of his past exposure to asbestos. In a situation of that kind, there may be very limited sources of exposures, and so there may be only one or two defendant companies, and a financial recovery (or not) will depend on the facts revealed by investigation. Probes also may be undertaken by government agencies.

An example of both arises from the use of vermiculite with plants; some sellers used vermiculite that was "contaminated" with asbestiform fibers (EPA 2009).

Persons with mesothelioma of course are heterogeneous in many ways, including their genetic characteristics, home environments, workplace surroundings, histories of asbestos exposure (or no exposure), and other possible contributory factors, ranging from cigarette smoking to exposures to other types of natural or man-made fibers. Also, many people have very little or no knowledge about (1) which products contain asbestos, (2) the types and amounts of asbestos in a product, (3) the industrial uses and OSHA practices related to such products, and/or (4) which products actually release asbestos fibers (some products may release few if any fibers because the fibers are encased in vinyl or other substances). Physicians and others also may well operate under misconceptions about the years in which different products contained asbestos. It is true that EPA and OSHA significantly limited some uses of asbestos-containing products as of the early 1970s. However, other products continued to contain asbestos well into the 1990s and early 2000s (e.g., brake and clutch linings made by some companies).

A first-of-its-kind May 2015 paper indicates that workplace asbestos fiber levels remained well above federal limits in some workplaces up through 2011. Interestingly, the paper was written by persons at Cardno ChemRisk, a consulting firm that works mainly for large companies. Some lawyers for plaintiffs accuse it and other similar firms of bias against persons seeking compensation for cancer. However, the data found and published runs contrary to assumptions and arguments asserted by some defendants. The abstract and Sect. 3.3 explain finding over limit exposures from 1984 to 2011 as follows:

> The United States Occupational Safety and Health Administration (OSHA) maintain the Chemical Exposure Health Data (CEHD) and the Integrated Management Information System (IMIS) databases, which contain quantitative and qualitative data resulting from compliance inspections conducted from 1984 to 2011. This analysis aimed to evaluate trends in workplace asbestos concentrations over time and across industries by combining the samples from these two databases. From 1984 to 2011, personal air samples ranged from 0.001 to 175 f/cc. Asbestos compliance sampling data associated with the construction, automotive repair, manufacturing, and chemical/petroleum/rubber industries included measurements in excess of 10 f/cc, and were above the permissible exposure limit from 2001 to 2011.
>
> ***
>
> Despite the fact that airborne concentrations as measured by OSHA decreased significantly after 1985, as of 2010, the OSHA asbestos sampling data indicated that exposures in certain industries (e.g., construction) still continue to exceed current occupational exposure guidelines. Therefore, exposures in excess of the OSHA regulatory limits may still be present in major industries such as construction and manufacturing and may present a public health challenge for those working in those industries when proper PPE [personal protective equipment] is not implemented, as required by Federal Regulations (Maylie et al., 2004). According to NIOSH, asbestosis-related mortality has continued to increase from 77 in 1968 to 1265 in 1999, suggesting that asbestos exposure continues to be an occupational health concern. (Cowan et al. 2015; underlined sentences indicate emphasis added by chapter authors)

17.2.5   Caution Is in Order at "Mesothelioma Information" Websites

Because so many people turn to the Internet for information, "mesothelioma information websites" are numerous and should be considered with some caution. In fact, some websites are mainly advertising "click bait" aimed at helping some law firms to recruit new clients. Indeed, some plaintiff law firms pay to sponsor or associate themselves with "mesothelioma information" websites they had built for recruiting. These and other firms pay high fees for "click through" traffic on phrases related to mesothelioma. The situation is not new. A *New York Times* article on the same topic revealed the prices prevailing at that time (Liptak 2007). A 2015 review of "click fees" explained the situation as follows:

> Way back in October 2009, AdGooroo found that the keyword 'mesothelioma' was the most expensive keyword in paid search, costing an average of $99.44 per click (Leichenko 2015). We recently returned to that subject and found things have both changed and stayed the same in the ensuing years. In analyzing the full year of 2014, we found that the term 'mesothelioma' per se was no longer the most expensive keyword in terms of cost per click and that it had actually dropped in price to an average CPC of $82.69. That being said, 13 of the top 20 most expensive keywords in 2014 were, in fact, related to mesothelioma, the cancerous tumor that is at the center of many asbestos-related lawsuits.

> Moreover, the price to sponsor these keywords has skyrocketed. The most expensive keyword term for 2014, 'mesothelioma attorneys tx', had an average cost per click of $319.34. The other 12 mesothelioma-related keywords in the top 20 averaged a $216.17 cost per click (Leichenko 2015).

In 2015, the firm identified the terms and prices for search terms related to mesothelioma. The findings are summarized in Table 17.2. These websites often include a wide but shallow amount of information about mesothelioma and are designed to show up at or near the top of a list of Internet search results. Some of the sites strive to attract mention by arranging links to other websites, mentioning college scholarships or mentioning the names of doctors, hospitals, or universities. Some of the sponsors also are said to have paid fees or other compensation to patients, family members, and/or physicians who write statements to be included on the websites or related blogs, thus adding to their look of legitimacy. For example, the website "asbestos.com" is sponsored by the Peterson Law Firm, which is disclosed on the site if one looks at the "about" page or looks thoroughly through other pages of the site.

Some plaintiff firms that sponsor such websites are not interested in actually filing a lawsuit or going to court. They instead prefer to recruit in potential clients, sign them to a contingency fee agreement (see below), and then refer the lawsuit to a different plaintiff firm for actual handling. The referrals usually involve "fee splitting," in which contingent legal fees are split between (1) the law firm that first recruited the plaintiff and (2) a law firm that will actually handle the case, perhaps including going to trial before a jury or judge. Such arrangements are legal in most states, but in general are economically wasteful because money may well be paid to

Table 17.2 Internet keyword terms and prices for search terms related to mesothelioma

Most expensive paid search keywords by average cost per click
US Google Desktop Text Ads, January–December 2014

Keyword	Cost per click	Spend	Impressions	Click-through rate	# of advertisers
Mesothelioma attorneys tx	$319.34	$47,420	3349	4.43%	134
Buying structured settlement annuities	$312.49	$16,005	793	6.46%	61
Alabama mesothelioma attorney	$291.93	$12,341	828	5.11%	71
Hawaii mesothelioma lawyers	$247.64	$10,239	811	5.10%	79
Mesothelioma attorneys California	$231.35	$13,994	1075	5.63%	68
Structured settlement industry	$230.04	$7388	631	5.09%	57
National structured settlement trade association	$229.33	$7962	446	7.79%	36
Cash structured settlements	$226.43	$65,712	6171	4.70%	91
Insurance structured settlements	$222.04	$9307	774	5.41%	57
Virginia mesothelioma attorney	$221.25	$9065	774	5.29%	68
Mesothelioma claim	$211.01	$179,634	25,067	3.40%	100
Mesothelioma attorney Washington	$206.13	$9160	817	5.44%	80
Virginia mesothelioma lawyers	$206.04	$8433	786	5.21%	69
Virginia mesothelioma lawyer	$203.54	$9086	896	4.98%	73
Maryland mesothelioma lawyers	$200.21	$8359	818	5.10%	62
A mesothelioma	$196.65	$3503	578	3.08%	64
Selling structured settlements	$189.78	$497,479	51,884	5.05%	73
Nevada mesothelioma attorney	$189.53	$7387	784	4.97%	77
Wisconsin mesothelioma attorney	$188.76	$8083	805	5.32%	81
Structured settlements annuities	$187.00	$47,429	4690	5.41%	95

Leichenko (2015)

a plaintiff's firm that is not situated to or capable of contributing real value to successful pursuit of the lawsuit. When multiple law firms are involved in a representation, the firms collectively tend to charge an overall larger fee, as further described below.

17.2.6 Contingent Fee Agreements

Virtually all plaintiff firms are hired based on a written "contingent fee agreement," which is simply a descriptive name for the contract for services between the law firm and the person with mesothelioma (or his/her estate). Different states have slightly different laws and rules applicable to contingent fee agreements, so they are not identical across the country. Under a typical agreement, the law firm agrees to pay the fees and costs incurred in order to investigate and then file a lawsuit seeking compensation for causation of mesothelioma (or other asbestos-related disease). The law firm also agrees to provide the legal services needed to handle the case from beginning to end. If the firm fails to recover money for the claimant, the firm loses the money and time invested in the investigation and the case. In return, the person with mesothelioma agrees that the law firm may keep a percentage of all monies recovered from defendants. That amount typically ranges from 33 to 40%, but some agreements exist at lower and higher amounts. Lower percentage amounts, for example, sometimes are available to union members if a law firm has strong ties to members of the union, perhaps based on personal relationships or perhaps based on prior lawsuits and good outcomes. However, when selecting a law firm, it is usually more important to focus on the actual, relevant skills of the firm, as opposed to trying to save a percentage point or two.

17.3 Financial Information on Asbestos Litigation and Claim Payments

17.3.1 Condensed Aggregate View of Data from Asbestos Compensation Systems

Asbestos claim data are provided below, subject to the caveat that datasets are generally from private sources because public datasets are nonexistent or poor. According to private data, during 2014 and 2015, approximately 2000 mesothelioma lawsuits were filed in the USA, with most lawsuits filed in a relatively few courts. During 2014–2015, well over 40% of mesothelioma lawsuits were filed in state court in Madison County, Illinois (east of St. Louis, MO). Currently, most other mesothelioma lawsuits will be filed in state or federal courts in the vicinity of major cities that had nearby shipyards, or industrial centers, or high-rise buildings built in the 1950s–1980s. For example, many cases are filed each year in courts in or near Baltimore, Chicago, Los Angeles, Miami, New York, Norfolk, Philadelphia, St. Louis, and San Francisco/Oakland. As of 2016, most mesothelioma lawsuits will require 1–2 years to reach an outcome against most defendants.

In aggregate terms, since its inception in 1967, asbestos litigation has generated something in the vicinity of $80 billion of expense, with over half of that amount paid out as fees to lawyers and other professionals as of the 2005 report by RAND Corporation. For a variety of historic reasons, the aggregate amount paid as compensation to persons with mesothelioma has been relatively modest when compared to amounts paid to persons with other asbestos-related diseases, such as asbestosis or lung cancers. One historic reason for this disparity is that many persons heavily exposed to asbestos also were smokers and were injured by or died of other diseases before mesothelioma could appear. Also, prior to about 2005, there were large sets of payments to persons with nonmalignant disease, due to developments in legal systems and the creation of asbestos trusts systems beginning in the late 1980s. As of the early to mid-2000s, much more attention was focused on prioritizing and increasing individual and aggregate payments to persons with mesothelioma. That change emerged due to bankruptcy cases filed in the early 2000s by several former defendant companies as well as proposed federal asbestos legislation in the mid-2000s. These and other events helped to generate some relatively unified efforts to focus more attention to prioritizing payments to persons with mesothelioma. The efforts involved some plaintiff lawyers with law firms focused on representing persons with cancer, some lawyers who are assigned to represent the interests of persons who will develop mesothelioma in the future, some insurance companies, and some lawyers and business persons from companies frequently sued in asbestos litigation.

17.3.2 Overview of Financial Recoveries Through Litigation and Asbestos Trust Claims

Through a lawsuit and/or claims submitted to "asbestos trusts," a person with mesothelioma may seek compensation based on the overall claim that asbestos caused her mesothelioma, in whole or in part, using the legal system definition of causation. As described below in more detail, the limited public data suggest that most *net recoveries* to a person with mesothelioma will fall in a range from perhaps $300,000 to $1.5 million, including recoveries from both lawsuits and claims submitted to asbestos trusts. There are of course outlier numbers, with many of the higher outlier recoveries due to unusual personal circumstances (e.g., death at a relatively young age or many dependent children), and/or the ability and willingness of a person and/or their family to endure pursuit of a compensation claim up through the uncertainty of jury verdicts. The *net recovery* amounts are the amounts remaining *after* payment of contingent attorneys' fees and expenses for evidence and expert witnesses. Currently, such expenses typically consume 33%–50% of gross recoveries.

17.3.3 Asbestos Trust Overview

Compensation claims to asbestos trusts involve administrative claiming processes, with some possibilities to move to litigation if dissatisfied with an administrative outcome. Claims may be asserted against both old and new trusts. The older trusts, however, in general have relatively less money left to pay current or future claims. The first trust claiming processes were created in the late 1980s to in effect serve as replacements for lawsuits against some of the major sellers of asbestos products, which had become "bankrupt" entities due to thousands of asbestos disease lawsuits on behalf of persons seriously harmed or killed by their products. Throughout the 1980s, asbestos litigation was very much reshaped by the use of bankruptcy court processes to create the Johns-Manville trust to replace the global set of Johns-Manville companies. From the late 1800s through the early 1980s, the Johns-Manville companies had mined asbestos fibers in Canada, had imported to the USA and Europe other asbestos fibers from Africa and Australia, and had sold around the globe many hundreds of types of asbestos-containing products used by millions of people, often tradesmen working at shipyards, power plants, large industrial operations, and large buildings. The same bankruptcy process (known as "Chap. 11") was used by more companies in the 1990s, and several additional and large asbestos trusts were created between 2005 and 2010. More trusts are in creation today through ongoing Chap. 11 bankruptcy proceedings. Overall, there have been approximately 100 "asbestos bankruptcies," and the trusts distributed approximately $13.5 billion from 2007 to 2011. As of year-end 2011, data by Bates White show that the trusts held approximately $18 billion of assets (cash or investments) (Scarcella and Kelso 2012). As of year-end 2013, the trusts still held approximately $18 billion of assets, and another $10 billion was expected (Scarcella and Kelso 2015).

Many thousands of asbestos trust claims are filed each year, but the overall numbers can be misleading in the sense that 4–30 different trust claims may be filed on behalf of a single person. Thus, the number of claims asserted will far exceed the number of persons stricken by mesothelioma. The timing of claims to mesothelioma trusts varies due to case-specific facts and strategic decision-making by both plaintiff and defense lawyers. In general, the simplest and easiest form of trust claim can be asserted and resolved within 4–6 months. Some persons with mesothelioma may be able to assert their own claims to trusts, with assistance from family members, especially if the person's work history was simple, such as 30 years spent working at one location. However, the incentive to do so is often limited, because many persons with mesothelioma will at least consider filing a lawsuit, and so will talk to and/or hire a law firm to investigate the historic facts and to make decisions, including whether and when to assert claims to asbestos trusts. In most but not all instances, retaining a well-qualified plaintiff lawyer will produce a better financial outcome for the person with mesothelioma. Expert advice also may well be needed to understand and plan for "medical liens" that may well be imposed to take away some of the money paid out by a trust or through a lawsuit. Medical liens can be and often are imposed by health insurers, hospitals, or other service providers in order to ensure that they are fully paid for their services related to the disease.

17.3.4   Asbestos Trusts Are Paying Out Less and Less to Individual Claimants

It also is important to understand and plan for the fact that the vast majority of asbestos trusts are running low on money, and payouts are being reduced dramatically. The point that trusts are running out of money is simple to illustrate. Indeed, data published by Bates White show that asbestos trust payment percentages keep falling as trusts perceive they are running out of money (Scarcella and Kelso 2012; available online at bateswhite.com). Their compilations show that most asbestos trusts are paying less than 50% of the amount originally planned. Indeed, 13 of the trusts are paying out less than 10% of the amount originally planned. Looking further ahead, even those substantially reduced payments may be further reduced if annual mesotheliomas in the USA continue to exceed past projections. The payment percentages also will be further in jeopardy if trusts receive and pay larger volumes of claims for non-mesothelioma lung cancers and/or claims for other cancers sometimes linked to asbestos intake, such as laryngeal and ovarian cancers.

17.4   Genetics and Precision Medicine

17.4.1   Will Inherited Mutations Lead to Precision Legal Analysis of Relative Risk?

Another topic to consider is whether the arrival of genetics in toxic tort claiming will mean that judges will adopt new principles of "precision toxic tort litigation," just as physicians have adopted new principles for "precision medicine." To use a cancer example, precision medicine can refer to a situation in which a specific drug is provided to a patient because the drug is known to target a genetic "driver" of the tumor, which was identified using genomic analysis. By analogy, "precision toxic tort litigation" could arise through courts accepting "relative risk" calculations specific to persons with (1) particular genetic mutations and (2) intake of one or more specific toxins.

The concept of precision toxic tort litigation could specifically apply with respect to the concept of "relative risk" and its application in tort litigation. More specifically, the relative risk principle often is associated with the Texas Supreme Court's decision in *Merrell Dow Pharm. Corp. v. Havner*, 953 S.W.2d 706 (Tex. 1997), a case about Vioxx allegedly causing heart attacks. In this case, the court required that a plaintiff prove "general causation" through at least two statistically significant epidemiological studies showing that Vioxx more than doubled the risk of heart attack. In short, the Texas Supreme Court held that a tort claim is proper only if there is a showing of a relative risk of 2.0, meaning that exposure to a toxin results in at least a doubling of the usual relative risk of 1.0.

To date, relative risk calculations have almost always been based on generic populations (cohorts) of individuals exposed to a drug or toxin. However, in a world of "precision toxic tort litigation," would courts accept or require "precision" relative risk calculations focused on the relative risk experience of only persons with a particular genetic mutation and intake of a particular toxin? If so, perhaps larger or smaller populations of individuals would become eligible to assert toxic tort claims. Issues of this sort will be relevant for mesothelioma lawsuits. As pointed out elsewhere in this book, there is a continuing stream of research papers showing both biologic and statistical reasons for concluding that the persons with germ line *BAP1* mutations are more susceptible to mesothelioma. Moreover, when compared to genetically normal mice, sibling animals with a germ line mutation of *BAP1* have been shown to have increased susceptibility to mesothelioma following injection of asbestos into the abdomen, and development of the disease can occur at much lower doses of crocidolite fibers than in genetically normal mice.

The fact that older risk estimation methods are imperfect was highlighted in a 2015 invited commentary by Moolgavkar, who has testified several times for defendants in asbestos personal injury litigation. He explained:

> It is becoming increasingly clear that summary measures of exposure, such as cumulative exposure, cannot capture the impact of complex temporal patterns of exposure on disease risk, and that the relative hazard, which is the target of estimation with the proportional hazards model, has serious limitations .... [A]nother equally important factor in the misinterpretation of epidemiological data is the ubiquitous and often inappropriate application of the proportional hazards model for analysis and the virtually universal use of the relative risk as a measure of effect (Moolgavkar 2015).

Moolgavkar's paper further pointed out that the disease risks for a particular individual can vary many fold if testing shows a particular inherited frailty, such as a significant gene mutation. Moreover, many disease risks (including cancer risks) also are age dependent. Thus, Moolgavkar stated:

> I would use the term frailty only when there is clear biological evidence that a fraction of the population is either exclusively at risk, or at vastly increased risk compared with the general population of contracting a disease. An example of the former situation is cystic fibrosis, an autosomal recessive condition, which is caused only by inherited mutations in a single gene; an example of the latter is familial adenomatous polyposis (FAP) of the colon, a dominantly inherited condition that greatly increases the risk of colon cancer. Although there is no direct estimate of the relative hazard associated with FAP, it can be surmised to be several thousand and strongly age-dependent.

Similar analysis suggests courts and experts will be facing future questions regarding "relative risk," asbestos intake, and "other cancers." Questions will arise because there are debates regarding whether there is a relative risk of 2.0 or greater for intake of asbestos to cause some of the categories of cancer presently defined based on the organ of origin. Consider, for example, the situation with ovarian cancer and asbestos intake. The scientific literature includes articles on both sides of the issue; some find a relative risk above 2.0 and others find a relative risk below 2.0. The relative risk calculation, however, could change if analyses were focused on the incidence of ovarian cancer in persons with asbestos intake and a germ line *BAP1* mutation. This particular hypothetical is now somewhat moot as to ovarian cancer, because IARC and the Helsinki Conference recently concluded the better view is that at least some ovarian cancers are linked to asbestos intake (Wolff et al. 2015).

The same line of analysis can be applied to colorectal and stomach cancer. For both of these cancers, the IARC and the Helsinki Conference recently concluded that an association with asbestos intake remains open to debate as to whether the relative risk is above or below 2.0 (Wolff et al. 2015). These examples illustrate ways in which either defense and plaintiff interests could gain or lose a case depending on the results of further investigation into relative risks and familial tumor susceptibility disorders, such as mesothelioma cases from BAP1 cancer syndrome families.

17.4.2 The Possibility of Mesothelioma Susceptibility Genes in Addition to BAP1

Some lawyers also are aware that *BAP1* may just be one part of a broader story regarding individual susceptibility to mesotheliomas and other cancers. On this topic, lawyers and others were alerted to the issues when some BAP1 researchers (Testa et al. 2011) stated reasons to think other genetic mutations may also induce susceptibility to mesothelioma. Thus, Testa et al. stated:

> Our results provide the first demonstration that genetics influences the risk of mesotheli-oma, a cancer linked to mineral fiber carcinogenesis. As observed for *BRCA1* and *BRCA2*, which account for only some hereditary breast carcinomas, it appears likely that in addition to *BAP1*, more genes will be found associated with elevated risk of mesothelioma. Indeed, among our 26 sporadic mesotheliomas – and excluding malignancies common in the 6th-8th decades of life, such as skin and prostate carcinomas – nine had been diagnosed with one or more additional tumors. …. Seven of 26 were females, and 2/7 also had uterine leiomyo-sarcoma, a malignancy with an incidence of ~$10/10^6$ per year in the U.S.; one of them had also uveal melanoma, an unlikely coincidence.

17.4.3 Some Lawyers Are Following Research Seeking Somatic Mutation "Signatures," and Others Are Seeking Such Signatures for "Asbestos-Caused" Lung Cancers

One of the drivers of asbestos litigation is the strong association between mesothe-lioma and intake of asbestos fibers. This association provides a "signature" that most lawyers credit for increasing the litigation. With "signatures" in mind, some lawyers are following research on somatic mutation patterns that may provide some degree of a "fingerprint" for the disease source. A general example cited at litigation conferences is a study in which lung cancers were induced in mice either by exposure to two different toxins, methyl-nitrosourea (MNU) and urethane, both well-known for causing tumors in mice, or by genetic activation of *Kras* (a cancer driver mutation). The researchers used whole-exome sequencing to determine the gene expression profiles of the lung cancers that arose in the mice. Overall, the authors found that tumors from the *Kras*-mutant mice exhibited a significantly higher level of aneuploidy and chromosome copy number alterations compared to toxin-induced tumors. In contrast, tumors that arose from the toxin exposures produced myriad non-synonymous (mutant), somatic single nucleotide variants (SNVs), and the SNVs correlated with previously observed SNVs in exposed animals that developed tumors (Westcott et al. 2015). Overall, the exome-wide mutation spectra in the toxin-induced tumors exhibited genomic signatures of the initiating toxin.

17.4.4 Possible Somatic Signatures for Lung Cancers Caused by Asbestos

Several studies arising from laboratories in Finland have assessed lung tumor somatic mutation patterns seeking to find one or more mutation patterns associated with asbestos intake. The research appears to be driven to some degree by a desire to find a biomarker useable for purposes of decision-making regarding compensation programs similar to the process known as "workers compensation" in the USA. In general, the lung cancer somatic mutation studies have been the product of work from Nymark and collaborators working with patients with lung tumors after known exposures to asbestos. Again in general terms, the data suggest that specific chromosomal aberrations found in lung tumors may be useful in distinguishing between asbestos-related and non-asbestos-related lung cancers.

The work of Nymark and others extends back for several years. In 2009, two groups independently reported finding an association between asbestos intake and genomic alterations involving chromosomal locations known as 2p16, 9q33.1, and 19p13 (Nymark et al. 2009). In performing these studies, the teams sought to correlate mutation patterns to objective measures of asbestos fibers in the lungs, such as amount of fibers per gram of tissue. This group then extended some of their previous analyses of tumor tissue to evaluate DNA copy number alterations and combinations of allelic imbalances in the previously identified chromosomal regions (19p13, 2p16, and 9q33.1). The investigators reported that looking at the combined set of genomic alterations identified asbestos-exposed patients' lung tumors better than looking only at the results for one of the chromosomal regions. Thus, they proposed that the combination of alterations can form the basis for the development of a genomic test potentially useful for the identification of asbestos-related lung cancers (Nymark et al. 2013).

Another study (Wikman et al. 2007) used gene expression arrays from lung tumor samples from heavily asbestos-exposed and non-exposed patients (the two sets of patients were matched for other characteristics). The authors identified 47 genes that could differentiate the tumors of asbestos-exposed patients from those of non-exposed patients. Further, the gene expression data were combined with comparative genomic hybridization microarray data. According to the authors, a combinatory profile of DNA copy number aberrations and expressional changes was significantly associated with asbestos exposure. Changes related to asbestos exposure were detected in multiple chromosomal regions, the most prominent being 19p13, which also was a location identified by Nymark and colleagues.

In sum, research to date has identified multiple genetic alterations that may be associated with exposure to asbestos. Further research is ongoing. Over time, these somatic mutation patterns could prove accurate in distinguishing asbestos-related lung cancer from non-asbestos-related lung cancer. If that were to happen, the results could drive significant change in litigation and claiming depending on the numbers of persons found to have (or not have) the relevant patterns of mutations or gene expression.

17.4.5   The 2014 Helsinki Asbestos Gathering Addressed the Nymark Lung Cancer Findings

The potential lung cancer tumor signature findings of Nymark et al. were highlighted at the 2014 iteration of the ongoing series of "Helsinki Conferences" focused on asbestos diseases. The initial Helsinki Conference, *Asbestos, Asbestosis, and Cancer*, was held in 1997. The conference focused on an examination of disorders associated with asbestos, as well as on developing criteria to appropriately diagnose and surveil asbestos-related diseases. The meeting produced a consensus report known as *Asbestos, asbestosis, and cancer: the Helsinki criteria for diagnosis and attribution*. Subsequently, experts convened in Helsinki in 2000 to discuss new advances in screening of asbestos-related disorders and updated the criteria accordingly (Wolff et al. 2015). Given the great advances in the field, the expert group convened again in 2014 and provided an update to the 1997 and 2000 Helsinki criteria documents.

Regarding the work of Nymark et al. on potential signatures in somatic mutation patterns, the group noted two related but different points. For one, the group noted that findings regarding homozygous deletion of the tumor suppressor gene *p16INK4A* show promise for use as a biomarker to distinguish between benign and malignant mesothelial pleural proliferations. With regard to lung cancer and asbestos-related molecular changes, the group also discussed Nymark's findings regarding allelic imbalances in 2p16, 9p33.1, and 19p13. The consensus group concluded that the biomarker triplet should not yet be considered sufficient proof of asbestos causation in a given cancer patient, without independent confirmation by international multicenter studies with standardized methodology for molecular assays and exposure assessment (Wolff et al. 2015).

17.4.6   Possible Litigation Consequences of Biomarkers

Biomarkers may be relevant both to causation and damages. As to causation, plaintiff lawyers may (or may not) see screenings using biomarkers as a way to increase the speed and accuracy of a lung cancer or mesothelioma diagnosis of a potential plaintiff. Biomarkers also are relevant to damages. For example, relatively early detection of a mesothelioma may result in prolonged survival, potentially leading to additional treatment, higher patient costs, and added pain and suffering. Longer survival also may result in more "living meso" trials in which a jury will hear firsthand from the person who has been through the horror of a cancer diagnosis and treatment. A living plaintiff also may recover punitive damages, but that remedy often (not always) ends if the person has died. Therefore, punitive damages could increase for some defendants. Earlier detection and more effective treatments could also mean that a person is alive for a personal injury trial, and then later the death of the same person may give rise to a second trial for wrongful death. In California, some law firms have more than once managed to take both such cases to trial. For example, two multimillion dollar verdicts were entered against a defendant after trials for the personal injury and then wrongful death claims related to one patient (Heather Isringhausen Gvillo, Legal Newsline 2014b), and the same firm obtained two trials and verdicts for claims arising from a second person (http://www.kazanlaw.com/verdicts/4055000-verdict-for-automobile-serviceman/).

17.4.7   Is It a Mesothelioma or Not: miRNAs

As of 2014, microRNAs (miRNAs) have made their way into asbestos trials and diagnoses and no doubt will appear again. In both instances, they were used to evaluate whether a tumor was, or was not, a mesothelioma. In addition, miRNA analysis also can be used to answer the question a jury wants to know: if it is not a mesothelioma, what is it?

miRNAs are small, noncoding RNA molecules (containing roughly 21–25 nucleotides). As of now, researchers think that more than 2000 different miRNAs exist, and they all have names based on a convention that resembles the following: mirXYZ. These short molecules function primarily as regulators of messenger RNA (mRNA), which is responsible for protein production in the cell (Cannell et al. 2008). However, miRNAs have also been shown to have other functions, including a significant role in the control of epigenetic regulation and chromosomal dynamics (Bernstein and Allis 2005). Scientists continue to unravel the mechanistic features of these molecules. Nonetheless, at this point, miRNAs have emerged as important diagnostic biomarkers and prognostic factors for use in diagnosing cancer types, including mesothelioma. Specifically, miRNAs are useful for identifying different types of tumors because different levels of specific miRNAs are found in different tumor types. One commercially available diagnostic known as the *Rosetta*

Mesothelioma Test™ is available from Rosetta Genomics. The test provides a quantitative and objective diagnosis of mesothelioma with high sensitivity and specificity. In a study by Rosetta Genomics, miRNA biomarkers for the differential diagnosis of mesothelioma were identified and developed into a standardized miRNA-based test. Using formalin-fixed, paraffin-embedded samples, the authors identified miRNAs differentially expressed between mesothelioma and various carcinomas. The diagnostic assay based on the expression of a number of specific miRNAs reached a sensitivity of 100% and a specificity of 94% in a blinded validation set of 68 samples from the lung and pleura (Benjamin et al. 2010). More recent work identified miRNAs as potential prognostic factors (Ak et al. 2015). For lawyers, the technology was explored in depth in an online webinar (Perrin Conferences.com 2014).

17.5   Looking Ahead: Asbestos Fibers and Epigenetic Alterations

Some lawyers also are watching developments involving epigenetics and intake of asbestos fibers. Epigenetic alterations are less known than gene mutations, but they can be of equal or greater importance than mutations because they can switch genes on or off without actually altering the DNA sequence. Thus, an epigenetic change can affect the expression of a cancer-related gene, making the likelihood of cancer more or less likely. This process is often referred to as epigenetic regulation, and there are two broad types of epigenetic regulation: (1) DNA methylation and (2) histone modifications (histones are proteins that intersect with DNA in a "complex" to form chromatin). In brief, these two forms of epigenetic alterations are objective, observable changes that can be investigated and measured.

Among other things, some lawyers wonder whether additional research may show that epigenetic alterations can potentially serve as biomarkers for past intake of asbestos. An emerging body of mechanistic data suggests that asbestos may induce mesothelioma by causing epigenetic alterations. In particular, a number of studies have supported the view that certain methylation signatures (i.e., the methylation pattern observed across a number of genes) can differentiate asbestos-induced mesothelioma from non-asbestos-induced mesothelioma. For example, one study showed that methylation profiles can differentiate malignant pleura from non-tumor pleura and that asbestos burden and methylation profiles are independent predictors of mesothelioma patient survival (Christensen et al. 2009).

Another study revealed a significantly higher asbestos fiber burden in patient lungs when they also found methylation of any of a number of cell cycle genes, i.e., *APC, CCND2, CDKN2A, CDKN2B, HPPBP1,* and *RASSF1.* The same investigation revealed a significant trend of increasing lung asbestos body burden (counts) as the number of methylated cell cycle pathway genes increased from 0 to 1 to greater than 1 (Christensen et al. 2008).

In the context of litigation, speed and expense matter. In contrast to lung fiber burden studies that draw notable amounts of time and cost by pathologists, DNA methylation profiles can be obtained using high-speed sequencing equipment and software. Therefore, developments in this area are potentially significant because observable, objective epigenetic changes may become an effective means for diagnosing mesotheliomas, as well as for determining whether an individual actually took in asbestos and, if so, how much.

We hope the information presented in this chapter assists patients, family members, and physicians in reducing the stress that arises from simultaneously coping with the demands of mesothelioma therapy and litigation. Both are daunting processes outside the range of day-to-day life experiences, and they create unfamiliar events and demands for information, some of which may feel very personal. We have spent many years participating in our respective roles in the processes and therefore have seen the wide range of events and demands that may arise. We emphasize it is normal for both patients and professionals to experience stress and uncertainty in these processes and encourage reducing uncertainty and stress by asking questions before making decisions, especially when seeking legal counsel. We suggest that institutions develop ethical guidelines for those practicing in the field from both a medical and legal aspect. Too often the lines are crossed and the patient and their family members are shortchanged in the process.

Declaration of Interests   K.H. is involved in asbestos litigation and consulting for former manufacturers of asbestos-containing products. M.H. is the Executive Director of the Mesothelioma Applied Research Foundation, an advocacy group.

References

Ak G, Tomaszek SC, Kosari F et al (2015) MicroRNA and mRNA features of malignant pleural mesothelioma and benign asbestos-related pleural effusion. Biomed Res Int 2015:635748

Benjamin H, Lebanony D, Rosenwald S et al (2010) A diagnostic assay based on microRNA expression accurately identifies malignant pleural mesothelioma. J Mol Diagn 12:771–779

Bernstein E, Allis CD (2005) RNA meets chromatin. Genes Dev 19:1635–1655

Cannell IG, Kong YW, Bushell M (2008) How do microRNAs regulate gene expression? Biochem Soc Trans 36:1224–1231

Christensen BC, Godleski JJ, Marsit CJ et al (2008) Asbestos exposure predicts cell cycle control gene promoter methylation in pleural mesothelioma. Carcinogenesis 29:1555–1559

Christensen BC, Houseman EA, Godleski JJ et al (2009) Epigenetic profiles distinguish pleural mesothelioma from normal pleura and predict lung asbestos burden and clinical outcome. Cancer Res 69:227–234

Cowan DM, Cheng TJ, Ground M et al (2015) Analysis of workplace compliance measurements of asbestos by the U.S. Occupational Safety and Health Administration (1984–2011). Regul Toxicol Pharmacol 72:615–629

EPA (2009) Investigation of asbestos-contaminated vermiculite; available online at: http://nepis.epa.gov/Exe/ZyPDF.cgi/P10014IJ.PDF?Dockey=P10014IJ.PDF

Harding AH, Darnton A, Osman J (2012) Cardiovascular disease mortality among British asbestos workers (1971-2005). Occup Environ Med 69:417–421

Heather Isringhausen Gvillo, Legal Newsline (2014a) Napoli leaders talk about past mistakes, future plans for firm's asbestos lung cancer cases (September 2014); available online at: http:// madisonrecord.com/stories/510556698-napoli-leaders-talk-about-past-mistakes-future-plans- for-firm-s-asbestos-lung-cancer-cases

Heather Isringhausen Gvillo, Legal Newsline (2014b) Calif. jury awards mesothelioma victim's family $11 M in wrongful death lawsuit (February 2014); available online at: http://legalnews- line.com/issues/asbestos/246991-california-jury-awards-mesothelioma-victims-family-11m- in-wrongful-death-lawsuit-previously-awarded-4m-in-personal-injury-suit

Leichenko J (2015) The most expensive keywords in paid search, by cost per click & spend; avail- able online at: https://www.adgooroo.com/resources/blog/the-most-expensive-keywords-in-- paid-search-by-cost-per-click-and-ad-spend/#sthash.nd4gjVbt.dpu

Liptak A (2007) Competing for clients, and paying by the click. New York Times (October 15, 2007); available online at: http://www.nytimes.com/2007/10/15/us/15bar.html

Moolgavkar SH (2015) Commentary: frailty and heterogeneity in epidemiological studies. Int J Epidemiol 44:1425–1426

Napoli P, Crosby B (2011) Compensation through legislation for 9/11 responders and victims: an analysis of Zadroga. Westlaw J Toxic Torts 29:3–8

Nymark P, Kettunen E, Aavikko M et al (2009) Molecular alterations at 9q33.1 and polyploidy in asbestos-related lung cancer. Clin Cancer Res 15:468–475

Nymark P, Aavikko M, Makila J et al (2013) Accumulation of genomic alterations in 2p16, 9q33.1 and 19p13 in lung tumours of asbestos-exposed patients. Mol Oncol 7:29–40

Perrin Conferences.com (2014) MicroRNA tools for trial use for evaluating asbestos-related can- cers and other non-asbestos cancers; available at: "Previous Events" tab. at https://www.per- rinconferences.com/html/Previous_2014/webinar-application-of-microrna.shtml

Potter M (2016) Updated asbestos litigation data (presented at Perrin Conference: March 2016); avail- able online at: http://riskybusiness.kcic.com/presenting-perrin-updated-asbestos-litigation-data/

Scarcella MC, Kelso PR (2012) Asbestos Bankruptcy Trusts: a 2012 overview of trust assets, com- pensation & governance, 11 Mealey's Asbestos Bankruptcy Report, No. 11; see Figure 1

Scarcella MC, Kelso PR (2015) A reorganized mess: the current state of the asbestos bankruptcy trust system, 14 Mealey's Asbestos Bankruptcy Report, No. 7; and A reorganized mess: the current state of the Asbestos Bankruptcy Trust System, 30 Mealey's Litigation Report: Asbestos (March 2015); see Figure 4

Terrell J (2015) KCIC's "Asbestos Litigation: 2015 Year in Review" Report; available online at: http://riskybusiness.kcic.com/kcics-asbestos-litigation-2015-year-in-review-report/

Testa JR, Cheung M, Pei J et al (2011) Germline *BAP1* mutations predispose to malignant meso- thelioma. Nat Genet 43:1022–1025

Westcott PM, Halliwill KD, To MD et al (2015) The mutational landscapes of genetic and chemi- cal models of Kras-driven lung cancer. Nature 517:489–492

Wikman H, Ruosaari S, Nymark P et al (2007) Gene expression and copy number profiling sug- gests the importance of allelic imbalance in 19p in asbestos-associated lung cancer. Oncogene 26:4730–4737

Wolff H, Vehmas T, Oksa P et al (2015) Asbestos, asbestosis, and cancer, the Helsinki criteria for diagnosis and attribution 2014: recommendations. Scand J Work Environ Health 41:5–15

Chapter 18
The Patient's Experience of Malignant Mesothelioma

William M. Buchholz

Abstract Much of our understanding of malignant mesothelioma (MM) is from the perspective of the scientist and physician, focusing on the etiology, biology, and treatment for the disease. Clinicians caring for persons with this cancer have to be prepared to go beyond biology and examine the patient's experience. The human experience of MM is complex and extends into the realms of psychology, sociology, communication styles, and personal identity. Understanding the elements of that experience allows the care team to respond skillfully to patients. Often patients' distress can be prevented and treated if the nature of suffering is recognized. Unfortunately, much of that suffering goes unrecognized and untreated. Treatment guidelines in major medical organizations such as ASCO, NCCN, and British Thoracic Society now include specific recommendations to remedy this. Case studies demonstrate how to recognize the circumstances that require such interventions and ways to integrate care into a comprehensive treatment strategy. In this review, ways to prevent distress are explored from both patient and physician perspectives.

Keywords Malignant mesothelioma • Patient and family experiences • Team approach • Strategic treatment plan • Mesothelioma case studies

18.1 Principles of a Patient's Experience of Malignant Mesothelioma

Successful care of a patient with malignant mesothelioma (MM) requires both medical treatment of the disease and understanding the experience of the patient. Both disease and its treatment have associated symptoms that compromise a patient's life span as well as their quality of life. A comprehensive treatment strategy looks at the psychosocial context and needs of the patient (Hawley et al. 2004). It leads to a

W.M. Buchholz (✉)
Buchholz Medical Group, 1320 Sunrise Ct, Los Altos, CA 94024, USA
e-mail: drbill@buchholzmedgroup.com

© Springer International Publishing AG 2017
J.R. Testa (ed.), *Asbestos and Mesothelioma*, Current Cancer Research,
DOI 10.1007/978-3-319-53560-9_18

better experience for patients and a more rewarding one for medical professionals caring for them. Several principles provide the basis for understanding the person and developing an integrated treatment plan.

18.1.1 Largeness of Life

The goals of treatment go beyond curing the disease and extending life. From the patient's perspective, simply living more days is not sufficient. Length of life is only one dimension. Another dimension is the height of quality of life (QOL). Prolonging a miserable existence or painful death is of little value to the patient. Medical success, however, is generally measured in the time dimension as disease-free survival or survival from time of diagnosis to death. Health-related quality of life (HRQOL), the vertical dimension, might not be a specified goal though validated measures do exist (Hollen et al. 2006; Mollberg et al. 2012). Even HRQOL, however, does not capture the true extent of a patient's experienced QOL, since other unmeasured factors are equally important (Salmon et al. 1996; Clayson et al. 2005).

Patients' daily experience of life includes health-related symptoms but also issues of satisfying social roles, pleasant or unpleasant emotional states, and an intact or damaged sense of self. Quality of life can be measured by the balance between painful or unpleasant symptoms versus enjoyable experiences. Diminishing the distress of any symptom increases QOL.

The third dimension is the depth of meaning or sense of purpose. Without a reason or motivation to go through treatments that have significant side effects, patients may decline them. The intangible and difficult to measure *will to live* often depends upon having a reason to live. Sense of purpose or meaning in life is generally considered a spiritual issue, in or outside of religion. *Man's Search for Meaning* describes Viktor Frankl's experience in Nazi concentration camps and has led to a school of psychotherapy that emphasizes the importance of meaning in life for healthy survival (Frankl 1992). The association of meaning and well-being can be traced back to Aristotle (Ryff 2014). The ability to find meaning in difficult situations gives individuals greater resilience, the ability to cope with adversity and even to survive. Studies of people with cancer showed that in early stages of disease most were well adjusted. With disease progression, only one third remained well adjusted. Established meaning of life, value systems, and personal religion helped individuals adjust more successfully (Majkowicz et al. 2014).

Sense of purpose is created by the individual, but it can be supported or thwarted by others. Understanding what is important to the patient offers the medical team a window into that person's life. Taking into account what patients value helps the team make treatment decisions. When extending life is unlikely and there are few medical options to improve their quality of life, supporting patients' value system can still make their lives larger. Ways of doing this range from adjusting chemotherapy schedules to letting the patient visit a new family member or attend a wedding. End-of-life care may be organized around supporting patients and helping families find closure, which goes beyond just orders for comfort care. Questionnaires have been developed to measure the meaning of life for individuals. There are tools that allow meaning of life to be measured (Salmon et al. 1996).

Presenting the concept that the goal of treatment is based on a three-dimensional model, *largeness of life*, gives both patients and physicians a way to maintain a positive and valuable goal even as the focus of treatment changes. It maintains realistic hope that there is something good possible when prolonging life is a less obtainable goal. It also encourages patients to be active participants in their treatment. This perspective enhances the doctor-patient relationship and often makes a caregiver's job easier. The most important benefit of presenting care in this manner is that it avoids increasing patients' despair by being forced to tell them *there is nothing more we can do*. Rather, physicians can say *we can help you in a different way*.

18.1.2   Nature of Suffering

Eric Cassel's seminal article, *The Nature of Suffering and the Goals of Medicine* (Cassel 1982), defined suffering as a threat to the integrity of the person and occurs when an impending destruction of the person is perceived. Suffering can occur in relation to any aspect of the person, whether it is in the realm of social roles, group identification, the relation with self, body or family, or the relations with a transpersonal, transcendent source of meaning.

Suffering is distinct from pain, although it may include pain. This is particularly true under certain circumstances: *Patients feel out of control, when the pain is overwhelming, when the source of the pain is unknown, when the meaning of the pain is dire, or when the pain is chronic. Another aspect essential to an understanding of the suffering of patients is the relation of meaning to the way in which illness is experienced.*

To understand fully the patient's experience of MM, care providers must recognize that suffering goes beyond physical symptoms (Hughes and Arber 2008; Moore et al. 2010). Threats to self-identity, social and family roles, body image, loss of sovereignty, or autonomy can be just as debilitating as tumor invasion of ribs or costal nerves. Loss of self is a fundamental form of suffering in the chronically ill (Charmaz 1983). That kind of suffering does not respond to morphine and requires a different approach.

18.1.3   Family Experience

Persons are different from patients. The patient is described in the context of a disease. They have a relationship both with the disease and health professionals treating them. Becoming a patient does not replace being a person. That distinction may be lost when focus on treating the disease becomes so central and little attention is paid to other issues. Patients expect medical doctors to use all of their technical skills and concentrate on curing their cancer. They appropriately believe that is the doctor's job. Their wish for health professionals to treat them as persons is also strong. It is unspoken and often revealed only by their disappointment with care.

Persons live in the context of a family and social system that has their own expectations. Persons need psychological support as well as physical care. Persons are defined in many dimensions. They have families that have expectations and may have to make adjustments in their lives if the person is unable to go shopping or drive the children to soccer practice. They have jobs in which they earn the money to provide for their dependents. Persons have activities they enjoy such as playing golf, walking along a beach, playing the piano, and socializing with friends. When they become patients engaged in treatment of their MM, many of these activities are interrupted. Even a threat to such pursuits causes suffering if these things are important to that individual.

Family members often provide medical care for loved ones beyond simply driving them to an appointment. If the patient, for that is what they become to family members as well as nurses and doctors, is not eating enough, the spouse worries. Families have the same fears of the future that the patient does.

18.1.4 Team Approach

Patient care requires a team to provide solutions to the complex problems MM creates. This can be most obvious at tumor boards where medical oncologists, surgeons, radiotherapists, and other professionals confer and develop a treatment plan. Large medical centers have other resources available such as palliative care, nurse specialists, social workers, physical therapists, and support groups. Hospice organizations, for example, are required to provide spiritual care. Personnel trained specifically to do this are part of the team that already includes nurses, social workers, and a physician.

Developing a comprehensive care plan to address both the medical and psychosocial needs of patients and families requires a team. Not only are multiple perspectives needed to recognize all the problems, multiple personnel are needed to provide solutions. Not all physicians treating MM have these resources already available. It becomes necessary to network with other services in the community and form ad hoc teams. This is vital for both patients who need the services and caregivers who can be overwhelmed by trying to provide them.

18.2 Case Studies

The following case studies describe patient and family experiences of mesothelioma. They are seen thru the lens of the principles described in the section above. Information has come from interviewing patients and review of medical records.

The descriptions have been changed only to protect patient confidentiality. The person called Roger was my patient, and his family has given me permission to use him for this article.

18.2.1   Case Study: Roger

Roger was 78 years old when he died in the emergency room, having celebrated his 57th wedding anniversary 4 months earlier. He had been diagnosed with a malignant pleural effusion in 1994. It was diagnosed as adenocarcinoma of unknown origin at the time although MM was considered in the differential diagnosis. He had four cycles of carboplatinum and Taxol. Side effects of chest pain and peripheral neuropathy were finally resolved after 2 years. He was asymptomatic and in remission for 9 years until he developed exertional dyspnea and secondary polycythemia in 2003. At that time he was diagnosed with COPD and sleep apnea.

In 2005, he complained of left chest pain. He said he could live with the pain but was distressed at his limited ability to care for his wife. She had agoraphobia, a severe social anxiety disorder, and was reluctant to leave the house. His main concern was that if he could not take care of her, she would need to be placed in a care home. A PET scan of the left pleura was positive, and a biopsy revealed MM.

Treatment with cis-platinum and pemetrexed was started. Within 6 days, he developed severe left shoulder pain requiring higher doses of OxyContin. Nausea and anorexia became worse, and he had lost seven pounds by the time for the second dose of chemotherapy. The day after treatment, he had uncontrolled nausea and vomiting, requiring hospitalization in the ICU for dehydration and symptom control. He was discharged from the ICU 2 days later. He had to be readmitted the next day with profound weakness and chills without fever but still anorectic and dehydrated. In spite of how ill he was, his main concern was for his wife. Roger feared that he would not be able to care for her because he was too weak. He asked if the cis-platinum could be stopped.

Three weeks later, Roger remained weak and anorectic, spending most of the day in bed. He usually prepared lunch for his wife but was now unable to perform any of his customary jobs. His wife spent most of her time in her room on the second floor. Even if he moved slowly, he was too dyspneic to climb a single flight of stairs and could not even bring her a glass of milk. He was in a bind, wanting to stay alive but knowing he needed the chemotherapy. We jointly decided to hold off all chemotherapy until he improved. He had received only two cycles of cis-platinum and pemetrexed, seemingly not enough to make a difference.

Two months later, a PET scan did show improvement, but he wasn't encouraged. He was still short of breath and was not sure he could continue caring for his wife—the reason that sustained him and main focus of his life. We decided to resume pemetrexed, although both of us understood that the chances of a single drug working rather than a combination were less. He still wanted to try anyway. He tolerated the drug reasonably well and said that 75% of the days were "good." He added that when his energy dropped periodically, he became angry and doubtful. He was still in considerable pain and required significant doses of oxycodone around the clock.

A month after resuming chemotherapy, we had an hour-long discussion. I needed to understand his values and develop strategies to achieve his goals. By his sixth dose, it was clear that he was improving and gaining weight. He still described feeling poorly for a week after treatment. He did not feel strong enough to go ocean fishing, his favorite activity. He mentioned that he felt uncertain and wanted to know if he was winning his fight. After seven cycles, his CT scans showed no further improvement and chemotherapy was stopped.

Two months later, increasing chest pain and weight loss showed his MM was progressing. He was reluctant to take adequate doses of medicine to control the pain. He said he wanted to monitor the pain to know if the cancer was growing. Both he and his wife were so weak that they required having food brought in.

Although a repeat PET scan indicated that his disease was stable, he had more symptoms. He began to acknowledge his depression, so he was started on antidepressants. For the last 6 months of his life, he was on oxygen, continued to grow weaker, and, finally, accepted adequate doses of pain medications. Even though he swore he would never go back to the hospital, he was in such distress that his family brought him to the ER. Three hours after arriving, he died with his family around him, fighting literally to the last breath.

Roger was a full partner in his medical care. His values helped guide treatment decisions. What gave his life meaning was more than just an important dimension in the largeness of his life. It became the purpose of his treatment. His medical care gave him the highest quality of life possible under the circumstances. We both worked to give him the longest life obtainable. Being able to care for his wife and provide for her well-being gave him the sense of purpose that sustained him until the very end.

18.2.2   Case Study: Alan

Alan was an internationally ranked tennis player, twice married and twice divorced. At the time of the onset of illness, he was an industrial security consultant and life coach. He had served in the Middle East as an Army Ranger for 8 years before he became a consultant. His first symptoms were chest pain and shortness of breath. A chest X-ray showed a pleural effusion. Several thoracenteses were not diagnostic but he delayed the suggested pleural biopsy, because he wanted to keep playing tennis and continue working. After biopsy showed MM, he underwent an extrapleural pneumonectomy.

He described his reaction after being told of his diagnosis as follows:

My doctor told me there wasn't any cure for this. I was shocked, given the kind of shape I was in and how well I felt. Then the back started hurting me more. After the shock came despair and loss of hope. The next thing I knew, I was thinking that I'm going to die and I can't believe it. When the surgeon suggested surgery, he remembered thinking that he couldn't fathom any of the things she said, but if that's what we have to do, we've got to do it.

He had considerable pain postoperatively, which was unrelieved by PCA. Pulmonary therapy treatments were likewise painful. He started radiotherapy and chemotherapy with cis-platinum and pemetrexed 2 months later. He had significant side effects including marked dyspnea, fatigue, and weight loss of 40 pounds. He had an episode of neutropenic fever that interrupted both chemotherapy and radiation. There were multiple hospital admissions for dehydration and "failure to thrive." Chemotherapy was discontinued after two of the anticipated four cycles.

Poor family and social support complicated his home care. He lived with a nephew who worked and was home each night, but Alan was in bed almost 20 h per day. An ex-wife offered to help but could not be there daily either. He was left alone much of the time, too weak to walk very far and needing a wheel chair to go any distance. When he tripped and fell several times, it was very difficult to get up without help.

Following his abbreviated treatment, he became clinically depressed. Just as he was reluctant to acknowledge his pain because it might show weakness, he did not consider himself depressed *unless he was crying all the time and ready to jump off a bridge.* After being questioned by a physician, he did recognize that all his other symptoms, including feeling the bleakness of his future, did constitute depression. He accepted antidepressants, and his mood improved.

Alan was in remission for 10 months before a follow-up PET scan showed recurrence. Less than 2 years from surgery, he died at age 67. He was never able to return to his job as a security consultant, play tennis, or coach others on how to live their lives.

Alan's experience demonstrates the kind of suffering that occurs when there is both physical and psychological suffering. Every aspect of his life was affected. His identity as a strong, independent, active professional was destroyed. He could not do any of the things that defined his identity. He was cut off socially from people who knew and validated him. He could look in the mirror and see only a man who had lost more than 40 pounds, whose face was no longer tanned and robust, but pale and drawn instead. He was depressed and could not enjoy even the activities that remained.

Depression is three to five times more common in patients after the diagnosis of cancer than in the general public and may affect survival (Irwin 2007; Steel et al. 2007). Studies show from 25% to almost 40% of patients suffer from major depression, and up to 58% have a depression spectrum syndrome. Factors associated with an increased risk of depression include young age, a prior history of depression, advanced cancer, greater levels of disability, and the presence of uncontrolled symptoms such as cancer-related pain. Patients with cancer of the lung are more often affected than other types of cancer (Holland and Gooen-Piels 2003a, b; Massie 2004), and ASCO guidelines note that the physicians need to have a role in treating this.

Although clinicians may not be able to prevent some of the chronic or late medical effects of cancer, they have a vital role in mitigating the negative emotional and behavioral sequelae. Recognizing and treating effectively those who manifest symptoms of anxiety or depression will reduce the human cost of cancer (Andersen et al. 2014).

Alan could not tolerate effective doses of chemotherapy. He was physically weakened, but his depression and hopelessness may also have contributed. He lacked the motivation to continue more treatment and endure the side effects. It is possible that his suffering caused an early relapse and death. An EORTC-NCIC trial suggested that combined with a Prognostic Index, *pain and appetite loss may be independent prognostic factors in patients with advanced MM* (Bottomley et al. 2007). It is clear, however, that much of his suffering could have been ameliorated with more aggressive supportive therapy including counseling, nutritional support, and better pain control.

The British Thoracic Society Standards of Care Committee makes the following recommendation. *Most patients need symptom palliation from the time of diagnosis onwards. Palliative care should aim to provide relief from pain and other physical symptoms and to respond to emotional, psychological, social and spiritual needs* (British Thoracic Society Standards of Care Committee 2001).

Too often patients respond to the suggestion that palliative care consultation is needed with the comment, *You mean I need hospice?!* The word *hospice* is more familiar to patients. They associate it with the 6-month prognosis requirement and equate it with a death sentence. It is not clear whether palliative care was offered to Alan, but given his initial comments about dying, he might have had similar beliefs. Clarifying this misinformation and describing symptom palliation in a positive way reduces reluctance to receiving it. When palliative care is started at the time of diagnosis along with chemotherapy, survival is extended by almost 3 months in metastatic non-small cell lung cancer (Temel et al. 2010).

A team approach is necessary to provide this type of care. No single provider has the time or training to do all that is needed to treat a patient such as Alan. If treatment is given in a larger medical facility or cancer center, there may already be personnel who form such a team. Palliative care departments generally perform these services. If no such team is available, the treating physicians may need either to train existing nurses or technicians or develop a referral network of providers.

A physician who became a patient when he was diagnosed with MM offered his conclusions. *The requirement for an integrated multi-professional approach to management cannot be overstated. As active treatment options are limited in both choice and efficacy, and are associated with considerable morbidity, the role of active supportive care is paramount* (Sweeney et al. 2009).

Alan's personality, personal history, and social situation made his suffering more likely. As a competitive tennis player and Army Ranger, Alan defined himself as a fighter. He was accustomed to being respected as a knowledgeable professional consultant both for individuals, as a life coach, and for companies, as a security consultant. The diagnosis of MM, generally believed to be incurable, did not initially make him feel defeated. He chose aggressive therapy, taking the risk of side effects that he may not have understood. The physical impact of treatment was overwhelming for him. He could not maintain his identity as a strong, independent "warrior." His relative social isolation and dependency upon others for his basic needs left him with no acceptable alternative identity. It seems ironic that his professional roles were teaching others to be more successful as a life coach and more secure as an industrial security consultant.

18.2.3   Case Studies: Suicide

Not all patients with MM die from their disease. Some individuals take things into their own hands and end their lives before anything worse can happen. The following two cases show different pathways in which this can happen.

18.2.3.1   Larry

Larry was 68 years old when he shot himself 11 days after the diagnosis of sarcomatoid MM was confirmed. He dressed himself neatly, called 911 to make sure his wife would not be the first to find him, laid down on a blanket in his back yard, and put a 0.22 caliber automatic pistol in his mouth. The chest tube was still in his right chest when the police found his dead body.

Over the previous 4 months, Larry had increasing chest pain and recurrent bloody pleural effusion. This was drained three times in the emergency room without providing a diagnostic cytology. CT scans showed a 4.7 cm mass extending to the right pulmonary artery, and the radiology report suggested MM. He delayed the needle biopsy that ultimately confirmed the suspected diagnosis. The procedure was performed on December 26, because he did not want to receive bad news before Christmas.

Larry's health had been declining for several months. He was losing weight and becoming more short of breath. He had promised his wife to build a patio in the backyard, but he was unable to continue because he was growing weaker. He had given up his favorite sport, hockey, when the pain started. He was started on hydrocodone, but the pain control was poor. He began to have more neuropathic pain but could not tolerate effective doses of gabapentin.

He began to talk about knowing that he would die. He thought he would get worse regardless of diagnosis or treatment, yet he still wanted to be in charge of his life. Psychiatric consultation concluded: *He wants to maintain control over his situation, and in the future if things ever became too intolerable, he wanted to have the choice to 'opt out' and end his life on his terms.* The psychiatrist and social worker did not conclude he was actively suicidal but did have suicidal ideation. Since there were guns in the household, the recommendation was that they be removed and antidepressants started. Thirty years before he was diagnosed with MM, there was a family crisis and Larry had suicidal ideation. This resolved quickly, however, with counseling.

He was ambivalent about CPR. He stated that he wished to be a full code, but his advance directive stated that he did not want intubation or life support, even if he would die without them. He repeatedly indicated that *being in control over my own destiny* was very important. Even before he was told of his diagnosis, he said he would use a gun as an alternative to end his life if *things became intolerable and he would suffer too much.*

There was a note in his chart stating that his daughter had found the key to his gun safe and removed the weapons located there. Clearly, however, he was able to find another gun.

18.2.3.2 Dominic

Dominic and his girlfriend Naomi were enjoying their retirement. Three of his co-workers had developed MM, but they were diagnosed when they were in their 60s. He felt that he had "dodged the bullet," since he was now 75. At first his cough and chest pain were diagnosed as pneumonia, since these symptoms improved with anti-biotics. The pleural effusion did not resolve, however, so he underwent a pleural biopsy. When it showed MM, Dominic immediately became depressed, as his co-workers had all suffered miserable deaths.

Dominic's doctors began active measures to control his pain and depression. Pain management included both continuous-release analgesia to prevent pain and immediate-acting drugs to treat breakthrough pain. They were adjusted when measures did not give satisfactory pain relief. Drugs for neuropathic pain were added. Doses were increased or medications switched. Problems did occur when he ran out of drugs on one occasion and had to go to the emergency department to get relief. The main problem was not that the medication was failing, but that his cancer was growing. Similarly, when one antidepressant was not working or tolerated, another one was prescribed. Ultimately, he was referred to a pain clinic for a possible nerve block.

With the MM growing, Dominic continued to lose weight and became weaker. He had always been very active, going fishing and riding his Harley motorcycle across country with Naomi in the sidecar. He was a rancher with 120 head of cattle on his 200-acre farm. He described himself as *230 pounds of muscle* before his illness. He was now 170 pounds and having trouble getting out of bed. The "last straw" came when he lost control of his bowels in bed and was left lying in his own feces. His humiliation was complete when his girlfriend had to clean him. At this point, Dominic did not fear being disabled in the future. His worst fear had already come to pass. This previously strong, independent rancher was now so weak that he would need diapers. He took his only option: he shot himself when Naomi was outside walking the dog.

The first patient, Larry, took his life because he could not tolerate the thought of being helpless and out of control. His image of himself was incompatible with that of someone dying with cancer. Though he had pain, there were many things that could have relieved it. There may not have been adequate information to get involuntary admission to a psychiatric inpatient unit, but clearly he had a plan and an opportunity to carry out his threat to take matters into his own hands.

If he had lived in a US state that had aid in dying laws allowing physicians to prescribe medications to end life, Larry might have chosen that route. These laws have safeguards that prevent impulsive behavior. Patients must make at least two requests for such aid. There must also be at least two physicians certifying the patient has adequate mental capacity and judgment to request these medications. This process still keeps the patient dependent upon physicians to carry out their plans and places a time interval between request and action. Larry's strong need to be in control might also have made these restrictions unacceptable.

The second patient, Dominic, had no history of depression and did not have symptoms that would have justified that diagnosis. He did have a breaking point, however, and it is not clear that any proactive measure would have changed the outcome. He was on antidepressants, and his pain was being managed.

Depression is up to five times more common in patients with cancer than the general population (Pirl et al. 2009). Both Larry and Dominic had depression and took the option of ending their own lives. Depression may be present, but is not the only cause of suicide in cancer patients.

The risk of suicide is increased among cancer patients, more so in men than in women (Misono et al. 2008). A Scandinavian study showed that the relative risk was 1.55 for men and 1.35 for women and was higher in the first few months after diagnosis. Cancer of the respiratory organs had the highest relative risk, 4.08, followed by brain cancer with relative risk of 2.40. It was speculated that certain cancer types may have more profound effects on quality of life and induce stronger degrees of anxiety or fear because of symbolic values and difficulties in breathing or eating (Hem et al. 2004). Other studies have shown even higher suicide rates, with a relative risk of 12.6 for all cancer patients in the first week after diagnosis (Fang et al. 2012).

Other psychiatric diagnoses are more common in cancer patients than in the general public. Approximately half of cancer patients suffer from some form of depression, anxiety, or adjustment disorders. Persons without cancer may react to this information by projecting themselves into the patient's situation: *If I had cancer, I'd be depressed and anxious too*. This notion minimizes the degree of suffering that can be associated with comorbid depression and its impact upon quality of life. If physicians underestimate the morbidity caused by depression, they may not treat it as aggressively as they would with other symptoms (Roy-Byrne et al. 2016).

Physicians generally view suicide as a failure. They question what they might have done differently. Patients may see suicide as something that delivers an escape from intolerable situations. In several states, laws have been passed that allow physician-assisted death. While the public may describe it as assisted suicide, in California it is officially known as the End of Life Options Act.

Considered from this perspective, suicide is only one of several ways that patients can prevent future suffering. Adequate pain control and palliative care from the beginning can prevent the desperation that drives patients to view an early death as the only way to relieve suffering. Helping patients confront fears of death is often a job for spiritual care personnel. Helping patients confront fears of dying is a job for both medical and psychological caregivers. Supporting the family's needs so they can cope with their loved one's illness decreases their suffering and provides additional caregivers.

End-of-life care is complex. Trained palliative care staff can identify trouble points and prevent problems. Having patients and families communicate their wishes for medical care can prevent interventions that are not wanted. Advance directives may be effective ways to create consensus between patients, families, and physicians. Unfortunately, such directives may create more distress than they prevent. Doctors may not follow the directives if they are not properly signed, not available in crises when decisions are made, or when conflicting requests come from family members.

The most important part of an advance directive is not the written and signed document. It is the conversation between a patient and his or her family that reaches a consensus on what is to be done and whether the family will support the patient's wishes. Different scenarios must be considered, since not everyone dies after a lingering illness. The next important part of the process is the conversation between the physician and patient. Again consensus is important. Physicians might have to consider whether they are willing to agree to the limits patients place on what care they want and what care they refuse.

18.2.4 Case Study: Family

Sean was a 59-year-old contractor and the primary breadwinner for his family. After evaluation of chest pain and a bloody effusion, a pleural biopsy showed MM. Additional medical procedures showed he was a possible surgical candidate. He described himself as a fighter, so Sean and his son Martin concentrated on finding the best possible surgeon, even going outside his insurance provider and traveling to the East Coast. He was told that any surgery had potential problems, but he felt the risk was worth the chance of a cure. After having two courses of neo-adjuvant cis-platinum and pemetrexed without response, he underwent a very complicated extrapleural pneumonectomy. The operation took 10 h, required removing a rib, and had an estimated blood loss of 4.5 L.

Two days after discharge, Sean was readmitted with sepsis, empyema, and a bronchopleural fistula. He went back to the operating room where another rib was removed to facilitate drainage. Daily dressing changes were very painful, and he required several boluses of his hydromorphone PCA. During this time, his wife and son were quite anxious, and both were seeing social workers for support. Sean's wife Mary, now the only breadwinner, was very concerned about Sean going home, since she would have to do the dressing changes.

Sean still had significant pain and was apprehensive about his own future. He went home on oxygen and with a large cavity in his right chest, $11 \times 16 \times 31$ cm, and still draining malodorous material. His son had to quit his job to take over wound care when Sean's wife had to go back to work. Every member of the family was anxious. Curiously, they were worried more about other family members than themselves. Mary was frantic with worry about Sean. She confessed that she was unable to sleep at night and was near the end of her rope. Sean worried about Mary and Martin. He also worried about what the neighbors thought about him in his debilitated state and how his wife of 38 years would cope if he died. Mainly, he worried about finances. He had always been able to support his family. Now, they could not afford to hire extra help at home to take the burden from his son. Martin worried about both his father and mother and his wife and three school-age children.

Families as well as patients suffer with MM. Patients do sign consent forms for aggressive treatments after being informed of the risks. Family members do not do this, and yet they too must deal with the consequences of the treatments. This family's communication and coping skills were not very well developed. The stress of the diagnosis with its attendant psychological impact and physical complications overwhelmed the family. Even with additional support, they had a difficult time. Financial burdens and the limits of insurance coverage are common problems faced by such families. Other matters, e.g., getting transportation to doctors' offices and even walking the dog, create additional stress.

The NCCN distress scale (Holland and Alici 2010) is a useful means to measure and identify sources of distress for both patients and families. Distress has been proposed as the sixth vital sign. In circumstances like those encountered by Sean's family, measuring distress is critically important. Patients depend upon family caregivers. If the family is too stressed, they cannot assume the duties needed to keep patients in their home environment.

Family problems can have a profound impact on patient care and quality of life. There may be warning signs that additional resources are needed. Knowing that there are family members with drug abuse issues raises the question of possible drug diversion. If a spouse is an alcoholic or if family relationships are markedly dysfunctional, decisions about home care may need to be changed. If finances are poor or insurance coverage is inadequate, patients may not be taking the prescribed medications. When these problems occur, the care team has to create solutions that go far beyond treating the cancer.

18.3   Developing a Strategic Treatment Plan

In the life of patients diagnosed with MM, there are several points that offer opportunities for doctors to obtain information about patients and then guide them to better outcomes of the disease. By considering these points and asking patients the right questions, clinicians can intervene to prevent problems. Even if the patient dies, when they help patients maintain their quality of life, families see providers as caring people and doing the best job in a difficult situation.

18.3.1   Before Diagnosis

Even before the first encounter, patients have a history of prior experiences with illnesses and stories they have heard about other people's experience with cancer. Patients have already developed some ability to cope with significant events, established some kind of support system, and have defined who they are in terms of their roles and activities.

Patient histories customarily include past medical illness, family history, and sometimes social or lifestyle history. This information gives some picture of the person but is incomplete. The context of the person's life is also important. This includes occupational history, a description of the family and social environment in which they live, and their educational level. Additional information is needed about socioeconomic status, spiritual or religious practices, drug and alcohol use, and particularly the ways the person has responded to stress in the past. With this information, providers develop a more complete picture of the human being and can recognize areas of their strengths and vulnerabilities.

Clinicians also have their own history. Their training and prior experience with MM is likely to determine the treatment choices they prefer. Their prior experience with patients generally leads to certain expectations of patients. Their conscious and subconscious attitudes toward cultural, racial, gender, socioeconomic, and physical appearance of the patient can influence the way they treat certain individuals. The doctor's communication style including body language, style of interpersonal interactions, and her or his definition of the patient-physician relationship also affect how that patient will be treated.

Persons do not prepare to become patients, but physicians can and do prepare to care for them. Many elements of professional style are unconscious. Doctors' prior exposure to MM, and to patients generally, has already set some habits and affects current behavior. The attitudes toward patients as well as expectations of themselves are malleable and can be consciously modified. It is natural to want to repeat experiences that turned out well. The experiences that have created doubt, remorse, or a sense of failure can be starting points to develop other behaviors that are closer to clinicians' vision of what they want to become.

When subconscious behaviors are brought to awareness, they can be examined and future conduct modified. Optimally this is viewed as a part of continuing medical education. A potential danger of such self-examination can be unwarranted and sometimes brutal self-criticism. Too often doctors pass off their exemplary behavior as "just what is expected" and don't acknowledge the good they do. Calling attention to one's self might be viewed as bragging. Receiving praise from colleagues can become an occasion for brushing off compliments rather than simply saying thank you for the comment. Doctors strive to improve their medical skills. That same motivation can be used to develop more proactive and effective ways of working with patients.

18.3.2 At the Time of Diagnosis

Patient expectations of whether they will live or die are often set at the time of diagnosis. This is based on *how* they are told as well as *what* they are told. Previous experiences of illnesses affect their beliefs about what is likely or possible for themselves. This is particularly true for stories about other persons' experience with MM and other cancers.

A common presentation for pulmonary MMs is pain and shortness of breath with a chest X-ray showing a pleural effusion. A therapeutic thoracentesis may be done in the emergency department to relieve symptoms. Patient or family questions may lead the individual doing the procedure to mention the possibility of cancer. The mention of cancer can bring patients to the psychological edge of a cliff with a profound need for more information. The patient or family members may importune the provider with a barrage of questions. Their questions cannot be answered at this point, because the information is not available. Only their fear is present. Sensing that fear can pressure the provider to offer reassurance. If handled well, the patient may accept that there are several possibilities and that an organized diagnostic process is beginning. When told they will have to wait for answers, they may be left with more fear, more confusion, and sometimes less trust in the medical system.

Optimally the patient will be referred immediately to another clinician, either primary care or specialist, with experience in pulmonary disease. The prompt referral can prevent the patient from feeling completely helpless and adrift in a complex medical system without guidance.

The roles of the clinicians, as well as the sequence in which they see the patient, may determine how information is presented. The thoracic surgeon may be required to perform a biopsy if prior thoracentesis and cytologies were not diagnostic. They may then become the physician who first tells the patient the diagnosis. If someone else has already played that role, then the surgeon may be required to discuss both the surgical procedure and prognosis.

The first doctor to tell the patient they have MM is in a critical position to influence the patient's course. That clinician must assess where the patient and family are emotionally. Whether they are the provider who manages the patient's emotional needs or not, the way patients are first told their diagnosis has a profound effect on future encounters.

Some patients will be in such shock they are unable to process factual information. At the same time, accompanying family may have myriad questions and need or even demand answers that only lead to more questions. Acknowledging an individual's emotional state can help build trust. That person then feels recognized and their position legitimized. There are several ways this situation can be addressed.

This news must come as a shock. It can be hard to take in all the details. Many people have lots of questions. Tell me what you know about this rather rare type of lung cancer. Perhaps I can then answer your questions in an organized fashion. Depending upon the responses, clinicians can direct the conversation to the one in most distress while letting the others know they will have their questions answered later.

Until the most pressing emotional needs are addressed, there is little room for information about treatment or prognosis. Sometimes providing such information cannot wait until a later appointment and the physician must find out who is best equipped to receive it. An anxious patient still needs reassurance, but this may come from another person such as a nurse or family member. Letting them know you understand their situation and will address it as soon as you can may be enough to give them some relief.

Presenting the diagnosis in this way creates the basis for trust that the person is seen and important. That helps diminish the threat of being alone in a dangerous situation. Other areas of potential suffering can be addressed later as the clinician gets more detailed information about the patient's life. Such questioning builds further trust, because it indicates the clinician is interested in the person not just the disease. Other providers may ask the questions and gather information that can predict the patient's coping abilities, support resources, and areas of vulnerability where additional measures will be needed. The goal of this process is to develop a strategic treatment plan that prevents as much suffering as possible and empowers the patient and family as they go through treatment. Various approaches at this point may help.

> *Tell me what you understand of what you've been told.*
> *What have you heard or read about mesothelioma?*
> *Sometimes the statistics can seem pretty grim. Yet there are some people who unexpectedly do very well. Do you think you might be one of them?*
> *Most people will need help at home after surgery. Who can you call on to give you help while you're recovering?*
> *Everybody has been in situations where they felt overwhelmed. What helped you cope with things when you faced difficult situations before?*

Chemotherapy and radiotherapy may be considered along with surgery. Presenting the case at tumor board can help make such decisions, allowing integrated treatment. It is also an ideal time to involve social workers or other therapists who can provide patient and family support if care is needed.

Patients are confused if they hear markedly different views about the need for and success of various treatments. Developing and articulating a clear plan can prevent this. If there are multiple options or treatment pathways possible, acknowledging this ahead of time may help patients tolerate ambiguity or uncertainty. Maintaining dialogue with patients reassures them that their needs will be addressed and can help answer even unasked questions.

Patients are most vulnerable when discussing prognosis. They know their future is threatened but not the magnitude of the threat. Doctors likewise are vulnerable to the dilemma of giving unrealistic or false hope versus painting too bleak a picture and giving false despair. Care providers generally want to allay patient fears and maintain hope. One danger of giving too optimistic an outlook is damaging trust and the patient-physician relationship when adverse events happen. The danger of presenting too dismal a future is that false despair can destroy hope and decrease patients' motivations to receive possibly life-prolonging treatment (Buchholz 1988).

Evasive answers to patient questions about prognosis or just giving numbers without context is also unsatisfactory. Few patients understand the statistical concept of *median survival* and only hear that death is inevitable if numbers like *50% are alive at 1 year* are offered. It takes skill to tell patients that even if the glass isn't half full, there is still something at the bottom that is worthwhile. Acknowledging that prognosis is a statistical concept and doesn't apply to individuals can allow patients to consider they might be in the small group of longer-term survivors. At this point it is useful to ask patients more questions about how they see their future.

> *I recognize that only some people have prolonged survival. Do you think you might be one of them?*
> *What would you need to help you be in that group?*
> *If you don't think you'll be one of the lucky ones, what do you want to do? Would you want to try some treatment and discover whether it works for you?*
> *Should we try to help you live as best you can for the longest time you can?*

Some patients will make decisions because that is what their family wants, not what they want. Though that type of reasoning can be authentic for them, it raises the possibility that these patients may not be genuinely motivated to go through treatment and suffer side effects. It also raises the question about whether there will be family conflicts at the time that advance directives become a dominant issue.

Ethically, physicians have a fiduciary obligation to respect patients' requests. Pointing out that there might be conflicts between the patient's and the family's goals shifts the need to establish consensus back to the family, not to the doctor.

There can also be conflicts within the physician treating the patient. Doctors are trained to fix problems (Gawandi 2014). Specialists have developed skills in their particular field, surgery, chemotherapy, or radiotherapy. Doctors' desire to do something, especially the modality they do best, may influence the way they make decisions and present options to patients. Doctors need to be aware of their own bias to insure patients' needs are foremost.

18.3.3   During Treatment

Managing side effects, being aware of impact on family, and maintaining hope are the main issues during treatment. Each modality has its own constellation of side effects and impacts various individuals differently. The balance between patients' coping abilities, the intensity of side effects, and the success of supportive interventions determine both how much patients suffer at the time and how they view the future. The most common side effects are pain, breathlessness, fatigue or low energy, and limited activities. Pain and shortness of breath are most amenable to medical treatment.

Pain management is part of every doctor's responsibility. Complex pain syndromes, however, may require palliative care involvement. Not all pain responds to opioids. Fear of overdose often results in underdosing and unrelieved pain. Patients describe pain differently to doctors than they do to nurses and especially how they describe their pain to the family. Getting multiple assessments of the pain's intensity is often necessary. Oncology nurses (personal communication) have suggested that the pain scale from 0 to 10 is not linear but more S shaped. Values between 5/10 and 9/10 tend to be more proportional to actual differences in the degree of pain. Reports of pain at 9/10 or 10/10 often reflect anxiety. Pain reports of greater than 4/10 generally require treatment. Patients and family views on pain and pain management are often based on misinformation. Correcting such beliefs often can improve pain control, although not everyone will take the prescribed medicine to diminish their pain.

Fear amplifies almost any complaint, especially pain. Providing explanations before treatment, giving information on the expected duration of pain (e.g., postoperative pain), and exploring the meaning patients and families place upon pain can both reduce its intensity and strengthen coping skills. Correcting assumptions that any pain means the MM is growing diminishes the pain and makes it less frightening.

Families watching their loved ones in pain often feel helpless, and such experiences are very stressful to them. Teaching patients and families techniques such as guided imagery or meditation gives them some sense of control and empowers them. Teaching stress control techniques, e.g., mindfulness-based stress reduction (MBSR), addresses many of the global symptoms of being ill. Such courses are widely available in hospitals and other health systems.

Decreased energy and diminished capacity to maintain customary activities and roles is common with any treatment. Such inability to do what previously has defined their lives is a source of suffering beyond physical symptoms. Patients can no longer be the person they thought they were. Such interruptions in personhood cannot be prevented, but their impact can be mitigated. Often side effects are time limited, and patients can be reassured that their disabilities are temporary. They and their families can be creative and find substitutes for many activities. Cooking in the kitchen can become menu planning and having help while shopping. Supervising others doing the cooking may return a sense of agency and control. Managing business activities by phone or online seated at home is better than just watching TV. Colleagues and co-workers can visit and bring work with them.

The most difficult, yet most widely effective, is dis-identifying certain roles. We are foremost human beings and may perform in the role of parent, manager, salesperson, or teacher. The most common way we identify ourselves may be *I am a doctor*, although we are equally a *son* or a *sister* or a *parent*. Keeping this perspective opens up the possibility of deeper exploration of who they really are. This philosophical question may bring individuals to seek the help of others who have wrestled with such questions themselves. It also makes it more likely that substitutes for previously pleasurable activities can be found. If appropriate, guidance from clergy or counselors is possible.

The most useful measurement of the impact of treatment is functional status. Asking about broad areas of life including family activity, hobbies, and social events is just as important for measuring suffering as finding out how far a patient can walk without stopping or whether they get dressed and out of bed for most of the day.

The effect of treatments on families can be complex. A family member may be required to do technical things such as dressing changes or managing a chest tube. They may also need to clean up the bed if the patient is incontinent or interrupt their schedule to drive their father to doctors' appointments.

Both patients and families think about the future as well as cope with the present. While the patient deals directly with physical symptoms, families imagine what their loved one feels. Their imagination of how they would feel in the other's shoes may be much worse than what the patient is actually experiencing. Patients may have doubts about their future. Families have both doubts and are doing anticipatory grieving, even if only subconsciously. A spouse may be imagining life without their partner and perhaps feeling guilty for doing so.

Generally the care team focuses on the identified patient. Families and caregivers also have significant distress and needs of their own. Social workers and counselors can become important resources for everyone. There are specific tools to measure the degree of distress for all involved. The NCCN has published guidelines on distress management including a *Distress Thermometer* and a listing of various sources of distress ranging from physical symptoms to worries about childcare, dealing with a partner, and depression or anxiety. As with the pain scale, global distress numbers of 4/10 or greater require attention. The specific sources of distress can guide the type of referral needed. Studies show that more than 40% of lung cancer patients have significant distress (Holland and Alici 2010; Holland and Jacobsen 2016).

When patients are routinely screened for distress, physicians and other providers feel more confident in assessing and managing patients' medical and psychosocial problems. Care can become more efficient as physicians concentrate on medical issues such as pain control, and other members of the interdisciplinary care team manage other areas of need. The most appreciated outcome of this study was that staff saw a more comprehensive picture of their patients. Both patients and providers benefit when such distress measurements become routine (Tamagawa et al. 2016).

18.3.4   Living with Active Disease

Both patients and their families live now with the question "When?" rather than "If?" Depending upon the degree and type of denial, thoughts of death and dying are present in their minds. Appropriately used denial can be a useful coping strategy. Without acknowledging the total impact of an event, individuals can process parts of the situation by digesting smaller pieces and not become overwhelmed by the whole. This is the suggested strategy of *how to eat the elephant: one bite at a time*.

Unless this process becomes a way of avoiding preparing for the outcome, the care team can be patient and not confront the person. If certain actions or decisions must be made in a specified time frame, the care team has to find a way to let the individuals hold on to a portion of their denial and yet confront the other facts necessary for a decision. Doing this takes skill and practice. Some team members may be better at handling this task than others.

Pathologic denial presents a different problem. Clinicians must assess the probable consequences patients and families will face if they don't develop other coping strategies. During this active phase of the disease, the goals are to maintain the best global quality of life possible. If denial is creating more suffering, conversations about worst-case scenarios can be introduced. Even if it is presented as a theoretical problem or "what advice would you give another person?", suggesting additional ways of coping can be introduced and encouraged.

There are different styles of coping. Often physicians and nurses who must act or make treatment decisions will tend to confront problems directly. There can be a tendency to push this style on patients or families who are not yet prepared to adopt this style. Understanding that the person is actively chewing on the last bite of the elephant and intends to take another bite soon makes *expressive* denial acceptable. Expressive denial is what a person may say to others. It is the *internal* denial that prevents the person from taking necessary actions that becomes problematic.

Even if the most significant physical symptoms have diminished, patients still may be suffering. They have had to accept their *new normal* that does not include their previous activities and roles. The distress associated with this situation may not need formal psychological counseling. Talking with other respected individuals such as clergy, good friends, and family members or reading from the large selection of self-help books about coping with cancer may be sufficient.

Some physical symptoms may remain and need to be treated. Asking patients about symptoms that prevent certain activities allows focusing on the most important areas. A common complaint is low energy. Letting the patient know that simple walking rather than running, or that lifting small weights rather than heavy weights, can improve energy may take away the common psychological resistance to exercise which has been shown to improve both energy and mood.

Another common problem is persistent pain and misinformed beliefs about pain management. The fear of addiction or overdose has increased as there is more media attention to such issues. This can affect physicians as well as family members or patients and can lead to underdosing needed medications. Pain that prevents desired activities should be prevented or treated. Side effects like constipation can be easily avoided. Inappropriate beliefs about opioid toxicity can be addressed. Ultimately, the larger context of the problem as end of life care can put these issues in perspective.

18.4   End Game

There is no defined start to when the end game begins. Loosely, it is the time either professionals or patients realize they are nearing the end of life. Patients may not be actively dying, but they recognize that treatments are failing. Doctors may know that the life expectancy is short even while therapy continues to offer some chance of prolonging life. For patients, the end game has clearly begun when they decide to stop treatments to prolong life and concentrate on comfort care. The paradox is that they should already have been receiving measures to comfort them and prevent suffering long before this.

18.4.1   Physicians Recognize that Further Treatments Are Not Beneficial

Doctors are in a curious bind. They have several sets of values that conflict with each other. Medical ethics includes the principles of *Do No Harm, Beneficence or Do Good*, and *Patient Autonomy*. There are personal human values also. *Do the best I can* is expressed as not wanting to exclude a chance to help even if it is of low probability. *Avoid failure* is a value expressed as avoiding self-criticism or patient criticism for giving up. The expectations held by doctor and patient alike are never to stop trying for a cure or at least a longer life. If you do give up, you are somehow a bad person. *Maintain the doctor-patient relationship* is a value that is manifested by trying to give patients hope because this is what they need.

Conflict can occur when professional training and experience tells doctors that the patient is going to die regardless of treatment but makes them feel they *have to do something* and *they can't just stand there*. What doctors have been trained to do is to fix problems. Rarely are they trained to deal with situations they cannot fix (Gawandi 2014). Perceived patient expectations seem to demand that the doctor must do something to help them. Yet doctors do not feel they have anything to do that will truly be beneficial except perhaps to maintain the fiction of hope (Gilligan 2012).

Depending on whether the physicians' personal beliefs or the cultural ethical beliefs are stronger at the moment, treatment may be offered. To resolve cognitive dissonance, doctors support their decision by increasing the probability of success and decreasing the impact of side effects. Thus, the end game is delayed because there is something seen as beneficial to do.

Different outcomes are possible, however. Physicians can either be trained in other ways of helping patients or refer to those providers already trained. Sometimes this is a palliative care team or a hospice provider. In all situations, providers can use the existing doctor-patient relationship that has been built on trust. This relationship can be more powerful than doctors realize. Like other important relationships, it requires honesty, openness, and the willingness to be vulnerable. Patients do not always expect to be fixed. They may be more appreciative of the relationship than disappointed when even best efforts did not work. Physicians may confuse the fact that a treatment failed to produce the desired effect with a sense of personal failure.

18.4.2   Patients Recognize that Further Treatments Are Not Beneficial

Patients likewise are in a bind. What if they decide to forgo further treatment? The implications of disappointing family, doctor, and their own expectations can be overwhelming. Patients likewise want to do the best they can, avoid failure, and maintain relationships. In addition, they may begin to understand they are actually dying and that death is not far away. Practical and existential fears arise whether it is death itself or the process of dying that is most present.

Patients may long ago have reached the conclusion that treatments are not offering benefit commensurate with cost. Willingness to continue depends on hope that treatment will give something valuable. If the person's quality of life is too low and there is little expectation that it will improve, a *what's the use?* feeling develops. Something else that will provide better quality of life with fewer side effects becomes preferable. If there is no belief that something else will make life worth living, then allowing a natural death becomes an option.

In those situations, patients face the problem of telling family that they want to stop treatment. Patients may have gone past any sense of personal failure or disapproval for not trying harder, but families may not have accepted those conclusions. For them, patients stopping treatment can be perceived as a failure. The family *didn't do enough* and *they didn't try hard enough* and hence are to blame for the patient's decision. Though family may have witnessed the suffering, they have not experienced it personally and not reached the conclusion *that's enough!*

It's hard to face a disappointed or disapproving family. Patients are dependent on them for support. They may fear abandonment if they don't conform to family expectations. Depending on the communication style in the family, this process may be more or less difficult. If the care team perceives there is coercion, then someone may need to facilitate the conversation. This can be particularly important with end of life decisions in which patients may want to end life support and families cannot let go.

Patients fear abandonment by their doctors. *Will you still take care of me if I don't take the treatments?* There are times when doctors either directly or indirectly tell patients they cannot take care of them any longer. Patients may place more importance in the doctor-patient relationship than they express directly. Asking if their doctor will continue to care for them if they stop treatment makes them too vulnerable to rejection. Given the asymmetric relationship, the onus falls upon doctors to reassure patients they will not be abandoned. Even when patients are referred to other caregivers, it is a simple act of courtesy to send a note to patients letting them know the doctor is still thinking of them.

Only infrequently do doctors, patients, and families reach the conclusion simultaneously that there is no benefit from continuing treatments. Defining the goals of treatment as having the *largest life* possible at the beginning of treatment provides an opportunity to maintain hope, quality of life, and consensus between parties throughout the disease. Life-prolonging treatment can be presented as a balance between having a longer life but, at least temporarily, a decreased height of quality of life. Such a cost-benefit analysis is both truthful and accurate. Expressed this way, both caregivers and patients can be flexible in their assessment of benefit. Patients and families provide the source of adding the depth of purpose and meaning in life. Assistance from religious or spiritual advisers and counselors can also be important. Increasing sense of purpose or even legacy may remain a way to increase the largeness of life when nothing else will.

18.4.3 Difficult Conversations: Responding to Requests for Non-beneficial Treatment

In California, case law has determined there is no obligation for doctors to provide *non-beneficial* treatment. The choice of wording, *non-beneficial*, is important rather than *futile*. It is easier to define a specific treatment for a specific purpose as not having benefit if the ethical values of *doing good* and *avoiding harm* are considered. The ethical value of *patient autonomy* does not present a compelling reason to give such treatment, since the law does not require doctors to do so.

In spite of this analysis, conversations about refusing to accede to patient or family demands for treatment are still difficult. If they are handled sensitively, they need not result in angry denunciations of each other. It can prevent patients or families from storming out of the room to find another care provider who will agree with them. This situation can be defused if each party recognizes and acknowledges the feelings and points of view of the other. Patients or families may need to maintain hope to avoid dealing with fear of dying. Both hope and fear look at an imagined future. Hope sees a desired outcome, and fear sees an undesired outcome. Depending on the strength of individual coping styles, movement away from needing hope may not be possible. Nevertheless, dealing with emotions directly can allow parties to agree to disagree on a specific course of action.

18.4.4 Difficult Conversations: Discussing Changing Goals of Care

The immediate goals of care frequently change. An underlying long-term goal may remain, while decisions about doing surgery or changing chemotherapy shift the goals of care to postoperative recovery or weighing the chances of response versus side effects. The bigger goals of prolonging life or maintaining quality of life are not in conflict. Their immediate priority does change. Side effects are tolerated if a longer life is the highest goal. Patients' needs for comfort remain; there is just a bargain between one goal and another.

For both patients and doctors, there may be a sense that accepting quality of life as the highest goal means eliminating treatments that prolong life. Defining hospice as the treatment for *less than 6 months life expectancy* has made hospice seem like a place you only go to die. Hospice in some minds means abandonment and hopelessness. Palliative care, which may be less widely available than hospice care, is given regardless of life expectancy. Nevertheless, it may carry the same stigma as does hospice. The belief may be that palliative care is given when there is nothing else to be done. Though incorrect, some physicians may still hold this view. Palliative care was recognized as a medical specialty with board certification in 2006 but is yet not familiar to the public.

The NCI dictionary of cancer terms defines palliative care as follows: *a multidisciplinary approach to specialized medical care for people with serious illnesses. It focuses on providing patients with relief from the symptoms, pain, physical stress, and mental stress of a serious illness—whatever the diagnosis. The goal of such therapy is to improve quality of life for both the patient and the family.* The word palliative is derived from the Latin word *pallium*, meaning to cloak or to mitigate. This broad definition corresponds to the concept that the goals of medicine are the relief of suffering (Cassel 1982). Palliation has always been part of medical care, whether given as willow bark tea or NSAIDs for arthritis. Oncologists offer palliative care when they use an antiemetic for chemotherapy-induced nausea, a standard practice.

More recently, palliative care has been shown to increase survival in advanced NSCLC when given at the time of diagnosis along with chemotherapy (Temel et al. 2010). When palliative care is presented from this perspective, it becomes a logical part of treatment rather than an abrupt change in treatment. If changing the goal of care to emphasize quality of life is presented not as a failure of prior treatments but of extension of treatment already given, patients may have less resistance. If they are reassured that this is continuity of care and not abandonment, the conversation becomes less difficult.

At times the conversation may be more difficult for doctors than patients. Physicians may identify their value to the patient in the surgery they perform or the chemotherapy they provide. They may not have the same training or skills to deal with this situation as they do in their specialty. Some individuals may have chosen to enter medicine to become a healer in the image of Marcus Welby, MD, the hero of the medical drama TV program in the 1970s. They may want to respond to the more human needs of patients but are disappointed when they become simply an interchangeable technician brought in only to do a technical job.

18.4.5 Avoiding Failure: Death Is Not the Enemy

In spite of patients fighting hard to *beat the cancer*, doctors doing everything they can to cure the disease, and families supporting their loved ones to the best of their abilities, median survival for pleural MM is about 1 year. With so much effort spent to extend survival, it is easy to perceive death as a failure. The culture supports this conclusion. If we think in terms of *waging a war on cancer*, when patients die, it means we have lost the war. After a diagnosis of cancer, dying means different things to different persons.

Cultural cancer mythology in the past has suggested that somehow patients were at fault for developing cancer if they did not handle stress effectively, did not find existential meaning in the disease, did not die heroically, or died without resolving life issues. Some patients have even felt they were being punished by getting cancer. Dying then became a spiritual as well as medical failure.

There can be shame attached to dying. Patients have their own expectations of themselves. When they cannot (literally) live up to these expectations, they may judge themselves harshly. If the failure is perceived more personally, patients may feel guilty. Cultural issues may have them lean more toward one emotional response than the other. The language of medicine also seems to blame patients, stating that they *failed treatment* if they did not respond, rather than that the treatment failed them.

One of the most painful losses is the loss of a dream. Death of the body may be more easily accepted than the loss of an imagined future. There is pleasure in planning a future retirement, seeing grandchildren grow up or anticipating the activities put off because there wasn't time. Dying takes away the enjoyment of such planning as well as the actual experience of these anticipated events. It is almost as if death has become a thief stealing the future.

Sometimes patients feel they have let their family down if they don't perform as expected. This dynamic often plays out over meals. When patients are not hungry and do not eat, families see the rejection of food as a rejection of their love. Family dynamics are complex. They are often filled with expectations arising from past history. When death cuts short the opportunity to fulfill such expectations, both family and patients may see the other as failing them.

There is no simple way for clinicians to discover all the psychodynamics involved. Sometimes opportunities occur when a well-chosen question may reveal critical information about what a patient expects. Counseling patients and families about other ways of perceiving events may relieve their sense of failure. Unspoken expectations may be apparent early in the course of the disease. Addressing them promptly may prevent future conflicts.

Physicians particularly may feel that death is a defeat. Medical training emphasizes interventions that change the outcome of the disease process. Cardiac arrest is treated with drugs and defibrillators to prevent death. Surgery is performed to remove localized cancers to extend lives. The medical profession seems to forget, however, that the death rate for persons being born is 100%.

This is the paradox that doctors face. They are trained to prevent or delay an inevitable outcome—death. When that outcome is taken personally, death is an enemy. Doctors can develop various coping strategies to face death without it becoming a failure.

18.5   Conclusion

Caring for the person with MM has great challenges as well as the possibility for doing great good. The complexity of understanding and responding to the human being who has this cancer requires a broad understanding of who that individual is and who the care provider is as well. An expanded model of how patients may be perceived allows the development of treatment strategies that prevent suffering and bring greater satisfaction to patients, families, and physicians alike.

Declaration of Interests   The author has been involved in asbestos litigation as an expert witness on cancer-related suffering.

References

Andersen BL, DeRubeis RJ et al (2014) Screening, assessment, and care of anxiety and depressive symptoms in adults with cancer: an american society of clinical oncology guideline adaptation. J Clin Oncol 32:1605–1619

British Thoracic Society Standards of Care Committee (2001) Statement on malignant mesothelioma in the United Kingdom. Thorax 56:250–265

Bottomley A, Coens C, Effiace F et al (2007) Symptoms and patient-reported well-being: do they predict survival in malignant pleural mesothelioma? a prognostic factor analysis of EORTC-NCIC 08983: randomized phase III study of cisplatin with or without raltitrexed in patients with malignant pleural mesothelioma. J Clin Oncol 25:5770–5776

Buchholz WM (1988) The medical uses of hope. West J Med 148:69

Cassel E (1982) The nature of suffering and the goals of medicine. N Engl J Med 306:639–645

Charmaz K (1983) Loss of self: a fundamental form of suffering in the chronically ill. Sociol Health Illn 5:168–195

Clayson H, Seymour J, Noble B (2005) Mesothelioma from the patient's perspective. Hematol Oncol Clin North Am 19:1175–1190

Fang F, Fall K, Mittleman MA et al (2012) Suicide and cardiovascular death after a cancer diagnosis. N Engl J Med 366:1310–1318

Frankl V (1992) Man's search for meaning. Beacon Press, Boston

Gawandi A (2014) Being mortal. Henry Holt, New York

Gilligan T (2012) If I paint a rosy picture, will you promise not to cry? J Clin Oncol 30:3421–3423

Hawley R, Monk A, Wiltshire J (2004) The mesothelioma journey: developing strategies to meet the needs of people with mesothelioma, their family carers and health professionals involved in their care. The University of Sydney, Sydney

Hem E, Loge JH, Haldorsen T et al (2004) Suicide risk in cancer patients from 1960 to 1999. J Clin Oncol 22:4209–4216

Holland JC, Jacobsen PB (eds) (2016) Distress Management Guidelines 2.2016. NCCN.org. Report; available online at: https://www.nccn.org/store/login/login.aspx?ReturnURL=https://www.nccn.org/professionals/physician_gls/pdf/distress.pdf/

Holland JC, Alici Y (2010) Management of distress. J Support Oncol 8:4–12

Holland JC, Gooen-Piels J (2003a) Psycho-oncology. In: Kufe DW, Pollock RE, Weichselbaum RR, Bast Jr RC, Gansler TS, Holland JF, Frei III E (eds) Cancer medicine, 6th edn. BC Decker, Hamilton, pp 1039–1053

Holland JC, Gooen-Piels J (2003b) Psycho-Oncology. In: Holland JC, Frei E (eds) Cancer medicine, 6th edn. BC Decker Inc, Hamilton, ON, pp 1039–1053

Hollen PJ, Gralla RJ, Liepa AM et al (2006) Measuring quality of life in patients with pleural mesothelioma using a modified version of the Lung Cancer Symptom Scale (LCSS): psychometric properties of the LCSS-Meso. Support Care Cancer 14:11–21

Hughes N, Arber A (2008) The lived experience of patients with pleural mesothelioma. Int J Palliat Nurs 14:66–71

Irwin MR (2007) Depression and risk of cancer progression: an elusive link. J Clin Oncol 25:2343

Majkowicz M, Pankiewicz P, Zdun-Ryzewska A et al (2014) Types of reactions to malignant disease in view of V.E. Frankl philosophy. J BUON 19:799–806

Massie MJ (2004) Prevalence of depression in patients with cancer. J Natl Cancer Inst Monogr 32:57–71

Misono S, Weiss NS, Fann JR et al (2008) Incidence of suicide in persons with cancer. J Clin Oncol 26:4731–4738

Mollberg NM, Vigneswaran Y, Kindler H et al (2012) Quality of life after radical pleurectomy decortication for malignant pleural mesothelioma. Ann Thorac Surg 94:1086–1092

Moore S, Darlison L, Tod AM (2010) Living with mesothelioma. A literature review. Eur J Cancer Care 19:458–468

Pirl WF, Greer J, Temel JS et al (2009) Major depressive disorder in long-term cancer survivors: analysis of the National Comorbidity Survey Replication. J Clin Oncol 27:4130–4134

Roy-Byrne PP, Silver JM, Solomon D (2016) Diagnosis of psychiatric disorders in patients with cancer. UpToDate.org. Accessed 18 Oct 2016

Ryff CD (2014) Self realization and meaning making in the face of adversity: a eudaimonic approach to human resilience. J Psychol Afr 24:1–12

Salmon P, Manzi F, Valori RM (1996) Measuring the meaning of life for patients with incurable cancer: the life evaluation questionnaire (LEQ). Eur J Cancer 32A(5):755–760

Steel JL, Geller DA, Gamblin TC (2007) Depression, immunity, and survival in patients with hepatobiliary carcinoma. J Clin Oncol 25:2397–2405

Sweeney K, Toy L, Cornwell J (2009) A patient's journey. Mesothelioma BMJ 339:511–512

Tamagawa R, Groff S, Anderson J et al (2016) Effects of a provincial-wide implementation of screening for distress on healthcare professionals' confidence and understanding of person-centered care in oncology. J Natl Compr Cancer Netw 14:1259–1266

Temel JS, Greer JA, Muzikansky A et al (2010) Early palliative care for patients with metastatic non–small-cell lung cancer. N Engl J Med 363:733–742

Printed in the United States
By Bookmasters